T. Rabe   K. Diedrich   T. Strowitzki (Eds.)

Manual on Assisted Reproduction

2nd updated Edition

Springer-Verlag Berlin Heidelberg GmbH

T. Rabe K. Diedrich T. Strowitzki
(Editors)

Manual on Assisted Reproduction

2nd updated Edition

With 143 Illustrations and 85 Tables

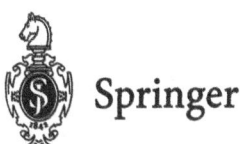 Springer

Professor Dr. med. Dr. h.c. Thomas Rabe
Division of Gynecology and Reproductive Medicine
University Women's Hospital
Voss-Straße 9
69115 Heidelberg, Germany

Professor Dr. med. Klaus Diedrich
Medical University Lübeck
Department Obstetrics and Gynecology
Ratzeburger Allee 160
23538 Lübeck, Germany

Professor Dr. med. Thomas Strowitzki
Division of Gynecology and Reproductive Medicine
University Women's Hospital
Voss-Straße 9
69115 Heidelberg, Germany

Umschlagabbildung: Blastomerenbiopsie, Abbildung freundlicherweise von Herrn Diplom-biologen M. Montag und Herrn Prof. Dr. med. H.H. van der Ven, Universitäts-Frauen-klinik Bonn, zur Verfügung gestellt.

ISBN 978-3-540-67299-9

Library of Congress Cataloging-in-Publication Data
Manual on assisted reproduction/[edited by] T. Rabe, K. Diedrich, T. Strowitzki. – 2nd ed.
    p. cm.
    ISBN 978-3-540-67299-9   ISBN 978-3-642-58341-4 (eBooK)
    DOI 10.1007/978-3-642-58341-4
    1. Human reproductive technology – Handbooks, manuals, etc. I. Rabe, T. (Thomas) II.
Strowitzki, Th. (Thomas), 1959–   III. Diedrich, Klaus, 1946–
    RG133.5.M364 2000
    618.1'7806–dc21   00-038608

© Springer-Verlag Berlin Heidelberg 2000
Originally published by Springer-Verlag Berlin Heidelberg New York 2000

Production: PRO EDIT GmbH, Heidelberg, Germany
Cover design: de'blik, Berlin, Germany
Typesetting: K+V Fotosatz GmbH, Beerfelden, Germany

Printed on acid-free paper   SPIN 10788448   22/3130/Di   5 4 3 2 1

Dedication

It was in 1978 when, as a young resident in Obstetrics and Gynecology, I heard for the first time the name of Professor Robert G. Edwards, on the occasion of the birth of Louise Brown, the world's first in vitro fertilization (IVF) baby, conceived from his collaboration with Patrick Steptoe. Thereafter, I had the opportunity to attend many of his exciting lectures, which were indeed opening a new world, and finally to meet him personally in 1984 at the 3rd World Congress of In Vitro Fertilization and Embryo Transfer in Helsinki. There, he proposed the founding of the European Society of Human Reproduction and Embryology (ESHRE), of which he became the first chairman. Within the context of ESHRE, I had the privilege of collaborating closely with him, and this enabled me to appreciate not only his immense scientific knowledge and restless mind, which is always open to new ideas and concepts, but also his warm and friendly personality and his strong desire to help young researchers to pursue and publish their scientific work.

With his extraordinary scientific and human qualities, Bob Edwards has influenced immensely my generation of physicians and scientists. Furthermore, his pioneer work has offered to millions of infertile couples around the world the most precious gift, a child. Thus, it is most appropriate to dedicate this *Manual of Assisted Reproduction* to Professor Robert Edwards, honoring his outstanding contribution in the field of reproductive medicine to the scientific community and to society at large.

Professor Robert Geoffrey Edwards was born on September 27, 1925 and grew up in Batley, Yorkshire, and in Manchester. Initially, he decided to study agriculture at the University College of North Wales (UCNW) in Bangor, but he soon realized that he was interested not so much in plants but rather in animal reproduction. Thus, he transferred to the Department of Zoology and received his B.Sc. in 1951 from UCNW; in 1962 the same institution offered him the degree of D.Sc.

After graduating, Bob won a scholarship to the Institute of Animal Genetics at the University of Edinburgh, where he worked for his PhD, which he received in 1955. It was there that he met his future wife, Ruth Fowler, who was also working for her PhD on mouse genetics. They were married in 1956, and their family was blessed with the birth of five daughters.

After working for 1 year at the California Institute of Technology, in Pasadena, with a grant from the Population Council, on the immunology of reproduc-

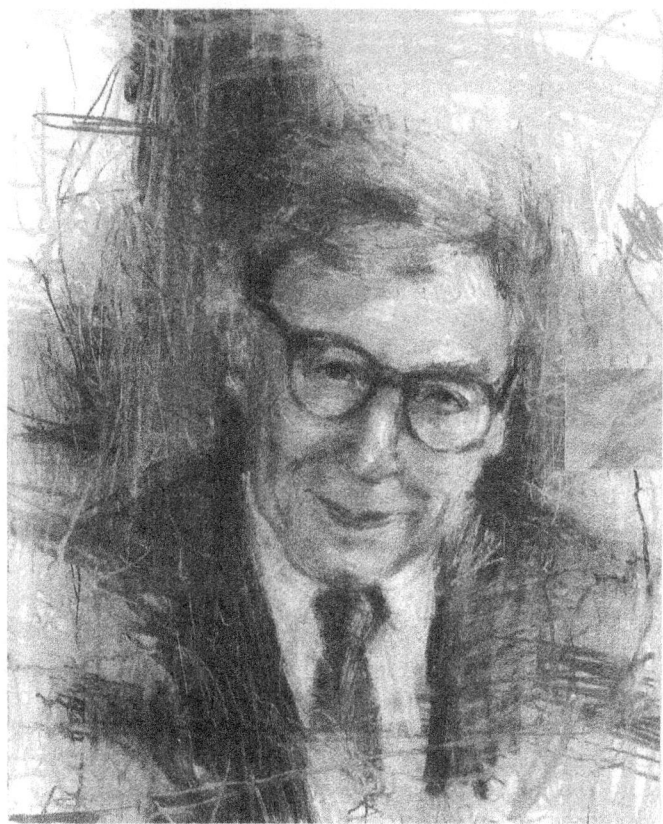

Professor Robert Geoffrey Edwards

tion, he returned to the UK and got a 5-year position at the National Institute for Medical Research in Mill Hill, London. There, he continued his research on oocyte maturation in a variety of animal species. Furthermore, he managed to obtain human ovarian tissue from the nearby Edgeware General Hospital, which gave him the opportunity to start working for the first time with human oocytes.

When his contract with the National Institute expired, Bob was appointed to the Physiological Laboratory in Cambridge. There, he continued his basic research but did not have access to human oocytes. Thus, he went for 6 weeks to the Johns Hopkins Hospital in Baltimore, Md., USA, where he collaborated with Howard and Georgeanna Jones in trying to mature and fertilize human oocytes in vitro, but with limited success.

The most important moment of Bob's career and in the evolution of human in vitro fertilization was when he attended a lecture at the Royal Society of Medicine in London given by Patrick Steptoe, a gynecologist, describing laparoscopy, a surgical technique that could give access to the ovaries, enabling the retrieval of eggs in order to be fertilized in vitro. Their collaboration started in

1968, but since Patrick Steptoe was working in the Oldham General Hospital, Bob had to travel 4 hours from Cambridge to Oldham whenever there were oocytes available. These difficulties did not deter him, and in 1969 he achieved normal fertilization and cleavage of human oocytes in vitro, using freshly ejaculated spermatozoa. The "real" success, however, came almost 10 years later, in 1978, when Bob and Patrick were able to report the first viable intrauterine pregnancy after IVF, which resulted in the birth of Louise Brown.

During these hard years, many new concepts, e.g., ovarian stimulation and embryo freezing, were explored. However, it is important to note that all this pioneer work was not funded by public UK funds. Hence, when Patrick Steptoe retired from Oldham, the work had to stop completely until they were able to open Bourn Hall Clinic in October 1980, which immediately became the leading IVF Institute in the world. In 1985, Bob became Professor of Human Reproduction at Cambridge until his retirement in 1989.

At the same time, together with other distinguished European colleagues, he founded the European Society of Human Reproduction and Embryology (ESHRE), of which he became the first Chairman (1985–1987) and an Honorary Member (1993). Furthermore, he launched the three journals of ESHRE, *Human Reproduction, Human Reproduction Update,* and *Molecular Human Reproduction,* which have grown under his editorship to be the leading journals in the field.

Bob's scientific work has been published in numerous journals and books and presented at meetings. However, his outstanding contribution, for which he has been honored by many scientific societies and universities around the world, was not exhausted in the scientific arena but also expanded in the social one, since he actively participated and sometimes stimulated the public debate about the ethical ramifications of these novel techniques. Thus, he contributed immensely not only to the enrichment of our knowledge in this field but also to the public awareness and acceptance of assisted reproduction techniques.

Now, more than 10 years after his official retirement, Robert Edwards remains as active as ever, exploring new ideas, delivering lectures and striving to make his journals even better. Thus, all of us, his friends, sincerely hope that he continues his activities with the same energy and enthusiasm for many more years to come.

Thessaloniki, February 2000

Basil C. Tarlatzis, M.D., Ph.D.
Associate Professor of 1st Department Ob/Gyn
Aristotle University of Thessaloniki, Greece
Past Chairman of the European Society of
Human Reproduction & Embryology (ESHRE)

Preface

Our knowledge of reproductive medicine has expanded rapidly since the birth of Louise Brown, the first baby to be conceived by in vitro fertilization, which was performed by Professors Patrick Steptoe and Bob Edwards in Oldham, England, in 1978. Hardly a year goes by without the development of a new or a modification of an existing method of assisted reproduction.

Within a relatively short period, in vitro fertilization has been introduced into the treatment of female infertility. Intracytoplasmic sperm injection has also created new opportunities for the treatment of male infertility.

The first edition of this book was published in 1996. In the second edition most of the chapters have been updated and additional interest is focused on intracytoplasmic sperm injection (ICSI) in view of the risk of malformations in newborns.

This manual addresses the techniques of assisted reproduction that are available today. Competent authors from various centers present, in a concise way, their tried-and-tested procedures, so that the latter can be readily implemented.

Due to different legal regulations, the scope of assisted reproduction is much more limited in Germany than in many other countries. For example, whereas only three embryos may be created and transferred in Germany, such restrictions do not exist in several other European countries and the United States. Furthermore, heterologous fertilization, oocyte donation, and surrogate motherhood are banned in Germany.

We are glad that many international experts present the various fields of assisted reproduction from their perspective. We hope this book will help to establish the various therapies and will achieve a wide distribution.

We would like to dedicate this manual to the pioneer and father of assisted reproduction Professor Bob Edwards, to whom we feel committed in friendship and gratitude.

Heidelberg and Lübeck, May 2000   Thomas Rabe
                                                   Klaus Diedrich
                                                   Thomas Strowitzki

Contents

Sperm Maturation and Oocyte Interaction 1
R. J. Aitken

Menstrual Cycle: Follicular Maturation 11
A. Hourvitz, E. Y. Adashi

Physiology of the Menstrual Cycle 23
K. Grunwald, Th. Rabe, B. Runnebaum

Human Gonadotropins 79
B. Lunenfeld, E. Lunenfeld, V. Insler

Gonadotropin-Releasing Hormone: Agonists and Antagonists 133
R. Felberbaum, Th. Rabe, K. Diedrich

Ovarian Stimulation for In Vitro Fertilization: Past and Present 165
J. Urbancsek, Th. Rabe, T. Strowitzki

Ovarian Hyperstimulation Syndrome 197
V. Insler, E. Lunenfeld, B. Lunenfeld

Luteal Phase: Physiology and Pharmacotherapy 215
H. W. Jones Jr., G. S. Jones

An Andrological Approach to Assisted Reproduction 223
F.-M. Köhn and W.-B. Schill

Mammalian Sex Preselection: Flow-cytometric Sorting of X and Y Spermatozoa
Based on DNA Difference 289
L. A. Johnson, G. R. Welch

Assessment of Oocyte and Early Embryo Morphology with Regard
to Embryonic Development and the Outcome of Assisted Reproduction 303
A. Herrler and H. M. Beier

Predicting Embryo Development 321
L. Scott

Cryoconservation: Sperms and Oocytes 339
G. Verheyen, J. Van der Elst, A. van Steirteghem

Microinjection 377
A. van Steirteghem, P. Devroey, I. Liebaers

In Vitro Fertilization 389
Th. Rabe, K. Diedrich, I. Eberhardt, S. Al-Hasani

Evolution of Pregnancies and Initial Follow-up of Newborns Delivered
after Intracytoplasmic Sperm Injection 449
G. D. Palermo, Q. V. Neri, R. Raffaelli, O. K. Davis, Z. Rosenwaks

Outcome of Children Born after In Vitro Fertilization (IVF) and Intracytoplasmic
Sperm Injection (ICSI) 461
M. Ludwig, K. Diedrich

Laser in Assisted Reproduction 473
M. Montag, K. Rink, G. Delacrétaz, H. van der Ven

Assisting Reproduction with the Use of Donor Eggs 489
J. A. Schnorr, J. P. Toner

Oocyte Maturation In Vivo and In Vitro: Principles of Regulation 503
W. Küpker, K. Diedrich

Preimplantation Diagnosis 517
I. Liebaers, W. Lissens, K. Sermon, E. van Assche, C. Staessen, H. Joris,
A. van Steirteghem

Genetics in Assisted Reproduction – Basic Aspects and Clinical Perspectives 529
M. Ludwig, K. Diedrich

The Role of Endoscopy in Congenital Abnormalities: Diagnosis and Treatment ... 549
J. Donnez, Michelle Nisolle

Endoscopic and Microsurgical Techniques in Reproductive Failure 561
M. Vandervorst, P. Devroey

Micro- and Macroconsequences of Ooplasmic Injections
of Early Haploid Male Gametes 575
N. Sofikitis, N. Kanakas, I. Miyagawa

Artificial Intrauterine Insemination: Noninvasive Management
of Subfertile Couples 601
G. Prietl, H. van der Ven, D. Krebs

Subject Index 657

Ein Hinweis für die deutschsprachigen Leser: Das Embryonenschutzgesetz ist im Internet unter der Adresse **http://www.bmgesundheit.de/gesetze/embryo/ aus.htm** abrufbar.

Contributors

Eli Y. Adashi, M.D., Professor and Chair
Department of Obstetrics and Gynecology, University of Utah, Health Sciences
Center, 50 North Medical Drive, Suite 2B200, Salt Lake City, UT 84132, USA

Robert John Aitken, FRSE, Professor
MCR Reproductive Biology Unit, Centre for Reproductive Biology,
37 Chalmers Street, Edinburgh EH3 9 EW, UK

Safaa Al-Hasani, Dr. med.
Medical University Lübeck, Department of Obstetrics and Gynecology,
Ratzeburger Allee 160, 23538 Lübeck, Germany

Henning M. Beier, Prof. Dr. med., Dr. rer. nat.
Institut für Anatomie und Reproduktionsbiologie, Universitätsklinik,
Wendlingweg 2, 52057 Aachen, Germany

Owen K. Davis
The Center for Reproductive Medicine and Infertility, The New York Hospital-
Cornell Medical Center, 505 East 70th Street, New York, NY 10021, USA

Guy Delacrétaz, Ph.D.
Institut d'Optique Appliquée, Ecole Polytechnique Fédérale de Lausanne,
1015 Lausanne, Switzerland

Paul Devroey, M.D., Ph.D.
Centre for Reproductive Medicine, Academisch Ziekenhuis, Vrije Universiteit
Brussel, Laarbeeklaan 101, 1090 Brussels, Belgium

Klaus Diedrich, Prof. Dr. med.
Medical University Lübeck, Department of Obstetrics and Gynecology,
Ratzeburger Allee 160, 23538 Lübeck, Germany

Jacques Donnez, M.D., Ph.D.
Department of Gynecology, Université Catholique de Louvain, Cliniques
Universitaires St-Luc, avenue Hippocrate 10, 1200 Brussels, Belgium

Inge Eberhardt, Dr. sc. hum.
Div. Gynecol. Endocrinol & Reprod. Medicine, University Women's Hospital,
Voss-Strasse 9, 69115 Heidelberg, Germany

Josiane van der Elst, M.D., Professor
Centre for Medical Genetics, Academisch Ziekenhuis, Vrije Universiteit Brussel,
Laarbeeklaan 101, 1090 Brussels, Belgium

Ricardo Felberbaum, Prof. Dr. med.
Medical University Lübeck, Department of Obstetrics and Gynecology,
Ratzeburger Allee 160, 23538 Lübeck, Germany

Klaus Grunwald, Dr. med.
RWTH Aachen, Abteilung Gynäkologie, Pauwelsstrasse 30, 52074 Aachen,
Germany

Andreas Herrler, Dr. med.
Institut für Anatomie und Reproduktionsbiologie, Universitätsklinik,
Wendlingweg 2, 52057 Aachen, Germany

Ariel Hourvitz, M.D.
Department of Obstetrics and Gynecology, University of Utah Health Sciences
Center, ARUP II, 546 Chipeta Way, Room 109, Salt Lake City, UTAH 84108,
USA

Vaclav Insler, M.D., Professor
Hebrew University Hadassah Medical School, Jerusalem, Israel

Lawrence A. Johnson, M.D., Professor, Research Leader
Germplasm and Gamete Physiology Laboratory, Agricultural Research Service,
U.S. Department of Agriculture, Building 200, BARC-EAST,
Beltsville, MD 20705, USA

Georgeanna Seegar Jones, M.D., Professor Emeritus
Obstetrics & Gynecology, Eastern Virginia Medical School, 601 Colley Avenue,
Norfolk, Virginia 23507, USA

Howard W. Jones, Jr., M.D., Professor Emeritus
Obstetrics & Gynecology, Eastern Virginia Medical School, 601 Colley Avenue,
Norfolk, Virginia 23507, USA

Hubert Joris, M.D., Professor
Centre for Reproductive Biology, Academisch Ziekenhuis, Vrije Universiteit
Brussel, Laarbeeklaan 101, 1090 Brussels, Belgium

Nikos Kanakas, M.D.
52 Kifisias Ave., 11526 Athens, Greece

Frank Michael Köhn, Priv.-Doz. Dr. med.
Department of Dermatology and Allergology, Technical University,
Biedersteiner Strasse 29, 80802 Munich, Germany

Dieter Krebs, Prof. Dr. med.
Universitäts-Frauenklinik, Sigmund-Freud-Strasse 25, 53105 Bonn, Germany

Wolfgang Küpker, Priv. Doz. Dr. med.
Medical University Lübeck, Department of Obstetrics and Gynecology,
Ratzeburger Allee 160, 23538 Lübeck, Germany

Ingeborg Liebaers, M.D., Ph.D., Professor
Centre for Medical Genetics, Academisch Ziekenhuis, Vrije Universiteit Brussel,
Laarbeeklaan 101, 1090 Brussels, Belgium

Michael Ludwig, Dr. med.
Medical University Lübeck, Department of Obstetrics and Gynecology,
Ratzeburger Allee 160, 23538 Lübeck, Germany

Bruno Lunenfeld, M.D., Professor
Department of Life Sciences Bar-Ilan University, Ramat Gan, Israel

Eitan Lunenfeld, M.D.
Department of Obstetrics and Gynecology, Soroka Medical Center, Ben Gurion
University of the Negev, Beer Sheva, Israel

Ikjo Miyagawa, M.D., Professor
Department of Urology, Tottori University, School of Medicine, Yonago 683,
Japan

Markus Montag, Ph.D., Dr. rer. nat.
Universitäts-Frauenklinik Bonn, Sigmund-Freud-Strasse 25, 53105 Bonn,
Germany

Quennie V. Neri, B.Sc.
The Center for Reproductive Medicine and Infertility, The New York Hospital-
Cornell Medical Center, 505 East 70th Street, New York, NY 10021, USA

Michelle Nisolle, M.D., Ph.D.
Department of Gynecology, Université Catholique de Louvain, Cliniques
Universitaires St-Luc, avenue Hippocrate 10, 1200 Brussels, Belgium

Gianpiero D. Palermo, M.D., Professor
Director, Assisted Fertilization and Andrology, The Center for Reproductive
Medicine and Infertility, The New York Hospital-Cornell Medical Center,
505 East 70th Street, New York, NY 10021, USA

Gernot Prietl, Priv.-Doz. Dr. med.
Universitäts-Frauenklinik, Sigmund-Freud-Strasse 25, 53105 Bonn, Germany

Thomas Rabe, Prof. Dr. med. Dr. h.c.
Division of Gynecology and Reproductive Medicine, University Women's
Hospital, Voss-Strasse 9, 69115 Heidelberg, Germany

Ricciarda Raffaelli, M.D.
The Center for Reproductive Medicine and Infertility, The New York Hospital-
Cornell Medical Center, 505 East 70th Street, New York, NY 10021, USA

Klaus Rink, Ph.D.
MTM Medical Technologies Montreux SA, 1815 Clarens, Montreux, Switzerland

Benno Runnebaum, Prof. Dr. med. Dr. h.c.
Wasserturmstrasse 71, 69214 Eppelheim, Germany

Zev Rosenwaks, M.D., Professor, Director
The Center for Reproductive Medicine and Infertility, The New York Hospital-
Cornell Medical Center, 505 East 70th Street, New York, NY 10021, USA

Wolf-Bernhard Schill , Professor, Dr. Dr. med.
Center of Dermatology and Andrology, Justus Liebig University,
Gaffkystrasse 14, 35385 Gießen, Germany

John A. Schnorr, M.D.
The Jones Institute for Reproductive Medicine, 601 Colley Avenue, Norfolk,
Virginia 23507-1627, USA

Lynette Scott, Ph.D.
The A.R.T. Institute of Washington, DC, Walter Reed Army Medical Centerm,
Box 59727, Washington, DC 20012, USA

N. Sofikitis, M.D., Ph.D., Professor
Department of Urology, Tottori University, School of Medicine, Yonago 683,
Japan

Catherine Staessen, MSc, Professor
Centre for Reproductive Biology, Academisch Ziekenhuis, Vrije Universiteit
Brussel, Laarbeeklaan 101, 1090 Brussels, Belgium

André van Steirteghem, M.D., Ph.D., Professor
Centre for Medical Genetics, Academisch Ziekenhuis, Vrije Universiteit Brussel,
Laarbeeklaan 101, 1090 Brussels, Belgium

Thomas Strowitzki, Prof. Dr. med.
Division of Gynecology and Reproductive Medicine, University Women's
Hospital, Voss-Strasse 9, 69115 Heidelberg, Germany

Basil C. Tarlatzis, M.D., Ph.D., Professor
1st Department of Obstetrics, Gynecology and Reproductive Medicine,
Aristotle University of Thessaloniki, Greece

Jim Toner, M.D., Ph.D., Associate Professor
The Jones Institute for Reproductive Medicine, 601 Colley Avenue, Norfolk,
Virginia 23507-1627, USA

Janos Urbancsek, M.D., Ph.D.
First Department of Obstetrics and Gynecology, Semmelweis University Medical
School, Baross utca 27, 1088 Budapest, Hungary

Mark Vandervorst, M.D., Professor
Centre for Reproductive Medicine, Academisch Ziekenhuis, Vrije Universiteit
Brussel, Laarbeeklaan 101, 1090 Brussels, Belgium

Hans van der Ven, Prof. Dr. med.
Universitäts-Frauenklinik Bonn, Sigmund-Freud-Strasse 25, 53105 Bonn,
Germany

Greta Verheyen, Ph.D., Professor
Centre for Reproductive Medicine, Academisch Ziekenhuis, Vrije Universiteit
Brussel, Laarbeeklaan 101, 1090 Brussels, Belgium

G.R. Welch, M.D., Professor
Germplasm & Gamete Physiology Laboratory, Agricultural Research Service,
U.S. Department of Agriculture, Building 200, BARC-EAST, Beltsville,
MD 20705, USA

Sperm Maturation and Oocyte Interaction

R. J. Aitken

Introduction

Testicular spermatozoa are not fully differentiated cells and must undergo a process of biochemical maturation before they gain the capacity to fertilize the ovum. The fact that viable human pregnancies can be generated following the direct injection of testicular spermatozoa, and even spermatids, into the ooplasm, indicates that this maturation process does not involve any genomic change [1]. The haploid genetic material carried in the sperm head must be fully imprinted and competent to orchestrate normal embryonic development by the beginning of spermiogenesis. Similarly, the sperm centriole that in the human, if not the mouse, is needed to organize cell division in the zygote, must be fully differentiated and functional by the spermatid stage of spermatogenesis [2]. Thus the maturation that testicular spermatozoa must undergo before they can acquire the capacity to fertilize the ovum must only involve those attributes of sperm biology needed to deliver the sperm nucleus and centriole into the cytoplasm of the oocyte.

In order to achieve fertilization, the spermatozoon must first ascend the female reproductive tract and locate the oocyte. A complex cascade of changes then ensues involving the tight binding of the spermatozoon to the surface of the ovum, the induction of the acrosome reaction, penetration of the zona pellucida, and ultimately fusion with the vitelline membrane of the oocyte. The biochemical basis of these changes is now being elucidated and, in the wake of this knowledge, a deeper understanding gained of the mechanisms responsible for failed fertilization, both in vivo and in vitro. The clinical implications of this research can be found in the development of rational diagnostic strategies for selecting between the various therapeutic options available for the treatment of the infertile couple. Moreover, a knowledge of the mechanisms responsible for failed fertilization in vitro may contribute to the development of modified in vitro fertilization protocols that would be more efficient than those used in current practice. By such means a technique that was originally pioneered by Steptoe and Edwards as a treatment for bilateral tubal occlusion could be optimized for the treatment of those infertility cases where defects in the male partner have been implicated in the failure to conceive. The purpose of this chapter is to consider the various attributes of sperm biology that are essential for fertilization and to examine how these properties are acquired, with particular emphasis on the role of the epididymis in the generation of a functionally competent spermatozoon.

Biology of Sperm Maturation

Motility

One of the most important properties that spermatozoa are known to acquire as they migrate through the epididymis is the capacity for movement. In animal models with highly differentiated epididymes the acquisition of motility occurs at a sharply defined area of this organ comprising the distal corpus in the rat and proximal cauda in the hamster. In such species spermatozoa from the caput epididymis are completely or virtually immotile [3]. In the human the situation is less clearcut. An analysis of fertile men undergoing vasectomy indicated that immature spermatozoa from the caput epididymis were immotile or exhibit nonprogressive twitching movements in a modified Tyrode's medium. In contrast, more than 60% of the spermatozoa recovered from the cauda epididymis exhibited progressive motility with straight line velocities exceeding 25 µm/s [4]. An increase in the percentage of progressively motile spermatozoa during epididymal transit is a common feature of all studies conducted on the functional competence of spermatozoa at different stages of maturation [4, 5]. However, differences exist between studies in the level of motility attained by spermatozoa in the caput epididymis [4–6]. It is clear that in patients exhibiting congenital absence of the vas deferens motility is present in spermatozoa aspirated from the caput epididymis, and ironically the greatest motility appears to be exhibited by spermatozoa recovered from the most proximal regions of the epididymis [6]. Notwithstanding the possibility that epididymal physiology may be profoundly altered in patients exhibiting congenital absence of the vas, these results would seem to imply that there are few obligatory contributions that the epididymis makes to the attainment of motility by human spermatozoa. Although the epididymis appears to increase the efficiency with which spermatozoa achieve the potential for movement, it is also evident that some spermatozoa can spontaneously initiate progressive motility without the need for specific factors generated by the epididymal epithelia [7]. In order to understand how the epididymis does contribute to the efficient expression of motility, the ontogeny of the cellular mechanisms controlling flagellar activity during sperm maturation (protein phosphorylation, cAMP, calcium, pH, and redox status) need to be elucidated.

Zona Binding

Another attribute of sperm function that is thought to be acquired during epididymal transit is the capacity of these cells to bind to the surface of the zona pellucida. This is an extremely important recognition event that initiates a cascade of interactions with the oocyte culminating in fertilization. Although mature spermatozoa from the cauda epididymis do bind to the zona pellucida in greater numbers than those recovered from the caput in all species examined including the primate [8], the interpretation of such data is complicated by two factors. First of all the binding of spermatozoa to the zona surface is highly correlated with motility and, as discussed above, motility is an independent biological function acquired by spermatozoa during epididymal passage. Thus, it is extremely difficult to dissect out the failure of caput epididymal spermatozoa to bind to the zona pellucida from their lack of movement.

Such an analysis might be possible if the biochemical basis of sperm-zona interaction were clearly understood, but unfortunately this is not the case. The only apparent certainty is that the target molecule on the surface of the zona pellucida is the zona glycoprotein, ZP3. The data to support this assertion derive largely from studies conducted in the mouse [9] although recombinant human ZP3 has been also been shown to induce the acrosome reaction in homologous spermatozoa [10]. However, ZP3 may not be the only zona glycoprotein involved in the primary binding of spermatozoa to the oocyte because in the pig the sperm receptor is a biochemical entity known as ZP3α, which is now known to be the molecular homologue of the murine structural glycoprotein, ZP1 [11, 12].

The nature of the complementary receptor(s) on the sperm surface is even less clear. Evidence has been presented recently suggesting that the human zona receptor is a 95-kDa tyrosine kinase receptor which, when aggregated by ZP3, induces an autophosphorylation event that leads to the initiation of a signal transduction cascade culminating in the acrosome reaction [13]. The aggregation-dependent mechanism of action typically exploited by tyrosine kinase receptors is in keeping with existing data on the nature of sperm-zona interaction. It is known, for example, that proteolytically generated fragments of this molecule do not induce the acrosome reaction in murine spermatozoa, in contrast to intact ZP3 [14]. However, if anti-zona IgG is added to the incubation mixture to cross-link the zona fragments on the sperm surface, then the spermatozoa are activated and the acrosome reaction is induced. If univalent Fab fragments of this antibody are used, acrosome reactions can only be induced following the addition of a secondary IgG antibody directed against Fab [14]. Thus ZP3 glycopeptides can induce the acrosome reaction in murine spermatozoa, but only after they have been cross-linked.

While this necessity for multiple associations with ZP3 is in keeping with the involvement of tyrosine kinases in the control of human sperm function there are other aspects of this association that are not typical of this class of receptor. In particular there is considerable evidence to suggest that spermatozoa recognize a particular class of O-linked oligosaccharides on ZP3, not the polypeptide core of this molecule [9]. This contrasts with classical tyrosine kinase receptors that generally target proteinaceous ligands. It is possible that sperm-zona interaction is a multicomponent process involving a preliminary recognition event mediated by the carbohydrate side chains of ZP3 followed by a more intimate contact with the polypeptide core of this molecule mediated by a tyrosine kinase type of receptor [15]. Sperm surface molecules that might be involved in the primary recognition event include sp56, a lectin-like protein located on the sperm plasma membrane that recognizes terminal galactose residues on the O-linked oligosaccharide side chains of ZP3 and is a member of a superfamily of "Sushi" receptors [16]. Unfortunately, no homologue for this molecule appears to exist on the surface of human spermatozoa. In contrast to the galactose residues recognized by sp56, another candidate ZP3 receptor is a membrane-bound β1, 4-galactosyl transferase that targets N-acetyl D-glucosamine residues on the ZP3 O-linked oligosaccharides [17]. In addition to these candidate ZP3 receptors in the mouse, a series of small molecular weight sperm "adhesins" have been implicated in sperm-zona interaction in the pig [18]. The latter are not integral membrane proteins and appear to be transferred to the surface of the spermatozoa as these cells pass through the rete testes [19]. The site of origin of the other candidate ZP receptors is unknown with the exception of sp56 which is an intrinsic component of the male germ cell which is expressed at the round spermatid stage of mouse spermatogenesis [16]. Biologically, it *is* known that if caput epididymal spermatozoa are carefully washed then some adhesion to the zona pellucida can be demonstrated [20]. Thus the available evidence suggests that spermatozoa in the proximal epididymis have already acquired the surface components needed to effect sperm-binding to the zona surface. Such a conclusion would also be in keeping with the clinical data indicating that IVF can be performed successfully with spermatozoa aspirated from the vasa efferentia and caput epididymis, without the need for epididymal transit. Although epididymal maturation certainly enhances sperm-zona interaction [21], it is probable that such effects are mediated by general changes in the biophysical properties of the plasma membrane and the capacity for movement, rather than the specific acquisition of a zona-binding protein.

The Acrosome Reaction

Since caput epididymal spermatozoa can be induced to bind to the zona pellucida by washing them free of epididymal plasma [20], it would be of interest to determine whether similar treatment could also induce such immature spermatozoa to acrosome react. Recent studies indicate that the addition of heat solubilized zona glycoproteins to spermatozoa isolated from the caput epididymis could not induce the acrosome reaction in unwashed cells even if they were incubated under capacitating conditions [22]. Under these circumstances only the ionophore A23187 can induce the acrosome reaction [23]. However, if such caput epididymal spermatozoa are washed before being capacitated, then physiological stimuli such as solubilized zonae pellucidae can induce the acrosome reaction [22]. These results suggest that the caput epididymis elaborates one or more factors that not only suppress the ability of spermatozoa to bind to the zona pellucida but also prevent the induction of the acrosome reaction. The nature of the suppressive factors have not yet been determined although proteinase inhibitors have been implicated [22]. Whatever the nature of the inhibitory factors present in the caput epididymis, these results clearly indicate that spermatozoa entering the epididymis already possess an intrinsic capacity to bind to the zona pellucida and respond to this recognition event by undergoing the acrosome reaction. In other words such apparently "immature" spermatozoa possess the complete assembly of receptor activation, signal transduction, and second messenger generation systems needed to effect the acrosome reaction in response to ZP3. Again, such results are in keeping with the ability of spermatozoa from the vasa efferentia or caput epididymes of patients exhibiting occlusion of the vas deferens to achieve fertilization in vitro [6]. Thus the epididymis does not appear to be a site where the cellular mechanisms necessary for fertilization are assembled; rather, it is the site where these systems are inhibited in preparation for sperm storage in the cauda.

Sperm–Oocyte Fusion

Whether spermatozoa from the caput epididymis that have been induced to acrosome react can also generate a fusogenic equatorial segment capable of initiating fusion with the vitelline membrane of the oocyte is not known. One of the key sperm surface molecules involved in fusion with the oocyte is PH30 or fertilin [24]. This molecule was first identified in guinea pig spermatozoa and is known to consist of a heterodimeric peptide comprising a- and β-subunits, both of which are type 1 integral membrane proteins. Fertilin β appears to be responsible for effecting the initial binding of the spermatozoon to the surface of the oocyte through an integrin recognition event. The latter involves a disintegrin domain on fertilin-β interacting with integrins on the oocyte surface, since short peptides mapping to the disintegrin region block sperm-oocyte interaction in vitro [25]. Fertilin-a may also be an integrin ligand but, in addition, is predicted to possess zinc-dependent metalloprotease activity and to promote membrane fusion through the mediation of a domain possessing a viral fusion motif [24]. Recent studies suggest that fertilin a and β are members of a large family of similar proteins that contain disintegrin and metalloprotease domains and an additional five sequence-similar proteins have been cloned from guinea pig and mouse testes [25]. The fact that the messenger RNA for these molecules exists in the testis indicates that spermatozoa entering the testis already possess their complement of fertilin(s). Although these molecules appear to undergo some processing during epididymal maturation, it is not known whether such processing is an obligatory requirement for fertilization. The fertilins must clearly undergo some terminal processing at the moment of the acrosome reaction because it is only after this event has occurred that the spermatozoon gains its capacity to recognize and fuse with the vitelline membrane of the oocyte. Such terminal processing of the fertilin molecule may involve proteases released from the acrosomal vesicle at the time of the acrosome reaction. What is *not* known at this stage is whether the induction of the acrosome reaction in immature caput epididymal spermatozoa would effect the necessary processing of fertilin such that acrosome reacted caput spermatozoa could initiate sperm-oocyte fusion. However, the fact that human spermatozoa from the vasa efferentia are competent to fertilize homologous oocytes in vitro suggests that either post-testicular processing of fertilin before the induction of the acrosome reaction is not needed to generate a fusogenic spermatozoon or is an inherent property of these cells that does not need to be promoted by specific epididymal factors.

Conclusion

Thus the fact that viable pregnancies have been established following in vitro fertilization with spermatozoa from the caput epididymis or vasa efferentia suggests that all elements of sperm maturation are intrinsic to the spermatozoa, including those involving the expression of hyperactivated motility, the binding of spermatozoa to the zona surface, the induction of the acrosome reaction and the generation of a fusogenic equatorial segment [6]. Furthermore, the documentation of pregnancies to male patients who had undergone surgical anastimoses of the vas deferens to the vasa efferentia suggests that spermatozoa that have not undergone epididymal transit are functionally competent in vivo as well as in vitro.

While it could be argued on the basis of such evidence that the epididymis does not make an obligatory contribution to the maturation of human spermatozoa. The efficiency of the maturation process is clearly enhanced by epididymal transit via mechanisms involving general changes in the phospholipid composition of the plasma membrane [26] and the progressive cross-linking of thiols in the sperm nucleus and possibly the tail [27]. In addition, as spermatozoa pass into the cauda epididymis, they undergo further changes that are not designed to promote their capacity for fertilization as much as to provide for their long term storage (Fig. 1). The latter involves poorly characterized changes in the spermatozoa including membrane stabilization [27]. The secretion of important antioxidant enzymes in the epididymis, such as superoxide dismutase or glutathione peroxidase [28, 29], are further expressions of the evolution of this structure as a storage organ designed to preserve spermatozoa in a stable state, without undergoing peroxidative damage.

The specialization of the epididymis as a storage organ may have necessitated the parallel evolution of mechanisms whereby the stabilization that spermatozoa undergo for storage, can be reversed in order to prepare these cells for the membrane fusion events associated with fertilization (Fig. 1). This reversal of a stabilized state conferred during epididymal storage may be one of the major purposes served by capacitation [27]. Components of this destabilization process involve the loss of (glyco)proteins from the sperm surface and the removal of membrane cholesterol using albumin as an acceptor molecule. The ease with which spermatozoa can be capacitated will clearly depend upon the degree to which they have been stabilized for the purpose of epididymal storage. In the case of human spermatozoa the storage function of the epididymis does not seem to be highly developed, possibly because of the continuity of re-

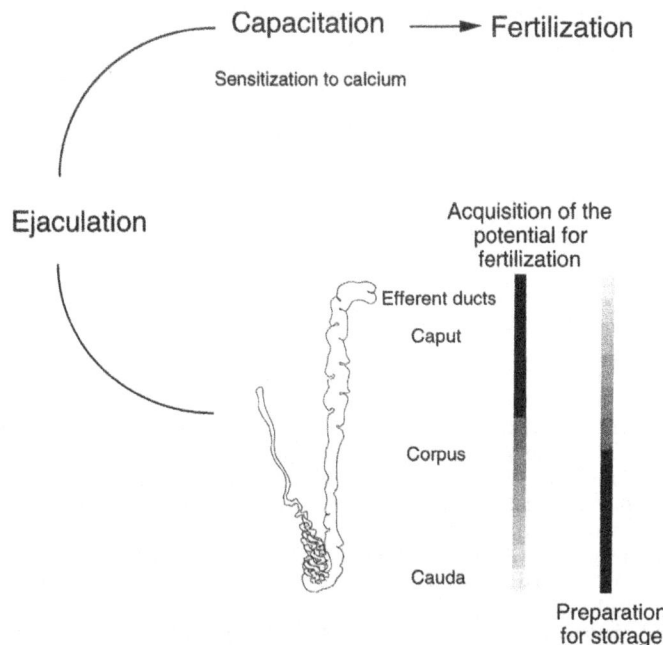

Fig. 1. One of the most important functions of the epididymis is to prepare the spermato-zoa for storage in the cauda. Several key aspects of sperm function, such as zona recogni-tion and the competence to undergo the acrosome reaction, are already established in sper-matozoa entering the epididymis. Acquisition of the potential for movement is achieved as the spermatozoa move through the epididymis although whether this change is an intrinsic property of the spermatozoa or conferred by specific constituents in the microenvironment generated by the epididymis is not certain. The stabilization of the spermatozoa for storage may have necessitated the parallel evolution of capacitation as a mechanism to destabilize these cells in preparation for the membrane fusion events associated with fertilization

productive activity in man. As a consequence, ejaculated human spermatozoa are not in a highly stabilized state and can be relatively easily capacitated. An important feature of capacitation is that it is not a synchronized process, and there is some heterogeneity between the individual members of an ejaculated sperm population in the rate at which this process proceeds. This is presumably a reflection of the differences between spermatozoa in the extent to which they have been stabilized for storage during epididymal transit. A small proportion of spermatozoa that have completed their journey through the epididymis with-out becoming highly stabilized are ready to fertilize the oocyte immediately after removal of the seminal plasma.

In the absence of a functional epididymis, as in cases exhibiting agenesis of the vas, a few spermatozoa may be able to complete their maturation sponta-neously. However, in the absence of a cauda epididymis these cells neither be-come stabilized for storage nor benefit from the protective functions afforded by the epididymal secretions, particularly in the context of oxidant damage. Two corollaries of these considerations are: (a) that in the absence of a cauda epididymis the spermatozoa quickly deteriorate, explaining why sperm quality appears to be reduced in spermatozoa recovered from the most distal regions of the epididymis in patients exhibiting agenesis of the vas, and (b) that those cells that are viable require a minimal degree of capacitation before they are competent to fertilize the ovum. Both of these predictions are borne out by the clinical experience of treating patients exhibiting vas occlusion and have clear implications for the treatment of patients exhibiting epididymal dysfunction and the potential of this organ as a site for contraceptive attack.

References

1. Tesarik J, Mendoza C, Testart J (1995) Viable embryos from injection of round spermatids into oocytes. New Eng J Med 333:525
2. Simerly C, Wu G-J, Zoran S et al (1995) The paternal inheritance of the centrosome, the cells microtubule-organizing center, in humans, and the implications for infertility. Nature Med 1:47–52
3. Yeung CH, Oberlander G, Cooper TG (1994) Maturation of hamster epididymal sperm motility and influence of thiol status of hamster and rat spermatozoa on their moility patterns. Mol Reprod Dev 38:347–355
4. Moore HDM, Hartman TD, Pryor JP (1983) Development of the oocyte penetrating capacity of spermatozoa in the human epididymis. Int J Androl 6:310–318
5. Yeung CH, Cooper TG, Oberpenning F et al (1993) Changes in movement characteristics of human spermatozoa along the length of the epididymis. Biol Reprod 49:274–280
6. Silber SJ (1994) The use of epididymal sperm in assisted conception. In: Tesarik J (ed) Male factor in human infertility. Ares-Serono Symposia, Rome, pp 335–368
7. Turner TT (1995) On the epididymis and its role in the development of a fertile ejaculate. J Androl 16:292–298
8. Mahony MC, Oeninger S, Doncel G et al (1993) Functional and morphological features of spermatozoa microaspirated from the epididymal regions of cynomolgus monkeys (Macaca fascicularis). Biol Reprod 48:613–620
9. Wassarman PM (1995) Towards molecular mechanisms for gamete adhesion and fusion during mammalian fertilization. Curr Opin Cell Biol 7:658–664
10. Van Duin M, Polman JEM, De Breet ITM et al (1994) Production, purification and biological activity of recombinant human zona pellucida protein, ZP3. Biol Reprod 51:607–617
11. Paterson M, Kerr L, Aitken RJ (1995) Progress in characterization of zona pellucida antigens as candidates for birth control vaccine. In: Kurpitz M, Fernandez N (eds) Immunology of human reproduction. BIOS Scientific, Oxford, pp 485–501
12. Yurewicz EC, Hibler D, Fontenot GK et al (1993) Cloning and sequence analysis of cDNA encoding ZP3-alpha, a sperm-binding glycoprotein from zona pellucida of pig oocyte. Biochim Biophys Acta 1174:211–214
13. Burks DJ, Carballada H, Moore HDM et al (1995) Interaction of a tyrosine kinase from human sperm with the zona pellucida at fertilization. Science 269:83–86
14. Bleil JD (1991) Sperm receptors of mammalian eggs. In: Wassarman PM (ed) Elements of mammalian fertilization, vol 1. CRC Press, Boca Raton, pp 133–152
15. Aitken RJ (1995) The complexities of conception. Science 269:39–40
16. Bookbinder LH, Cheng A, Bleil JD (1995) Tissue and species-specific expression of sp56, a mouse sperm fertilization protein. Science 269:86–89
17. Youakim A, Hathaway HJ, Miller DJ et al (1994) Overexpressing sperm surface β1,4-galactosyl transferase in transgenic mice affects multiple aspects of sperm egg interactions. J Cell Biol 126:1573–1583

18. Calvete JJ, Solis D, Sanz L et al (1993) Characterization of two glycosylated boar spermadhesins. Eur J Biochem 218:719–725
19. Sinowatz F, Amselgruber W, Töpfer-Peterson E et al (1995) Immunohistochemical localization of spermadhensin AWN in the porcine male genital tract. Cell Tiss Res 282:175–179
20. McLaughlin JD, Shur BD (1987) Binding of caput epididymal mouse sperm to the zona pellucida. Dev Biol 123:557–561
21. Ben Ali H, Guerin JF, Pinatel MC, Mathieu C, Boulieu D, Tritar B (1994) Relationship between semen characteristics, alpha-glucosidase and the capacity of spermatozoa to bind to the human zona pellucida. Int J Androl 17:121–126
22. Biegler BE, Aarons DJ, George BC et al (1994) Induction of physiological acrosome reactions in caput epididymal spermatozoa of mice. J Reprod Fertil 100:219–224
23. Lakoski KA, Carron CP, Cabot CL et al. Epididymal maturation and the acrosome reaction in mouse sperm: response to the zona pellucida develops coincident with modification of M42 antigen. Biol Reprod 38:221–223
24. Blobel CP, Wolfsberg TG, Turck CW et al (1992) A potential fusion peptide and an integrin ligand domain in a protein active in sperm oocyte fusion. Nature 356:248–252
25. Wolfsberg TG, Straight PD, Gerena RL et al (1995) ADAM, a widely distributed and developmentally regulated gene family encoding membrane proteins with a disintegrin and metalloproteinase domain. Dev Biol 169:378–383
26. Haidl G, Badura B, Hinsch K-D et al (1993) Disturbances of sperm flagella due to failure of epididymal maturation and their possible relationship to phospholipids. Human Reprod 8:1070–1073
27. Bedford JM (1994) The contraceptive potential of fertilization: a physiological perspective. Human Reprod 9:842–858
28. Perry ACF, Jones R, Hall L (1993) Isolation and characterization of a rat cDNA clone encoding a secreted superoxide dismutase reveals the epididymis to be a major site of its expression Biochem J 293:21–25
29. Ghyselinck NB, Dufaure I, Lareyre JJ et al (1993) Structural organization and regulation of the gene for the androgen-dependent glutathione peroxidase-like protein specific to the mouse epididymis. Molec Endocrinol 7:258–272

Menstrual Cycle: Follicular Maturation

A. Hourvitz, E. Y. Adashi

Introduction

As might be expected, the teleological underpinning of ovarian function draws on the fundamental need to preserve the species. Accordingly, the very existence of the ovary, and for that matter the very existence of the reproductive axis as a whole, is designed to subserve a single central objective, i.e., the generation of a mature fertilizable ovum. In this respect the ovary clearly need not be viewed as playing a secondary role in reproductive biology. Rather, it may be viewed as the "master gland" the very function of which is facilitated by the contribution of the various other components of the hypothalamic-pituitary-ovarian axis. This view differs of course from the more traditional outlook ascribing the role of a "master gland" to the pituitary, the workings of which are highly dependent on hypothalamic principles. However, current information would suggest that the ovary may in fact play an active rather than a passive role in the initiation and maintenance of reproductive cyclicity, the hypothalamus and pituitary being viewed as playing a permissive tonic role in this connection. Indeed, it is the changing tide of ovarian signals that appears to determine to a large extent the nature of the activities of the hypothalamic-pituitary unit. It is for these reasons that the ovary has often been likened to a pelvic clock ("zeitgeber") dictating in more ways than one the comings and goings of the reproductive process. Stated differently, consideration might be given to the argument that the ovary does, in effect, possess a "mind" of its own, as attested to by a multitude of putative intraovarian regulators, the very action of which is highly reminiscent of events previously viewed as the domain of the central nervous system.

Follicular Growth and Development:
Primordial Follicle, Recruitment, Selection, and Dominance

The primordial follicle consists of an oocyte arrested in the diplotene stage of the first meiotic prophase, surrounded by a single layer of granulosa cells. It is first noted at 16 weeks of intrauterine life, and it is generally accepted that its formation ends no later than 6 months post partum. It is quite certain that this stage of follicular development is entirely gonadotropin independent.

The preantral growth phase is the phase of follicular development and concerns the conversion of the primordial follicles (30 μm in diameter) to mature secondary follicles (120 μm in diameter). Initiated during the 5th–6th months of gestation, the process becomes evident when the granulosa cells undergo proliferation and differentiation, combined with thecal hypertrophy and the growth and differentiation of the oocyte, including the acquisition of the zona pellucida. The resulting mature secondary follicles constitute the pool of preantral follicles from which tonic, likely follicle-stimulating hormone (FSH=-dependent recruitment of follicles takes place [1–3].

The term recruitment has been used to indicate that a follicle has entered the so-called growth trajectory, i.e., the process wherein the follicle departs from the resting pool to begin a well-characterized pattern of growth and development. It is recognized that growing follicles are vulnerable to atresia and thus may leave the trajectory at any point. Consequently, recruitment, while obligatory, does not guarantee ovulation. Stated differently, recruitment is a necessary but not a sufficient condition for ovulation to occur. Recruitment is a "continuum" process [4] beginning at infancy and ceasing when the numbers of available oocytes is exhausted. It goes on at all times, at all ages, uninterrupted by pregnancy or other periods of nonovulation. The stimuli for follicle recruitment are unknown, but for the process to continue a favorable hormonal environment is needed. The absence of this environment will cause the atresia of most of the follicles. However, a favorable hormonal environment present at the beginning of the cycle, mostly the production of FSH, will enable the formation of a cohort of developing follicles [5]. Following recruitment, the flattened granulosa cells become cuboidal and small gap junctions are formed between the granulosa cells and the oocyte.

The term selection implies the final winnowing of the maturing follicular cohort (by atresia) down to a size equal to the species-characteristic ovulatory quota. Accordingly, selection is complete when the number of healthy follicles (i.e., with ovulatory potential) in the cohort equals the size of the ovulatory quota. As with recruitment, selection does not guarantee ovulation. However, given its greater temporal proximity to ovulation, selection may, with high probability, be expected to be followed by ovulation in a typical cycle.

It appears noteworthy that during the late luteal phase the largest healthy follicle cannot as yet be viewed as the one selected, since smaller follicles may harbor granulosa cells with a mitotic index greater than that of the presumably leading follicle. Consequently, the apparent growth delay of nonleading follicles could well be compensated for in a matter of days, the final selection occurring in the early part of the subsequent follicular phase. However, even in the early follicular phase no morphological differences exist between the selected follicle and other healthy members of the cohort. The above notwithstanding, the leading follicle can be distinguished from other members of the cohort by its sheer size and by the high mitotic index of its granulosa cells. Moreover, only the leading follicle can boast detectable levels of FSH in its follicular fluid at this point in time. It appears that this concentration of bioactive FSH within the follicular fluid is a major determinant of follicular fate. Once FSH exerts its inductive effect on the granulosa cells, as illustrated by the formation of the preantral follicle, the latter becomes strictly dependent on the continued presence of a favorable concentration of FSH in the follicular fluid. The presence of a critical level of FSH in the microenvironment is almost a guarantee that the sequence of selection will occur and that this follicle will become committed to growth and will become a dominant follicle. This same follicle also displays significant levels of estradiol. Indeed, it is generally agreed that the capacity to aromatize androgens efficiently is an important determinant of the chosen follicle. All told, the success of a follicle depends upon its ability to convert an androgen microenvironment to an estrogen microenvironment [6]. In contrast, the absence of adequate FSH leads to the cessation of proliferation and differentiation, followed by the progressive expression of apoptosis in the follicular wall. Most importantly, the follicle destined to ovulate displays a granulosa cell mitotic index high enough to ensure that smaller, albeit healthy follicles are unlikely to "catch up".

The term dominance refers to the status of the follicle destined to ovulate, given its presumed key role in regulating the size of the ovulatory quota. The selected follicle becomes dominant about a week prior to ovulation. Consequently, it must maintain its dominance during this week. Stated differently, the follicle selected for ovulation is functionally (not merely morphologically) dominant in that it is presumed to inhibit the development of other competing follicles on both ovaries. Inevitably, and for reasons not entirely clear, the dominant follicle (i.e., the sole follicle destined to ovulate) continues to thrive under circumstances which it itself has made inhospitable for others [7–9]. This dominant follicle has produced relatively more estrogen than the other follicles in its cohort. The dominant follicle thus enjoys an orderly sequence of events wherein FSH and estrogen stimulate growth, antrum formation, and the appearance of LH receptors. The dramatic increase in estrogen production by the dominant follicle, observable during the second half of the follicular phase is accompanied by falling levels of FSH [10]. As a result, the nondominant follicles fail to thrive. Apparently, the intrafollicular concentrations of gonadotropins and of steroids are central to the self-amplification process.

The preceding and related concepts were formulated in large measure in the course of the seminal work of Hodgen et al. [11, 12]. There is little doubt that this body of work profoundly affected the thinking of ovarian physiologists grappling with the difficult issues of ovarian cyclicity. Critical to these series of experiments were those by Goodman and Hodgen in which it was observed that cauterization of the largest visible follicle (days 8–12) delayed the expected time of the next preovulatory surge of pituitary gonadotropins [13] (Fig. 1). In contrast, luteectomy during the midluteal phase (days 16–19) advanced the expected time of the next preovulatory gonadotropin surge [14] (Fig. 2). Similar observations were made in women in whom the interval from ablation of the dominant follicle or corpus luteum to the next ovulation proved to be a fortnight [15]. As such, these findings are consistent with the possibility that the ovary itself may in fact play a "zeitgeber" (German for "time giver") role during the menstrual cycle, and that this time-keeping function is subserved by

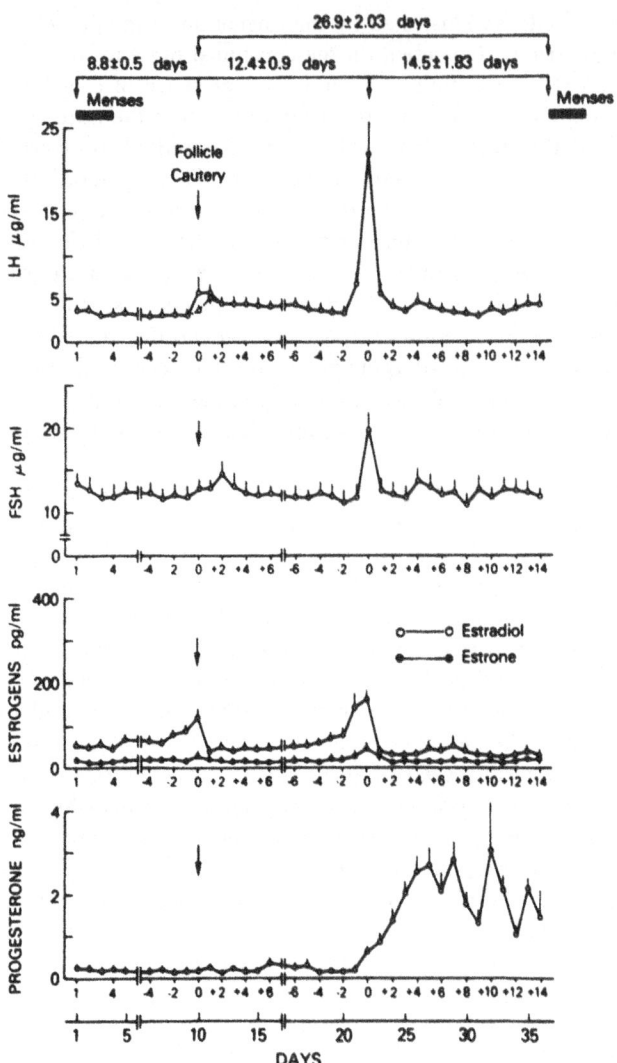

Fig. 1. Hormonal patterns before and after cautery of the largest visible follicle in rhesus monkeys. (Reproduced with permission from [11])

the activities of the cyclic structures of the dominant ovary. The 28-day menstrual cycle is thus the result of the intrinsic life span of the cyclic ovarian dominant structures and not of timed changes dictated by the brain or pituitary. The dominant follicle thus determines the length of the follicular phase, the corpus luteum determining the length of the luteal phase.

The preceding finding also suggested that the selection of the follicle destined to ovulate had already occurred by the time of cautery (i.e., by day 8 of the cycle). Indeed, it would appear that no other member of the follicular co-

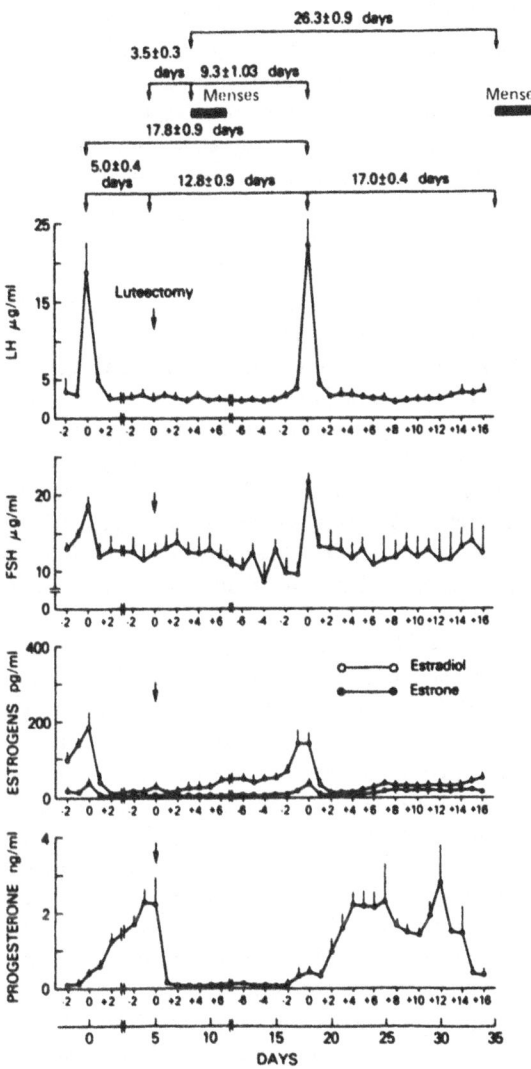

Fig. 2. Hormonal patterns before and after luteectomy in rhesus monkeys. (Reproduced with permission from [11])

hort was competent to serve as a surrogate for the cauterized follicle in order to achieve a timely, midcycle ovulation. Thus it could be suggested that the dominant follicle itself plays a key role in regulating the size of the ovulatory quota by inhibiting the development of any competing follicles in either ovary. A similar function is subserved by the corpus luteum. Therefore, the ovulatory follicle, once it is selected by midfollicular phase, and the corpus luteum are truly dominant ovarian structures. Accordingly, the next round of follicular growth occurs only after the interference by the cyclic structure is removed, either artificially, by experimental intervention, or naturally, after the demise of the corpus luteum. Further insight was gained from studies in which progesterone-replaced luteectomized primates were evaluated, revealing progesterone to be the principal luteal hormone responsible for the inhibition of luteal follicular growth. It is critical to note that circulating gonadotropin levels were apparently maintained after follicular or luteal ablation, and that follicle recruitment occurred without an attendant increment in circulating gonadotropins. Thus the inhibition of follicular growth by the cyclic structures of the ovary was not due to a decrease in the circulating levels of gonadotropins. Rather, it appeared to be due to local intraovarian influences. The above notwithstanding, reevaluation of these issues may well be warranted in that careful examination of the data suggests at least a slight, albeit transitory, increase in the circulating levels of FSH following ablation.

Further insight was derived from experiments revealing that the follicle destined to ovulate attains dominance 5–7 days after the demise of the corpus luteum. This conclusion was based on the observation that the levels of estradiol in ovarian venous serum were significantly different between ovaries as early as days 5–7 of the cycle. This difference in estrogen secretion between ovaries provides the earliest hormonal index attesting to the emergence of the dominant follicle.

Follicles with a diameter of less than 8 mm show a relatively low intrafollicular estrogen/androgen ratio. However, from the midfollicular phase onwards this ratio is reversed. With its increased capacity to aromatize androstenedione, the "chosen" follicle is able to synthesize estradiol in sufficient quantities; this results in appreciable passage of this hormone into the general circulation, thereby demonstrating (as early as days 5–7 of the cycle) the asymmetry of ovarian function [16]. In the late follicular phase the intrafollicular concentrations of estradiol are maximal at a time when the circulating estradiol levels surge to a peak. With the ovulatory LH surge the intrafollicular concentrations of estradiol decrease along with parallel drops in the intrafollicular concentrations of androstenedione. Concurrently, distinct progressive increments have been noted for the intrafollicular content of both progesterone and 17a-hydroxyprogesterone, reflecting early granulosa cell luteinization [17].

Antral fluid concentrations of estrone, estradiol, androstenedione, testosterone, and progesterone have been measured in specimens collected from ovarian follicles of women undergoing surgery [18–21]. Results of such studies have been reasonably consistent; data from one laboratory have been adapted for graphic display in Fig. 3. Despite large differences, the mean antral concentrations of steroid hormones tended to vary with the time in the cycle and with the size of the follicle. Throughout the cycle antral fluid levels of androgens and estrogens have varied independently, with higher ratios of androgens to estrogens in smaller than in larger follicles. The concentrations of progesterone were found to be elevated in large follicles sampled late in the follicular phase. Thus, higher antral concentrations of estrogens and progestogens and lower concentrations of androgens constitute a characteristic steroid hormone profile of preovulatory follicles [22]. In contrast, hormone profiles of smaller follicles

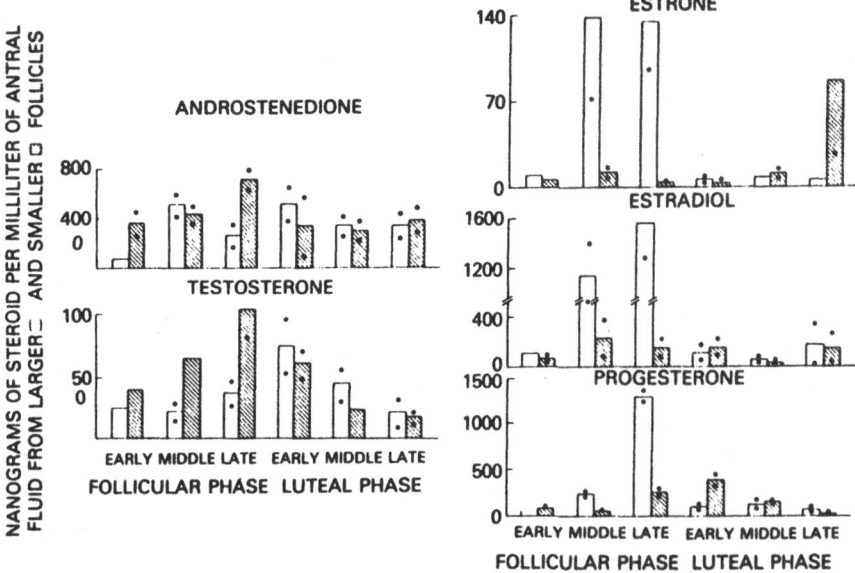

Fig. 3. Steroidal content of follicular fluid recovered from larger (*clear bars*) and smaller (*hatched bars*) antral follicles sampled at the indicated time during the menstrual cycle. (Adapted from [23])

sampled late in the follicular phase have been characterized by higher concentrations of androgens and lower concentrations of estrogens and progesterone. Although the data do not establish whether antral fluid steroid hormone profiles determine the ovulatory follicle, they do establish that the profiles of individual follicles are distinctive. In other words, mechanisms exist for regulating the antral fluid steroid hormone milieu in individual human ovarian follicles.

Since steroid hormone secretion depends on gonadotropic stimulation, the antral fluid levels of gonadotropin were also evaluated [23]. One study that determined antral fluid FSH, luteinizing hormone (LH), and prolactin noted evidence of differences related to follicle size and cycle time. LH was detected in the antral fluid of only 16% of smaller follicles but was detected in 70% of larger follicles around midcycle. FSH levels were measurable in antral fluid from both small and large follicles. However, in relation to prevailing serum FSH levels, antral FSH concentrations tended to be higher in larger follicles. It was also observed that estradiol levels were higher in antral fluids marked by measurable levels of FSH. Thus, antral fluid levels of FSH and estradiol are positively correlated. Moreover, incubation with FSH induces aromatase activity in granulosa cells recovered from follicles with low antral fluid estradiol levels, usually follicles less than 8–10 mm in diameter. It was therefore postulated that the presence or absence of measurable FSH was responsible for differences observed in antral fluid androgen-estrogen ratios. Taken together, these data are consistent with the concept that hormone concentrations are regulated in the microenvironment of individual follicles. Moreover, a functional role was imputed to the hormonal composition of the microenvironment when it was shown to affect progesterone synthesis by isolated granulosa cells in vitro. Thus, granulosa cells exposed to antral fluid containing FSH, LH, and estradiol in vivo secreted more progesterone than did cells isolated from follicles devoid of and thus unexposed to these hormones [24].

Ovulation

As midcycle approaches, there is a dramatic rise in estrogen followed by an LH surge and, to a lesser extent, an FSH surge which trigger the ovulation of the dominant follicle. For reasons not well understood, but possibly because of unique microenvironmental circumstances, one (rarely, more than one) follicle ovulates and gives rise to a corpus luteum during each menstrual cycle. In the human being, both LH and hCG have been shown to stimulate rupture of mature follicles. However, in hypophysectomized rats highly purified FSH can serve as the "ovulatory hormone" after follicular maturation has been stimulated by the administration of FSH and LH. Interestingly, inhibitors of prostaglandin synthesis (introduced systemically or locally into the antrum) have been shown to inhibit ovulation in rats and rabbits. Since LH has been shown to stimulate prostaglandin biosynthesis by ovarian follicles [25–33], increased prostaglandin synthesis might mediate the ovulatory stimulus of LH.

Mechanically, ovulation consists of rapid follicular enlargement followed by protrusion of the follicle from the surface of the ovarian cortex. Ultimately, rupture of the follicle results in the extrusion of an oocyte-cumulus complex. In the human ovary this sequence may well begin 5–6 days prior to the onset of the preovulatory LH surge. However, it is the latter event that marks the end of the follicular phase of the cycle and precedes actual rupture by as much as 36 h. Fortuitous endoscopic visualization of the ovary around the time of ovulation reveals that elevation of a conical stigma on the surface of the protruding follicle precedes rupture [34] (Fig. 4). Rupture of this stigma is accompanied by gentle, rather than explosive, expulsion of the oocyte and antral fluid, suggesting that the latter is not under high pressure [35, 36]. Indeed, direct measurements have demonstrated that intrafollicular pressure is low in the preovulatory follicle [37].

Several hypotheses have been advanced to account for the rapid increases in size and rupture of the follicle. For one, consideration was given to changes in the composition of the antral fluid during the period of rapid preovulatory follicular enlargement. In addition to changes in the steroid hormone content, an increase in colloid osmotic pressure has been noted. Although the granulosa cell-derived proteoglycans undoubtedly play a critical role in regulating the colloid osmotic pressure, little concrete information is in fact available as to the nature of their involvement [38–41]. Thus, a cause-effect relationship between the altered composition of antral fluid and the enlargement and rupture of the follicle remains to be established. Alternatively, stigma formation and rupture may reflect the effects of hydrolytic enzymes acting locally on protein sub-

Fig. 4. Ovulation of the cumulus-oocyte complex through the stigma. (Reproduced with permission from [3])

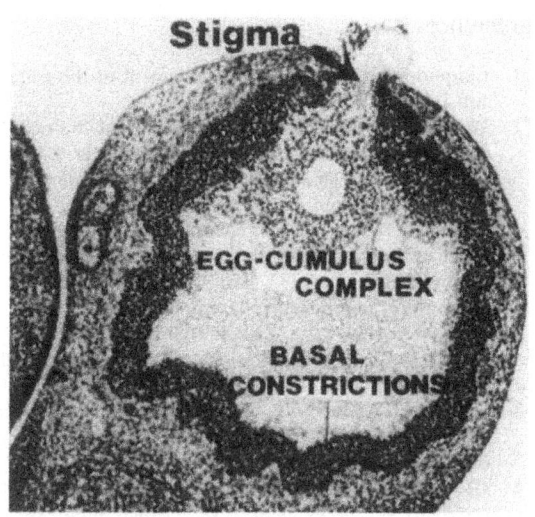

Stigma

EGG-CUMULUS COMPLEX

BASAL CONSTRICTIONS

strates in the basal lamina [42, 43]. In keeping with this notion, instillation of protease inhibitors into the antral fluid inhibits ovulation. One such proteolytic enzyme, plasminogen activator, has been localized in increasing concentrations in the walls of rat ovarian follicle just prior to ovulation [44]. Plasminogen activator, a serine protease, stimulates the conversion of plasminogen (a follicular fluid constituent) to the proteolytically active enzyme plasmin. The latter is known to activate collagenase, presumably an obligatory element in the dissolution of the basal membrane and the perifollicular stroma in the course of ovulation. It is thus generally presumed that plasminogen activator-mediated conversion of plasminogen to plasmin may contribute to the proteolytic digestion of the follicular wall as a prerequisite of follicular rupture. Consideration is also being given to the possibility that plasminogen activator may be involved in gap junction disruption and thereby in the delicate communication between the oocyte and the surrounding cumulus cells. Although the ultimate physiological significance of plasminogen activator remains a matter of study, there is little doubt as to the ability of somatic ovarian cells to produce this protease in measurable amounts in a manner subject to tight hormonal regulation. The FSH-dependent production of plasminogen activators by granulosa cells is particularly well documented. Recent studies have shown that prior to ovulation, while extracellular matrix degradation occurs within the mural granulosa at the site of follicle rupture, an expansive, viscoelastic extracellular matrix is synthesized and deposited around the oocytes by cumulus cells. Such matrix facilitates the extrusion of the oocyte through the rupture of the follicle at ovulation. It is suggested that the oocyte has a main role in promoting synthesis and preventing degradation of cumulus matrix by modulating cumulus cell response to an ovulatory gonadotropin stimulus [45].

References

1. Chiquoine HD (1960) The development of the zona pellucida of the mammalian ovum. Am J Anat 106:149
2. Weakly BS (1966) Electron microscopy of the oocyte and granulosa cells in the developing ovarian follicles of the golden hamster. J Anat 100:503
3. Erickson GF (1986) An analysis of follicle development and ovum maturation. Semin Reprod Endocrinol 4:233
4. Peters H, Byskov AG, Himelstein-Braw R, Faber M (1975) Follicular growth:the basic event in the mouse and human ovary. J Reprod Fertil 45:559
5. Vermesh M, Kletzky OA (1987) Longitudinal evaluation of the luteal phase and its transition into the follicular phase. J Clin Endocrinol Metab 64:653
6. Chabab A, Hedon B, Arnal F, Diafouka F, Bressot N, Flandre O, Cristol P (1986) Follicular steroids in relation to oocyte development and human ovarian stimulation protocols. Hum Reprod 1:449
7. DiZerega GS, Marrs RP, Roche PL, Campeau JD, Kling DR (1983) Identification of protein(s) in pooled human follicular fluid which suppress follicular response to gonadotropins. J Clin Endocrinol Metab 56:35
8. DiZerega GS, Goebelsmann U, Nakamura RM (1982) Identification of protein(s) secreted by the preovulatory ovary which suppresses the follicle response to gonadotropins. J Clin Endocrinol Metab 54:1091
9. DiZerega GS, Hodgen GD (1980) The primate ovarian cycle: suppression of human menopausal gonadotropin-induced follicular growth in presence of the dominant follicle. J Clin Endocrinol Metab 50:819
10. Fritz MA, Speroff L (1982) The endocrinology of the menstrual cycle, the interaction of folliculogenesis and neuroendocrine mechanisms. Fertil Steril 38:509
11. Goodman AL, Hodgen GD (1983) The ovarian triad of the primate menstrual cycle. Recent Prog Horm Res 89:1
12. Hodgen GD (1982) The dominant ovarian follicle. Fertil Steril 38:281
13. Goodman AL, Hodgen GD (1979) Between ovary interaction in the regulation of follicle growth, corpus luteum function, and gonadotropin in the primate ovarian cycle. II. Effects of luteectomy and hemiovariectomy during the luteal phase in cynomolgus monkeys. Endocrinology 104:1310
14. Goodman AL, Hodgen GD (1979) Between ovary interaction in the regulation of follicle growth, corpus luteum function, and gonadotropin secretion in the primate ovarian cycle. I. Effects of follicle cautery and hemiovariectomy during the follicular phase in cynomolgus monkeys. Endocrinology 104:1304
15. Nilsson L, Wikland M, Hamberger L (1982) Recruitment of an ovulatory follicle in the human following follicle-ectomy and luteectomy. Fertil Steril 37:30
16. DiZerega GS, Marut CK, Turner, Hodgen GD (1980) Asymmetrical ovarian function during recruitment and selection of the dominant follicle in the menstrual cycle of the rhesus monkey. J Clin Endocrinol Metab 51:698
17. Brailly S, Gougeon A, Milgram E, Bomsel-Helmreich O, Paiernik E (1981) Androgens and progestins in the human ovarian follicle: differences in the evolution of preovulatory, healthy nonovulatory, and atretic follicles. J Clin Endocrinol Metab 53:128
18. McNatty KP (1981) Hormonal correlates of follicular development in the human ovary. Aust J Biol Sci 34:249
19. McNatty KP, Baird DT, Bolton A, Chambers P, Corker CS, McLean H (1976) Concentration of oestrogens and androgens in human ovarian venous plasma and follicular fluid throughout the menstrual cycle. J Endocrinol 71:77
20. McNatty KP (1978) Cyclic changes in antral fluid hormone concentrations in humans. Clin Endocrinol Metab 7:577
21. McNatty KP, Moore-Smith D, Makris A, Osathanondh R, Ryan KJ (1979) The microenvironment of the human antral follicle: interrelationships among the steroid levels in antral fluids, the population of granulosa cells, and the status of the oocyte in vivo and in vitro. J Clin Endocrinol Metab 49:851

22. Sanyal MK, Berger MJ, Thompson IE, Taymor ML, Horne HW (1974) Development of graafian follicles in adult human ovary. I. Correlation of estrogen and progesterone concentration in antral fluid with growth of follicles. J Clin Endocrinol Metab 38:828

23. McNatty KP, Hunter WM, McNeilley AS, Sawers PS (1975) Changes in the concentration of pituitary and steroid hormones in the follicular fluid of human graafian follicles throughout the menstrual cycle. J Endocrinol 64:555

24. McNatty KP, Sawers RS (1975) Relationship between the endocrine environment within graafian follicle and the subsequent rate of progesterone secretion by human granulosa cells in vitro. J Endocrinol 66:391

25. Bauminger S, Lindner HR (1975) Periovulatory changes in ovarian prostaglandin formation and their hormonal control in the rat. Prostaglandins 9:737

26. Armstrong DT (1975) Role of prostaglandins in follicular responses to luteinizing hormone. Ann Biol Anim Biochim Biophys 15:181

27. Armstrong DT, Grinwich DL (1972) Blockage of spontaneous and LH-induced ovulation in rats by indomethacin, an inhibitor of prostaglandin synthesis. Prostaglandins 1:21

28. Armstrong DT, Zamecnik J (1975) Pre-ovulatory elevation of rat ovarian prostaglandin F, and its blockade by indomethacin. Mol Cell Endocrinol 2:125

29. Armstrong D, Grinwich D, Moon Y, Zamecnik J (1974) Inhibition of ovulation in rabbits by intrafollicular injection of indomethacin and prostaglandin F antiserum. Life Sci 14:129

30. Erickson GF, Challis JRG, Ryan KJ (1977) Production of prostaglandin F by rabbit granulosa cells and thecal tissue. J Reprod Fertil 49:133

31. Marsh JM, Yang NST, LeMaire WJ (1974) Prostaglandin synthesis in rabbit graafian follicles in vitro. Effect of luteinizing hormone and cyclic AMP. Protaglandins 7:269

32. Triebwasser WF, Clark MR, LeMaire WJ, Marsh JM (1978) Localization and in vitro synthesis of prostaglandins in components of rabbit preovulatory graafian follicles. Prostaglandins 16:621

33. Tsafriri A, Lindner HR, Zor U, Lamprecht SA (1972) Physiological role of prostaglandins in the induction of ovulation. Prostaglandins 2:1

34. Doyle JB (1951) Exploratory culdotomy for observation of tubo-ovarian physiology at ovulation time. Fertil Steril 2:475

35. Espey LL, Lipner H (1963) Measurements of intrafollicular pressures in the rabbit ovary. Am J Physiol 205:1067

36. Blandau R, Rumery R (1963) Measurements of intrafollicular pressure in ovulatory and preovulatory follicles in the rat. Fertil Steril 14:330

37. Blandau RJ (1969) Anatomy of ovulation. Clin Obstet Gynecol 10:347

38. Gebauer H, Lindner HR, Amsterdam A (1978) Synthesis of heparin-like glycosaminoglycans in rat ovarian slices. Biol Reprod 18:350

39. Bellin ME, Lenz RW, Steadman LE, Ax RL (1983) Proteoglycan production by bovine granulosa cells in vitro occurs in response to FSH. Mol Cell Endocrinol 29:51

40. Ax RL, Ryan RJ (1979) The porcine ovarian follicle. IV. Mucopolysaccharides at different stages of development. Biol Reprod 20:1123

41. Ax RL, Ryan RJ (1979) FSH stimulation of ^{3}H-glucosamine-incorporation into proteoglycans by porcine granulosa cells in vitro. J Clin Endocrinol Metab 49:696

42. Espey LL (1974) Ovarian proteolytic enzymes and ovulation. Biol Reprod 10:216

43. Bjersing L, Cajander S (1974) Ovulation and the mechanism of follicle rupture. IV. Ultrastructure of membrana granulosa of rabbit graafian follicles prior to induced ovulation. Cell Tissue Res 153:1

44. Beers WH, Strickland S, Reich E (1975) Ovarian plasminogen activator: relationship to ovulation and hormonal regulation. Cell 6:387

45. Tirone E, D'Alessandris C, Hascall VC, Siracusa G, Salustri A (1997) Hyaluronan synthesis by mouse cumulus cells is regulated by interactions between follicle-stimulating hormone (or epidermal growth factor) and a soluble oocyte factor (or transforming growth factor beta 1). J Biol Chem. 272:4787

Physiology of the Menstrual Cycle

K. Grunwald, T. Rabe, B. Runnebaum

Introduction

This chapter deals with the regulation of the menstrual cycle with a focus on endocrine control mechanisms. The morphological changes during the cycle are described in the chapter "Menstrual Cycle: Follicular Maturation" (Adashi, this volume). The regulatory processes are presented with a view to possible therapeutic consequences, which are described after the sections on the hypothalamus, the pituitary, and the ovaries.

The Darwinian principle states that individuals best adapted to their environment survive and with them the species to which the individuals belong. Since an adequate number of individuals must survive to ensure the preservation of a species (especially since evolution progresses through the survival of randomly better adapted individuals), one can appreciate the central importance of the reproductive system.

Since species with a flawed reproductive system cannot survive, the species alive today can be assumed to have a reproductive system that is optimum for their particular circumstances. All regulatory systems in reproductive biology can act via multiple pathways, so that when one system is lost, another can usually take over its functions. Human beings, currently at the apex of the evolutionary process, show many ontogenic traces of the phylogenic steps involved in the development of the human reproductive system. This pertains both to organ systems and to regulatory mechanisms.

Findings in laboratory animals do not necessarily apply to human beings. Regulatory systems that are of major importance in animals may be demonstrable in humans, but they may make little if any significant contribution to human functioning. The pineal gland, for example, evolved from the lateral parietal eye of reptiles to an organ that still utilizes light stimuli to modify reproductive processes. In humans, however, the pineal gland appears to perform no essential reproductive functions.

The three major organs that regulate human reproduction are the hypothalamus, the pituitary, and the ovary. It is believed that the pulse-generator function of the hypothalamus plays a central role in directing the ovulatory cycle. The pulsatile secretion of GnRH into the hypophyseal portal circulation is essential for sustaining the metabolic processes that periodically culminate in ovulation (Fig. 1). At the same time, a normal menstrual cycle would be impos-

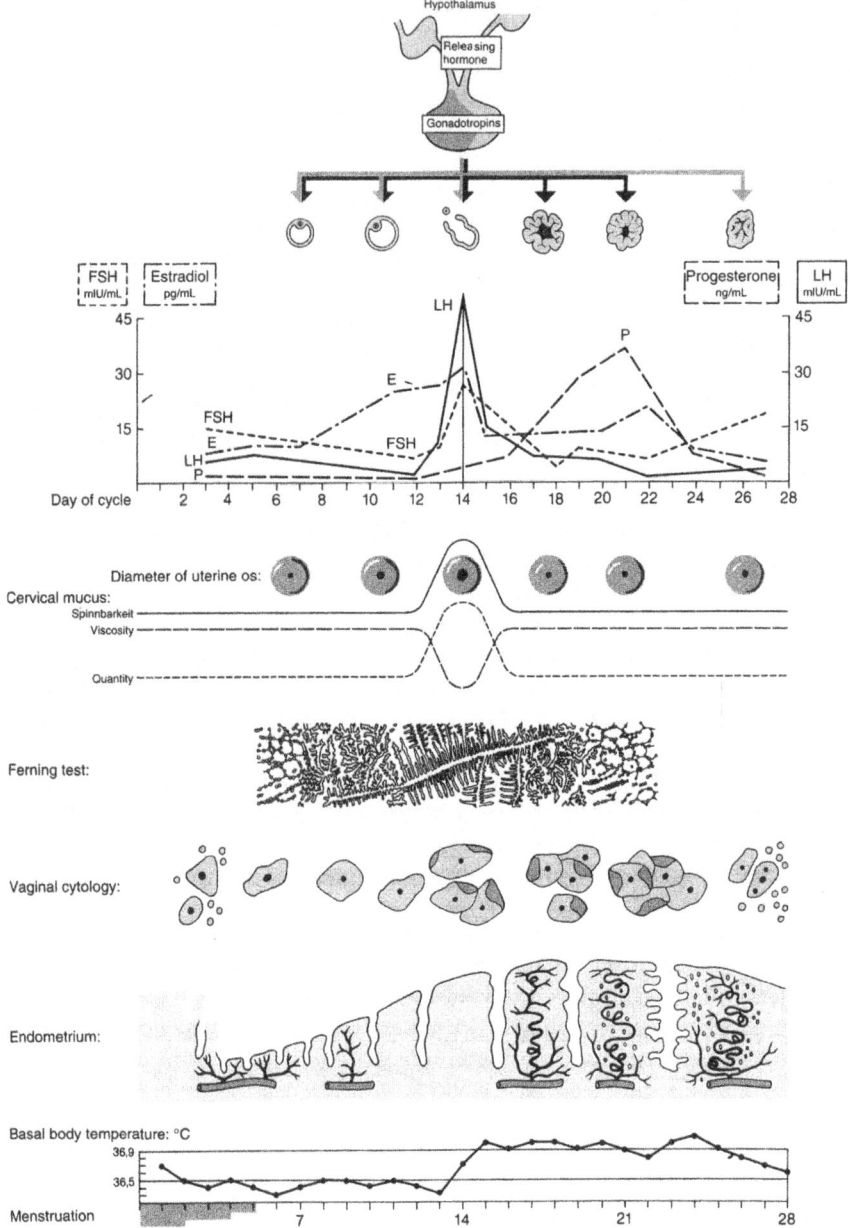

Fig. 1. Cyclic changes in the blood levels of sex hormones and their biological effects. (From Schmitt-Mathiesen 1991)

sible without the peripheral signals from ovarian steroids and other substances as well as input from higher and lower brain centers. The regulation of oocyte maturation, the timing of ovulation, and the function and regression of the corpus luteum are controlled by the ovaries through multiple feedback mechanisms. Both steroidal and nonsteroidal mechanisms act on the hypothalamus and pituitary in a way that adapts gonadotropin function to meet ovarian demands and ensure optimum oocyte maturation. The ovaries also influence gonadotropin secretion by modulating the frequency and amplitude of their pulsatile release. Thus the ovaries function as the central organs for regulation of the menstrual cycle in order to establish the conditions necessary for optimum oocyte maturation.

In many cases it is unclear how the connections between the hypothalamus and other brain areas described in this chapter contribute to physiological regulation of the human menstrual cycle. From a teleological standpoint, they provide a means of moderating or augmenting the reproductive potential in accordance with the environment as it is perceived by the sensory organs. The ability to recognize environmental conditions that are favorable in terms of temperature, light, nutritional sources, and other factors and to determine the moment that offers the best chances of offspring survival is crucial to the survival of the species. The degree to which these mechanisms are still active in human reproduction, rather than phylogenetic relics, remains unclear. It may be that modern environmental stresses in the form of diverse toxic agents are driving a new type of "natural selection" process.

The existence of a neuroendocrine (i.e., hypothalamic-anterior pituitary) chemotransmitter system was first postulated by Green and Harris in 1949. Many other organs and tissues also take an active or passive part in the cyclic hormonal changes, most notably the vagina, cervix, endometrium, uterine tubes, and breasts. The fluctuating hormone levels can also produce changes in psychological state, mood, and autonomic nervous activity that vary markedly from one individual to the next. The reproductive potential is also subject to modulation by environmental influences (light-dark cycle) acting via the sensory organs. Stressful situations can directly influence the control of the reproductive cycle by their effects on hypothalamic function.

Central Nervous System

The central nervous system (CNS) influences the reproductive system in a variety of ways. These include regulation via direct neural connections and by humoral control. The hypothalamus acts as the integrator of neuronal and endocrine functions, using feedback control to regulate processes such as appetite, osmoregulation, secondary sexual development, and reproductive functions. The present section details the various regulatory mechanisms of the menstrual cycle that are operative at the level of the CNS.

Hypothalamus

From the standpoint of menstrual regulation, the hypothalamus forms the connecting link between the cerebrum and the anterior lobe of the pituitary, i.e., between neural and endocrine regulation. Additionally, the hypothalamus has numerous afferent (arising from the hypothalamus) and efferent (acting on the hypothalamus) connections with other portions of the brain.

The relay of neuronal impulses through the hypothalamus is accomplished by the release of five hypophysiotropic hormones: thyrotropin-releasing hormone (TRH), gonadotropin-releasing hormone (GnRH), corticotropin-releasing hormone (CRH, CRF), growth hormone (GH)-releasing hormone (GRH), and somatostatin (SS; somatotropin release inhibiting factor) – which are released into the portal circulation in the median eminence.

Hypothalamic Hypophysiotropic Hormones

The hormonal control of the anterior pituitary by the hypothalamus was first documented by studies with brain extracts (Guillemin and Rosenberg 1955) and confirmed by identification of the hypothalamic releasing hormones TRH (Burgus et al. 1970), GnRH (Schally et al. 1971; Matsuo et al. 1971), CRH (Vale et al. 1981), and GRH (Guillemin et al. 1982). Only in recent decades has the development of assay methods for steroid and peptide hormones enabled a more precise investigation of the underlying mechanisms. More recently, techniques in molecular biology have made it possible to isolate the genes of most of the releasing hormones and pituitary hormones and investigate the control of transcription and translation.

The Neuronal GnRH System

The regulation of pituitary luteinizing hormone (LH) and follicle-stimulating hormone (FSH) secretion is mediated by the stimulatory action of GnRH. GnRH is a decapeptide derived from a large precursor molecule, pre-pro-GnRH (92 amino acids). The last 56 amino acid sequence, termed GnRH-associated peptide, can inhibit prolactin (PRL) secretion. The synthesis of GnRH follows the classic pathway from high-molecular polypeptide precursors. The gene sequence for GnRH was elucidated by Seeburg and Adelman in 1984.

The biological activity of GnRH is very short, with a half-life of 4–6 min. Degradation occurs by cleavage of the peptide bonds at positions 6 and 7, yielding biologically inactive peptides. Degradation is effected by specific peptidases whose activity is regulated by steroids and released LH.

The GnRH-secreting cells have been identified as neurons of the arcuate nucleus whose axons traverse the median eminence of the mediobasal hypothalamus (MBH). GnRH is synthesized in the neurons, stored in granules, and transported to the portal capillaries via the neural axons.

Age-Related Changes in GnRH Secretion

Fetal Period. GnRH can be detected in the fetal hypothalamus between the 14th and 16th weeks of gestation. Also, in vitro studies have shown that the isolated MBH of the human fetus secretes GnRH in a pulsatile pattern between weeks 20 and 23 of gestation (Rassmussen et al. 1989). Moreover, the fetal gonadotroph (the LH- and FSH-secreting cell of the pituitary) at this stage can respond to GnRH stimulation by secreting LH under in vivo and in vitro conditions (Rossmanith et al. 1990). This means that a functioning hypothalamic-pituitary unit is present in the fetus as early as the middle of the second trimester, and that this unit is capable of sustaining gonadotropin secretion. The secretory output of GnRH during fetal development is comparable in the male and female hypothalamus, but during the second trimester the concentration of LH in the pituitary and serum is significantly higher in female human fetuses than in males (Reyes et al. 1974). This could be due to negative feedback from fetal testicular hormones. Studies in fetal pituitaries have shown that repeated GnRH pulses evoke a six times greater pituitary release of LH in female fetuses than in male fetuses.

Neonatal Period. A pulsatile pattern of GnRH secretion is evident during the neonatal period. Pituitary sensitivity to exogenous GnRH declines during the first years of childhood.

Childhood. The GnRH frequency in early childhood is approximately 1 pulse/h in boys and 1 pulse/3–4 h in girls. The serum level of gonadotropins (especially LH) gradually falls during this period and remains at a low level during the first 10 years, with an elevated FSH:LH ratio. Pituitary resposiveness to exogenous GnRH is low during this time.

Puberty. The onset of puberty is marked by a renewed increase in GnRH secretion, which is associated with a change in the opioid tone. The increased frequency and amplitude of the GnRH pulses initially occurs at night but later is maintained throughout the day. The mechanisms underlying this change are poorly understood. Animal studies suggest that a fall in endogenous opioid levels is responsible, but this mechanism appears questionable in humans, especially since opiate antagonists in prepubertal children do not evoke an increase in LH secretion. Another important development during puberty is reflected in the altered sensitivity of the neuroendocrine system to steroidal effects. Initially the nocturnal rise in GnRH secretion augments the release of FSH, which is suppressed by the increase in estrogen production. The further increase in the frequency and amplitude of the GnRH pulses is associated with a preferential increase in the secretion of LH. Rising estrogen production further stimulates LH release as pituitary sensitivity to GnRH pulses is enhanced. Estradiol in early puberty cannot reduce the GnRH pulse frequency.

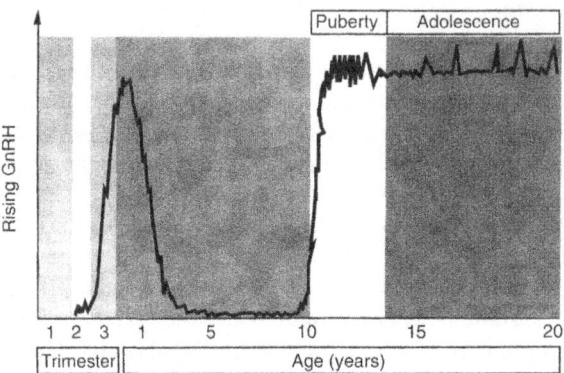

Fig. 2. Pattern of GnRH secretion up to age 20 years

Reproductive Period. GnRH secretion during the reproductive years is subject to the cyclic influences of ovarian steroids and other factors (see "The Ovaries").

Postmenopause. Ovarian quiescence is associated with a disinhibition of GnRH secretion, leading to a rise in the frequency and amplitude of LH and FSH secretion (Fig. 2).

Pulse Generator

In a series of studies by Knobil and coworkers (Knobil et al. 1980; Wilson et al. 1984; Knobil 1989) rhythmic electrical impulses were recorded from GnRH neurons in the MBH. These rhythmic discharges show a definite synchronicity with GnRH secretion into the hypophyseal portal blood and with peripheral LH pulses.

The pulse generator for the rhythmic action potentials is very likely located in or near the arcuate nucleus in the MBH. Experiments in primates whose arcuate nucleus had been destroyed by stereotactic surgery demonstrated a rapid cessation of pulsatile GnRH and gonadotropin secretion (Wildt et al. 1981). It remains unclear whether the rhythmic electrophysiological discharges are an intrinsic property of the GnRH neurons or arise in association with nearby neurons by a mechanism that is still unknown.

Pulsatile Secretion

The electrophysiological action potentials occur in the MBH at intervals of 60–90 min. The rhythmic activity in the MBH and the release of GnRH from neurosecretory granules into the portal circulation give rise to peak concentrations of gonadotropins in the serum. The importance of pulsatile LH and FSH secretion for the ovaries is unclear, since ovarian steroid secretion is maintained even during the continuous exogenous administration of gonadotropins. It may be that with a pulsatile secretory pattern smaller amounts of gonadotropins are needed to produce the same amount of steroids than with a tonic pattern of gonadotropin secretion (Rossmanith et al. 1987).

Changes in the frequency of GnRH secretion, and thus of the gonadotropin pulses, disrupt the normal course of an ovulatory menstrual cycle:

- High GnRH pulse frequencies lead preferentially to the expression of LH α-mRNA but not to that of LH β-mRNA or FSH-β-mRNA.
- Low GnRH pulse frequencies selectively induce the expression of FSH β-mRNA.
- Only physiological GnRH pulse patterns can allow the synthesis of both gonadotropins in the gonadotroph.
- An increase or decrease in the pulse frequency leads to the disruption of physiological menstrual function (Fig. 3).

Gonadotropin secretion also appears to depend on the concentration of GnRH in the portal venous blood: high concentrations stimulate secretion while low concentrations produce only a priming effect. As a result, even low GnRH am-

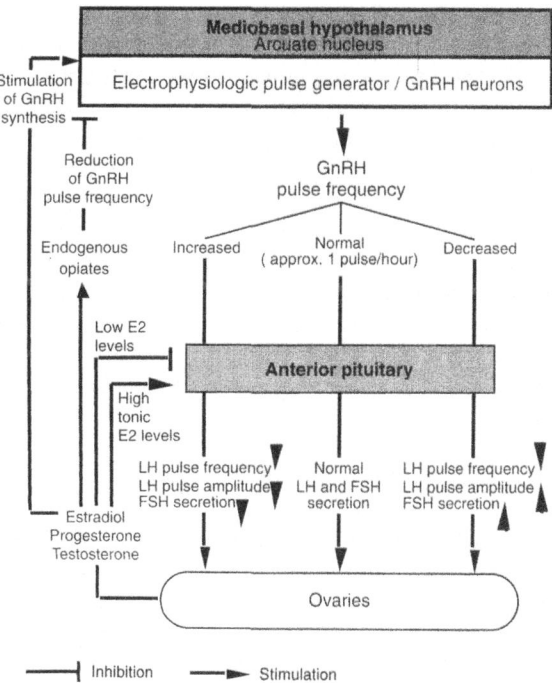

Fig. 3. GnRH pulse frequency: effect on LH and FSH secretion. The secretion of LH and FSH is modulated (usually suppressed) by the steroids, and the action of GnRH alone has virtually no effect on the pituitary in vivo. The postmenopausal increase in LH and FSH secretion is due to the lack of steroid suppression

plitudes induce an up-regulation of GnRH receptors after a latent period of about 4 h, enabling the generation of higher-amplitude LH pulses.

While the pulse generator controls GnRH secretion, and thus the secretion of gonadotropins, it performs only a permissive function with regard to the menstrual cycle. Ovarian steroids play the key role in regulating the frequency and possibly the amplitude of GnRH secretion. Moreover, a variety of factors are involved in the modulation of GnRH and gonadotropin secretion.

Rhythmic, short-term, pulsatile LH fluctuations occur at different frequencies in different animal species. The average intervals between successive pulses are as follows (Knobil 1974): rat, 20 min; monkey, 60 min; and human, ca. 90 min. This provides a rationale for intermittent GnRH replacement in patients with deficiency symptoms and in the treatment of infertility.

Regulation of GnRH Secretion

With regard to the modulation of gonadotropin secretion, one way in which gonadotropin secretion can be influenced is by altering the frequency of the pulse generator. A second approach is to modulate the reaction of the GnRH neurons to generator impulses in terms of the storage and secretion of GnRH. Other possible sites of action are the release of GnRH into the portal circulation (negative short-loop feedback from increased levels in the portal blood), the GnRH receptor on the gonadotrope, postreceptor mechanisms, and the storage of gonadotropins and their release into the circulation.

Agents with a modulatory action are neurotransmitters (e.g., a-adrenergic, serotoninergic, and dopaminergic neurons); the endogenous opiate system, which can be stimulated and inhibited by various other neuromodulators; and especially the steroids (estrogens, progesterone, androgens), which exert permissive, direct and indirect actions on the frequency of GnRH pulses and on gonadotropin release at various levels (Fig. 4). Three major classes of neurochemical transmitters are known: (a) biogenic amines (e.g., norepinephrine, epinephrine, dopamine, serotonin); (b) amino acids (e.g., γ-aminobutyric acid, glycine); and (c) neuropeptides (e.g., opioids, neuropeptide Y).

Endogenous Opioids

The hypothalamic opioid system forms a well-defined neuronal network within the MBH that has close anatomic and functional associations with the GnRH neurons. Endogenous opioids play a central role in gonadotropin secretion through their inhibitory effect on hypothalamic GnRH secretion (Yen et al. 1985).

Action. Endogenous opioids can suppress the hypothalamic GnRH pulse frequency. The action of the opioid system cannot be considered separate from the steroid milieu; however, as its activity is regulated by steroids, especially es-

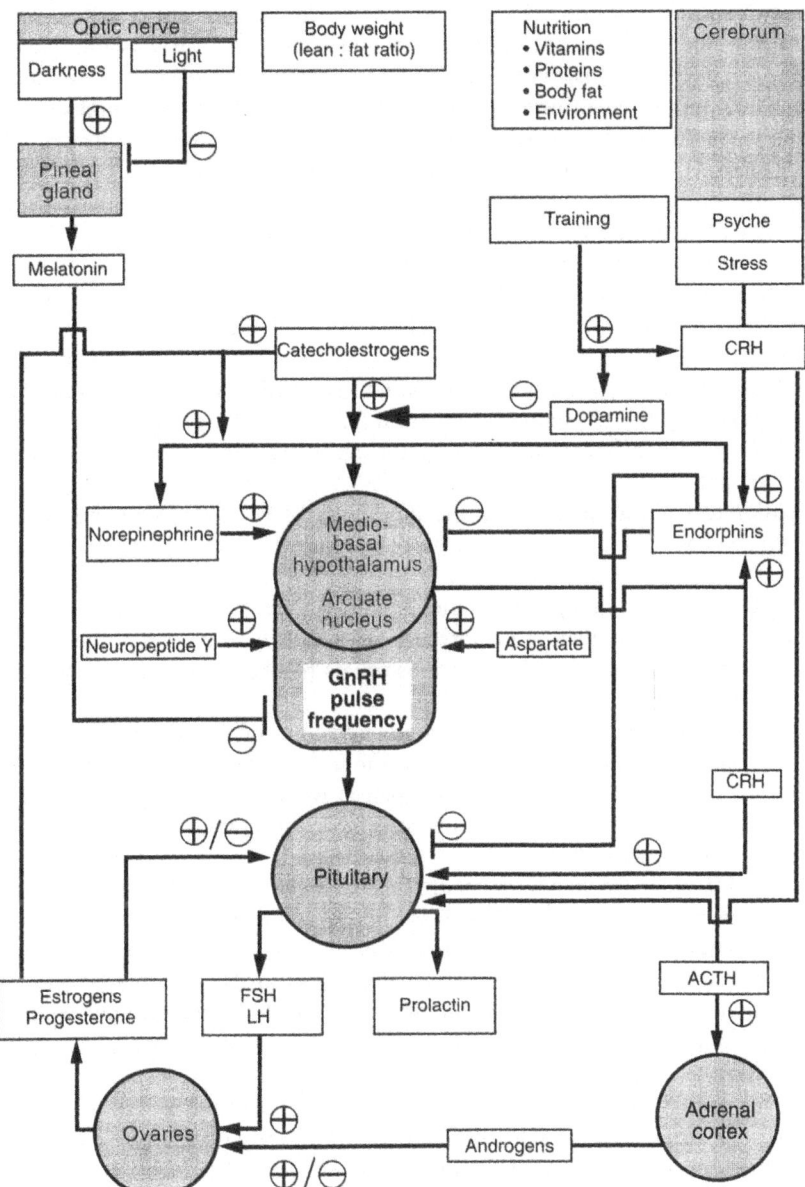

Fig. 4. Factors that affect pulsatile GnRH secretion

tradiol and progesterone (Melis et al. 1988). The hypothalamic content of β-endorphin and pre-pro-opiomelanocortin messenger RNA varies with changes in steroid concentrations, with low opioid concentrations occurring in the early follicular phase (when estradiol levels are low) and high concentrations occurring in the luteal phase (Wehrenberg et al. 1982). Accordingly, a blockade of endogenous opioids in the late follicular phase and luteal phase has the effect of stimulating gonadotropin release. This effect is not elicited when estrogen levels are low (in the early follicular phase and after menopause).

Rossmanith et al. (1988) performed studies with opiate antagonists to investigate endogenous opiate activity during the menstrual cycle. They observed the following effects produced by 8-h infusion of the opiate antagonist naloxone:
- Early follicular phase: no change in GnRH and LH secretion during the day; blockade of the physiological noctural fall in GnRH secretion.
- Late follicular phase: increase in the frequency and amplitude of LH and FSH pulses.
- Midluteal phase: increase in the amplitude of LH pulse with no change in frequency.

The blockade of endogenous opioids in the late follicular phase and luteal phase tends to stimulate gonadotropin release. It also increases the sensitivity of gonadotropin release to endogenous opiate blockade from the early follicular phase to the luteal phase.

It has been shown that intravenous infusions of β-endorphin significantly lower the serum levels of LH in the midfollicular phase (Reid et al. 1981). The absence of this response in postmenopausal women implies that estrogens and progestins not only regulate the expression of the opioids but can also control opioid receptor activity.

The LH pulse frequency normally falls at night during sleep in the early follicular phase. In the early luteal phase opiate antagonists have no effect on the pulse frequency in the waking state during the day, although the opiate antagonist naloxone can abolish the nocturnal changes in the pulsatile pattern of LH secretion (Rossmanith et al. 1987). This may relate to a circadian rhythmicity of opioid binding sites – a phenomenon that has been demonstrated in rats (Jacobson et al. 1986).

The endogenous opioid system also may be involved in initiating the LH midcycle surge. It is thought that opioidergic activity declines at midcycle, lifting the suppressive action of the opioids on LH and FSH secretion. A 24-h infusion of naloxone leads to an increase in pulsatile LH and FSH secretion that corresponds to the spontaneous LH peak (Rossmanith et al. 1988). It remains unclear, however, whether a decline in opioidergic activity is due to a decrease in receptor activity or density or to reduced concentrations of opioids at sites of neuronal regulation (Jacobson and Kolra 1989). Opiate neurons are known to possess estradiol receptors, and a change in endogenous opiate activity therefore leads to a feedback effect of ovarian steroids on the hypothalamus and pituitary.

Dopaminergic Modulation

Despite comprehensive research the role of dopamine in the regulation of GnRH secretion remains controversial. Dopamine can exert a stimulatory or inhibitory action on GnRH secretion, depending on the experimental conditions. The identity of dopamine as PRL-inhibiting factor is well established. An absence of dopamine in the region of the substantia nigra leads to Parkinson's disease. The following actions of dopamine have been demonstrated:
- Inhibition of PRL secretion.
- Stimulation of β-endorphin secretion, causing indirect inhibition of GnRH secretion.
- β-Endorphins inhibit the release of dopamine in the hypothalamus.
- Findings on the effect of dopamine on GnRH pulse frequency are controversial. Dopamine may exert a direct stimulatory action and indirect inhibitory action (opioid-mediated) on the pulse generator.

Estrogens

Estrogen-binding neurons are found predominantly in the preoptic and hypothalamic regions of the brain. The greatest density of binding sites for estradiol occurs in the periventricular region between the preoptic area and the lower part of the arcuate nucleus. Only 1 in 500 GnRH neurons contains estrogen receptors, however (Shivers et al. 1983).

Animal studies have shown that estrogens can stimulate GnRH secretion (Rudenstein et al. 1979) or inhibit it (Gross 1980) depending on the dose and duration of the exposure. There is evidence that direct control of the GnRH gene by estrogens can produce a slight stimulatory effect (Pfaff 1986). It is more likely, however, that estrogenic effects are mediated indirectly by adjacent neurons that secrete such compounds as γ-aminobutyric acid, opioids, dopamine, or adrenergic agents.

Mediation of the steroidal effect by opioidergic neurons is evidenced by the fact that a significant percentage of the opioidergic neurons have receptors for estradiol (about 20%) and progesterone (about 30%). Some 20% of the dopaminergic neurons contain estrogen receptors, and 90% contain progesterone receptors (Sar 1984; Romano et al. 1989; Fox et al. 1990; Hoffman et al. 1990). As in other tissues, estrogens can induce progesterone receptors on neurons of the MBH.

The following actions of estrogens on hypothalamic GnRH secretion are known:
- Activation of β-endorphin secretion.
- Activation of the dopaminergic system.
- β-Endorphins inhibit both dopamine secretion and GnRH secretion.
- Dopaminergic activation inhibits GnRH secretion by the activation of β-endorphins.

Because neuropeptides exert stronger and longer-lasting effects than amines, the β-endorphin-mediated suppressive effect is usually predominant (Rasmussen et al. 1987). Estradiol can induce the formation of progesterone receptors in neurons of the MBH (Romano et al. 1989). GnRH neurons in the arcuate nucleus have few if any progesterone and estradiol receptors (Fox et al. 1990).

Progestins

Progesterone binding occurs in the MBH and the region about the median eminence. Progesterone receptors have not been found on GnRH neurons in the arcuate nucleus, but they have been detected on about 90% of dopamine neurone in the arcuate nucleus and about 30% of β-endorphin neurons.

Progestins, as with estrogens, can exert stimulatory or inhibitory effects on the neuroendocrine axis depending on their concentration and time of action. These effects are not produced directly via GnRH neurons; they occur indirectly and depend on the estradiol concentration. Both dopaminergic and opioidergic neurons have axo-axonal synapses with GnRH neurons, enabling them to influence the GnRH pulse generator. At the same time, progesterone reduces the frequency and increases the amplitude of LH pulses during the luteal phase and after estrogen treatment. Progesterone can release GnRH from the hypothalamus and inhibit its degradation. This effect, too, is mediated by the opioid system. The neuromediators involved in this process include β-endorphin, norepinephrine, and as recent studies indicate neuropeptide Y.

Progesterone has been confirmed to stimulate both dopaminergic and opioidergic neurons in the arcuate nucleus of the MBH, with the result that (a) β-endorphin inhibits both dopamine and GnRH secretion and (b) dopamine stimulates both β-endorphin and GnRH secretion. Thus, the actions of progesterone on the hypothalamus are regulated with the aid of autoregulatory dopamine and opioid secretion, which have opposite effects on GnRH secretion.

Androgens

Androgen binding is evidenced by very high receptor densities in the hypothalamus, the amygdala, and to a lesser degree the septum and hippocampus. Androgen concentrations are lower than estrogen concentrations in all areas of the brain. It is thought that a significant percentage of circulating androgens are converted to estrogens by aromatization and thus exert estrogenic effects. Studies indicate that the morphological differentiation of the male brain depends partly on the capacity for androgen aromatization in the hypothalamus and forebrain. On the whole, the impact of androgens on GnRH secretion remains unclear. By their aromatization in the brain, androgens may support estrogen-mediated effects. It is also likely that they exert effects on the hypothalamus analogous to those of estradiol.

Corticotropin Releasing Hormone

CRH-binding neuron systems occur in various hypothalamic and extrahypothalamic regions as well as outside the brain. It is thought that CRH also functions as a stimulatory neurotransmitter. In this way the CRH system could contribute significantly to the linkage of the brain-pituitary-adrenal axis and to stress-related autonomic reflexes and behaviors such as pain perception, arousal, and motivation.

Actions on the Reproductive System

By inducing the secretion of β-endorphins, CRH exerts a suppressive effect on the GnRH pulse generator. CRH exerts a direct suppressive effect on the electrophysiological activity of the pulse generator. The actions of CRH can be summarized as follows:
- Activation of the pituitary-adrenal axis (pituitary adrenocorticotropin secretion)
- Increased activity of the sympathetic nervous system
  - Elevation of blood glucose
  - Increase in oxygen consumption
  - Rise in cardiac output
  - Blood pressure elevation
- Reduced activity of the reproductive system
  - Suppression of GnRH secretion
  - Decreased sexual activity
- Suppression of gastrointestinal function
  - Anorexia
  - Reduced gastric acid secretion
- Stimulation of respiration
- Alteration of immunological and inflammatory responses
  - Antipyretic action
- Behavior changes (arousal, locomotor activity).

Growth Hormone Releasing Hormone

Secretion. The episodic secretion of pituitary GH is subject to regulation by two hypothalamic peptides: SS and GRH. The pulsatile secretion of pituitary GH results from the alternating secretion of SS and GRH, with SS exerting an inhibitory action and GRH a stimulatory action (Tannenbaum and Ling 1984). GRH is secreted into the median eminence and portal circulation from axons of neurons residing in the MBH, especially the posterior portion of the arcuate nucleus. There are also stimulatory connections with the somatostatin neurons that create a negative feedback mechanism.

GRH regulates only the secretion of GH. Aside from this, it has been found in other intra- or extracerebral tissues only in cases of ectopic GRH production in the setting of acromegaly. Circulating insulin-like growth factors (IGFs), whose secretion is induced by GH, exert a negative long-loop feedback effect on GRH secretion. GRH itself has no known physiological functions in terms of regulating the menstrual cycle. The actions of GRH-induced IGF-I are discussed under the appropriate heading.

Thyrotropin-Releasing Hormone

TRH is not known to have a physiological effect on human menstrual regulation.

Pathophysiology of Hypothalamic Function

Disorders of hypothalamic function are summarized in Table 1.

Hyperprolactinemia (reduced or absent hypothalamic prolactin-inhibiting factors), visual field disorders (compression of the chiasma opticum), and diabetes insipidus (destruction of nervous connections between the hypothalamus and the posterior pituitary) are signs of hypothalamic dysfunction. Since the hypothalamus forms a link between the nervous and the humoral regulation of the reproductive function, all clinically manifest disorders except tumors and Kallman's syndrome are the result of disturbed feedback with upstream and downstream organs (higher brain functions, pituitary, ovaries, thyroid, adrenal).

Table 1. Causes of hypothalamic disorders

Organic Hypothalamic Disorders
  Kallman's syndrome
  Craniopharyngeoma
  Germinoma (ectopic pinealoma)
  Glioma of the chiasma opticum or of the hypothalamus
  Hand-Schüller-Christian syndrome
  Dermoid cysts, teratomas
  Endodermal sinus tumor (yolk sac carcinoma)
  Tuberculosis, sarcoidosis
  Metastases
  Skull trauma
  Radiotherapy

Functional Hypothalamic Disorders
  Pseudogravidity
  Anorexia nervosa
  Stress, depression
  Competitive sports
  Malnutrition
  Drug abuse (morphine derivatives)
  Pharmaceuticals
  Hypermelatoninemia

Kallman's syndrome is a genetic disorder which may be caused by at least three different genetic defects. Inheritance may be autosomal recessive, dominant, or via the X chromosome. It is caused by a disturbed migration of GnRH neurons, which normally migrate along with olfactory nerves from the olfactory placode to the brain. Causative treatment of the disease is not possible. If the patient wishes to conceive, ovulation and pregnancy can be achieved by pulsatile GnRH or gonadotropin stimulation. Nearly all follicles found in the ovaries are at the primordial stage because the later stages are gonadotropin dependent.

Tumors in the *hypothalamic region* lead to the partial or complete breakdown of hypothalamic functions and, depending on the extent of the tumor, to symptoms of intracranial neoplasia. Therapy is according to the type of the tumor. In most cases, a cautious surgical approach combined with radiotherapy is required. Replacement therapy is needed along with vasopressin to treat diabetes insipidus.

Functional disorders of the hypothalamus result from multiple changes in the brain sections and peripheral organs involved. However, it is usually not possible to identify a single cause because of the way the hypothalamus is integrated into regulatory systems. Hypothalamic interaction with the limbic system (amygdala, hippocampus, neocortex, and midbrain), which is involved in processing many external and internal mental stimuli, makes it possible for the individual to adjust to different environmental conditions.

The reaction to excessive stress of a mental or physical nature (decompensated stress reaction) can cause the impairment or breakdown of the reproductive function. Clinically, the patient presents with amenorrhea. Table 1 lists the causes of hypothalamic dysregulation.

Pseudogravidity (pseudocyesis) is a typical example of the interaction between the psyche and the reproductive function. The exact mechanisms leading to the manifestation of unambiguous symptoms of pregnancy are not fully known. Clinically, an increased amplitude of the pulsatile secretion of prolactin and LH is found. Serum levels of estradiol and progesterone are increased so that luteal function is maintained. FSH secretion is suppressed. After the patient is informed that she is not pregnant, the central changes normalize rapidly. In many cases, however, the patient will need psychological or psychiatric support.

Functional hypothalamic amenorrhea of psychogenic origin: one of the most frequent forms of amenorrhea is menstrual failure without any apparent disorder of the pituitary-ovarian axis. The changes include activation of the hypothalamic-pituitary axis and hypersecretion of CRF and cortisol, while the diurnal rhythm is maintained. A central opioid-mediated inhibition of GnRH secretion can be identified, which causes an impairment of ovarian function ranging from luteal phase disorders to amenorrhea. Factors such as CRH and dopamins have an additional inhibitory effect on GnRH secretion. The best option for therapy is psychological support. If no improvement is seen after 6–8 months, combined estrogen and gestagen may be successful in many cases. If the patient wishes to conceive, stimulation treatment with antiestrogens, gonadotropins, or a GnRH pump should be attempted. In cases of hypogonadotropic amenorrhea, therapy with pulsatile GnRH (GnRH pump) or stimulation with human chorionic gonadotropin (HMG) should be tried.

One from between 200 and 500 adolescent girls suffers from *anorexia nervosa*. They try to become as slim as possible by fasting. The fasting phases may be punctuated by episodes of voracious eating (bulimia). Frequently, vomiting is induced after eating. This can result in life-threatening weight loss with the need for intravenous feeding. The typical symptoms include hypothermia, hypotension, the growth of lanugo hair, and amenorrhea. The personality profile of these patients is characterized by ambition, hyperactivity, and impulsiveness. The disease occurs mainly in upper middle class girls with a dominating or insensitive parent. Patient history frequently reveals emotional or sexual abuse or incest. The patients present with a suppressed hypothalamic function with varying degrees of reduced GnRH secretion. Further findings are increased serum levels of cortisol and CRH with no disruption of the diurnal rhythm. The negative feedback of cortisol is intact at the pituitary but disturbed at the hypothalamic level. Similarly, the regulation of TRH (and, consequently, GH) and ADH (mild diabetes insipidus due to a disturbed influence of the hypothalamus on the posterior pituitary) may be impaired. Along with the life-saving measures of intravenous feeding, therapy is mainly based on psychological/psychiatric support.

Women engaging in *competitive sports* and those taking exercise for recreation may show impaired cyclic function because of a hypothalamic dysfunction. The incidence of amenorrhea varies, depending on the sport: it is much higher in ballet dancers and runners than in swimmers. One factor is the body fat ratio, which is higher in swimmers than in runners or ballet dancers. However, this is neither the only nor the most frequent factor in the genesis of cyclic disorders. The type, duration, and intensity of the sport, body composition, psychological status, and individual stress factors are just some of the factors contributing to the development of amenorrhea. Therapy is based on a controlled and optimized diet, psychological support, changes in the training program and possibly replacement therapy with a combination of estrogens and gestages to counteract osteoporosis caused by hypoestrogenemia. If the patient wishes to conceive, the question is whether such a wish is reconcilable with the continued practice of the sport.

Pineal Gland

The secretory product of the pineal gland is melatonin, whose secretion responds to the presence or absence of light. Melatonin exerts a suppressive effect on the GnRH pulse generator. In animals, seasonal changes in the reproductive system represent an important adaptation to a hostile environment.

Endocrine Function

The major product of the pineal gland is melatonin (5-methoxy-N-acetylserotonin), a tryptophan derivative that is synthesized in the gland. The secretion of melatonin in all mammals, including man, follows a definite circadian rhythm with a nocturnal peak. The stimuli for the circadian rhythm depends on endogenous mechanisms and lighting. Exposure to light inhibits melatonin secretion, while darkness promotes it. Melatonin counteracts pituitary melanocyte-stimulating hormone in the skin and tends to reduce skin pigmentation.

It is believed that information on ambient light exposure is conveyed to the paraventricular nucleus via the retinohypothalamic tract and suprachiasmatic nucleus. Axons from neurons of the paraventricular nucleus terminate in the superior cervical ganglion. In darkness, sympathetic neurons from this ganglion activate pituitary secretion.

Melatonin exerts a suppressive effect on the GnRH pulse generator, lowering the GnRH pulse frequency and thereby suppressing reproductive function in animals and humans (Dailey and Neill 1981; Hutz et al. 1985). This is clearly evident in sheep, whose estrus is timed to ensure that lambs are born at a time that is favorable for survival. The importance of light-dependent effects on the GnRH pulse generator in humans is subject to marked individual variations. Generally no definite seasonal increase in human birth rates can be demonstrated. Melatonin is currently being investigated for its contraceptive efficacy and its importance in breast carcinoma.

Pituitary

The first speculations on the importance of the pituitary were those of by Galen in the second century A.D., who believed that "waste products" from the brain collect in the pituitary and are filtered, yielding nasal mucus. This idea persisted into modern times and is reflected in the term "pituitary" (from the Latin *pituita* = phlegm). The pituitary consists of two functionally and anatomically distinct components:
- The anterior pituitary (anterior lobe, adenohypophysis), which is subdivided into:
  - A distal part (pars distalis, prehypophysis), which comprises most of the anterior lobe
  - An intermediate part (pars intermedia), consisting of a narrow zone bordering the posterior pituitary
  - An infundibular part (pars infundibularis, pars tuberalis)
  - The posterior pituitary (posterior lobe, neurohypophysis), which is attached to the hypothalamus by the infundibulum (pituitary stalk).

The glandular portion of the pituitary, the anterior lobe, accounts for approximately 80% of the total pituitary volume.

The anterior pituitary responds to hypothalamic releasing hormones by secreting the appropriate glandotropic hormones: thyrotropin, LH, FSH, adrenocorticotropin, and melanocyte-stimulating hormone. Various inhibitory and stimulatory feedback mechanisms serve to regulate the secretion of the releasing hormones as well as the synthesis, secretion, and storage of the corresponding glandotropic hormones.

Anterior pituitary cells were formerly classified as chromophobes, acidophils, and basophils by the staining affinity of their secretory produces - a classification that is no longer adequate today. A more useful classification is based on the specific secretory products of the cells as determined by electronic microscopic studies of secretory granules and especially by immunofluorescent analysis. Today the following cell types have been positively identified: corticotropes, somatotropes, lactotropes, thyrotropes, and gonadotropes.

Anterior Pituitary Hormones

The anterior pituitary secretes thyrotropin, LH, FSH, adrenocorticotropin, and melanocyte-stimulating hormone.

Gonadotropins

LH and FSH have many chemical and structural features in common. They are dimers composed of two glycosilated polypeptide subunits (a- and β-subunits). The a-subunit is the same for LH, FSH, thyrotropin, and human chorionic gonadotropin; the β-subunit of each hormone has a specific amino acid sequence that determines the hormonal activity. Studies of the LH content of human pituitaries have shown lower levels at the start of the follicular phase and a steady rise until ovulation, followed by a rapid decline and a renewed rise. A similar, less pronounced pattern has been observed for FSH.

The response of LH to GnRH infusions is biphasic: (a) an initial release of LH that is maximal at 30 min and (b) a second rise at 90 min that persists for 4 h. This biphasic pattern implies the presence of two LH compartments in the human pituitary (Naor et al. 1982). Estradiol increases the degree of the second LH surge, and progesterone increases both the first and second surges after previous estrogen treatment. In contrast to this biphasic pattern, the release of FSH shows only the second, later increase.

GnRH Receptors

Hypothalamic GnRH reaches the pituitary cells via the hypophyseal circulation and binds to specific cell membrane receptors (Clayton and Catt 1981). The occupation of these receptors leads to clustering and activation of the GnRH-receptor complexes. The pituitary cell membrane has two bindings sites for the GnRH molecule. The high-affinity binding sites for GnRH are the actual receptors, while the low-affinity binding sites represent endopeptidases. The GnRH receptor is a glycoprotein (MW 60000) that contains sialic acid residues.

It is believed that receptors are distributed uniformly on the cell surface. Once binding occurs, the hormone-receptor complex moves along the cell membrane in a process known as lateral migration. This migration ends at a specialized region called the coated pit. Coated pits are lipid vesicles that are bound to a "basket" of specific latticelike proteins. Approximately 500–1500 such sites are present on the cell surface. Lateral migration carries multiple hormone-receptor complexes into the coated pit in a process called clustering. Finally, the coated pit invaginates and is internalized in the process of endocytosis. Some of the receptors undergo degradation into lysosomes, and others are returned to the cell membrane. The concentration of cell membrane receptors is subject to physiological regulation aimed at providing a maximum number of receptors prior to the midcycle LH surge (Clayton and Catt 1981). The receptor concentration decreases with advancing age and during lactation, and increases after ovariectomy.

Binding of the GnRH molecule to its highly specific receptor initiates a process of clustering, receptor protein activation, and internalization of the hormone-receptor complex. The hormone-receptor complex then undergoes degradation, and a significant number of the receptors are quickly reinserted into the cell membrane. This retransfer to the cell surface is based on the capacity of GnRH to up-regulate its own cell membrane receptors. (a) Up-regulation. Little is known about the mechanism of up-regulation. Presumably it involves an accelerated recycling of internalized receptors (Hazum and Conn 1988) and the synthesis of new receptors. (b) Down-regulation. The GnRH polypeptide receptor appears to have two binding sites: an external site for the polypeptide hormone and an internal site that has a role in internalization. Internalization effects down-regulation by the degradation of receptors in lysosomes (Fig. 5).

Second Messengers of Gonadotropin Secretion

Binding of the GnRH molecule to receptors on the gonadotrope leads to stimulation of the biosynthesis, secretion, and storage of pituitary gonadotropins. The GnRH receptor is a class I receptor, i.e., the cellular response occurs without internalization of the hormone-receptor complex. Internalization of the hormone-receptor complex does occur on gonadotrophs, but the hormonal action does not depend on it.

The binding of GnRH to the receptor initiates a complex series of reactions leading to the secretion of gonadotropins, the biosynthesis of α- and β-subunits for LH and FSH, and the dimerization and glycosylation of these subunits. Gonadotropin release is induced by metabolic pathways that depend on extracellu-

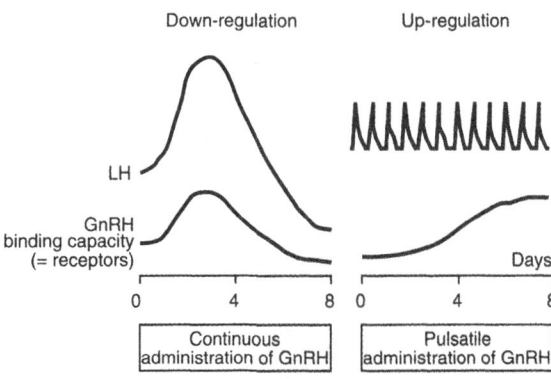

Fig. 5. Up- and down-regulation of LH secretion and GnRH binding capacity in response to the continuous and intermittent administration of GnRH

lar calcium and by pathways that are independent of extracellular calcium (Kiesel and Catt 1984; Kiesel et al. 1984a,b).

The clustering of cell membrane receptors that follows GnRH binding leads to an influx of calcium from the extracellular space and to an enzymatic second-messenger cascade. The calcium influx leads in turn to an increased intracellular calcium concentration that activates the exocytotic release of secretory granules containing LH and FSH. The action of calcium on gonadotropin release is mediated by calmodulin, an intracellular calcium-binding protein.

Further transmission of the GnRH signal relies on the sequential interaction of three membrane-bound proteins: (a) receptors for extracellular binding, (b) a GTP-binding protein (G protein) that allows the exchange of tightly bound cGDP (inactive ligand) for cGTP (active ligand), and (c) cGTP-bound G protein activates phospholipase C.

Four mechanisms are ultimately responsible for the secretion of gonadotropins:

- The influx of extracellular calcium ions inducing the release of stored gonadotropins.
- The activation of intracellular calcium by inositol triphosphate, inducing the discharge of gonadotropin stores.
- Arachidonic acid metabolites: leukotrienes lead to the secretion of gonadotropins.
- Protein kinase C: protein phosphorylation leads to the synthesis and secretion of gonadotropins.

These mechanisms have been elaborated during evolution and are important for species survival, for if one metabolic pathway is lost, the other pathways can take over its role.

Regulation of Gonadotropin Secretion

As in all biocybernetic systems the regulation of pituitary hormone secretion relies on various mechanisms of feedback control. Three types of feedback loop are recognized, each of which may produce inhibitory or stimulatory effects (Fig. 6): (a) long feedback loop, (b) short feedback loop, and (c) ultrashort feedback loop.

In the long feedback loop signals are transmitted from the ovary to the hypothalamus and pituitary by circulating ovarian steroids. Positive feedback is illustrated by the midcycle effect of estradiol (and progesterone) on pituitary LH secretion, negative feedback by the effect of inhibin on pituitary FSH secretion.

The short feedback loop refers to the feedback of gonadotropins on the pituitary secretion of LH and FSH. Again, the regulation occurs via the bloodstream but does not involve another stimulatory or inhibitory factor. The feedback effect may be positive or negative, but most of the feedback is negative. The significance of the short-loop feedback control of LH and FSH warrants further study. The

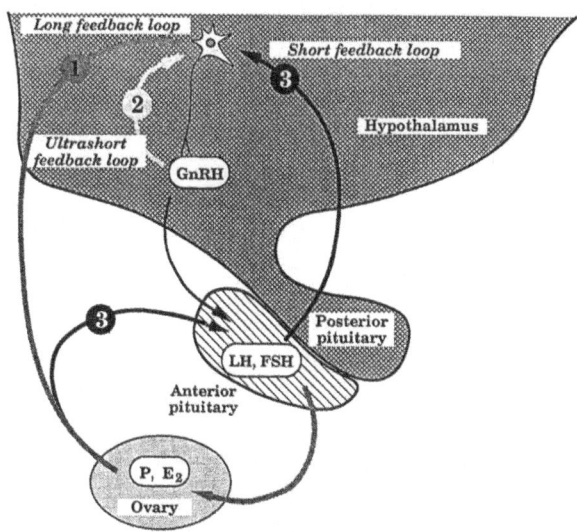

Fig. 6. Feedback loops on the neuroendocrine axis. E_2, 17β-Estradiol; P, progesterone

administration of human menopausal gonadotropin in ovariectomized women inhibits the secretion of endogenous gonadotropins (Szontagh 1973).

The ultrashort feedback loop involves inhibition by the hypothalamic releasing hormone of its own synthesis, storage, and release. Additionally there are pituitary autocrine and paracrine factors that perform a modulatory function.

The frequency and amplitude of gonadotropin secretion are regulated by the hypothalamus (via GnRH secretion) and by effects on the pituitary production, secretion, and storage of gonadotropins. The amplitude of the gonadotropin pulses depends both on the quantity of GnRH that acts on the gonadotrope and on the sensitivity of the gonadotrope itself. The pulse and amplitude characteristics of gonadotropin secretion are critically influenced by gonadal function, with various substances having the capacity to produce modulatory effects (Fig. 7).

Ovulatory women with normal menstrual cycles display a high frequency and low amplitude of LH pulses during the follicular phase. Toward the middle of the cycle the pulse amplitude increases while the frequency declines. The pulse amplitudes are variable during the luteal phase, giving rise to "large" and "small" LH pulses. Pulse amplitudes are higher in the late luteal phase than in the early part of the phase, and the pulse frequency is low (Fig. 8).

The midcycle preovulatory LH surge is itself pulsatile and contains LH pulses of high amplitude compared with the pulses during the preovulatory phase. The frequency pattern of LH secretion remains unchanged during the preovulatory phase and LH surge (Fig. 9). It is currently thought that pituitary sensitivity to GnRH (including exogenously administered GnRH) increases markedly toward the middle of the cycle. It is conceivable, however, that increased amounts of GnRH are released at that time by the GnRH neuronal system.

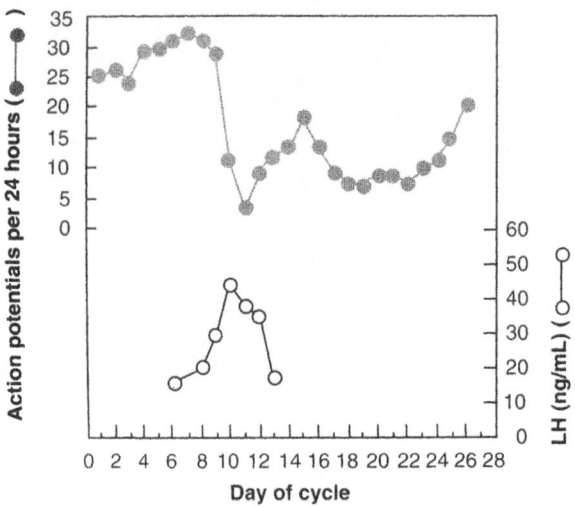

Fig. 7. GnRH pulse-generator frequency (elemetric measurements in rhesus monkeys) and LH serum concentrations during the menstrual cycle. (From Yen 1991)

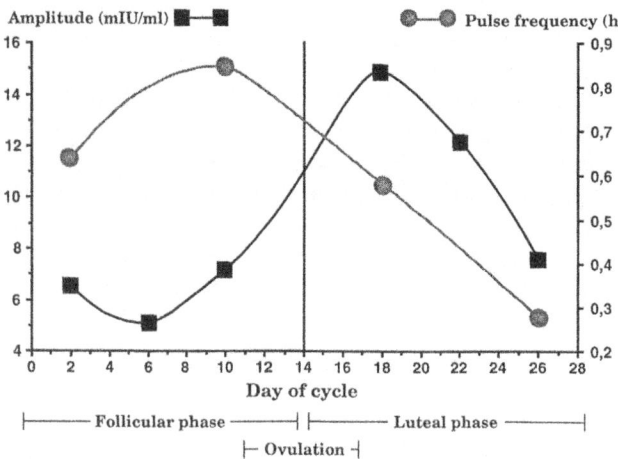

Fig. 8. Changes in the LH pulse frequency during the menstrual cycle. (Based on data from Speroff et al. 1989)

Estrogens

Estradiol exerts both stimulatory and inhibitory effects on pituitary LH and FSH secretion and storage (Knobil 1980).

A positive feedback of estrogens on LH secretion is observed in both prepubertal and adult (normal and ovariectomized) animals and humans (Knobil 1974; Yen and Tsai 1972). This positive effect of estrogens plays a physiological

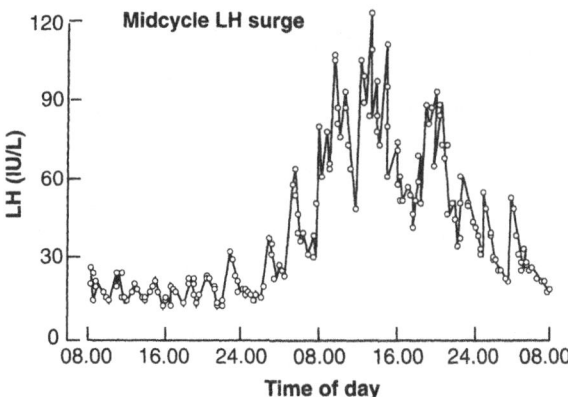

Fig. 9. Midcycle pulsatility of LH. Serum concentrations of LH in an ovulatory cycle were measured at 15-min intervals (*circles*) over a 24-h period during the midcycle LH surge. (From Roseff et al. 1989)

role in the induction of female puberty and in triggering the preovulatory LH surge. The positive feedback mechanism in women becomes operative when the serum estradiol level reaches about 250–300 pg/ml. The exogenous administration of estradiol over a 3-day period under experimental conditions was found to induce a rise of gonadotropins in hypogonadal women (Liu and Yen 1983). There is evidence that this positive feedback mechanism acts on sites in both the hypothalamus and the pituitary. In the pituitary, estrogens increase the pituitary response rate to GnRH stimulation when present in sufficient concentration and duration of effect.

The negative feedback effects of estrogens are seen most clearly in ovariectomized and postmenopausal women. Estrogens are the most potent inhibitors of gonadotropin secretion; usually FSH is more easily suppressed than LH (Zanisi and Martini 1975a,b). Estrogens in the follicular phase reduce pituitary secretions while increasing the synthesis and storage of gonadotropins. Thus, rising estrogen levels during the follicular phase create a gonadotropin reservoir that can be discharged at midcycle. Estrogens mainly exert an inhibitory effect on hypothalamic GnRH secretion.

In summary, estrogens are known to exert the following actions on the pituitary: (a): the midcycle LH surge is initiated by higher estradiol levels over a longer period of time, with release of stored gonadotropins (positive feedback) and (b): low estrogen levels negatively affect the secretion of gonadotropins and positively affect the synthesis and storage of gonadotropins (negative feedback).

Progesterone

Progesterone also gives rise to positive and negative feedback effects on the pituitary. In terms of positive feedback, the administration of progesterone is followed by a rise of LH in ovariectomized rats previously treated with estrogen.

This positive feedback effect of progesterone is probably mediated in part by the hypothalamus and occurs only after prior treatment with estradiol. As with negative feedback, the systemic administration of progesterone alone cannot suppress LH and FSH levels (Zanisi and Martini 1975b), but this effect can be achieved in synergy with estrogens. Progesterone exerts its negative feedback effect on the anterior pituitary and, indirectly, on the hypothalamus. In summary, (a) progesterone acts synergistically with estrogens to influence pituitary gonadotropin secretion, and (b) the specific actions of progesterone and estradiol on the pituitary are not yet known.

Inhibins and Activins

Inhibins exert a regulatory effect on FSH secretion via the hypothalamic-pituitary axis and also produce autocrine and paracrine effects in the ovary. The physiological importance of the activins with regard to the menstrual cycle is still unclear since changes in activin serum levels have not yet been detected during the cycle (Batista et al. 1993). Activins and inhibins are known to produce a variety of extraovarian effects (Vale et al. 1990). The paracrine and autocrine actions of inhibin and activin are discussed in connection with ovarian regulation.

Inhibins are very potent and selective inhibitors of pituitary FSH synthesis and secretion in vitro and in vivo. Inhibin acts on the pituitary via its own receptors. Its action does not involve GnRH receptors. Activin has an equally strong stimulatory effect on the pituitary in vitro, but is does not appear to influence FSH regulation in vivo (Demura et al. 1993) since peripheral activin levels do not change during the menstrual cycle. Neither substance has an apparent effect on LH-β mRNA expression (Gharib et al. 1990). In summary, inhibin has the following established endocrine actions on the pituitary in vivo: (a) inhibition of pituitary FSH secretion via its own receptors (negative long feedback loop), and (b) autocrine and paracrine actions as described in the section "Development of the Ovaries."

Paracrine and Autocrine Modulators

The cells of the anterior pituitary are not only subject to control by hypothalamic hormones and the hormones of the target organs (steroids, thyroid hormones) but are also influenced by substances that are synthesized in the pituitary. A cell secretes a compound that may act on an adjacent cell (paracrine regulation) or on the secreting cell itself (autocrine regulation).

Various peptides of the CNS and gastrointestinal tract (e.g., dynorphin, angiotensin II, vasopressin, gastrin, substance P, motilin) and growth factors (e.g., epidermal growth factor, fibroblast growth factor, IGF) that can act as paracrine and/or autocrine factors have been demonstrated in pituitary cells. It is possible that pituitary cells have a mechanism of intercellular communication that acts through the aid of paracrine substances. Pituitary cells may influence their hormone secretion or their own receptors for hypothalamic hormones by secreting factors with autocrine activity. Here we can consider only the possible effects of substances that have been identified. It remains largely unclear whether and to what degree these compounds are important for the physiology of the menstrual cycle.

Prolactin

The PRL receptor of the rat was cloned in 1988 (Boutin et al. 1988). Its close resemblance to the human GH receptor underscores the close relationship between the two hormones. Specific PRL receptors in women have been found in the liver, lungs, adrenals, breasts, and ovaries. The hepatic PRL receptors show a definite steroid dependence; they are induced by estrogens and by PRL itself, and they are reduced by androgens. These receptors are called lactogenic because they bind PRL, placental lactogen, and GH, which also has lactogenic activity. They differ from GH receptors, which bind GH but not PRL and are not steroid-dependent.

The synthesis and release of PRL are influenced by inhibitory (PRL-inhibiting factor) and stimulatory factors (PRL-releasing factor) at the hypothalamic and pituitary levels. Physiological PRL secretion, unlike most other forms of endocrine hormone secretion, requires continuous suppression. The secretion follows a pulsatile pattern, with pulses of varying amplitude superimposed upon a constant basal secretion. Serum levels of PRL are higher during sleep than in the waking state. The cause of the circadian rhythmicity of PRL is unclear.

Dopamine is the principal inhibitor of PRL secretion at the hypothalamic level. Its effect is mediated by dopamine receptors on the lactotropic cell. Various observations suggest that γ-aminobutyric acid is another inhibitor of PRL secretion, though it is far less potent than dopamine (Vincet et al. 1982; Gudelsky et al. 1983; Melis et al. 1988).

Hypothalamic TRH exerts a strong stimulatory action on the release of PRL. Other stimulators of PRL secretion are vasopressin and vasoactive gastrointestinal peptide (VIP; Abe et al. 1985; Said and Porter 1979). VIP stimulates the secretion of PRL, mediated by the release of oxytocin (Samson et al. 1989). Additionally, VIP appears to cause an autocrine stimulation of PRL secretion from lactotrophs. Other compounds that have a stimulatory effect on PRL secretion are angiotensin II, serotonin, endogenous opioids, histamine, neurotensin, and substance P. Physiological states that are associated with increased PRL secretion are listed in Table 2.

The secretion of PRL is not controlled by negative feedback from peripheral target organs. It is regulated by short feedback loops at the hypothalamic level, i.e., by the retrograde action of secreted PRL on hypothalamic PRL receptors. The secretion of PRL into the portal circulation produces a local rise in the dopamine concentration and a decrease in vasopressin secretion (Gudelsky and Porter 1980; Sarkar 1989). GnRH can act by a paracrine mechanism to produce pulsatile stimulation of PRL secretion concurrently with LH secretion. This interaction is promoted by the close anatomic association of lactotropic and gonadotropic cells in the pituitary.

Table 2. Physiological prolactin increases

Condition	Prolactin level
Menstrual cycle	Increased in the late follicular and throughout the 'luteal phase
Coitus	Strong increase during orgasm
Pregnancy	10-fold increase around birth
Amniotic fluid	Peak in the second trimester
Puerperium	Increased in the first 3–4 weeks
Breastfeeding	Short-term increases
Fetus	Prolactin levels higher than in the mother at birth
Newborn	Increased 2–3 weeks after birth
Sleep	Endogenous rhythm; increase begins 10–60 min after falling asleep
Eating	High-protein food, especially around lunchtime
Exercise	Unclear mechanism

The third gonadotropin, PRL, exerts a variety of metabolic effects relating to osmoregulation, general metabolism, and reproduction. It is an important modulator of fertility and lactation. PRL exerts a luteotropic and luteolytic action on the ovaries of rodents and various other species. Its effects on the human ovary are not yet clearly understood. The fact that elevated PRL levels have often been found in women with galactorrhea and in about one-third of all women with secondary functional amenorrhea suggests that abnormally elevated PRL levels can affect reproductive functions. The suppressive effect of hyperprolactinemia on gonadal function is due largely to a reduction in gonadotropin secretion. This reduction is attributed to dopamine secretion in the hypothalamus inhibiting the secretion of GnRH. The prompt restoration of normal menstrual cycles after the administration of bromoergocryptine and the direct inhibitory effect of PRL on progesterone production by human granulosa cells suggest that PRL exerts regulatory effects on the pituitary-ovarian axis (Table 2).

Posterior Pituitary

In addition to the hormones vasopressin and oxytocin, the neurons of the paraventricular nucleus and the supraoptic nucleus (SON) synthesize the transport proteins neurophysin I and neurophysin II. Vasopressin and oxytocin pass through the median eminence to the posterior pituitary, where they are released into the circulation as well as the CSF and the portal venous system. The concentration of these hormones in the portal vessels is about 50 times higher than in the peripheral circulation. Oxytocin and vasopressin are the only peptide hormones that are synthesized together, stored together in granules, and secreted together in a fixed ratio along with specific carrier proteins.

Oxytocin can inhibit human chorionic gonadotropin stimulated progesterone secretion from human luteal cells in vitro. Oxytocin induces the uterine secretion of prostaglandin $F_{2\alpha}$, leading to a rise in intraovarian oxytocin levels. This may represent a local feedback mechanism that increases the contractility of the uterine tubes. The role of oxytocin in luteolysis is not fully understood (see below). The importance of the expression of posterior pituitary hormones in the organs of the reproductive system remains unclear.

The presence of vasopressin in reproductive organs implies that it exerts paracrine or autocrine functions in those regions. It is thought that the vaso-constrictor properties of vasopressin, along with other vasoactive peptides and growth factors, play a role in regulating the ovarian microculation. It is unclear whether vasopressin additionally performs a physiological endocrine function.

Pathophysiology of the Pituitary Function

Apart from the Sheehan and the Empty sella syndromes, primary disorders of the pituitary are limited to various (rare) tumors of both the anterior and the poste-rior pituitary. Other dysfunctions are pituitary infarction, lymphocytic hypophy-sitis, nonsecreting adenomas (ACTH, TSH, LH, FSH) and secreting tumors (pro-lactin, growth hormone) of the anterior pituitary, craniopharyngeomas, and me-tastases. The most frequent tumors are prolactin-secreting adenomas.

Prolactinomas are the most common adenomas. They can be subdivided into micro- and macroprolactinomas. In the case of microadenomas, serum concen-trations will not exceed 250 ng/ml. In macroadenomas, serum levels will nor-mally range between 250 and 1000 ng/ml. Therapy depends on concomitant symptoms (other pituitary functions, compression of the chiasma opticum). In many cases of microprolactinoma, treatment with dopamin agonists is suffi-cient. For macroprolactinomas, transphenoidal adenomectomy or hypophysect-omy may be required.

Latent or manifest hypothyroidism is a frequent cause of *functional hyperpro-lactinemia* (mostly < 50 ng/ml). For this reason, the thyroid function should be normalized before dopamin agonists are administered. This is particularly impor-tant if cyclic disorders, i.e., anovulation or luteal phase disruption, are present.

Sheehan syndrome, named after the physician who first described it, is char-acterized by acute necrosis of the anterior pituitary due to postpartal bleeding as a result of shock. In most cases, the posterior pituitary is involved. However, manifest diabetes insipidus is rarely found. Symptoms are very varied and de-pend on the extent of pituitary dysfunction. Spontaneous improvement of the resulting hypopituitarism has been described. The individual dysfunctions of the pituitary can be tested by stimulation with the corresponding releasing hor-mones (GnRH, TRH, CRH).

The Ovaries

Morphology of the Ovaries

The reproductive function of the ovaries is critically influenced by three mor-phologically and functionally distinct compartments: the granulosa cell compartment, the theca cell compartment, and the immune system (third compartment).

The granulosa cell compartment is a multifunctional heterogeneous system. A basement membrane separates the oocyte and surrounding granulosa cells from the surrounding stroma and the theca cell compartment. The granulosa cell layer does not have a direct vascular supply (at least until a few hours before ovulation). Communication and interchange among the cells of this compartment take place through numerous gap junctions. Additionally, the granulosa cells have cytoplasmic extensions that form gap-junction-like connections with the oocyte plasma membrane. Granulosa cells are functionally and morphologically diverse. Three layers of granulosa cells surround the oocyte: the mural cells, the antral cells, and the cumulus cells. The mural cells are closest to the basement membrane and display the highest metabolic activity, as indicated by activity studies of 3β-hydroxysteroid dehydrogenase, glucose-6-phosphate dehydrogenase, and cytochrome P450 (Zoller and Weisz 1979a,b). The mural granulosa cells also are rich in LH receptors. The cumulus cells, by contrast, have no cytochrome P450 activity and thus have no aromatase activity. The relative paucity of LH receptors and low LH reactivity of the cumulus cells compared with the mural granulosa cells suggests that the cumulus cell mass may function as a stem cell reservoir. This view is supported by the fact that cumulus granulosa cells replicate in a very undifferentiated state. The antral cells (granulosa cells lining the antrum) have not been associated with a specific function.

The capacity of the theca cell layer for androgen production was first demonstrated by Falck et al. (1962). The de novo synthesis of androgens by theca cells has been confirmed by subsequent investigations (Ryan and Petro 1966; Rice and Savard 1966). Androgen-producing cells occur in the loose connective tissue of the ovarian cortex and medulla.

Macrophages constitute the third cellular component of the human ovary (Hume et al. 1984). They are constantly present and do not vary with the phases of the cycle. Although the importance of this third compartment is still unclear, studies indicate that the macrophages may provide for additional local regulation by the secretion of cytokines such as interleukin-1 and tumor necrosis factor α (Adashi 1989). Moreover, macrophages can secrete growth factors such as basic fibroblast factor and transforming growth factor α and β. These substances are produced by granulosa cells and can exert autocrine and paracrine actions.

Macrophages are virtually the only components of the leukocyte series that are present during the early phase of follicular development. This changes quickly when a massive infiltration of the ovarian stroma by leukocytes occurs in the preovulatory phase (Parr 1974). Studies have shown that mast cells accumulate rapidly in the late follicular phase and then degranulate at a point coinciding with the LH surge (Krishna and Terranova 1985; Murdoch and Cavendar 1987). The resulting follicular hyperemia (Szego and Pitin 1964; Krishna et al. 1986) not only appears to play a role in the subsequent luteal phase (Cavendar and Murdoch 1988) but also initiates a sequence of events that are similar to an inflammatory response (Espey 1980), marked by an influx of eosinophils and T-lymphocytes. The follicular hyperemia is initiated by histamine (Morikawa et al. 1981) and intensified by prostaglandin E_2. Both substances cause an increase in vascular dilatation and permeability.

It has been shown in laboratory animals that the corpus luteum secretes a chemotactic agent that attracts infiltration by eosinophilic leukocytes (Murdoch 1987; Murdoch and Cormick 1989). Murdoch et al. (1988) postulate an immunological induction of luteolysis in which degeneration of the corpus luteum is effected by cytotoxins secreted by eosinophilic leukocytes.

Most observations pertaining to cells of the immune system indicate that these cells have a significant potential for exerting regulatory, initiatory, and modulatory effects on processes during the menstrual cycle. However, it is very likely that these cells are targets for steroidal and peptidergic influences. Moreover, it has been shown in animal studies that macrophages, for example, can influence steroid metabolism by their ability to synthesize steroids (Reynolds et al. 1981; Milewich et al. 1982).

Recent discoveries support the view that endocrinological processes cannot be considered separately from immunological changes. It appears that profound mutual effects take place between the endocrine and immune systems even in physiological regulatory processes.

Development of the Ovaries

Embryonic Development

The primordial germ cells originate in the endoderm of the yolk sac at the caudal end of the embryo. Staining techniques can demonstrate primordial cells at this site by only the third week of gestation (Baker 1963). These cells migrate to the genital ridge by means of pseudopid-assisted ameboid movements (Witschi 1948). It appears that germ cells are unable to exist outside the genital ridge. Apparently this is the only body region that is capable of gonadal development. Moreover, germ cells are essential for inducing the formation of gonads; a gonad does not form in the absence of germ cells.

Number of Germ Cells in Various Stages of Development

The premeiotic germ cells that arrive at the genital ridge by about 5 weeks' gestation are termed oogonia (Baker and Franchi 1962). For the next 2 weeks (the indifferent stage) the gonad is a mere prominence in the medial part of the urogenital ridge. It develops from proliferating germinal epithelium and mesenchyme and by the division of oogonia. By the 6th or 7th week of gestation approximately 10,000 oogonia are present in the primitive gonad. The oogonia multiply entirely by mitosis. The initial structures of the future gonads become apparent at this stage, with differentiation of the gonadal cortex and medulla.

There are approximately 600 000 oogonia by about the 8th week of gestation (Ohno et al. 1962). From this point on the fate of the germ cells depends on three concomitant processes: mitosis, meiosis, and oogonal atresia. This means that the onset of oogonal meiosis and atresia overlaps with mitotic divisions. The maximum number of germ cells, approximately 7 million, is reached by the 20th week. Thereafter the rate of mitosis steadily declines until the 7th month of pregnancy, when mitosis ceases to occur. Meanwhile, oogonal atresia increases and becomes maximal in about the 5th month.

Oogonal atresia ceases by the 7th month, and oogonia are no longer present in the ovary after that time. All surviving oogonia undergo meiosis, leading to the development of primordial follicles. At this time follicular atresia supersedes oogonal atresia. The process of follicular atresia reduces the germ cell population to about 1–2 million by birth. This number declines further with aging, reaching about 300 000 at puberty (i.e., at the start of the reproductive period). Thus, the female has already lost 80% of her germ cells while still in utero.

Meiosis starts in about the 8th week of intrauterine life when the cells, now called primary oocytes, arrest in the prophase of the first meiotic division. A primordial follicle thus consists of an oocyte that is surrounded by a single layer of granulosa cells and is arrested in the prophase of meiosis. The exact cause of the arrested meiosis is unknown, but it is assumed that among others a factor produced by the granulosa cells (meiosis inhibitor) is responsible. This hypothesis is based on the observation in in vitro fertilization programs that oocytes that have been freed from the surrounding granulosa cells resume meiosis spontaneously.

The onset of meiosis does not coincide in all oogonia and offers protection from degeneration through oogonal atresia. A distinction is drawn between oogonal atesia and follicular atresia, with the development to a primordial follicle providing a safeguard against oogonal atresia. This protection is only temporary, however. With meiosis and the development of granulosa cells around the primary oocyte, primordial follicles are generated whose numbers are further reduced by follicular atresia. Oogonia that do not undergo meiosis by the 8th month of gestation are lost to atresia, so the adult ovaries are completely devoid of oogonia. Ultimately only about 400–500 oocytes ovulate during a woman's reproductive years. This is less than 1% of the original population of germ cells (Table 3).

Development of Follicles from the Primordial to the Mature Stage

Gougeon (1986) states that ovarian follicles can be divided into classes based on the number of granulosa cells (Table 4, Fig. 10), and that these classes correspond to the various stages of follicular development. Analysis further shows that follicles of any size and granulosa cell content can be found at any given point in the cycle, and that the numbers of preantral follicles are more or less constant, implying that the entry of follicles into this class occurs in a succession of waves or cohorts (Fig. 9).

Table 3. Number of germ cells from the embryonic stage to puberty. In the reproductive years of a woman, only 400–500 oocytes reach ovulation

Week of gestation	Stages	Number of germ cells	Author
3/4	Primordial germ cells in the entoderm of the yolk sac		Baker et al. 1963
5–6	Premeiotic cells: oogonia	~10 000	Baker and Franchi 1962
8	Propagation by mitosis	600,000	Ohno et al. 1962
8–20	Mitosis, meiosis, atresia, Maximum at week 20	6–7 000 000	
20–40	Reduction of oozytes (80% of germ cells are lost)	1–2 000 000	Himelstein-Braw et al. 1976
Birth to puberty	Further oocytes are lost by atresia	300 000	Franchi et al. 1962

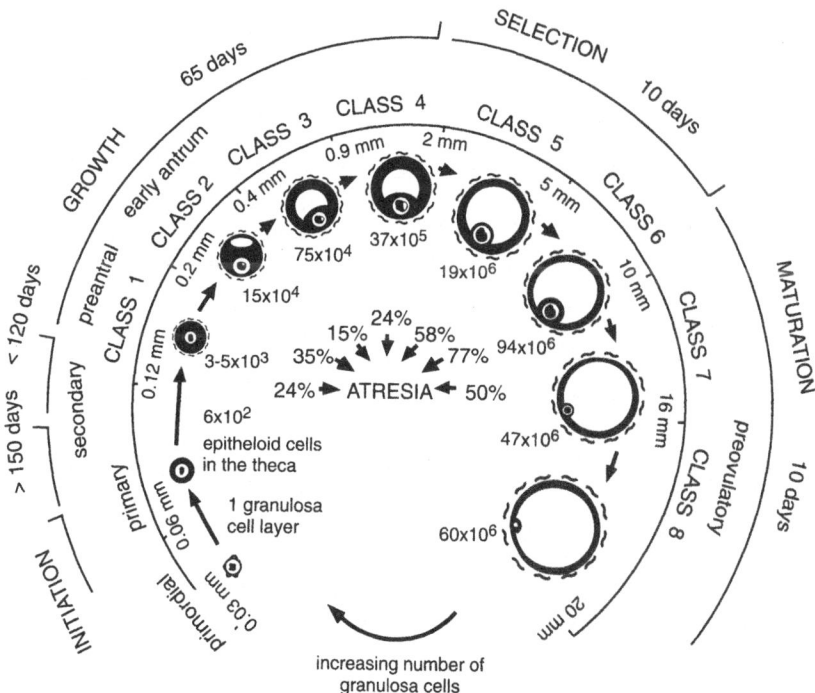

Fig. 10. Stages of folliculogenesis from the primordial to the preovulatory follicle. The follicles are divided into eight classes based on the number of granulosa cells. (From Gougion 1986)

Table 4. Folliculogenesis: definitions (from Gougeon 1986)

Name	Size (mm)	Stage of development
Primordial germ cell		Original cell from the entoderm (detectable from the 3rd week of pregnancy) migrates to genital ridge
Oogonium		Arrival in genital ridge (5th week of pregnancy)
Primordial follicle and oocyte	0.03–0.06	Oogonium enters meiosis I (oocyte) and a single layer of epithelial cells forms around the oocyte
Primary/secondary follicle	0.06–0.12	Single epithelial cell layer differentiates into single-line, cubic layer of epithelial cells around oocyte
Preantral follicle (Class 1)	0.12–0.2	Formation of multiple layers of epithelial cells by mitotic activity and beginning differentiation of the epitheloid theca interna; gonadotropins begin to have an effect Formation of a liquid-containing cavity: antrum (liquor folliculi)
Early antral follicle (Class 2)	0.2–0.4	Gradual emergence of a cumulus oophorus on the margin of the follicle and increase in antral size
Class 3 follicle	0.4–0.9	Continued development of theca and granulosa cell layers and of the antrum
Class 4 follicle	0.9–2	Continued development of theca and granulosa cell layers and of the antrum
Class 5 follicle	2–5	Continued development of theca and granulosa cell layers and of the antrum
Class 6 follicle	5–10	Follicle size at the time of recruitment in the late luteal/early follicular phase
Class 7 follicle	10–16	Dominant preovulatory follicle
Class 8 follicle	16–20	Ovulatory follicle

The development of oocytes in the ovary is partly gonadotropin-dependent and partly gonadotropin-independent. The gonadotropin-independent process concludes as the epitheloid cell layer around the follicle differentiates into the theca interna, marking the progression of the secondary follicle to the preantral stage. With the development of the thecal layer, the follicle is able to respond to gonadotropin stimulation and becomes subject to the effects of cyclic gonadotropin changes (Fig. 11, Table 4).

This entry of follicles into the preantral stage (class 1) occurs several days after ovulation in the early luteal phase (days 15–19) following high midcycle serum levels of estrogens and gonadotropins. It is known that these hormones promote the differentiation of the theca interna (Rao et al. 1978). Twenty-five days later,

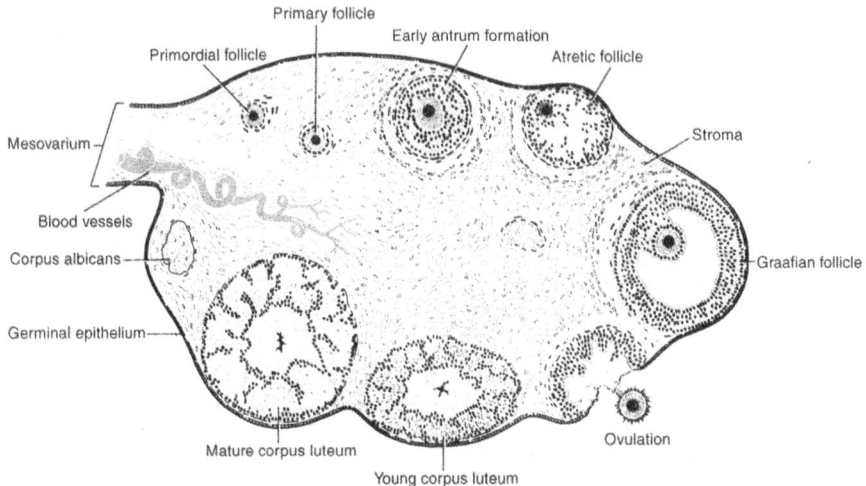

Primary follicle

Early antrum formation

Primordial follicle

Atretic follicle

Mesovarium

Stroma

Blood vessels

Corpus albicans

Graafian follicle

Germinal epithelium

Mature corpus luteum

Ovulation

Young corpus luteum

Fig. 11. Ovarian morphology and cyclic changes. (From Adashi et al. 1991)

between days 11 and 14 of the next cycle, this cohort of follicles enters into class 2 (0.2–0.4 mm), accompanied by the initial appearance of an antrum. This transition occurs simultaneously in both ovaries. Elevated serum levels of estradiol and FSH promote the initation of antrum formation (Goldenberg et al. 1972; Richards 1975).

Further follicular growth after this stage becomes more complex due to differences between the ovary bearing the corpus luteum of the previous cycle and the contralateral ovary. Due to the higher mitotic index in the ovulatory ovary, the transit to the next class occurs about 5 days later in this ovary (late luteal phase, days 25–28) than in the contralateral ovary (early follicular phase, days 1–5 of the next cycle; Gougeon 1986). As a result, follicles take 20 days to pass through class 2 in the ovulatory ovary and about 25 days in the opposite ovary. This asynchrony explains the alternating ovulation in the right and left ovaries.

The remaining stages progress simultaneously in both ovaries, with follicles passing through class 3 (0.3–0.9 mm) in 15 days, class 4 (0.9–2.0 mm) in 10 days, class 5 (2–5 mm) in 5 days, class 6 (6–10 mm) in 5 days, and class 7 (10–16 mm) in 5 days. The follicle cohort enters class 5 in the late luteal phase (days 25–28). Here they enter into the cycle in which one follicle in the cohort becomes the dominant follicle that is destined to ovulate. The further process of recruitment, selection, and dominance is described in the last section of this chapter (Fig. 12).

Oocyte

The primary oocyte remains in the prophase of the first meiotic division until the LH surge prior to ovulation. In response to the LH surge the first maturation division proceeds to completion, and the first polar body is formed. This marks the transition from the primary to the secondary oocyte.

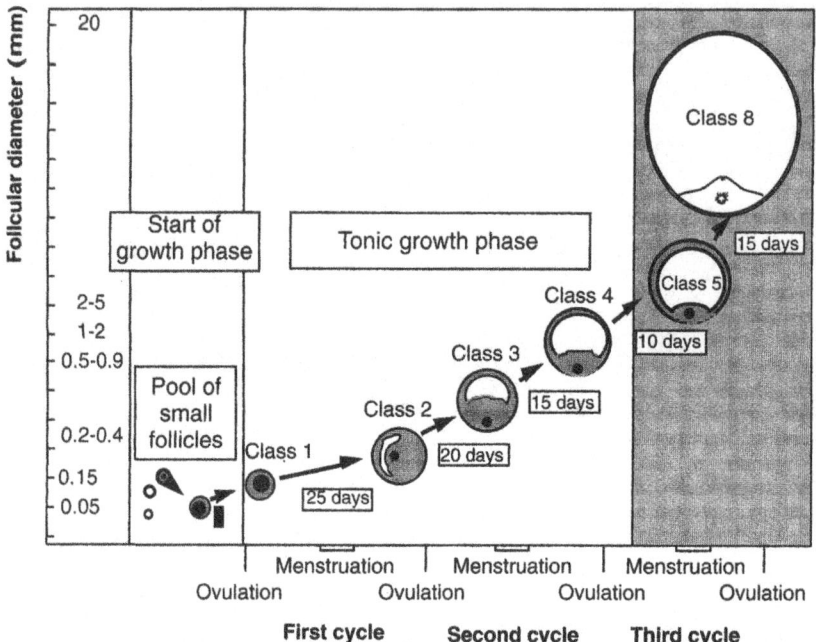

Fig. 12. Folliculogenesis. The progression from a preantral to a preovulatory follicle spans three menstrual cycles, the transition from one class to the next always occurring in particular phases of the cycle. The diagram traces the development of a single cohort of follicles, with one cohort entering the growth phase in each cycle. This explains why all developmental stages (classes) of follicles are found in histological examinations of premenopausal ovaries. (From Gougeon 1986)

Ovulation

When ovulation occurs, the oocyte with its surrounding granulosa cell mantle is expelled and picked up by the uterine tube. The penetration of a spermatozoon induces a second meiotic division of the oocyte, leading to release of the second polar body and the formation of a true haploid oocyte, whose genetic material forms the female pronucleus.

Regulation of Ovarian Activity

The selection of a single follicle for ovulation relates closely to its capacity for gonadotropin-induced estrogen biosynthesis (Hillier et al. 1981). The integrity of this follicular estrogen production depends on the interaction between the theca and granulosa cells. The function of both cell types is controlled by endocrine, paracrine, and autocrine mechanisms (Erickson 1982; Hsueh et al. 1983). As tropic hormones, LH and FSH can influence the timing of growth and maturational processes in the ovary and thus can modify the ovarian microenvironment (Goodman and Hodgen 1983).

Two-Cell Theory

The two-cell or two-compartment theory correctly describes the interaction between thecal interstitial cells and granulosa cells, and thus between gonadotropins and steroids, but it is incomplete because it disregards various paracrine and autocrine factors that were discovered in recent years. This section completes the model by adding to it the various new regulators. The "third compartment," which is still being investigated, consists of immunological elements that establish a functional link between endocrine processes and the immune system.

The sole target of FSH is the granulosa cell. By contrast, LH has multiple sites of action depending on the phase of the cycle: theca cells, stromal cells, granulosa cells, and luteal cells (Erickson 1982).

Follicular development relies on a synergistic interaction of gonadotropins (FSH and LH), steroids (androgens and estrogens), and autocrine and paracrine factors that exert their effects through specific receptors on the theca and granulosa cells.

Actions of FSH

The effects of FSH are strongest at the end of the previous cycle and for the first days of the follicular phase. The granulosa cells of the ovarian follicle have receptors for FSH. The importance of FSH for follicular growth is based on various concurrent actions:

- The main action of FSH is to induce the aromatase activity of the granulosa cell (Dorrington et al. 1975). In the presence of aromatizable androgens (androstenedione, testosterone) this leads to a rise of the estradiol level first in the follicle and then in the peripheral blood.
- Rising intraovarian and peripheral FSH levels lead to an up-regulation of FSH receptors on granulosa cells (positive feedback; Dorrington and Armstrong 1979).
- FSH promotes the proliferation of granulosa cells (Peluso and Steger 1978). The estrogenic environment induced by FSH (rising estradiol) exerts the strongest mitogenic action on the granulosa cells. This leads to a further overall rise in aromatase activity and an expotential rise in peripheral estradiol concentrations.
- FSH induces the formation of LH receptors on granulosa cells (Erickson et al. 1979). This action is intensified by estradiol, progesterone, testosterone, androstenedione, and LH (Rani et al. 1981). The LH receptor requires the constant presence of FSH.
- The pituitary secretion of FSH is regulated by negative feedback from the rising serum levels of estradiol and inhibin.

Estradiol stimulates all FSH functions through a paracrine action (Hsueh et al. 1983), including the increase of aromatase activity (Adashi and Hsueh 1982).

Initially, FSH stimulates a progressive increase in the number of FSH receptors but has no effect on the LH receptor concentration. However, as FSH receptors are exposed to a rising concentration of endogenous estradiol, the number of FSH receptors increases more rapidly. This is followed by a delayed but significant induction of LH receptors. Thus estradiol promotes the ability of FSH to increase the concentration of its own receptor and, later, that of LH (Figs. 13, 14). The synergistic relationship between FSH and estradiol creates a positive intraovarian autoregulatory mechanism that stimulates the rapid division of granulosa cells and thus is responsible for follicular growth.

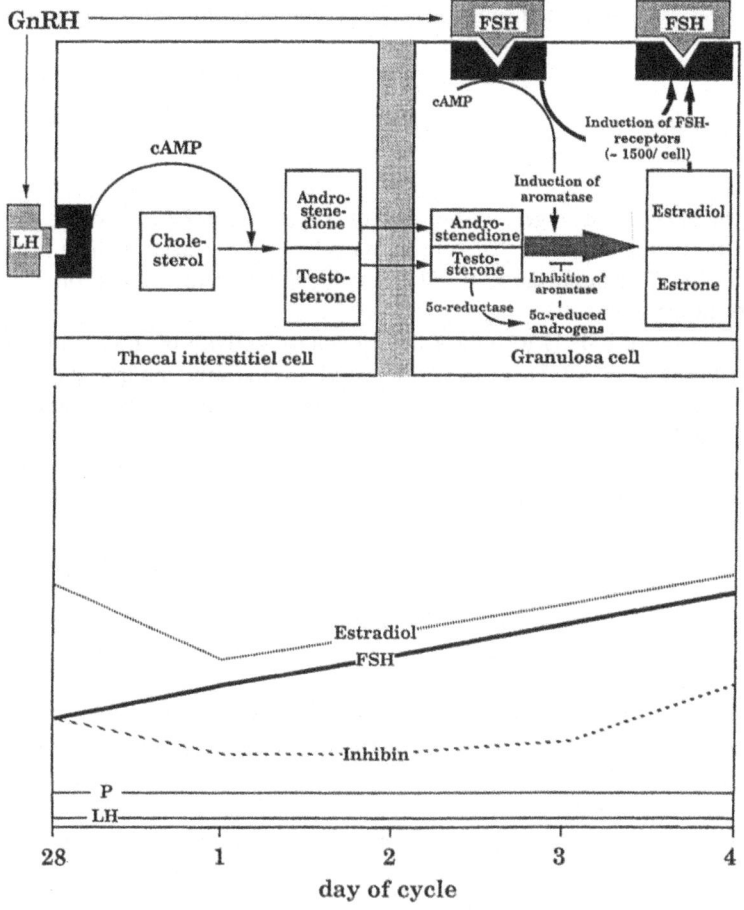

Fig. 13. Serum concentrations of LH, FSH, inhibin, and progesterone. Intracellular mechanisms in the theca and granulosa cell: luteal-follicular transition and early follicular phase

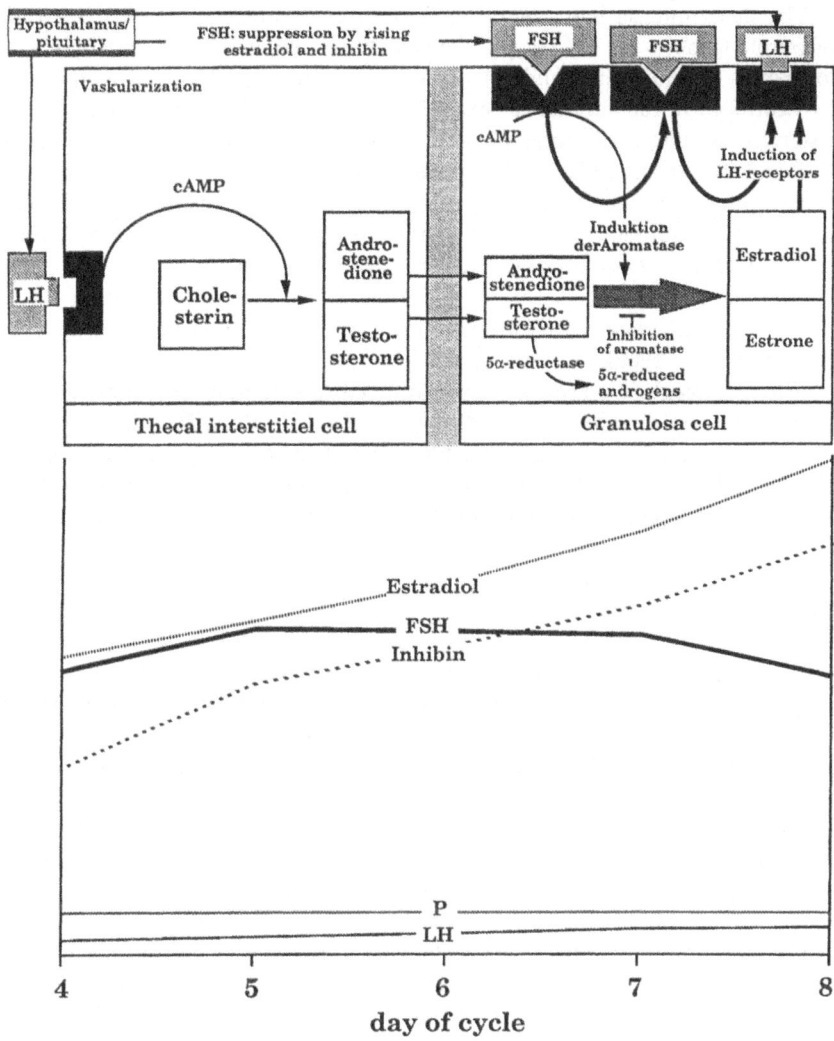

Fig. 14. Selection of the dominant follicle

Actions of LH

LH is important for all phases of the menstrual cycle. In the follicular phase androgens are secreted under the influence of LH to provide a substrate for estrogen production by the theca cells. Animal studies have shown that LH is necessary for the progression of small antral follicles to the preovulatory stage (Richards et al. 1980; Richards and Bogvich 1982). The LH surge at midcycle induces completion of the first meiotic division of the oocyte. Following its peak, LH maintains the luteal production of progesterone.

The theca interna has specific receptors for LH but not for FSH. Activation of steroidogenesis via LH receptors on the theca cell leads predominantly to the formation of androgens (androstenedione, testosterone). Much as with adrenocorticotropin in the adrenal cortex, LH catalyzes side chain cleavage of the cholesterol molecule. LH induces the key enzymes of steroidogenesis: 17a-hydroxylase and 17, 20-desmolase. The increased androgen production by the theca compartment provides a substrate for aromatization. The androgens diffuse into the follicular fluid and are aromatized by the granulosa cells to estrogens (Erickson 1982; Dorrington and Armstrong 1979; McNatty et al. 1979a). Minimal aromatization can also occur in the theca cells. The interaction of the two cell types is necessary for estrogen secretion to occur (McNatty et al. 1979a; Ryan and Petro 1966).

The LH receptors present on granulosa cells are responsible for progesterone production (Welsh et al. 1983; McNatty et al. 1979a). While FSH, in the presence of estradiol, increases the receptors for FSH and LH in the granulosa cells of the growing follicle, LH leads to a reduction in the number of receptors for FSH, LH, and estradiol in connection with the luteinization process (Richards et al. 1976).

Estrogens and Androgens

The androgens in the granulosa cell undergo either aromatization or 5a-reduction. It appears that the interaction between the granulosa and theca cell compartments in the follicle leading to accelerated estrogen production is not fully operative until the late stage of antral development. Granulosa cells from human preantral follicles show a higher 5a-reductase activity than aromatase activity, with the result that predominantly 5a-reduced androgen metabolites (e.g., 5a-dihydrotestosterone) are produced (McNatty et al. 1979b). Granulosa cells from large antral follicles, on the other hand, have substantial aromatase activity.

The establishment of an estrogenic intrafollicular milieu appears to be an essential factor in the autoregulation of the follicle. The fate of the follicle depends largely on its ability to produce estrogens, especially in terms of the selection and maintenance of a dominant follicle (McNatty et al. 1979b; Hillier et al. 1980; Fig. 15).

The increasing estrogen production suppresses FSH secretion and thereby inhibits the maturation of other follicles (Zeleznik 1981). At this time the number of FSH receptors per cell and the number of granulosa cells (i.e., the ability of the follicle to secrete estrogens) have a critical bearing on further follicular growth. By chance, one of the recruited follicles acquires a growth advantage (more FSH receptors, greater ability to aromatize androgens), and through higher estrogen and inhibin secretion and other paracrine and endocrine factors it creates intraovarian hormonal conditions that promote a wave of atresia among the lesser follicles due to deficient aromatization.

The continuation of estrogen secretion by the dominant follicle despite a falling peripheral FSH concentration may result from a compensatory ability of intrafollicular estrogen to increase FSH-induced aromatase activity. This autoregulatory role of intrafollicular estrogen is based largely on the results of in vitro studies

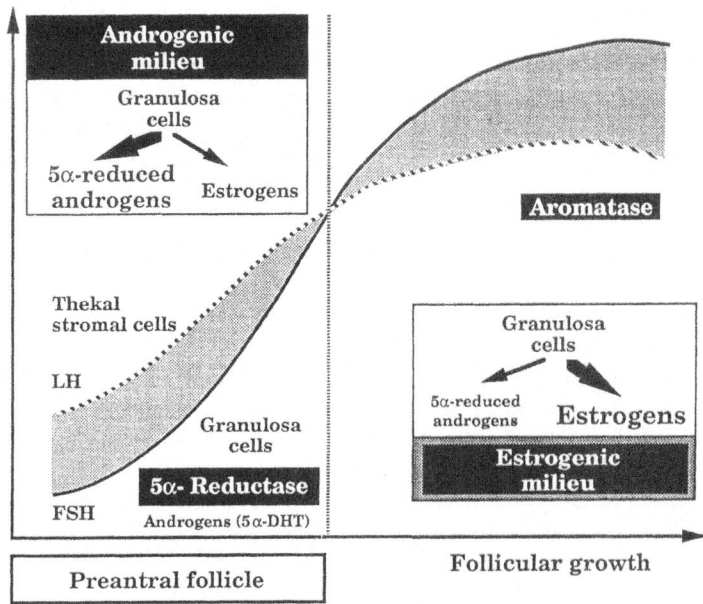

Fig. 15. Intrafollucular estrogen-androgen shift in the follicular phase

showing that follicular estrogens exert a paracrine action. Of special importance is local positive feedback from the estrogens, which sustain the dominance of the selected follicle by stimulating an increase in their own production (Hsueh et al. 1983). The role of androgens in early follicular development is complex. Because nonaromatized androgens such as 5α-dihydrotestosterone inhibit aromatase activity (Hillier et al. 1980), a more androgenic milieu leads to atresia in a portion of the recruited follicles. The fate of the preantral follicle, then, depends critically on the balance of the local androgen and estrogen concentrations, which is determined by the ratio of the 5α-reductase and aromatase activities.

Androgens, in addition to their importance as a substrate for aromatization, exert a number of receptor-mediated effects on the granulosa cells:

– Low androgen concentrations can enhance the FSH-mediated induction of aromatase (Daniel and Armstrong 1980; Hillier and DeZwart 1981).
– High intrafollicular concentrations of 5α-reduced androgens act as potent inhibitors of aromatase activity (Hillier et al. 1980).
– The administration of 5α-dihydrotestosterone in vitro or in vivo abolishes the ability of FSH to induce LH receptors (Farookhi 1980).
– Androgens promote progesterone biosynthesis (Armstrong and Dorrington 1976; Lucky et al. 1977).

On the whole, androgens play an important regulatory role in the process of follicular development, although we do not yet fully understand the manner in which their various effects are produced.

Progesterone

Serum progesterone levels are low before the preovulatory LH surge. Progesterone secretion can be detected in ovarian venous effluent on about day 10 of the menstrual cycle. With the onset of the LH surge a slight rise in progesterone is also observed. The preovulatory progesterone rise not only supports the positive feedback effect of estrogens on LH secretion but is also responsible for the midcycle rise in FSH (Batista et al. 1993).

Although peripheral progesterone levels remain constant during the follicular phase, the progesterone concentration in the follicular fluid starts to rise in the midfollicular phase. It is thought that the granulosa cells secrete progesterone into the follicular fluid in response to LH stimulation. This does not change the preovulatory peripheral concentration of progesterone. Progesterone levels are about 290 ng/ml in the fluid of the tertiary follicle and about 7000 ng/ml in the fluid of the mature follicle (Breitenecker et al. 1978).

The peripheral progesterone level starts to rise one day before ovulation. It attains a broad-based peak during the luteal phase, reaching serum levels higher than 10 ng/ml. This is more than 20 times the average basal progesterone serum level measured in the follicular phase.

The serum levels closely mirror the development and regression of the corpus luteum and are subject to circadian variations (Runnebaum et al. 1972). The peripheral serum concentrations of 17a-hydroxyprogesterone and 20a-dihydroprogesterone are higher in the luteal phase than in the follicular phase.

Insulin-Like Growth Factors

IGF-I and IGF-II are two homologous, single-chain polypeptides of low molecular weight. They display remarkable structural and functional similarities to insulin (see Aitken et al., this volume).

IGF-I is synthesized in the liver under the control of GH but is also found in many extrahepatic tissues including the ovaries. The secretion of IGF-I from the liver has been demonstrated by clinical studies in humans (Takano et al. 1977; Bala et al. 1981). A GH-dependent site of synthesis has not yet been identified for IGF-II. IGF-I and IGF-II are bound with high affinity to specific binding proteins, which thus regulate their bioavailability.

IGF-I and IGF-II have been detected in human follicular fluid (Geisthoevel et al. 1989, 1990). Various studies suggest that human ovaries synthesize IGF-I, IGF-II, and binding proteins, have receptors for these factors, and also function as a site of action for the IGFs (Geisthövel et al. 1990; Voutilainen and Miller 1987; Suikkari et al. 1989a,b; Koistinen et al. 1990). Human preovulatory granulosa cells appear to express IGF-II but not IGF-I (Geisthövel et al. 1990), while theca cells synthesize IGF-I (Hernandez et al. 1988).

Receptors for IGF-I, IGF-II, and insulin have been demonstrated in human ovaries (Poretsky and Kalin 1987). IGFs cross-react with one another and with insulin.

The serum concentrations of IGF-I are subject to pituitary control by GH secretion. Its bioavailability is regulated by binding proteins. The synthesis of these binding proteins concides with IGF synthesis to a degree, while some of their synthesis is independent of the IGFs. In contrast to IGF-I, the secretion of IGF-II does not appear to be growth-hormone-dependent (Zapf et al. 1981).

IGFs can exert endocrine, paracrine, and autocrine actions on the ovary. Growth-hormone-stimulating IGF-I synthesized in the liver can act via receptors on granulosa and theca cells (Geisthövel et al. 1990). The ovarian action of IGFs is regulated by locally produced IGF binding proteins. Recent studies (Geisthövel et al. 1990) suggest that IGF-I has mainly endocrine activity while IGF-II exerts endocrine, paracrine, and autocrine actions. IGF-I exerts its effects in human granulosa cells by binding to insulin and IGF-I receptors (Portesky and Kalin 1987). IGFs produce the following effects in theca and granulosa cells (Erickson et al. 1989; Zhiwen et al. 1987; Geisthövel et al. 1990):

- Increase the FSH-induced up-regulation of LH receptors on the granulosa cell
- Enhance the aromatase activity of the granulosa cell
- Directly increase progesterone synthesis by the granulosa cell
- Increase inhibin secretion by the granulosa cell.

In summary, as a general rule, IGFs act to increase both FSH- and LH-mediated actions on granulosa and theca cells. Almost all studies to date have dealt with granulosa cells in rats or swine. The degree to which the results of these (in vitro) studies can be applied to humans is unclear. It is also unclear whether the action of IGFs is necessary for normal reproductive function. Women with Laron-type dwarfism, which is caused by an absence of IGF secretion with normal levels of GH, have normal menstrual cycles.

Pathophysiology of the Ovarian Function

Ovarian function is inextricably linked to the hypothalamic-pituitary-ovarian feedback mechanism. In nearly all cases, disorders of ovarian function are secondary in nature or the exact cause cannot be determined. The only primary ovarian disorder leading to anovulation is premature ovarian failure, which is only pathological in that it occurs earlier than normally, i.e., before the age of 50.

The *polycystic ovarian syndrome* (PCO) is a very heterogeneous condition. The only invariable presentation is subcortical ovarian cysts confirmed on ultrasound, combined with a central stroma of higher than normal echogenicity. The syndrome was originally described by Stein and Levethal in 1935 as a triade of obesity, amenorrhea, and enlarged ovaries, and it has still not been possible to arrive at a uniform definition it. Women with polycystic ovaries as seen on ultrasound may either have ovulatory cycles with a normal luteal function or suffer from secondary amenorrhea. Hyperandrogenism is nearly always found in patients with oligo- or amenorrhea. Some of the patients are insulin resistant. In patients with PCO, the primary disorder may originate from the hypothalamus (increased LH/FSH ratio) or the adrenal (adrenal hyperandrogenism due to late-onset enzyme defects), or it may be of a peripheral nature (insulin resistence) or of ovarian origin (disturbed auto- or paracrine regulation). In many oligoamenorrheic patients with PCO, however, changes in all these organ systems are found.

Patients with PCO who have completed their family are treated with estrogen-antiandrogen combinations to prevent progression of the disease. In anovulatory patients with PCO who desire to have children, stimulation with clomiphene or low-dose gonadotropins is recommended. Especially low-dose stimulation with pure FSH (37.5 I.U. from days 3-4 of the cycle) is suitable for patients with an increased LH/FSH ratio. If the serum levels of LH are elevated, pretreatment with GnRH analogues for 3 months can improve the pregnancy rate by suppressing serum LH. It is assumed that increased LH has a negative impact on oocyte maturation, leading to lower pregnancy and higher abortion rates.

If drug treatment has failed, laparoscopic procedures such as the cauterization of ovarian cysts or laser coagulation may be used. Recent studies show a very high success rate, but the mechanism of action is not fully understood. The innervation of the ovaries, which has been known for a long time to be vegetative, may play a role. Further, the internal hormonal milieu of the ovaries may be improved by reducing the androgen-producing tissue and/or the evacuating multiple cysts.

The provocation of adhesions (bleeding, peritoneal injury) must be strictly avoided during the operation. During stimulation treatment, patients with hyperandrogenism and particularly those with hyperandrogenemic ovarian insufficiency are at an increased risk of hyperstimulation, multiple pregnancy, and early abortion. Even under therapy, pregnancy rates are significantly lower than in patients with hypogonadotropic ovarian insufficiency.

Especially PCO patients with hyperandrogenemic amenorrhea are susceptible to cardiovascular disease.

Summary of Findings Relevant for Reproductive Medicine

There are only a few measurable serum parameters which are important for fertility therapy (Table 5).

Pituitary/Hypothalamus. In order to diagnose hypothalamic/pituitary disorders, it is normally sufficient to measure LH, FSH and prolactin in the early follicular phase. Increased serum concentrations are either due to ovarian insufficiency or hyposensitive ovaries. An increased LH/FSH ratio is common in patients with polycystic ovaries associated with oligo- or amenorrhea.

When the patient is found to have increased prolactin levels, the first question to ask is whether she is taking any prolactin-increasing drugs. In addition, (latent) hypothyroidism should be excluded using a TRH test. If it is diagnosed, it should be treated first. Dopamin agonist therapy should only begin if prolactin levels fail to return to normal after normalization of the thyroid function.

Table 5. Important findings for therapy of patients with ovulatory and cyclic disorders. The normal ranges specified vary between laboratories

Organ	Diagnostic measure	Finding	Consequence
Hypothalamus	No specific diagnosis	–	–
Anterior pituitary	LH	Normogonadotropic	Normal
		Hypogonadotropic	Hypothalmic-pituitary disorder
		Hypergonadotropic	Ovarian insufficiency, hyposensitive ovaries
	FSH	Normogonadotropic	Normal
		Hypogonadotropic	Hypothalmic-pituitary disorder; stimulation with HMG
		Hypergonadotropic	Ovarian insufficiency, hyposensitive ovaries
	LH/FSH	< 1.5–2	No intervention
		> 1.5–2	preferably stimulation with FSH, ovarian ultrasound
	Prolactin	Normal	No intervention
		Elevated	Further diagnosis TRH Test Dopamin agonists Surgery
Posterior pituitary	No specific diagnosis	–	–
Hypothalamus/ thyroid	TSH at baseline and after TRH T3, T4		Normal; no intervention
		Latent hypothyroidism	L-Thyroxin
		Manifest hypo-/ hyperthyroidism	Further diagnosis, referral to internal specialist
Pineal gland	No specific diagnosis	–	–
Ovaries	Estradiol (days 3–5 of cycle)	> 40–50 pg/ml	Normal
	Progesterone luteal phase	> 10 ng/ml	Normal
	(2–3 measurements)	< 10 ng/ml	Luteal phase disorder
	Testosterone	Normal	No intervention
		< 1.5 ng/ml	Ovarian ultrasound
		≥ 1.5 ng/ml	Suspicion of tumor, further diagnosis
	Ultrasound	Normal	No intervention
		Polycystic	Further diagnosis, lowdose FSH-Stimulation
Adrenal	DHEAS	< 5 µg/ml	No intervention
		5–7 ng/ml	Adrenale hyperandro-genemia, low-dose corticoids
		> 7 µg/ml	Suspicion of tumor, further diagnosis

Serum prolactin levels between 50 and 250 ng/ml suggest a microprolactinoma, while levels above 250 ng/ml are indicative of a macroprolactinoma of the pituitary. Most patients with hypothyroidism have serum prolactin levels below 50 ng/ml. Prolactin should be measured in the early follicular phase. Stimulation tests, e.g., with TRH or metoclopramide, are not necessary.

Thyroid. Although it is assumed that patients with latent or manifest hypothyroidism (baseline TSH levels normal but increased after TRH) suffer from reduced fertility, there are not many studies on this subject, so that no definitive conclusions can be drawn at the moment. However, the available data suggest an increased incidence of early abortion in patients with latent hypothyroidism (Gerhard et al. 1991). For this reason, a TRH test is recommended before starting any infertility treatment or when the patient suffers from habitual abortion. T3 and T4 must be measured only if the TRH test is pathological. In all cases of hyperthyroidism or manifest hypothyroidism, treatment should be dispensed by or in cooperation with an internal specialist.

Ovaries. Measurement of estradiol between days 3 and 5 of the cycle in combination with LH and FSH measurements will show whether estradiol secretion is adequate and the hypothalamic-pituitary-ovarian interaction is normal. Progesterone measurements in the luteal phase will help to determine the quality of the corpus luteum and should be made at least twice between the fourth and eighth hyperthermic day.

Adrenal. Testosterone and DHEAS should be measured between days 3 and 5 of the cycle. These measurements allow the exclusion of hyperandrogenism and are especially useful in patients showing signs of virilism. An ACTH stimulation test is also suitable for further diagnosis of the adrenal, since an adrenal 21-hydroxylase defect can be discovered by measuring 17α-hydroxyprogesterone. Hyperandrogenemic patients wishing to conceive should be given low-dose corticoids (e.g., 0.25–0.5 mg dexamethasone).

References

Abe H, Engleer D, Molitch ME, Bollinger-Gruber J, Reichlin S (1985) Vasoactive intestinal peptide is a physiological mediator of prolactin release in the rat. Endocrinolgy 116:1383
Adashi EY (1991) In: Yen SCC, Jaffee RB (eds) The ovarian cycle Reproductive endocrinology. Saunders, Philadelphia, pp 181–237
Adashi EY, Hsueh AJ (1981) Stimulation of β2-adrenergic responsiveness by follicle-stimulating hormone in rat granulosa cells in vitro and in vivo. Endocrinology 108:2170
Adashi EY, Hsueh AJW (1982) Estrogens augment the stimulation of ovarian aromatase activity by follicle-stimulating hormone in cultured rat granulosa cells. J Biol Chem 257:6077
Adashi EY, Resnick CE, Croft CS, May JV, Gospodarowicz D (1988) Basic fibroblast growth factor as a regulator of ovarian granulosa cell differentiation: a novel non-mitogenic role. Mol Cell Endocrinol 55:7–14
Adashi EY, Resnick CE, D'Ercole AJ, Svoboda ME, Van Wyk JJ (1985) Insulin-like growth factors as intraovarian regulators of granulosa cell growth and function. Endocr Rev 6:400

Adashi EY, Resnick CE, Hernandez ER, May JV, Purchio AF, Twardzik DR (1988) Ovarian transforming growth factor-d (TGF-β): cellular sites(s), and mechanism(s) of action. Mol Cell Endocrinol 61:247

Adashi EY, Resnick CE (1986) Antagonistic interactions of transforming growth factors in the regulabon of granulosa cell differentiation. Endocrinology 119:1243

Adashi EY (1989) Cytokine-mediated regulation of ovarian function: encounters of a third kind. Endocrinology 124:2043-2045

Aedo AR, Pederson PH, Pederson SG, Diczfalusy E (1980) Ovarian steroid secretion in normally menstruating women. II. The contribution of the corpus luteum. Acta Endocrinol 95:222-231

Ali SM, McMurtry JP, Bagnell CA, Bryant Greenwood GD (1986) Immunocytochemical localization of relaxin in corpora lutea of sows throughout the estrous cycle Biol Reprod 34:139-143

Armstrong DT, Dorrington JH (1976) Androgens augnent FSH-induced progesterone secretion by cultured rat granulosa cells. Endocrinology 99:1411

Baker BL, Jaffe RB (1975) The genesis of cell types in the adenohypophysis of the human fetus as observed with immunocytochemistry. Am J Anatomy 143:137

Baker TG, Franchi LL (1967) The fine structure of oogonia and oocytes in human ovaries. J Cell Sci 2:213

Baker TG (1963) A quantitative and cytological study of germ cells in human ovaries. Proc R Soc Lond (Biol) 158:417

Bala RM, Lopatka J, Leung A, McCoy E, McArther RG (1981) Serum immunoreactive somatomedin levels in normal adults, pregnant women at term, children at various ages, and children with constitutionally delayed growth. J Clin Endocrinol Metab 52:508-512

Balboni GC, Vannelli GB, Barni T, Orlando C, Serio M (1987) Transferrin and somatomedin C receptors in the human ovarian follicles Fertil Steril 48:796-801

Barreca A, Minuto F, Volpe A, Cecchelli E, Cella F, Del Monte P, Artini P, Giordano G (1990) Insulin-like growth factor-I (IGF-I) and IGF-I binding protein in the follicular fluids of growth hormone treated patients Clin Endocrinol 32:497

Batista MC, Cartledge TP, Zellmer AW, Nieman LK, Merriam GR, Loriaux DL (1993) Evidence for a critical role of progesterone in the regulation of the midcycle gonadotropin surge and ovulation. J Clin Endocrinol Metab 74:565-570

Beers WH (1975) Follicular plasminogen and plasminogen activator and the effect of plasmin on ovarian folliclilar wall. Cell 6:379

Behrman HR, Romero RJ (1991) Prostaglandins and prostaglandin-like product in reproduction: eicosanoids, peroxides and oxygen radicals In: Yen SCC, Jaffee RB (eds) Reproductive endocrinology. Saunders, Philadelphia, pp 238-272

Blandau R, Rumery R (1963) Measurements of intrafollicular pressure in ovulatory and preovulatory follicles in the rat Fertil Steril 14:330

Bloom FE (1991) Neuroendocrine mechanisms: cells and systems In: Yen SCC, Jaffee RB (eds) Reproductive endocrinology. Saunders, Philadelphia, pp 1-25

Boutin JM, Jolicoeur C, Okamura H, Gagnon J, Edery M, Shirota M, Banville D, Dusanter-Fourt I, Dijane J, Kelly PA (1988) Cloning and expression of the rat prolactin receptor, a member of the growth hormone/prolactin receptor family. Cell 53:69

Breckwoldt M, Neumann F, Bräuer H (1993) Exempla endokrinologica: Bildatlas zur Physiologie und Morphologie des endokrinen Systems. Schering AG, Medical Service, Munich

Breitenecker G, Friedrich F, Kemeter P (1978) Maturation and degeneration of human ovarian follicles and their oocytes. Fertil Steril 29:336-341

Brown JB (1955) A chemical method for the determination of oestriol, oestrone and oestradiol in human urine. Biochem J 60:185-190

Brück K (1980) Funktionen des endokrinen Systems In: Schmidt RF, Thews G (eds) Physiologie des Menschen, 20th edn, Springer, Berlin Heidelberg New York, pp 722

Bulmer D (1964) The histochemistry of ovarian macrophages in the rat. J Anat 98:313

Burger HG, Findlay IK (1989) Potential relevance of inhibin to ovarian physiology. Semin Reprod Endocrinol 7:69

Burgus R, Butcher M, Amoss M, Ling N, Monahan MW, Rivier J, Fellows R, Blackwell R, Vale W, Guillemin R (1972) Primary structure of the ovine hypothalamic luteinizing hormone-releasing factor (LRF). Proc Natl Acad Sci USA 69:278–282

Burgus R, Dunn TF, Desiderio D, Ward DN, Vale W, Guillemin R (1970) Nature (London) 226:321–325

Carmichael MS, Humbert R, Dixen J, Palmisano G, Greenleaf W, Davidson JM (1987) Plasma oxytocin increases in the human sexual response. J Clin Endocrinol Metab 64:27

Carr BR, Sadler RK, Rochelle DB, Stalmach MA, MacDonald PC, Simpson ER (1981) Plasma lipoprotein regulation of progesterone synthesis by human corpus luteum tissue in organ culture. J Clin Endocrinol Metab 62:875

Catt JC, Dufau ML (1991) Gonadotropic hormones: biosynthesis, secretion, receptors and actions. In: Yen SCC, Jaffee RB (eds) Reproductive endocrinology. Saunders, Philadelphia, pp 105–155

Cavender JL, Murdoch WJ (1988) Morphological studies of the microcirculatory system of periovulatory ovine follicles. Biol Reprod 39:989

Childs GV, Hyde C, Naor Z, Catt RJ (1983) Heterogenous luteinizing hormone and follicle-stimulating hormone storage patterns in subtypes of gonadotropes separated by centrifugal elutriation. Endocrinology 113:2120–2128

Christie JE (1987) Classical Transmitters and Neurotransmitters. In: Flückinger E, Müller EE, Thorner MO (eds) Transmitter molecules in the brain. II. Function and dysfunction. Springer, Berlin Heidelberg New York, pp 46–54

Clayton RN, Catt KJ (1981) Gonadotropin-releasing hormone receptors: characterization, physiological regulation and relationship to reproductive function. Endocr Rev 2:186–209

Collins A, Eneroth P, Lalldgren B-M (1983) Psychoneuroendocrjne stress responses and mood as related to the menstrual cycle. Psychosom Med 47:512

Dailey RA, Neill JD (1981) Seasonal variation in reproductive hormones of rhesus monkeys: Anovulatory and short luteal phase menstrual cycles. Biol Reprod 25:560

Daniel SAJ, Armstrong DT (1980) Enhancement of folliclestimulating hormone-induced aromatase activity by androgens in cultured rat granulosa cells. Endocrinology 107:1027

Davoren JB, Hsueh AJW (1986) Growth hormone increases ovarian levels of immunoreactive somatomedin C/insulin-like-growth factor I in vivo. Endocrinology 118:888–890

Demura R, Suzuki T, Tajima S, Mitsuhashi S, Odagiri E, Demura H, Ling N (1993) Human plasma free activin and inhibin levels during the menstrual cycle. J Clin Endocrinol Metab 76:1080–1082

Dennerstein L, Abraham SF (1982) Affective changes and the menstrual cycle. In: Beumont PJV, Burrows GD (eds) Handbook of psychiatry and endocrinology. Elsevier, Amsterdam, pp 367–400

DiZerega GS, Mam RP, Roche PL, Campeau JD, Kling DR (1983) Identification of protein(s) in pooled human follicular fluid which suppress follicular response to gonadotropins. J Clin Endocrinol Metab 56:35

DiZerega GS, Tonetta SA, Westhof GJ (1987) A postulated role for naturally occurring aromatose inhibitors in follicle selection Steroid Biochem 27(1–3):375–383

Dluzen DE, Ramirez VD (1989) Receptive female rats stimulate norepinephrine release from olfactory bulbs of freely behaving male rats. Neuroendocrinology 49:28

Dorrington JH, Armstrong DT (1979) Effects of FSH on gonadal functions. Rec Prog Horm Res 39:301

Dorrington JH, Armstrong DT (1975) Follicle-stimulating hormone stimulates estradiol-17β synthesis in cultured Sertoli cells. Proc Natl Acad Sci USA 72:2677

Erickson GF (1982) Follicular maturation and atresia. In: Flamigni C, Givens JR (eds) The gonadotropins: basic science and clinical aspects in females. Academic, New York, pp 171–186

Erickson GF, Garzo VG, Magoffin DA (1989) Insulin-like-growth-factor-I regulates aromatase activity in human granulosa and granulosa luteal cells. J Clin Endocrinol Metab 69:716

Erickson GF, Hseuh AJW (1978) Secretion of "inhibin" by rat granulosa cells in vitro. Endocrinology 103:1960

Erickson GF, Wang C, Hsueh AJW (1979) FSH induction of functional LH receptors in granulosa cells cultured in a chemically defined medium. Nature 279:336

Espey L (1974) Ovarian proteolytic enzymes and ovulation. Biol Reprod 10:216

Espey L (1980) Ovulation and an inflammatory reaction – a hypothesis. Biol Reprod 22:73

Espey LL, Coons PJ, Marsh JM, LeMaire WJ (1981) Effect of indomethacin on preovulatory changes in the ultrastructure of rabbit graafian follicles. Endocrinology 108:1040–1048

Falck B, Menander K, Nordanstedt O (1962) Androgen secretion by the rat ovary. Nature 193:593

Farookhi R (1980) Effects of androgen on induction of gonadotropin receptors and gonadotropin-stimulated adenosine 3',5'-monophosphate production in rat ovarian granulosa cells. Endocrinology 106:1216

Feldman E, Haberman S, Abisogun AO (1986) Arachidonic acid metabolism in human granulosa cells: evidence for cyclooxygenase and lipoxygenase activity in vitro. Hum Reprod 1:353–356

Fisher DA (1983) Maternal-fetal neurohypophyseal system. In: Yen SSC Clin Perinatol 10:695

Fox SR (1990) Harlan RE, Shivers BD, Pfaff DW (1990) Chemical characterization of neuroendocrine targets for progesterone in the female rat brain and pituitary Neuroendocrinology 51:276

Fukuda M, Miyamoto K, Hasegawa Y, Normura M, Igarashi M, Kangawa K, Matsuo H (1986) Isolation of bovine follicular fluid inhibin of about 32 kDA. Mol Cell Endocrinol 44:55

Geisthövel F, Moretti-Rojas I, Asch RH, Rojas FJ (1990) Expression of insulin-like-growth-factor-II (IGF-II)-messenger ribinucleic acid (mRNA), but not IGF-I-mRNA, in human preovulatory granulosa cells. Hum Reprod 4:899–902

Gemzell CA, Li CH (1958) Estimation of growth hormone content in a single human pituitary. J Clin Endocrinol 18:146

Gharib SD, Wierman ME, Shupnik MA, Chin WW (1990) Molecular biology of the pituitary gonadotropins. Endocr Rev 11:177

Going JJ, Anderson TJ, Battersby S, Maclntyre CCA (1988) Proliferative and secretory activity in human breast during natural and artificial menstrual cycles. Am J Pathol 130:193

Goldenberg RL, Vaitukaitis JL, Ross GT (1972) Estrogen and follicle stimulating hormone interactions on follicle growth in rats. Endocrinology 90:1492–1498

Gong EJ, Garrel D, Calloway DH (1989) Menstrual cycle and voluntary food intake. Am J Clin Nutr 49:252

Goodman AL, Hodgen GD (1983) The ovarian triad of the primate menstrual cycle. Rec Prog Horm Res 39:1

Goodman AL, Hodgen GD (1979) Between-ovary interaction in the regulation of follicle growth, corpus luteum function, and gonadotropin secretion in the primate ovarian cycle. Effects of luteectomy and hemiovariectomy during the luteal phase in cynomolgus monkeys Endocrinology 104:1310

Gospodarowicz D (1989) Fibroblast growth factor: involvement in early embryonic development and ovarian function. Semin Reprod Endocrinol 7:21

Gospodarowicz D, Bialecki H (1979) Fibroblast and epidermal growth factors are mitogenic agents for cultured granulosa cells of rodent, porcine, and human origin. Endocrinology 104:757

Gospodarowicz D, Ferrara NJ (1989) Fibroblast growth factor and the control of pituitary and gonad development and function Steroid Biochem 32:183–191

Gougeon A (1986) Dynamics of follicular growth in the human: a model from preliminary results. Hum Reprod 1:81–87

Green ID, Harris GW (1949) Observation of the hypophyseal-portal vessels in the living rat. J Physiol (London) 108:359

Gross DS (1980) Effect of castration and steroid replacement on immunoreactive gonadotropin-releasing hormone in the hypothalamus and preoptic area. Endocrinology 106:1442–1450

Gudelsky GA, Apud JA, Masotto C, Locatelli V, Cocchi D, Racagni G, Muller EE (1983) Etha-nolamine-O-sulfate enhances α-aminobutyric acid secretion into hypophysial portal blood and lowers serum prolactin concentrations. Neuroendocrinology 37:397

Gudelsky GA, Porter JC (1980) Release of dopamine from tuberoinfundibular neurons into pituitary stalk blood after prolactin or haloperidol administration. Endocrinology 106:526

Guillemin F (1978) Peptides in the brain: the new endocrinology of the neuron. Science 202:390

Guillemin R, Brazeau P, Böhlen P, Esch F, Ling N, Wehrenberg WB (1982) Growth hor-mone-releasing factor from a human pancreatic tumor that caused acromegaly. Sience 218:585–587

Guillemin R, Brazeau P, Bohlen P (1984) Somatocrinin the growth hormone releasing factor. Recent Pro Horm Res 40:233

Guillemin R, Rosenberg B (1955) Humoral hypothalamic control of anterior pituitary a study of combined tissue cultures. Endocrinology 57:599–607

Guler HP, Zapf J, Froesch ER (1987) Short term metabolic effects of recombinant human in-sulin-like growth factor-I in healthy adults N Engl J Med 317:137

Hampson E (1990) Estrogen-related variations in human spatial and articulatory-motor skills. Psychoneuroendocrinology 15:97

Hardouin S, Gourmelen M, Noguiez P, Seurin D, Roghani M, LeBouc Y, Povoa G, Merimee TJ, Hosenlopp P, Binoux M (1989) Molecular forms of serum insulin-like growth factor (IGF-)-binding proteins in man: relationship with growth hormone and IGFs and physi-ological significance. J GClin Endocrinol Metab 69:1291

Hazum E, Conn PM (1988) Molecular mechanism of gonadotropin releasing hormone (GnRH) action. I. The GnRH receptor. Endocr Rev 9:379

Heinonen PK, Metsa Ketela T (1988) Prostanoids and cyclic nucleotides in malignant and benign ovarian tumors. Med Oncol Tumor Pharmacother 5:11–15

Henkin RI (1974) In: Ferin M, Halberg F, Richart R, Vande Wiele RL (eds) Biorhythms and human reproduction. Wiley, New York. pp 277–285

Hernandez ER, Jimenez IL, Payne DW, Adashi EY (1988) Adrenergic regulation of ovarian androgen biosynthesis is mediated via β-adrenergic theca-interstitial cell recognition sites. Endocrinology 122:1592–1602

Hillier SG, DeZwart FA (1981) Evidence that granulosa cell aromatase induction/activation by follicle-stimulating hormone is an androgen receptor-regulated process in vitro. En-docrinology 109:1303

Hillier SG, Reichert LE Jr, Van Hall EV (1981) Control of preovulatory follicular estrogen biosynthesis in the human ovary. J Clin Endocrinol Metab 52:847

Hillier SG, van den Boogaard AMJ, Reichert LE, van Hall EV (1980) Intraovarian sex steroid hormone interactions and the regulation of follicular maturation: aromatization of an-drogens by human granulosa cells in vitro. J Clin Endocrinol Metab 50:640

Hodgen GD (1982) The dominant ovarian follicle. Fertil Steril 38:281–300

Hoffman GE, Lee W-S, Attardi B, Yann V, Fitzsimmons MD (1990) Luteinizing hormone-re-leasing hormone neurons express c-fos antigen after steroid activation. Endocrinology 126:1736

Hsueh AIW, Dahl KD, Vaughan 1, Tucker E, Rivier J, Bardin CW, Vale W (1987) Heterodi-mers and homodimers of inhibin subunits have different paracrine action in the modula-tion of luteinizing hormone-stimulated androgen biosynthesis. Proc Natl Acad Sci USA 84:5082

Hsueh AJW, Jones PBC, Adashi EY, Wang C, Zhuang L-Z, Welsh TH Jr (1983) Intraovarian mechanisms in the hormonal control of granulosa cell differentiation in rats. J Reprod Fertil 69:325

Hume DA, Halpin D, Charlton H, Gordon S (1984) The mononuclear phagocyte system of the mouse defined by immunohistochemical localization of antigen F4 t 80: macrophages of endocrine organs. Proc Natl Acad Sci USA 81:4174

Hutchinson LA, Handlay IK, Devos FL, Robertson DM (1987) Effects of bovine inhibin, transforming growth factor-β and bovine activin-A on granulosa cell differentiation. Bio-chem Biophys Res Commun 146:1405

Hutz RJ, Dierschke DJ, Wolf RC (1985) Seasonal effects on ovarian folliculogenesis in rhesus monkeys. Biol Reprod 33:653

Ichikawa F, Yoshimura Y, Oda T, Shiraki M, Maruyama K, Kawakami S, Nakamura Y, Fukushima M (1990) The effects of lipoxygenase products on progesterone and prostaglandin production by human corpora lutea J Clin Endocrinol Metab 70:849–855

Illingworth DR, Corbin DK, Kemp ED, Keenan EJ (1982) Hormone changes during the menstrual cycle in abetalipoproteinemia: reduced luteal phase progesterone in a patient with homozygous hypobetalipoproteinemia. Proc Natl Acad Sci 79:6685

Ivell R, Richter D (1984) The gene for the hypothalamic peptide hormone oxytocin is highly expressed in the bovine corpus luteum: biosynthesis, structure and sequence analysis. EMBO J 3:2351

Jacobson W, Kalra SP (1989) Decreases in mediobasal hypothalamic and preoptic area opioid ([3H]naloxone) binding are associated with the progesterone-induced luteinizing hormone surge. Endocrinology 124:199

Jacobson W, Wilkinson M (1986) Association of diurnal variations in hypothalamic but not cortical opiatenaloxone binding sites with the ability of naloxone to induce LH release in the prepubertal female rats. Neuroendocrinology 44:132

Jänig W (1980) Das vegetative Nervensystem. In: Schmidt RF, Thews G (eds) Physiologie des Menschen, 1980, 20. Auflage, Springer, 142–144

Kaufman JM, Kesner JS, Wilson RC, Knobil E (1985) Electrophysiological manifestations of luteinizing hormone-releasing hormone pulse generator activity in the rhesus monkey: Influence of adrenergic and dopaminergic blocking agents. Endocrinology 116:1327

Kaverne EB, de la Riva C (1982) Pheromones in mice: Reciprocal interaction between the nose and brain. Nature 296:148

Kazer R, Mais V, Cetel N, Rivier J, Vale W, Yen SSC (1985) Inhibition of follicular maturation and induction of luteolysis by an antagonistic analog of GnRH in normal cycling women. Abstract No. 237. Society for Gynecologic Investigation. Phoenix, April 9

Kiesel L, Catt KJ (1984) Phosphatidic acid and the calcium-dependent actions of gonadotropin-releasing hormone in pituitary gonadotrophs. Arch Biochem Biophys 231:202–210

Kiesel L, Loumaye E, Catt KJ (1984a) Receptors and action of gonadotropin releasing hormone (GnRH) in the anterior pituitary. In: Runnebaum B, Rabe T, Kiesel L, Merz WE (eds) Secretion and action of gonadotropins. Springer, Berlin Heidelberg New York

Kiesel L, Rabe T, Hauser G, Runnebaum B (1984b) Stimulation of luteinizing hormone release by phospholipases and melittin in rat pituitary cells. Acta Endocrinol (Suppl 267)108:9–10

Knecht M, Catt KJ (1983) Modulation of cAMP-mediated differentiation in ovarian granulosa cells by epidermal growth factor and platelet-derived growth factor. J Biol Chem 258:2789

Knecht M, Feng P, Catt KJ (1986) Transforming growth factor-beta regulates the expression of luteinizing hormone receptors in ovarian granulosa cells. Biochem Biophys Res Commun 139:800

Knobil E (1974) On the control of gonadotropin secretion in the rhesus monkey. Recent Prog Horm Res 30:146

Knobil E, Plant TM, Wildt L et al. (1980) Control of the rhesus monkey menstrual cycle: permissive role of hypothalamic gonadotropin-releasing hormone. Science 207:1371–1373

Knobil E (1989) The electrophysiology of the GnRH pulse generator. J Steroid Biochem 33:669

Koistinen R, Kalkkinen N, Huhtala ML, Seppala M, Bohn H, Rutanen EM (1986) Placental protein 12 is a decidual protein that binds somatomedin and has an identical N-terminal amino acid sequence with somatomedin-binding protein from human amniotic fluid. Endocrinology 118:1375–1378

Koves K, Gottschall PE, Gorcs T, Scammell JG, Arimura A (1990) Presence of immunoreactive vasoactive intestinal polypeptide in anterior pituitary of normal male and long term estrogen-treated female rats: A light microscopic immunohistochemical study Endocrinology 126:1756–1763

Krishna A, Terranova PF, Maneri RL, Papkoff H (1986) Histamine and increased ovarian blood flow mediate LH-induced superovulation in the cyclic hamster. I Reprod Fertil 76:23

Krishna A, Terranova PF (1985) Alterations in mast cell degranulation and ovarian histamine in the proestrous hamster. Biol Reprod 32:1211

Laessle RG, Tuschl RJ, Schweiger U, Pirke KM (1990) Mood changes and physical complaints during the normal menstrual cycle in healthy young women. Psychoneuroendocrinology 15:131

Ledwitz-Rigby F, Rigby BW, Gay VL, Stetston M, Young I, Channing CP (1977) Inhibitory action of porcine follicular fluid upon granulosa cell luteinization in vitro. l'Endocrinol 74:175

Ling N, Ying SY, Ueno N, Shimasaki S, Esch F, Hotta M, Guillemin R (1986) Pituitary FSH is released by a heterodimer of the β-subunits from the two forms of inhibin. Nature 321:779

Liu JH, Yen SSC (1983) Induction of midcycle gonadotropin surge by ovarian steroids in women A critical evaluation. J Clinical Endocrinol Metab 57:797

Lloyd RV, Anagnostou D, Cano M, Barkan AL, Chandler WF (1988) Analysis of mammosomatotropic cells in normal and neoplastic human pituitary tissues by the reverse hemolytic plaque assay and immunocytochemistry. J Clin Endocrinol Metab 66:1103

Longacre TA, Bartow SA (1986) A correlative morphologic study of human breast and endometrium in the menstrual cycle. Am J Surg Pathol 10:382

Lucky AW, Rebar RW, Rosenfield RL, Roche-Bender N, Helke J (1977) Reduction of the potency of luteinizing hormone by estrogen. N Engl J M

Magoffin DA, Kurtz KM, Erickson GF (1990) Insulin-like growth factor-I selectively stimulates cholesterol side-chain cleavage expression in ovarian theca interstitial cells. Mol Endocr 4:489

Massague J, Czech MP (1982) The subunit structures of two distinct receptors for insulin-like growth factor I and II and their relationship to the insulin receptor. J Biol Chem 257:5038–5045

Matsuo H, Baba Y, Nair RM, Arimura A, Schally AV (1971) Structure of the porcine LH- and FSH-releasing hormone. I. The proposed amino acid sequence. Biochem Biophys Res Commun 43:1334–1339

McDonough PG (1991) Molecular Biology in reproductive endocrinology In: Yen SCC, Jaffee RB (eds) Reproductive endocrinology. Saunders, 65–104

McLachlan RI, Cohen NL, Dahl KD, Bremner WJ, Soules MR (1990) Serum inhibin levels during the periovulatory interval in normal women throughout the menstrual cycle. Clin Endocrinol 32:39

McNatty KP, Makris A, DeGrazia C, Osathanondh R, Ryan KJ (1979a) The production of progesterone, androgens, and estrogens by granulosa cells, thecal tissue, and stromal tissue from human ovaries in vitro. J Clin Endocinol Metab 49:687–699

McNatty KP, Makris A, Reinhold VN, DeGrazia C, Osathanondh R, Ryan KJ (1979b) Metabolism of androstenedione by human ovarian tissues in vitro with particular reference to reductase and aromatase activity. Steroids 34:429

McNatty KP, Smith DM, Makris A, Osathanondh R, Ryan KJ (1979c) The microenvironment of the human antral follicle: Interrelationships among the steroid levels in antral fluid, the population of granulosa cells, and the status of the oocyte in vivo and in vitro. J Clin Endocrinol Metab 49:851

McQueen JK (1987) Classical Transmitters and Neurotransmitters. In: Flückinger E, Müller EE, Thorner MO (eds) Transmitter molecules in the brain. I. Biochemistry of transmitter molecules. Springer, Berlin, 7–26

Melis GB, Cagnacci A, Gambacciani M, Paoletti AM, Caffi T, Fioretti P (1988) Chronic bromocriptine administration restores luteinizing hormone response to naloxone in postmenopausal women. Neuroendocrinology 47:159

Melmed S, Braunstein GD, Horvath E, Ezrin C, Kovacs K (1983) Pathophysiology of acromegalie Endocr Rev 4:271

Milewich L, Chen G, Lyons C, Tucker T, Uhr J, MacDonald P (1982) Metabolism of andros-tenedione by guinea-pig peritoneal macrophages: Synthesis of testosterone and 5α-re-duced metabolites. J Steroid Biochem 17:61

Morales TI, Woessner JF Jr, Marsh JM, LeMaire WJ (1983) Collagen, collagenase and col-lagenolytic activity in rat graafian follicles during follicular growth and ovulation. Bio-chim Biophys Acta 756:119–122

Morikawa H, Okamura H, Takenaka A, Morimoto K, Nishimura T (1981) Histamine concen-tration and its effect on ovarian contractility in humans. Int J Fertil 26:283

Murdoch WJ, McCormick RJ (1989) Production of low molecular weight chemoattractants for leukocytes by periovulatory ovine follicles. Biol Reprod 40:86

Murdoch WJ, Steadman LE, Belden EL (1988) Immunoregulation of luteolysis. Med Hypo-theses 27:197

Murdoch WJ (1987) Treatment of sheep with prostaglandin F2 alpha enhances production of a luteal chemoattractant for eosinophils. Am J Reprod Immunol Microbiol 15:52

Murdoch Wl, Cavender IL (1987) Mechanism of ovulation. Adv Contra Delv Sys 3:353

Nagy G, Mulchaney JJ, Neill JD (1988) Autocrine control of prolactin secretion by vasoac-tive intestinal peptide. Endocrinology 122:364

Naor Z, Katikineni M, Loumaye E, Garcia Vela A, Dufau ML, Catt KJ (1982) Compartmenta-lization of luteinizing hormone pools: dynamics of gonadotropin releasing hormone ac-tion in superfused pituitary cells. Mol Cell Endocrinol 27:213–220

Ohashi M, Carr BR, Simpson ER (1982) Lipoprotein binding sites in human corpus luteum membrane fractions. Endocrinology 110:1477

Ohno S, Klinger H, Atkin N (1962) Human oogenesis. Cytogenetics 1:42

Olasov B, Jackson J (1987) Effects of expectancies on women's reports of moods during the menstrual cycle. Psychosom Med 49:65

Parr EL (1974) Histological examination of the rat ovarian follicle wall prior to ovulation. Biol Reprod 11:483

Peluso IJ, Steger RW (1978) Role of FSH in regulating granulosa cell division and follicular atresia in rats. J Reprod Fertil 54:275

Pfaff DW (1986) Gene expression in hypothalamic neurons: luteinizing hormone-releasing hormone. J Neurosci Res 16:109–115

Pliner P, Fleming AS (1983) Food intake, body weight, and sweetness preferences over the menstrual cycle in humans. Physiol Behav 30:663

Plotsky PM, Cunningham ET Jr, Widmaier EP (1989) Catecholaminergic modulation of cor-ticotropin-releasing factor and adrenocorticotropin secretion. Endocr Rev 10:437

Poretsky L, Kalin MF (1987) The gonadotropic function of insulin. Endocr Rev 8:132

Ramirez VD, Feder HH, Sawyer CH (1984) The role of brain catecholamines in the regula-tion of LH secretion: A critical inquiry. In: Martini L, Ganong WF (eds) Frontiers in neuroendocrinology, Vol 8. New York, Raven Press, p 27

Rani CSS, Salhanick AR, Armstrong DT (1981) Follicle stimulating hormone induction of luteinizing hormone receptor in cultured rat granulosa cells: an examination of the needs for steroids in the induction process. Endocrinology 108:1379

Rao MC, Midgley AR, Richards JS (1978) Hormonal regulation of ovarian cellular prolifera-tion. Cell 14:71–78

Rasmussen DD, Gambacciani M, Swartz W, Tueros VS, Yen SSC (1989) Pulsatile gonadotro-pin-releasing hormone release from the human mediobasal hypothalamus in vitro: Opi-ate receptor-mediated suppression. Neuroendocrinology 49:150

Rasmussen DD, Liu JH, Swartz WH, Tueros VS, Yen SSC (1986) Human fetal hypothalamic GnRH neurosecretion: dopaminergic regulation in vitro. Clin Endocrinol (Oxf) 25:127

Rasmussen DD, Liu JH, Wolf PL, Yen SSC (1987) Neurosecretion of human hypothalamic immunoreactive β-endorphin: In vitro regulation by dopamine. Neuroendocrinology 45:197

Rasmussen DD, Liu JH, Wolf PL, Yen SSC (1983) Endogenous opioid regulation of gonado-tropin-releasing hormone release from the human fetal hypothalamus in vitro. J Clin En-docrinol Metab 57:881

Reid RL, Hoff JD, Yen SSC, Li CH (1981) Effects of exogenous β-endorphin on pituitary hormone secretion and its disappearance rate in normal human subjects. J Clin Endocrinol Metab 52:1179

Reyes RI, Boroditsky RS, Winter JSD, Faiman C (1974) Studies on human sexual development: Il. Fetal and maternal serum gonadotropin and sex steroid concentrations. J Clin Endocrinol Metab 38:612

Reynolds H, Nathan P, Srivastava L, Hess E (1982) Release of estradiol from fetal bovine serum by rat thymus spleen, kidney, lung and lung macrophage cultures. Endocrinology 110:2213

Rice BF, Savard K (1966) Steroid hormone formation in the human ovary. IV. Ovarian stromal compartment; formation of radioactive steroids from acetate-1-'4 C and action of gonadotropins. J Clin Endocrinol Metab 26:593

Richards JS (1975) Estradiol receptor content in rat granulosa cells during follicular development; modification by estradiol and gonadotrophins. Endocrinology 97:1174–1184

Richards JS, Bogvich K (1982) Effects of human chorionic gonadotropin and progesterone on follicular development in the immature rat. Endocrinology I 11:1429

Richards JS, Jongssen JA, Kersey KA (1980) Evidence that changes in tonic luteinizing hormone secretion determine the growth of preovulatory follicles in the rat. Endocrinology 107:641

Richards JS, Ireland JJ, Rao MC, Bernath GA, Midgley AR Jr, Reichert LE Jr (1976) Ovarian follicular development in the rat: hormone receptor regulation by estradiol, follicle-stimulating hormone and luteinizing hormone. Endocrinology 99:1562

Rivier C, Rivier J, Vale W (1986) Inhibin-mediated feedback control of follicle-stimulating hormone secretion in the female rat. Science 234:205

Robertson DM, Foulds LM, Leversha L (1985) Isolation of inhibin from bovine follicular fluid. Biochem Biophys Res Commun 126:220

Robertson DM, Klein R, Vos FLD, McLachlan Rl, Wettenhall REH, Hearn MTW, Burger HG, de Kretser DM (1987) The isolation of polypeptides with FSH suppressing activity from bovine follicular fluid which are structurally different to inhibin. Biochem Biophys Res Commun 149:744

Rodgers KE, Marks JF, Ellefson DD, Yanagihara DL, Tonetta SA, Vasilev SA, Morrow CP, Montz FJ, DiZerega GS (1990) Follicle regulatory protein: a novel marker for granulosa cell cancer patients. Gynecol Oncol 37:381–387

Romano GJ, Krust A, Pfaff DW (1989) Expression and es trogen regulation of progesterone receptor mRNA in neurons of the mediobasal hypothalamus: an in situ hybridization study. Mol Endocrinol 3:1295

Roseff SJ, Bangah ML, Kettel LM, Vale W, Rivier J, Burger HG, Yen SSC (1989) Dynamic changes in circulating inhibin levels during the luteal-follicular transition of the human menstrual cycle. J Clin Endocrinol Metab 69:1033

Rosenberg (1992) Postrezeptormechanismen der GnRH-induzierten Gonadotropinsekretion und ihre Interaktionen, Promotionsarbeit, Abt. Gynäkologische Endokrinologie und Reproduktionsmedizin, Universitäts-Frauenklinik Heidelberg, Univeristät Heidelberg

Rosenblatt H, Dyrenfurth 1. Ferin M, Vande Wiele RL (1980) Food intake and the menstrual cycle in rhesus monkeys. Physiol Behav 24:447

Rossmanith WG (1990) Neuroendokrine Steuerung der menschlichen Reproduktion: Regulation der Gonadotropinfreisetzung durch Neurotransmitter und ovarielle Steroide. Habilitationsschrift.

Rossmanith WG, Laughlin GA, Mortola JF, Johnson ML, Veldhuis JD, Yen SSC (1990) Pulsatile cosecretion of estradiol and progesterone by the midluteal phase corpus luteum: Temporal link to luteinizing hormone pulses. J Clin Endocrinol Metab 70:990

Rossmanith WG, Mortola JF, Yen SSC (1988) Role of endogenous opioid peptides in the initiation of the midcycle luteinizing hormone surge in normal cycling women. J Clin Endocrinol Metab 61:695

Rossmanith WG, Yen SSC (1987) Sleep-associated decrease in LH pulse frequency during the early follicular phase of the menstrual cycle: evidence for an opioidergic mechanism. I Clin Endocrinol Metab 65:715

Rudenstein RS, Bigdeli H, Mc Donald MH, Snyder PJ (1979) Administration of gonadal steroids to the castrated male rat prevents a decrease in the release of gonadotropin-releasing hormone from the incubated hypothalamus. J Clin Invest 63:262–267

Runnebaum B, Rieben W, Bierwirth, von Münstermann AM, Zander J (1972) Circadian variations in plasma progesterone in the luteal phase of the menstrual cycle and during pregnancy. Acta Endocrinol 69:731–738

Ryan KJ, Petro Z (1966) Steroid biosynthesis by human ovarian granulosa and thecal cells. J Clin Endocrinol Metab 26:46

Ryan RJ, Petro Z (1966) Steroid biosynthesis by human ovarian granulosa and thecai cells. J Clin Endocrinol Metab 51:1286

Said SI, Porter JC (1979) Vasoactive intestinal polypeptide: release into hypophysial portal blood Life Sci 24:227

Saint-Andre JP, Rohmer V, Alhenc-Gelas F, Menard J, Bigorgne JC, Corvol P (1986) Presence of renin, angiotensinogen- and converting enzyme in humanpituitary lactotroph cells and prolactin adenomas J Clin Endocrinol Metab 63:231

Salomon F, Cuneo RC, Hesp R, Sonksen PH (1989) The effects of treatment with recombinant humal growth horrnone on body composition and metabolism in adults with growth horrnone deficiency. Engl J Med 321:1797

Samson WK, Bianchi R, Mogg RJ, Rivier J, Vale W, Melin P (1989) Oxytocin mediates the hypothalamic action of vasoactive intestinal peptide to stimulate prolactin secretion. Endocrinology 124:812

Sano Y, Suzuki K, Okinaga S, Taaoki BI (1981) Changes in enzyme activities related to steroidogenesis in human ovaries during the menstrual cycle. J Clin Endocrinol Metab 52:994

Sar M (1984) Estradiol is concentrated in tyrosine hydroxylase containing neurons of the hypothalamus. Science 223:938

Sarkar DK (1989) Evidence for prolactin feedback actions on hypthalamic oxytocin, vasoactive intestinal peptide and dopamine secretion. Neuroendocrinology 36:27

Schaeffer JM, Liu J, Hsueh AJ1 V, Yen SSC (1984) Presence of oxytocin and arginine-vasopressin in human ovary, oviduct and follicular fluid. J Clin Endocrinol Metab 59:970

Schally AV, Arimura A, Baba Y, Nair RMG, Matsuo H, Redding TW, Debeljuk L, White WF (1971) Isolation and properties of the FSH and LH-releasing hormone. Biochem Biophys Res Commun 43:393–399

Schmidt CL, Black VH, Sarosi P, Weiss G (1986) Progesterone and relaxin secretion in relation to the ultrastructure of human luteal cells in culture: effects of human chorionic gonadotropin Am J Obstet Gynecol 155:1209–1219

Schramme C, Denef C (1983) Stimulation of prolactin release by angiotensin II in superfused rat anterior pituitary cell aggregates. Neuroendocrinology 36:483

Seeburg PH, Adelman JP (1984) Characterization of cDNA for precursor of human luteinizing hormone releasing hormone. Nature 311:666

Sheehan KL, Casper RF, Yen SSC (1982) Introduction of luteolysis by luteinizing hormone releasing factor (LRF) agonist: sensitivity, reproducibility and reversibility. Fertil Steril 37:209

Sherman TG, Akil H, Watson SJ (1989) The Molecular biology of neuropeptides. Geneva. Fondation pour l'Etude du Systeme Nerveux, Elsevier. Vol VI, No. 1

Shivers BD, Harlan RE, Morell JI, Pfaff DW (1983) Absence of oestradiol concentration in cell nuclei of LHRH-immunoreactive neurones. Nature 304:345–347

Simpson ER, Rochelle DBJ Carr BR, MacDonald PC (1981) Plasma lipoproteins in follicular fluid of human ovaries. J Clin Endocrinol Metab 51:1469

Skinner MK, Keski-Oja J, Osteen KG, Moses HL (1987b) Ovarian thecal cells produce transforming growth factor-β which can regulate granulosa cell growth. Endocrinology 121:786

Sommer B (1983) How does menstruation affect cognitive competence and psychophysiological response? In: Gotub S (ed) Lifling the curse of menstruation. New York, Hawworth Press, pp 53–90

Speroff L, Glass RH, Kase NG (1989) Neuroendokrinologie In: Gynäkologische Endokrinologie & steriles Paar (Hrsg deutsche Ausgabe Bohnet H), Diesbach Verlag Berlin, 49–85

Suikkari AM, Jalkanen J, Koistinen R, Butzow R, Ritvos O, Ranta T, Seppala M (1989a) Human granulosa cells synthesize low molecular weigt insulin-like growth factor-binding protein Endocrinology 124:1088

Suikkari AM, Ruutiainen K, Erkkola R, Seppala M (1989b) Low levels of low molecular weight insulin-like growth factor-binding protein in patients with polycystic ovarian disease. Hum Reprod 4:136–139

Szego CM, Pitin ES (1964) Ovarian histamine depletion during acute hyperaemic response to luteinizing hormone. Nature 201:682

Szontagh FE (1973) Short-loop ("internal") pituitary-hypothalamus gonadotropin feedback in the human. Endocnnol Exp 7:65

Takano K, Hizuka N, Shizume K, Hayashi N, Motoiko Y (1977) Serum somatomedin peptides measured by somatomedin A radioreceptor assay in chronic liver disease J Clin Endocrinol Metab 45:828–832

Tan GJS, Tweedale R, Biggs JSG (1982) Oxytocin may play a role in the control of corpus luteum. Endocrinology 95:65

Tannenbaum GS, Ling N (1984) The interrelationship of growth hormone (GH)-releasing factor and somatostatin in generation of the ultradian rhythm of GH secretion. Endocrinology 115:1952

Tonetta SA, DeVinna RS, diZerega GS J (1988) Effects of follicle regulatory protein on thecal aromatase and 3 beta hydroxysteroid dehydrogenase activity in medium- and large-sized pig follicles Reprod Fertil 82:163–171

Tonetta SA, Stone BA, Marrs RP, DiZerega GSJ (1990) Concentrations of follicle regulatory protein, steroids and gonadotrophins in antral fluids from women stimulated with metrodin and hCG Reprod Fertil 88:389–397

Too CKL, Bryant Greenwood GD, Greenwood FC (1984) Relaxin increases the release of plasminogen activator, collagenase, and proteoglycanase from rat granulosa cells in vitro Endocrinology 115:1043–1050

Too KLC, Greenwood FC (1981) The effect of relaxin on rat uterine collagenase activity. Biol Reprod 24:267

Ueno N, Lins N, Yins SY, Esch F, Shimasaki S, Guillemin R (1987) Isolation and partial characterization of follistatin: A single-chain Mr 35000 monomeric protein that inhibits the release of follicle-stimulating hormone. Proc Natl Acad Sci USA 84:8282

Vale W, Spiess J, Rivier C (1981) Characterization of a 41-residue ovine hypothalamic peptide that stimulates secretion of corticotropin an β-endorphin. Science 213:1394

Vale W, Hsueh A, Rivier C, Yu J (1990) The inhibin/activin family of hormones and growth factors. In: Sporn MB, Roberts AB (eds) Peptide growth factors and their receptors II. New York, Springer, 211–248

Vale W, Rivier J, Vaughan J, McClintock R. Corrigan A, Woo W, Karr D, Spiess J (1986) Purification and characterization of an FSH releasing protein from porcine ovarian follicular fluid. Nature 321:776

VandeWiele R, Bogumil J, Dyrenfurth I, Ferin M, Jewelewicz R, Warren M, Rixhallah T, Mikhail G (1970) Mechanisms regulating the menstrual cycle in women. Rec Prog Horm Res 26:63–92

Vierling JS, Rock J (1967) Variations in olfactory sensitivity to exaltolide during the menstrual cycle. J Appl Physiol 22:311

Vincent S, Hokfelt T, Wu JY (1982) GABA neuron systems in the hypothalamus and the pituitary gland. Neuroendocrinology 34:117

Voutilainen L, Miller WL (1987) Coordinate tropic hormone regulation if mRNAs for Insulin-like-growth factor II and the cholesterol side-chain cleavage enzyme P450scc, in human steroidogenic tissues Proc Natl Acad Sci USA 84:1590

Wehrenberg WB, Ling H, Bohlen P, Esch F, Brazeau P, Guillemin R (1982) Physiological roles of somatocrinin and somatostatin in the regulation of growth hormone secretion. Biochem Biophys Res Commun 109:562

Weingartner H, Gold P, Ballenger JC, Smallberg SA, Summers R, Rubinow DR, Post RM Goodwin FK (1981) Effects of vasopressin on human memory function. Science 211:601

Welsh TH Jr, Zhuang L-Z, Hsueh AJW (1983) Estrogen augmentation of gonadotropin-stimulated progestin biosynthesis in cultured rat granulosa cells. Endocrinology 112:1916

Wildt L, Hausler A, Marshall G, Hutchison IS, Plant TM, Belchetz PE, Knobil E (1981) Frequency and amplitude of gonadotropin-releasing hormone stimulation and gonadotropin secretion in the rhesus monkey. Endocrinology 109:376

Wilkes MM, Yen SSC (1980) Reduction by β-endorphin of efflux of dopamine and DOPAC from superfused medial basal hypothalamus. Life Sci 27:1387

Witschi E (1948) Migration of the germ cells of human embryos from the yolk sac to the primitive gonadal folds. Contrib Embryol 32:67

Yen SCC (1988) Reproductive strategies in women: Neuroendocrine basis of endogenous contraception. In: Roland R (ed) Neuroendocrinology of reproduction. Amsterdam, Excerpta Medica, 231–239

Yen SCC (1991) The human menstrual cycle: Neuroendocrine regulation In: Yen SCC, Jaffee RB (eds) Reproductive endocrinology. Saunders, 273–308

Yen SCC (1991) The hypothalamic control of pituitary hormone secretion In: Yen SCC, Jaffe RB (eds) Reproductive endocrinology. Saunders 1–25

Yen SSC, Quigley ME, Reid RL, Cetel NS (1985) Neuroendocrinology of opioid peptides and their role in the control of gonadotropin and prolactin secretion. Am J Obstet Gynecol 152:485

Yen SSC, Rebar RW (1972) Endocrine rhythms in gonadotropins and ovarian steroids with reference to reproductive processes. In: Krieger DT (ed) Endocrine rhythms. New York, Raven Press

Yen SSC, Tsai CC (1972) Acute gonadotropin release induced by exogenous estradiol during the mid-follicular phase of the menstrual cycle. J Clin Endocrinol Metab 34:298–305

Yen SSC (1983) Pituitary hormone release in response to food ingestion: Evidence for neuroendocrine signals from gut to brain. J Clin Endocrinol Metab 57:1111

Ying SY (1988) Inhibins, activins, and follistatins: Gonadal proteins modulating the secretion of follicle-stimulating hormone. Endocr Rev 9:267

Ying SY, Becker A, Swanson G, Tan P, Ling N, Esch F, Ueno N, Shimasaki S, Guillemin R (1987) Follistatin specifically inhibits pituitary follicle stimulating hormone release in vitro. Biochem Biophys Res Commun 149:133

Zanisi M, Martini L (1975a) Effects of progesterone metabolites on gonadotrophin secretion. J Steroid Biochem 6:1021

Zanisi M, Martini L (1975b) Differential effects of castration on LH and FSH secretion in male and female rats. Acta Endocrinol 78:683

Zapf J, Walter H, Froesch ER (1981) Radioimmunological determination of insulin-like growth factors I and II in normal subjects and in patients with growth disorders and extra-pancreatic tumor hypoglycemia J Clin Invest 68:1321–1330

Zhiwen Z, Carson RS, Herington AC, Lee VWK, Burger HG (1987) Follicle stimulating hormone and somatomedin-C stimulate inhibin production by rat granulosa cells in vitro. Endocrinology 120:1633

Zimmermann EA, Defendini R, Frantz AG (1974) Prolactin and growth hormone in patients with pituitary adenomas: a correlative study of hormone in tumor and plasma by immunoperoxidase technique and radioimmunoassay. J Clin Endocrinol Metab 38:577

Zoller LC, Weisz J (1979a) A quantitative cytochemical study of glucose-6-phosphate dehydrogenase and $/\sim 53\beta$-hydroxysteroid dehydrogenase activity in the membrana granulosa of the ovulable type of follicle of the rat. Histochemistry 62:125

Zoller LC, Weisz J (1979b) Identification of cytochrome P450, and its distribution in the membrana granulosa of the preovulatory follicle using quantitative cytochemistry. Endocrinology 103:310

Human Gonadotropins

B. Lunenfeld, E. Lunenfeld, V. Insler

Historical Perspective

The road from the first recognition of the physiological role of gonadotropic hormones to the development of preparations applicable for treatment of human infertility was long, difficult, and full of intellectual challenges and technical obstacles. In the mid 1920s Zondek and Smith independently but almost simultaneously discovered that gonadal function was controlled by the pituitary gland.

Zondek (1926) and Zondek and Ascheim (1927) demonstrated that implantation of anterior pituitary caused a rapid development of sexual organs in immature animals. At approximately the same time, Smith and his group showed that hypophysectomy resulted in a failure of sexual maturation in immature animals and in a rapid regression of sexual characteristics in adult animals (Smith 1926; Smith and Engle 1927).

During the 1930s and 1940s, gonadotropin extracts from various animal materials were prepared and applied for stimulation of ovarian function in human beings. It quickly became clear, however, that these preparations were of very limited clinical value because nonprimate gonadotropins produced a rapid immunological response in the human being, neutralizing their therapeutic effect (Zondek and Sulman 1942; Leethem and Rakoff 1948). This focused scientific and technological efforts on the extraction and purification of gonadotropins from human sources. During the years 1953–1955, Borth et al. (Borth et al. 1954, 1957) demonstrated that extracts from human menopausal urine stimulated spermatogenesis and folliculogenesis in rodents and speculated that these preparations might have important therapeutic applications. Thereafter, intensive research in this area was carried out simultaneously in Italy, England, Scotland, Germany, Switzerland, and Sweden. In the late 1950s and early 1960s these efforts were crowned by success. Gemzell and his co-workers reported the first successful induction of ovulation using human pituitary gonadotropin (hPG) in 1958 and the first pregnancy in 1960 (Gemzell et al. 1958, 1960). These results were confirmed by Bettendorf (Bettendorf et al. 1961).

Unfortunately, hPG preparation had to be withdrawn in the late 1980s because of the appearance of Creutzfeldt-Jacob disease (Cochius 1990; Dumble and Klein 1992). In 1960 Lunenfeld and his group (Lunenfeld et al. 1960; Lunenfeld 1963) reported follicular stimulation, ovulation, and pregnancies in anovulatory women using human menopausal gonadotropin (hMG). The hMG preparations avail-

Table 1. Milestones in developments leading to efficient treatment of female infertility

Year	Development
1926–1927	Discovery of the pituitary hormone controlling ovarian function
1955	Clinical use of urinary hormone assays (steroids and gonadotropins)
1959	Extraction and purification of gonadotropins from human pituitaries and menopausal urine
1961	Introduction of clomiphene citrate
1965	Wide-scale clinical use of gonadotropins and clomiphene
1968	First therapeutically oriented classification of anovulatory states
1970	Routine use of radioimmunoassays to estimate hormone levels
1971	Isolation, determination of structure, and laboratory synthesis of GnRH
1972	Introduction of prolactin assays
1973–1976	Reports on pregnancies induced by GnRH therapy
1974	Development of prolactin-inhibiting drugs
1978	Discovery of pulsatile nature of GnRH secretion
1979	Ultrasound imaging of ovarian follicles Introduction of pulsatile GnRH therapy Delivery of first "test-tube" baby
1982	Introduction of GnRH analogues for clinical use Introduction of purified FSH for ovulation-inducing therapy
1984	Routine clinical use of IVF-ET and GIFT programs
1985	Application of combined pituitary suppression/ovarian stimulation therapy to treat different types of fertility disturbances
1989	New therapeutically oriented classification of anovulatory states
1991	Trials of combined growth hormone/gonadotropin therapy in poor responders to ovulation induction
1993	Empirical introduction of micromanipulation procedures on gametes and zygotes
1994	Introduction of recombinant gonadotropins for clinical trials

able had only about 5% purity and contained both FSH and LH. However, since there was no alternative, they were accepted both by the regulatory agencies and the scientific community. Large-scale clinical studies were then undertaken at numerous centers throughout the world and their results reported in the literature. Of particular significance were the reports of Bettendorf (1963) and Gemzell (1964), who were able to induce ovulation and pregnancy in hypophysectomized women. The introduction of rapid and reliable hormonal assays, and later the availability of ultrasound scanners enabling visualization and measurement of ovarian follicles, made monitoring of gonadotropin therapy more accurate and objective and improved the results of treatment.

In the 1980s, the large-scale in vitro fertilization (IVF) programs used the principles developed for and the experience gained from induction of ovulation in anovulatory women and added important new insights to the understanding of the mechanism of controlled ovarian hyperstimulation (COH) induced by gonadotropins. Table 1 describes briefly the most important milestones along the tedious path from the discovery of the gonadotropic principle to controlled hyperstimulation as a unrivalled tool for the treatment of infertility.

Induction of ovulation with human gonadotropins has been an integral part of the routine work of many fertility clinics for more than 30 years. During this time, numerous reports describing in great detail all aspects of gonadotropin therapy have been published (Thompson and Hansen 1970; Insler and Lunenfeld 1974; Lunenfeld and Insler 1978; Brown 1986).

Experimental and clinical data obtained over the years also showed that FSH is capable of increasing recruitment of small antral follicles, of maintaining the normal development of multiple follicles to the preovulatory stage, and, consequently, of enlarging the yield of fertilizable eggs. These findings prompted the use of gonadotropins as the preferred treatment modality in most in vitro fertilization programs.

The use of gonadotropins for induction of superovulation in normally ovulating women necessitated conceptual changes in the monitoring schemes. The principal aim of inducing ovulation in anovulatory women is to attain the development of a single dominant follicle. This approach has been taken to achieve ovulation and pregnancy in many patients while preventing multiple follicular growth, multiple pregnancies, and hyperstimulation in most of them. In contrast, the concept of IVF, gamete intrafallopian transfer (GIFT), tubal embryo transfer (TET) or intracytoplasmic sperm injection (ICSI) programs is to use a super-physiological dose in order to obtain a large number of fertilizable eggs. For this purpose many different protocols have emerged, each with its own merits and disadvantages and all using ultrasonographic scanning to estimate both number and size of the growing follicles and estradiol assays to assess their functional integrity.

Human urinary follicle-stimulating hormone (FSH) as an alternative to hMG became commercially available in the late 1980s. It offers theoretical advantages over hMG when used in induction of ovulation, particularly in patients with polycystic ovarian disease (PCOD). Because PCOD is characterized by abnormally elevated serum LH levels, the use of purified FSH is attractive since it contains very little LH. During the past few years FSH has been used either in combination with hMG or as an alternative to hMG in many ovulation induction protocols and in assisted reproduction programs. Although many reports describing and comparing the clinical characteristics of ovulation induction with hMG and FSH have appeared in the literature, it is still not clear whether pure FSH is significantly more effective than hMG in inducing ovulation. However, there is consensus today that elevated levels of LH during the mid and late follicular phase may have adverse effects on fertilization and nidation, and it seems that preparations devoid of LH activity may increase live birth rates (Daya et al. 1994, personal communication). In the early 1990s a highly purified FSH preparation became available. This can be injected subcutaneously, can be self-administered, and has a higher safety profile in that it is practically devoid of urinary proteins, which contaminated the earlier hMG and FSH preparations by up to 95%. We are now witnessing the appearance of recombinant FSH, LH, and hCG preparations (rFSH, rLH, and rhCG) which will definitely replace urinary extracts in the near future.

In this chapter we will discuss the main principles of administering and monitoring gonadotropin treatment and summarize the results and complications of this therapy.

Chemistry, Pharmacokinetics, and Clearance

During the past 30 years, the major elements of the mechanism of action, control, and regulation of secretion of gonadotropins have been elucidated, and more recently, their structure has been determined. Gonadotropins are glycoproteins with molecular weights of around 30000 Daltons and contain about 20% carbohydrates. The carbohydrate moieties in their molecules are fucose, mannose, galactose, acetylglucosamine, and N-acetylneuraminic acid (Butt and Kennedy 1971). The sialic acid content varies widely among the glycoprotein hormones, from 20 residues in human chorionic gonadotropin (hCG) to five in FSH and only one or two in human luteinizing hormone (hLH). These differences are largely responsible for the variations in the isoelectric points of gonadotropins.

Different sialic acid content accounts for differences in the molecular weight of the hormones isolated from various sources and in differences in biological activity determined in in vivo assays. The higher the sialic acid content, the longer the biological half-life. Thus, the increased carbohydrate component in hCG is responsible for its significantly longer half-life than that of LH or FSH. Whereas the beta subunit of LH contains only one carbohydrate group, the beta subunit of hCG contains six. The function of the carbohydrates is not fully known, except for the fact that removal of the terminal neuraminic acid (sialic acid) residues drastically shortens the half-lives of the circulating hormones in blood. For this reason desialiated preparations of hLH, hCG, and hFSH show considerably reduced biological activity in vivo but retain activity in specific in vitro biological assays employing membrane receptors or isolated target cells. Measurement of these hormones by immunoassays or by the in vitro bioassay procedure therefore does not express their actual bioactivity in vivo. Deglycosylated hormones can act in vitro as competitive antagonists of the actions of the intact hormone upon the cyclic AMP production and, to a lesser extent, on steroid hormone biosynthesis.

The gonadotropic hormones consist of two hydrophobic noncovalently associated alpha and beta subunits. The three-dimensional structure of each subunit is maintained by internally cross-linked disulfide bonds. Gonadotropic hormones can be dissociated into the individual subunits by denaturing agents (De la Llosa and Jutisz 1969). The subunits are practically without biological activity, but the hormonal activity is regenerated by recombination of the subunits. All the gonadotropins, as well as thyroid-stimulating hormone (TSH) share a common alpha subunit of 92 amino acid residues in the same sequence, with five disulfide bonds and two carbohydrate moieties. The beta subunits (of FSH, LH, and hCG) are unique to each hormone and determine their biologic specificity. They have amino acid chains of varying length (116–147 amino acid residues) and contain six disulfide bonds.

There is only one known gene that codes for the beta chain of LH and one gene coding for each alpha and beta FSH subunit, while as many as six to eight genes or pseudogenes have been identified for the beta chain of chorionic gonadotropin (CG) (Talmadge et al. 1983). It is not known how many of these CG genes are translated.

Methods which allow analysis of the genes and gene products have shown that the two subunits of the gonadotropic hormones are translated from separate messenger RNAs (Fiddes and Goodman 1979), and both are synthesized as precursors. The nascent polypeptide alpha and beta subunits are then glycosylated in the Golgi apparatus by en bloc attachment of high mannose complex type oligosaccharides to two asparagine residues of each subunit (Fig. 1). Excess mannose and glucose residues are trimmed from the intermediates. Thereafter, the peripheral monosaccharides N-acetylglucosamine, galactose, and N-acetylneuraminic acid are attached sequentially to complete the oligosaccharide structures (Hussa 1980).

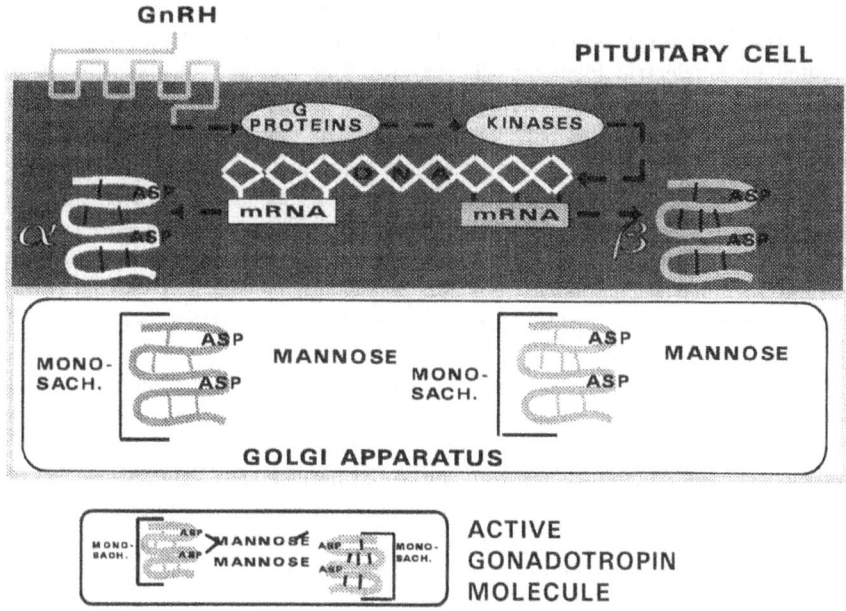

Fig. 1. Gonadotropin synthesis in the pituitary (gonadotrope) cell. A molecule of GnRH binds to a seven-arm membrane receptor and transmits a specific signal which initiates the function of G proteins, phospholipases, and kinases. Intracellular calcium ions are mobilized and calcium channels are opened to enable intake of extracellular calcium. Specific regions of the nuclear DNA of the pituitary cell are activated. Subsequently, mRNA specific for synthesis of the protein core of a- and β-subunits of gonadotropins is completed in the rough endoplasmic reticulum. The a-subunit of gonadotropins contains 92 amino acid residues with five disulfide bonds. The β-subunit (unique to FSH and LH) contains six disulfide bonds. The nascent polypeptide subunits are then transferred into the Golgi apparatus where en bloc attachment of high mannose complex-type oligosaccharide to two asparagine (*ASP*) residues is performed. Peripheral monosaccharides (*monosach.*) are then sequentially attached to complete the molecular structure. The integral FSH (LH) molecule is then stored in secretion granules until extruded by exocytosis

Table 2. Microheterogeneity of FSH: characteristics of basic and acidic isoforms[a]

	Basic isoform	Acidic isoform
Activity		
In vitro	High	Low
In vivo	Low	High[a]
Sialic acid content	Low	High
Clearance	Rapid	Slow
Half-life	Short	Long
Receptor binding	High	Low
Signal transduction	High	Low

[a] Gonadal steroids and GnRH affect pituitary neuraminidase and sialyltransferase activity to generate changes in isoforms.
[b] The overall in vivo bioactivity is higher due to its longer half-life and slower clearance.

It has been shown that both pituitary FSH and LH exist in several different forms (iso-hormones) which exhibit charge heterogeneity and may thus be separated by isoelectric focusing. The various FSH and LH species differ from one another not only in their isoelectric point but also in their relative abundance, receptor-binding activity, biological activity, and plasma half-life (Ulloa-Aguirre et al. 1988). Table 2 demonstrates schematically the different characteristics of acidic and basic isoforms of FSH. Cook et al. (1988) showed that also hMG consists of up to five different FSH iso-hormones and up to nine LH species. These differences may cause variations in patients' response, sometimes observed when several lots of the same preparation are used. These lot differences disappear when specific clones of highly purified FSH or rFSH, rLH, or rhCG are used.

FSH, a dimeric glycoprotein hormone composed of an alpha subunit (identical to the subunit of LH) and a beta subunit that confers biological specificity binds almost exclusively to the large N-terminal extracellular segment of a "seven-arm" transmembrane receptor on the granulosa cells. High-affinity binding requires a specifically charged amino acid in one of the peptide loops of the beta subunit (beta arg 35) (Flack et al. 1994).

Effective signal transduction requires a specific oligosaccharide in position 52 of the alpha chain (alpha 52; Flack et al. 1994), which induces granulosa cell multiplication and stimulates biochemical processes mediated through specific kinases and transcription factors. The LH receptor on thecal cells is also composed of a large N-terminal extracellular segment responsible for hormone binding and constituted of repeated leucine-rich motifs. It is followed by a segment spanning seven times the membrane, characteristic of G-protein coupling receptors, and by a short C-terminal domain (Milgrom 1993). LH binding to this receptor stimulates thecal cell development and androgen production.

Information regarding the metabolism of gonadotropic hormones is scarce. It has been shown that purified preparations of hFSH, hLH, and hCG injected intravenously into human subjects had serum half-lives (as determined by bioassays) of 180–240 min, 38–60 min, and 6–8 h, respectively. The half-life of the alpha and beta subunit of LH was found to be only 16 min. The higher carbohydrate content of hCG (10%) is responsible for its significantly longer half-life as compared with hFSH (5%) and hLH (2%).

Following intramuscular administration of Pergonal (containing FSH and LH derived from human menopausal urine) daily for 8 days and testing of blood levels twice a day, no increase in LH levels was observed. FSH, which has an intermediate half-life longer than that of LH but shorter than that of hCG, even when given in a low dose (150 IU), accumulated in the plasma and was still elevated above baseline level 3 days after the last injection (Diczfalusy and Harlin 1988). After i.m. administration of hCG, peak serum levels were observed at 6–8 h. The level of the hormone was reduced to about 50% after 36 h, and it was still discernible after 6 days. It is thus clear that hCG, when given as a substitution for LH, exerts a stronger and more prolonged biological effect due to its significantly longer half-life.

When hMG (150 IU FSH and 150 IU LH) was injected i.m. and FSH and LH were measured in serum at hourly intervals, it was demonstrated that hMG induced an increase of LH within 3 h that persisted for about another 5 h (Anderson et al. 1989). This increase, albeit short, could suffice to create an androgenic milieu which may impair follicular development.

Furthermore when pure FSH is administered, endogenous LH is inhibited and remains reduced for approximately 24 h (Anderson et al. 1989). This effect can be explained as follows: FSH stimulates production of inhibin, leading to a reduction of both endogenous FSH and endogenous LH. However, because only FSH is being administered exogenously, only the decrease in LH is apparent.

The mean metabolic clearance rate (MCR) of hFSH has been determined as 14 ml/min in women; it has not been determined in men. The MCR of hLH is 25–30 ml/min in women regardless of their ovulatory state and is almost 50% higher in normal men. The disappearance curves for both hormones are multiexponential, indicating a distribution of these hormones in more than three mathematical compartments. In premenopausal women daily production rates of hLH are 500–1000 IU with a marked preovulatory rise, whereas production rates in postmenopausal women are 3000–4000 IU/day. These values indicate that the pituitary content of hLH (and probably of hFSH) is turned over once or twice daily, and that rapid biosynthesis of gonadotropins is necessary to maintain the normal levels of pituitary storage and secretion. Only 3–10% of the daily production of FSH and LH is excreted in the urine in a biologically active form; nevertheless, this reflects the rate of gonadotropin secretion under physiologic and pathologic conditions. The recovery of exogenous gonadotropins in the urine of normal and infertile subjects is 10–20% of the administered hormone. Urinary excretion of gonadotropins accounts for only 5% of the MCR. The MCR of hMG in hypogonadotropic subjects is 0.4–1.7 ml/min.

Recent technological advances have made it possible to replace polyvalent antibodies with highly specific monoclonal antibodies. Previously, the production of "FSH (Metrodin)" was essentially a passive process, in which LH was separated from bulk material and the FSH, together with urinary proteins, was collected and lyophilized for use.

The "third-generation product" FSH HP results from a more direct process. In this procedure highly specific monoclonal antibodies selectively bind the FSH molecules in the hMG bulk material during their pass through the affinity column. The unbound urinary proteins pass through the column along with the LH and are removed. The column then contains pure FSH. This is extracted from the column as a highly purified product, devoid of both LH and contaminating urinary proteins. As a result of this improved processing, this FSH preparation (Metrodin HP) contains less than 0.1 IU of LH activity and less than 5% of unidentified urinary proteins. The specific activity of the FSH has been increased, from approximately 100–150 IU/mg of protein for "Metrodin" to about 9000 IU/mg protein for "Metrodin HP". The purity is also increased from 1–2% in Metrodin to 95% in Metrodin HP.

Due to its enhanced purity the total amount of injected proteins is very small, and Metrodin HP is therefore suitable for subcutaneous administration. Batch-to-batch variability is practically eliminated and the product lends itself to a detailed analysis by physicochemical methods in addition to the classical in vivo bioassay. This purified preparation also permits assessment of the pharmacodynamics and pharmacokinetics of FSH.

The technical developments which have led to the production of highly purified FSH (Metrodin HP) and to a deeper understanding of the pharmacodynamics and pharmacokinetics of these preparations have made it possible to redesign ovulation-inducing protocols (for example, low-dose regimens, low-dose increments, subcutaneous injection route). With the use of highly purified FSH preparation, it may be necessary to re-evaluate the role of estrogen as a marker of ovulation induction.

Now that highly purified urinary FSH preparations with about 9000 IU FSH/ mg protein) are available, we have to ask whether it is ethically admissible to continue using earlier preparations with 100–200 IU FSH/mg protein, containing 95% various urinary proteins.

Human pituitaries in the distant past and postmenopausal urine later on were the sole source for production of gonadotropin preparations. The detailed information regarding the physiological processes involved in the synthesis of gonadotropins by pituitary cells and development of recombinant DNA technology now make it possible to produce pharmacologically active FSH preparations in huge quantities.

The future of infertility therapy clearly relies on the capacity to produce pharmaceutical-grade gonadotropins in sufficient quantities to meet the ever increasing worldwide demand and to reduce the risk of biological contamination, small as it may be. Thus, the manufacture of gonadotropin compounds using recombinant technologies has become an important challenge for the treatment of infertility.

The production of recombinant gonadotropin molecules has proven to be difficult. Whereas bacteria efficiently synthesize nonglycosylated peptides such as insulin, and yeast has been cloned for the production of certain vaccines, prokaryotic cells are incapable of correctly glycosylating the peptide subunits to produce biologically active gonadotropins. The complex sugars are important for proper folding of the polypeptide backbone. The sites and extent of glycosylation determine tertiary structure, length of degradation time, the regions of the molecule exposed to target cell receptors, and exposure of the molecule to mechanisms that regulate metabolism in vivo. Recombinant glycosylated peptides may be synthesized by certain mammalian cell lines. Chinese hamster ovary cells are known to be suitable host cells for the production of glycosylated recombinant proteins. Such cell lines were chosen for the expression of recombinant human FSH and LH. The expression of human FSH dimer was achieved by transfecting Chinese hamster ovary cells with a genomic clone containing the complete FSH beta coding sequence together with the alpha subunit minigene. Stable cell lines expressing FSH dimer in relative abundance were selected. The resulting recombinant FSH was more homogeneous than the most purified pituitary FSH preparations, providing a basis for clinical use. Specific cell clones have now been selected for large-scale production of recombinant FSH. The resultant preparations are very pure and have a high biologic potency (>10000 IU/mg protein). r-hFSH is structurally identical to native pituitary hFSH, demonstrating a range of FSH isoforms similar to that found during the natural menstrual cycle. However, unlike u-hFSH, r-hFSH shows a low level of degradation and/or oxidation (typically less than 10% versus 30–40% for the former.

There have been numerous reports of ovulation induction followed by pregnancies when such recombinant FSH was used (Germond et al. 1992; Devroey et al. 1992, 1994; Homburg et al. 1994; Loumaye et al. 1994; Out et al. 1995). With recombinant DNA technology and highly defined cell culture techniques recombinant DNA gonadotropins are now being prepared on an industrial scale. What would currently require 30 million liters of urine per year can now be produced by genetically engineered cells in defined chemical-culture medium comprising only a small fraction of that volume. It is our hope that in the not too distant future DNA technology will provide an almost endless supply of human gonadotropins and totally replace urinary products.

Moreover, recombinant DNA technology permits the design of potential therapeutically active gonadotropin agonists and antagonists by altering key proteins and carbohydrate regions in the alpha and beta subunits of FSH and LH (Boime et al. 1990). FSH has a relatively short half-life and hCG a relatively long one.

The long half-life of hCG is due in part to the presence of four serine O-linked oligosaccharides attached to an extended hydrophilic carboxy terminus. Using site-directed mutagenesis and gene transfer techniques, it was possible to fuse the carboxy terminal extension of hCG beta (CTP) to the 3' end of the FSH coding sequence. The FSH-CTP fusion protein retained the same biologic activity as native FSH in vivo but had a prolonged circulating half-life. This resulted in a significantly higher in vivo potency than that of native FSH and may make the fusion product an obvious candidate for a long-acting FSH agonist (Fares et al. 1992).

Alternatively, deglycosylated mutants of this chimera can be engineered and, together with deglycosylated alpha subunit, could, by competitive binding to gonadotropin receptors, result in potent gonadotropin antagonists (Boime et al. 1990).

Better understanding of gonadotropin-receptor interaction combined with crystallography and sophisticated computer techniques will make it possible to design proteinomimetic, orally active gonadotropin agonists and antagonists. The current challenge in biotechnology is to reduce the size of these proteins by developing small, functional, mimetic synthetic molecules that can be administered through the oral or transdermal route.

To achieve this objective for gonadotropins one must develop (a) a working model to explain how gonadotropin activates its receptor, as well as (b) a high throughput assay specific for each gonadotropin, and (c) create a large number of molecules with possible agonistic or antagonistic activity to be tested.

Advances in the field of molecular reproductive endocrinology and the development of a number of molecular tools permitted the identification of low-molecular-weight FSH agonistic molecules that were able to interact with a catalytic region of the FSH receptor that controls G protein coupling and adenylate cyclase activation. With better understanding of FSH receptor activation it was possible to create small molecules predicted to induce gonadotropic signal transduction without the necessity to bind to the extracellular domains of the membrane protein. A number of such molecules are already being actively tested. Such molecules will ultimately be converted into high-potency, orally active therapeutic preparations to replace the dimeric glycoprotein hormones or to act as antagonists.

Classification of Patients

Gonadotropin treatment is primarily a substitution therapy and as such should be applied to patients lacking appropriate gonadotropin stimulation but having target organs (gonads) capable of normal response. In 1968, Insler et al. proposed a simple treatment-oriented classification of patients selected for gonadotropin therapy. This classification was modified and adopted by the WHO Scientific Group (World Health Organization, Technical Report Series, No. 514, 1976) and is still used in many centers today.

According to this classification, gonadotropin treatment is applied to two main groups of women:
- Group I: Hypothalamic-pituitary failure - amenorrheic women with no evidence of endogenous estrogen production, nonelevated prolactin levels, usually low FSH levels, and no detectable space-occupying lesion in the hypothalamic-pituitary region
- Group II: Hypothalamic-pituitary dysfunction - women with a variety of menstrual cycle disturbances including amenorrhea, with evidence of endogenous estrogen production, and normal levels of prolactin and FSH
  Patients with PCOD represent a distinctive variant of group II, both because of the possible difference in the underlying pathophysiological mechanism(s) of the disease and because of some differences in response to ovarian stimulation. In group II, gonadotropins are usually applied after other types of ovulation-inducing therapy have failed. It is theoretically plausible and clinically prov-

en that the results of gonadotropin treatment are significantly better in group I than in group II (Insler and Lunenfeld 1977). Amenorrheic women of group I, however, represent only a small and ever-diminishing proportion of the infertility clinic population (Bettendorf et al. 1981).

In recent years another, steadily growing group of patients has been treated with human gonadotropins – women undergoing in vitro fertilization or intrauterine insemination (IUI) combined with ovarian stimulation. Obviously, these patients differ from both group I and group II in having completely normal hormone levels and competent hypothalamic-pituitary-ovarian feedback mechanisms.

The general principles of gonadotropin therapy applied to the above-mentioned three groups of patients are similar, but the intensity of stimulation, course of treatment, and hormonal patterns differ significantly. It may thus be summarized that, at present, four modes of gonadotropin treatment are used:
– Substitution therapy – for patients of group I
– Stimulation therapy – given to patients of group II
– Regulation therapy – employed for women with PCOD
– Hyperstimulation therapy – used in IVF, GIFT, TET, ICSI, and IUI
  Each of the above therapeutic schemes may be used in conjunction with additional pharmaceutical agents to enhance the effect of gonadotropins or attenuate disturbing influences stemming from the ovary, the pituitary, the adrenal glands, or other sources. The combined therapies will be discussed in another section of this chapter.

Theoretical Basis and Clinical Goals of Gonadotropin Therapy

The comprehensive basis of gonadotropin therapy is, of course, the knowledge of the physiology of the reproductive ovulatory cycle. A detailed discussion of the principles of ovarian response to exogenous stimulation must, however, be focused on the events taking place in the ovary itself.

The experimental work of Hodgen and his group on primates (Goodman et al. 1977, Hodgen 1983), the introduction of sonography for monitoring follicular size, and the IVF programs allowing for observation of the size and appearance of ovarian follicles concomitant with the appreciation of the maturity of ova all established a firm core of data concerning the sequence of ovarian changes leading to ovulation.

Recruitment

About 3 months prior to ovulation, 30–300 follicles are recruited for growth and development. This initial recruitment of follicles and the early replication of granulosa cells is gonadotropin independent. Gougeon (1986) determined that in the human being, the progress from primordial to graafian follicle takes at least 10 weeks.

Rescue

Rescue of a follicular cohort is brought about by a slight but significant FSH rise observed during the preceding late luteal phase. This process is completed by the third day of the cycle.

Selection

Selection of the dominant follicle is a process by which one follicle of the cohort is endowed with the ability to mature earlier and/or more quickly than all others. The mechanism of the selection process is controlled by autocrine, paracrine, and endocrine factors. Important elements in this process are inhibin and activin. Baird (1987) stated that "the follicle of the month" is selected by chance because it is at the right place at the right time. Our experimental work in the rat indicated that the "assignment" of the follicle to be selected as the dominant one in the subsequent cycles is instigated by the rescuing action of the mid-cycle FSH peak in three consecutive previous cycles (Insler et al. 1990). The process of selection of the dominant follicle is completed by the seventh cycle day.

Dominance

Dominance is that part of the cycle when all the events such as the exponential rise of estrogen, negative feedback action upon the hypothalamus, modulation of pituitary secretion of gonadotropins, reduction of FSH secretion by inhibin, and positive feedback evoking the mid-cycle LH surge are subordinated to the developmental rhythm of the dominant follicle. This controlling action of the dominant follicle lasts from the eighth cycle day until ovulation and persists also during the corpus luteum phase (Fig. 2a–d).

The basic principles of gonadotropin therapy were proposed by Insler and Lunenfeld (1974, 1977) following observation of the course of treatment in several hundreds of patients. Ovarian response can be elicited only when a certain dose of FSH-like material has been administered. This amount of gonadotropin is called the "effective daily dose" (threshold principle): Administration of gonadotropins at levels significantly below the effective daily dose does not evoke any measurable effect even when therapy is prolonged.

Following the administration of the effective daily dose of gonadotropins a number of ovarian follicles are stimulated to begin growth and maturation. This period of gonadotropin therapy is called the "clinical latent phase". Since at this stage of follicular development appreciable amounts of estrogen are not yet secreted, the latent phase of therapy is clinically "mute". The latent phase begins with the administration of the effective daily dose of gonadotropins and ends with the appearance of measurable ovarian response, i.e., rising estrogen levels and increasing follicular diameter.

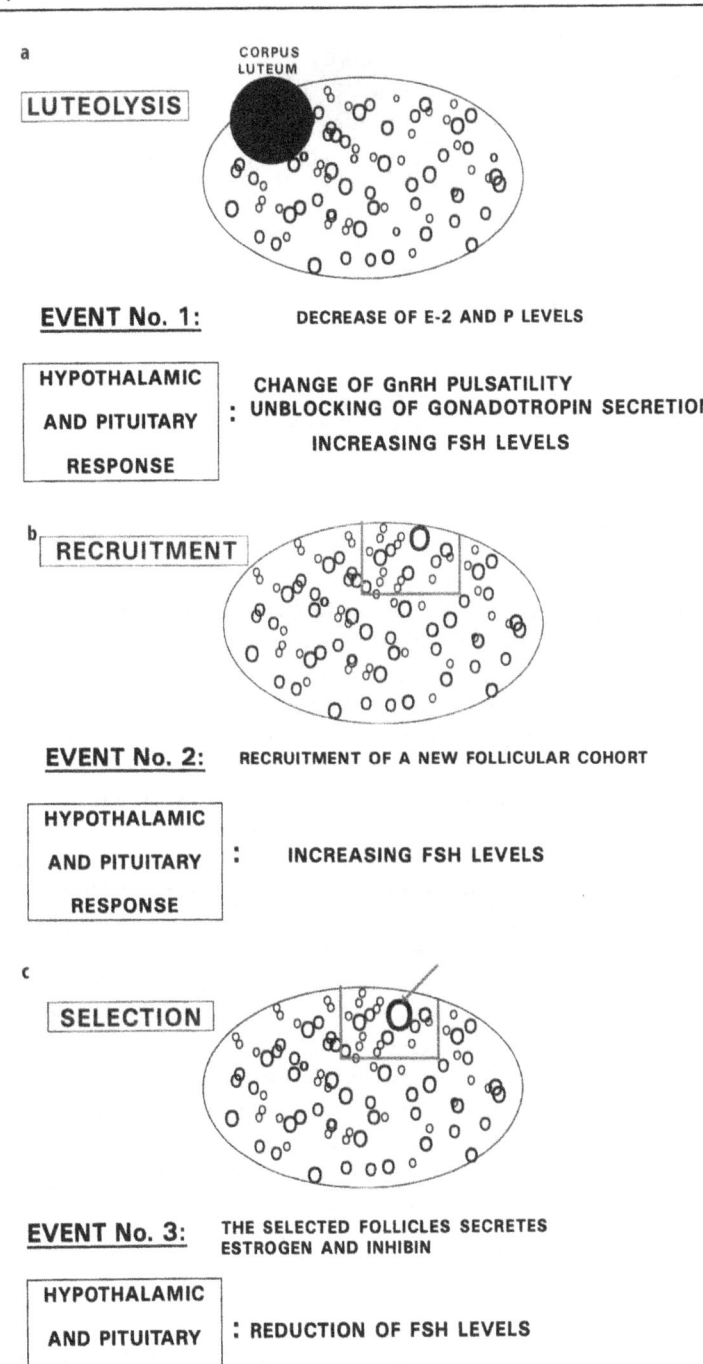

a

CORPUS
LUTEUM

LUTEOLYSIS

EVENT No. 1:   DECREASE OF E-2 AND P LEVELS

HYPOTHALAMIC   CHANGE OF GnRH PULSATILITY
AND PITUITARY   : UNBLOCKING OF GONADOTROPIN SECRETION
RESPONSE   INCREASING FSH LEVELS

b RECRUITMENT

EVENT No. 2:   RECRUITMENT OF A NEW FOLLICULAR COHORT

HYPOTHALAMIC
AND PITUITARY   :   INCREASING FSH LEVELS
RESPONSE

c

SELECTION

EVENT No. 3:   THE SELECTED FOLLICLES SECRETES
                ESTROGEN AND INHIBIN

HYPOTHALAMIC
AND PITUITARY   : REDUCTION OF FSH LEVELS
RESPONSE

Fig. 2a–d. The sequence of events in the ovary during a normal ovulatory cycle. a Luteoly-sis, b recruitment, c selection, d dominance

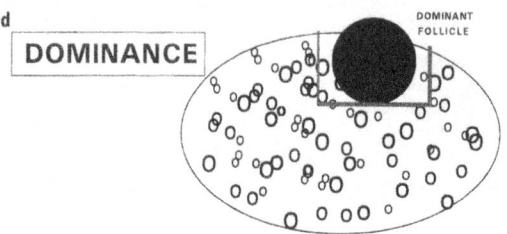

EVENT No. 4:   DOMINANT FOLLICLE AND OVUM MATURATION
PARACRINE BLOCKING OF SURROUNDING FOLLICLES

HYPOTHALAMIC

AND PITUITARY   :

RESPONSE

GnRH PULSATILITY AND GONADOTROPIN
SECRETION CONTROLLED
BY THE DOMINANT FOLLICLE

Fig. 2 d.

The second part of gonadotropin therapy, called the "active phase", lasts from the initial estrogen rise until ovulation induction. It is characterized by an exponential rise of estrogen levels and a steady increase in follicular diameter. The latent phase lasts 3–7 days and is significantly longer in patients of group I than in women of group II. The active phase lasts 4–6 days and is similar in all patients.

The above principles, based on clinical observation and thorough analysis of patients' response, actually preceded by several years the theoretical considerations of the physiological events produced by experimental work (see above). The latent phase of gonadotropin therapy represents a "telescoped" version of the rescue and selection phases of the spontaneous cycle. The active phase of therapy corresponds to the period of dominance.

The question of differences of response observed in patients of group I as compared with those of group II must now be briefly addressed. It is well known that in patients of group II the effective daily dose is smaller, the latent phase shorter, and the response to treatment less uniform (Insler and Lunenfeld 1977). It seems that these differences in response to stimulation with exogenous gonadotropins may be explained by the state of the ovary at the beginning of treatment. This is probably due to a particular endogenous gonadotropin stimulation and an individual ovarian response.

In women of group I, at the initiation of each treatment course the ovaries contain small preantral gonadotropin-independent follicles at different stages of development and degeneration. The pharmacologic dose of gonadotropins administered acts on a relatively uniform substrate. Not so in patients of group II; in this group endogenous gonadotropins may cause a certain follicular development before or between treatments. Gonadotropin therapy is thus administered to an ovary already containing scores of follicles at various stages of development, provoking further growth of some of them and recruitment of additional ones, and possibly preventing atresia of others. It is no wonder that the response to treatment is less uniform and more prone to hyperstimulation.

Gonadotropin therapy poses several interesting theoretical problems. The exact size of the follicular cohort rescued in each cycle in the woman is variable. Whatever the size of the initial cohort recruited, it seems that during the course of gonadotropin therapy more follicles are rescued from atresia and stimulated to undergo partial or full maturation by a sustained high level of FSH. This process results in the development of several dominant follicles that reach full maturation hours or maybe even days apart from one another.

As indicated by the very low efficiency of single-dose or "trigger" schemes to ensure follicular maturation during gonadotropin therapy, the FSH concentration must be sustained above threshold levels throughout the treatment. Despite the rather high levels of estrogen occurring relatively early in the treatment, premature LH surges are rather rare (Garcia et al. 1983) in patients with hypothalamic-pituitary failure. In women with hypothalamic-pituitary dysfunction or PCOD, or in spontaneous ovulators undergoing superovulation therapy, the premature luteinization episodes are much more frequent, however (Fleming and Coutts 1990). The exact role of the gonadotropin surge-attenuating factor (GnSAF) produced by follicles of certain size in spontaneous and stimulated cycles (Sopelak and Hodgen 1984) has yet to be established.

When human gonadotropins are used for induction of ovulation, it must be accepted that some features of the spontaneous ovulatory cycle cannot be manipulated in gonadotropin-induced cycles. These features are:

• Early gonadotropin-independent follicular development
• Premenstrual recruitment and initial selection of follicles
• Feedback control of gonadotropin levels
• Balanced effect of intraovarian sex steroids and growth factors and their binding proteins
• Full maturation of one follicle only
• Exact synchronization of structural functional and hormonal events throughout the entire genital system.

The ideal rationale for gonadotropin treatment of anovulatory patients is to provide gonadotropin levels of magnitude and timing similar to those observed in a normal ovulatory cycle and, consequently, to evoke recruitment of a follicular cohort, selection and full maturation of at least one dominant follicle, ovulation, and sustained corpus luteum function. Unfortunately, this goal has never been fully achieved. The FSH and LH levels and their ratios during gonadotropin-stimulated cycles are quite different from normal (Wu 1977, Healy and Burger 1983). Estrogen levels and their daily rate of ascent as well as progesterone values are not identical to those observed in spontaneous cycles (Insler and Potashnik 1983). The follicular fluid levels of estradiol and progesterone are lower and the level of inhibin is higher in gonadotropin-stimulated cycles than in the dominant follicle of the natural cycle (Seegar-Jones et al. 1985).

Moreover, the pregnancy rate in gonadotropin-induced cycles with steroid profiles closely resembling those found in spontaneous ovulations is dismally low

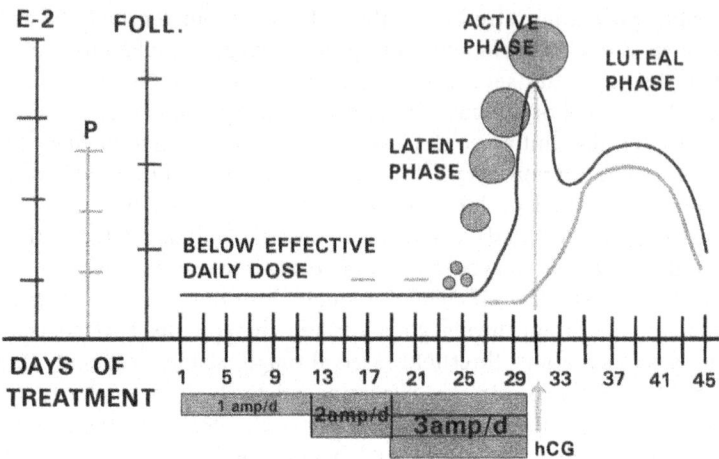

Fig. 3. Principles of gonadotropic therapy. Recruitment of a gonadotropin-dependent follicular cohort and initiation of follicular growth require that the amount of FSH at the ovarian plane reach a threshold level (effective daily dose). Following latent phase, which is clinically "mute", ovarian follicles continue an exponential growth accompanied by a corresponding increase in estrogen secretion (active phase lasting 4–5 days)

(Insler and Lunenfeld 1977). Thus, the theoretical rationale for gonadotropin therapy must be subordinated to its clinical aim, which is to obtain ovulation and pregnancy in all suitable cases while avoiding hyperstimulation (Fig. 3).

Large-scale clinical experience indicates that this goal can be practically achieved. The unequivocal proof of the clinical efficiency of gonadotropin therapy is the thousands of babies born following gonadotropin-induced ovulation and conception.

Treatment Schemes

A whole array of treatment schemes for gonadotropin therapy have been proposed and employed over the years. There are, however, only three essentially different types of therapy:
1. Fixed-dose regimes
2. Individually adjusted schemes
3. Combined therapy.

When clinical trials began, two types of gonadotropin preparations were used: human pituitary gonadotropins (hPG) and human menopausal gonadotropins (hMG). Due to the scarcity of human pituitaries and the appearance of Creutzfeldt-Jacob disease (Cochius et al. 1990, Dumble and Klein 1992) HPG preparations were abandoned, and since the late 1970s mainly hMG preparations have been employed. In the 1980s an FSH preparation containing a negligible amount of LH was introduced.

This preparation was used for the same indications as hMG and has also been proposed as the treatment of choice for patients with PCOD (Johnson and Pearce 1990). All these preparations were only partially purified (3%–5%) and contained 95% of various urinary proteins. Since the early 1990s highly purified FSH preparations either from urine or using recombinant technology have become available and have replaced the older ones, due mainly to increased safety, batch-to-batch consistency, and the possibility of self-administration.

In the fixed-dose regimens, a certain amount of hMG (or FSH) is administered on predetermined cycle days, followed by hCG given one or more days after the last injection of hMG. Although the dosages of gonadotropins and the days on which it was administered differed in various reports (Butler 1970, Crooke 1970, Marshall and Jacobson 1970), the general principle was identical. By using a fixed dose in each cycle, the patient's gonadotropin requirement (i.e., the effective daily dose) could be met only by successively increasing the dose in consecutive cycles.

The individually adjusted treatment scheme (Rabau et al. 1971) allows for successive increments of the gonadotropin dose according to the patient's response during the same cycle. It actually combines the tests courses with the treatment course in one cycle, thus significantly increasing the efficiency of treatment (mean number of treatment courses per pregnancy). In some particularly sensitive cases, the individually adjusted treatment may sometimes, by reducing the daily dose, avoid hyperstimulation which would have been brought about by using the fixed-dose schedule.

The size of the initial dose of hMG (or FSH) and of its increments, as well as the ideal estrogen level to be arrived at before commencing with the administration of hCG, is still a matter of discussion. We usually start with two ampules of hMG (150 IU) per day in patients of group I and with one ampule in women belonging to group II. The successive dose increments are usually one ampule each, and hCG is administered when urinary estrogen reaches a level of 75–300 μg/24 h or plasma estradiol attains a level of 300–1200 pg/ml, and when at least one follicle with a diameter exceeding 16 mm is observed on ultrasonography. In women with high ovarian sensitivity to stimulation (PCOD) successive dose increments of half an ampule (25–35 IU) are often used.

It is interesting to note that with the advent of IVF programs, the whole circle of trial and error regarding the safest and most efficient treatment schemes of hMG (or FSH) was repeated. Different groups proposed fixed-dose schedules not much different from those which had been tried and discarded years earlier. Recently, however, more and more groups seem to have adopted the individually adjusted treatment scheme, using some modifications suitable for the special purposes of an IVF program (Quigley 1985, Lopata et al. 1986). For the sake of completeness, one additional mode of ovulation induction using human gonadotropins should be mentioned here. In 1983 Kemmann et al. described their initial experience with a portable infusion pump delivering subcutaneously a constant amount of hMG over a period of 18 h/day. The authors claimed that a better response was obtained with this method of delivery than with the standard i.m. injection of hMG. This treatment modality did not receive widespread acceptance, but with the new, highly purified FSH preparations which, according to prescriber information, can be administered subcutaneously, this therapeutic modality could be reinvestigated.

Combined Therapy

In the past, most IVF programs used a combination of clomiphene citrate and hMG to stimulate a crop of follicles large enough and ready for ovum pick-up. The claim was that this combination produced better, or at least more uniform, ovum maturation than hMG alone. In addition, the clomiphene/gonadotropin combination required smaller hMG doses, thus reducing the cost of treatment. This mode of treatment is being abandoned due to the long half-life of clomiphene citrate, the high incidence of untimely LH surges, the relatively low pregnancy rate, and the relatively high abortion rate.

It is well known that patients of group I respond better to gonadotropin therapy than women of group II. The efficiency of treatment (mean number of treatment courses per pregnancy) and the pregnancy rate are significantly better in the former group as compared with the latter (Lunenfeld and Insler 1978).

Some of the reasons for this discrepancy are obvious. First, patients of group II receive gonadotropin therapy only after they have failed to conceive when treated with other ovulation-inducing drugs. Second, the frequency of additional disturbances possibly affecting fertility, such as endometriosis and polycystic ovaries, are much more frequent in group II.

There are, however, differences in response to stimulation between patients of group I and those of group II which seem to be inherent to the functional characteristics of the hypothalamic-pituitary-ovarian axis. In other words, with regard to gonadotropin therapy, the presence of a functioning pituitary gland may be a disadvantage rather than an asset. Even with the best protocols for inducing ovulation in anovulatory patients and superovulation in in vitro procedures, a number of patients may not ovulate. Of those who do, some produce poorly fertilizable eggs and in others poor implantation may be observed. It is conceivable that inappropriate endogenous LH secretion may be the dominant cause of failure in the majority of patients belonging to group II. This disturbance may appear in two main forms: (a) elevated LH levels during the follicular phase and (b) ill-timed LH surges.

The Effects of Excessive LH in the Follicular Phase

It has been suggested that a high concentration of LH through the follicular phase causes early maturation of the developing oocyte, producing at ovulation an egg that is physiologically aged (Homburg et al. 1988a). These oocytes are unlikely to be fertilized or, if conception is achieved, may fail to implant, or an early abortion may result. Several authors have reported that in IVF programs high concentrations of LH in the few days before oocytes were collected were associated with reduced rates of fertilization and conception (Stanger and Yovitch 1985, Howles et al. 1987, Punnonen et al. 1988, McFaul et al. 1989). McFaul et al. (1989) and Mcnamee (1990) also demonstrated that if conception is achieved in a cycle in which the oocyte is prematurely exposed to elevated LH there is a significantly higher probability that an early abortion will result. This situation is particularly frequent in patients diagnosed with PCOD, where ovulation rates following ovulation induction are relatively high but the live birth rate is low.

Johnson and Pearce (1990) support this concept and conclude that pituitary suppression by GnRH analogues before induction of ovulation (reducing LH levels) reduces the risk of spontaneous abortion in women with PCOD and primary recurrent spontaneous abortion following induction of ovulation. Spontaneous abortion occurred in 11 of 20 women given clomiphene citrate, compared with only two of 20 who had pituitary suppression with buserelin followed by administration of pure FSH. It may be argued that the negative effects suspected to be due to LH may in fact be due to an ovarian disorder which also causes elevated LH levels. This was tested in a study in which patients with normally appearing ovaries (at ultrasonography) and a normal FSH/LH ratio were given clomiphene citrate (Shoham et al. 1990). This study demonstrated that the adverse effect of an excess of LH in mid and late follicular phase can also be observed when an attempt is made to induce ovulation with clomiphene citrate (CC). When FSH and LH are measured in anovulatory women with no detectable features of PCOD who are undergoing ovulation induction with CC, two hormonal patterns can be seen. One group exhibits an excessive LH secretion and in the second group the LH/FSH ratio never exceeds 1.7. Not a single clinical pregnancy occurred in the group of women with an excessive LH response. Furthermore, the estrogen secretion pattern in this group was reminiscent of that seen in PCOD patients. All the pregnancies occurred in the group of patients who did not exhibit an excessive LH response. These observations indicate that also an iatrogenically induced excess of LH in mid and late follicular phase can adversely affect the outcome of the treatment cycle. In addition, this study indicates that determination of FSH and LH 1 or 2 days following termination of CC administration may help to select patients either for continuation of CC therapy or (those with excessive LH) for FSH therapy.

The Effects of an Untimely LH Surge

Premature luteinization is a specific category of anovulation. This entity is frequently unrecognized, or it is misdiagnosed as unexplained infertility or luteal phase defect.

This situation can occur if an untimely LH surge ensues in response to rising estrogen at a time when the follicle is still immature. It can be diagnosed if an LH peak is detected in the presence of relatively small (< 14 mm) follicles demonstrated by ultrasonography.

It is possible that the etiology of this entity is an exaggerated sensitivity of the pituitary to estrogen. Rising, but relatively low, estradiol (E-2) levels may trigger an LH surge. This could explain the failure of clomiphene citrate or hMG to restore ovulation in such cases. Both agents cause multiple follicular development with an exaggerated estrogen rise, making the appearance of a premature LH peak even more likely.

A similar situation exists in ovulatory women with a normal pituitary-ovarian axis undergoing IVF, GIFT, ZIFT, IUI, or AID procedures. They receive pharmacological doses of hMG (FSH) to induce superovulation. The exaggerated estradiol levels in response to this therapy provoke, in about 15% of treatment cycles, an untimely spontaneous LH surge, leading to cancellation of ovum pick-up or of the insemination procedure.

To overcome the possible interference of unbalanced and/or untimely endogenous gonadotropin secretion, combined therapy using agents suppressing hypothalamic-pituitary function together with a purified FSH preparation was recommended. Ben-Nun et al. (1984) generated pharmacological (drug-induced) hyperprolactinemia, causing a significant reduction of secretion and/or release of endogenous gonadotropins, and then stimulated the ovaries with exogenous hMG. They claimed that with this type of combined treatment, ovulation and pregnancy were obtained in several patients of group II who had previously failed to conceive when treated with hMG/hCG alone.

Laboratory synthesis of potent and/or long-acting analogues of gonadotropin-releasing hormone (GnRHa) makes it possible to efficiently reduce (downregulate) the production and release of pituitary gonadotropins (Crawley et al. 1982, Meldrum et al. 1982, Yen 1983). Treatment schemes combining pituitary suppression by GnRH analogues with ovarian stimulation by exogenous gonadotropins therefore seemed particularly attractive (Fleming et al. 1985, Shadmi et al. 1987, Insler et al. 1989).

Several different protocols for the combined GnRHa and gonadotropins have been proposed. In the "short" (Fig. 4) or "ultrashort" protocols the GnRHa is administered either together with gonadotropins or only a few days before the first gonadotropin dose and continued until indicated. This makes it possible to utilize the initial "flare-up" effect of the analogue, i.e., elevation of endogenous gonadotropin secretion. The treatment is shorter and the cost is lower, since fewer gonadotropins are required. On the other hand, the initial relatively high LH levels (particularly in women with PCOD) may create a hormonal environment unfavorable to follicular development.

The long protocols are based on the concept that ovarian stimulation should begin only after the pituitary gland has been adequately suppressed by an GnRH agonist. This effect can be achieved in the majority of cases within 14–21 days, depending on the type of GnRHa and the patient's response.

Two main types of long protocols are used. In one, GnRH agonists are started in the mid luteal phase and gonadotropins (hMG or FSH) are added after 10–14 days (Fig. 5). It is claimed that this protocol is preferable, since in the hormonal environment of the luteal phase (relatively high estrogens and progesterone) the initial stimulatory effect of the agonist is attenuated and thus

Fig. 4. The short protocol of combined GnRH analogue/gonadotropin therapy. GnRHa is administered together with gonadotropins and continued until indicated. This enables use of the initial "flare-up" effect of the analogue. When FSH reaches the threshold level follicular development is initiated. *Broken line*, estradiol levels

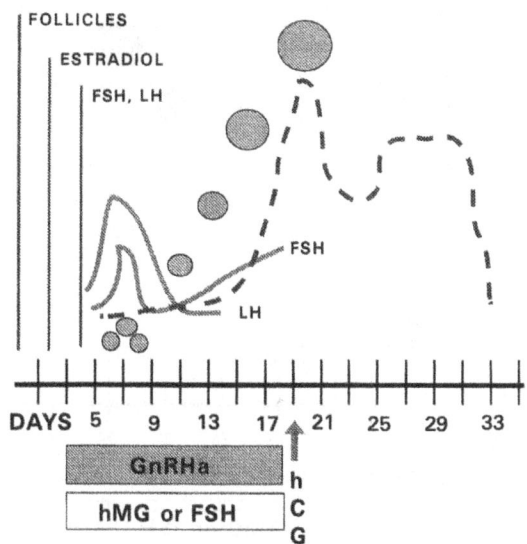

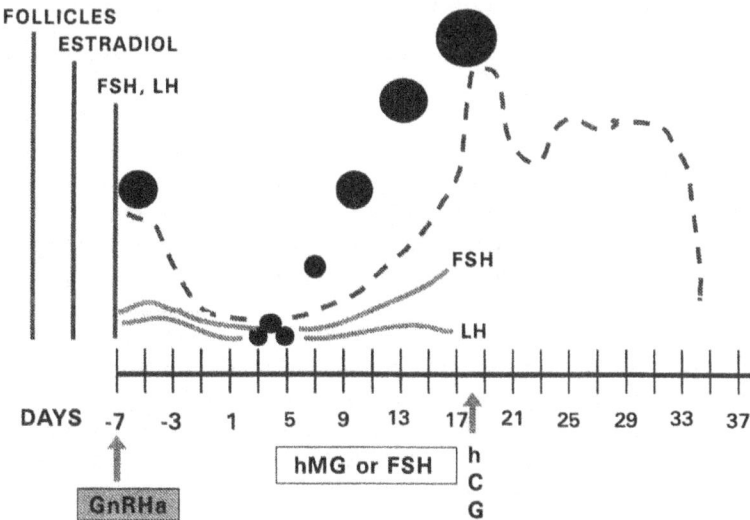

Fig. 5. The long (luteal phase) protocol of combined GnRH analogue/gonadotropin therapy. GnRH agonists are started in the mid luteal phase and gonadotropins (hMG or FSH) are added after 10–14 days. The initial stimulatory effect of the agonist is attenuated and thus the LH levels and, consequently, androgen production are diminished. Following exogenous FSH administration the FSH level rises, while LH levels remain suppressed. When FSH reaches the threshold level follicular development is initiated. *Broken line*, estradiol levels

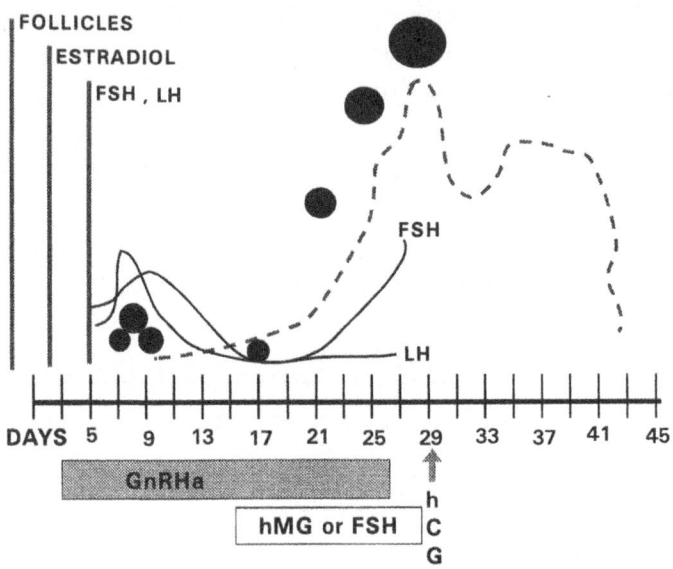

Fig. 6. The long protocol of combined GnRH analogue/gonadotropin therapy. After initial flare-up of gonadotropin levels both FSH and LH are suppressed, Following exogenous FSH administration the FSH level rises while LH levels remain suppressed. When FSH reaches the threshold level follicular development is initiated. *Broken line*, estradiol levels

the LH levels and, consequently, androgen production are diminished. The major problem with this protocol is the possibility of inadvertent administration of GnRHa to patients with early pregnancy. From preliminary data on 139 patients who inadvertently received GnRH-A during early pregnancy, it appears that no adverse affects upon pregnancy in the blastocyst or early nidation stage were noted (Roux et al. 1993).

In the second long protocol (Fig. 6) the GnRHa is started on the first days of menstruation and gonadotropin stimulation is begun when pituitary and ovarian function are suppressed, as indicated by low FSH and LH levels and/or by E-2 values below 50 pg/ml and/or lack of presence of antral follicles (with diameter exceeding 4 mm) on a sonographic ovarian scan. FSH/hMG administration in conjunction with the agonist is continued until at least one follicle reaches maturation, as judged by ultrasonography and estrogen levels. hCG is then administered to induce ovulation.

With either version of the long protocol of combined GnRHa/gonadotropin therapy premature endogenous LH peaks are rare (in less than 1% of cycles). The gonadotropin dosage necessary for ovulation or superovulation induction and the duration of treatment are significantly increased, however.

Both variants of the long protocol have already proven their merits. By simplifying logistics and by significantly reducing cancellation rates in IVF programs, the overall success rate has been increased. The combined therapy allows the design of stimulation protocols creating a predominantly FSH environment during the recruitment phase and eliminating the interference of endogenous gonadotropins during the dominance and periovulatory phase. However, the temporary functional gonadotropin-specific hypophysectomy has introduced new challenges. Inhibition of endogenous gonadotropins following ovulation induced by hCG may, if not properly monitored, result in an inadequate luteal phase. This situation can usually be prevented by postovulatory periodic administration of hCG (Blumenfeld and Nahhas 1988).

The choice of the GnRH analogue to be used should be based on a combination of factors including its delivery system, its mode of administration, and its biological half-life. All of the criteria above must be considered in designing a subsequent gonadotropin treatment protocol competent to stimulate follicular recruitment and development, timely ovulation induction, and adequate corpus luteum function.

Third-generation GnRH antagonists are already on the market. Due to their high affinity for the GnRH receptors, these compounds lead to a suppression of gonadotropin secretion within hours. They act through competitive binding, and the duration of their effect is dose dependent. Their immediate inhibition of gonadotropins without the flare-up effect may have a profound influence on their use in ovulation induction and assisted reproduction procedures.

They can be administered either daily for several days during the late follicular phase (usually from day 6 of stimulation onwards), i.e., the "multiple-dose protocol (Diedrich and Felberbaum 1998), or just at the moment when the LH surge is expected, i.e., the "single-dose protocol" (Oliviennes et al. 1997). Since GnRH antagonists cause a quicker and better-controlled pituitary (and ovarian) suppression they may be administered later during the treatment and for a shorter period of time. This will mean a reduction in the stimulatory dose of gonadotropins, thus lowering the cost of superovulation induction.

Combined Growth Hormone/Gonadotropin Therapy

Even with the best protocols for inducing ovulation in anovulatory patients or with superovulation for in vitro procedures, some patients require excessive amounts of gonadotropins and some remain "poor" responders despite the administration of extremely high doses.

During the past few years the importance of intraovarian regulation via the potentiating effects of growth hormone-releasing hormone, growth hormone, growth factors, and insulin on both the thecal cell response to LH and the granulosa cell response to FSH has been demonstrated (Adashi et al. 1985a–c, 1990, Jia et al. 1986, Davoren and Hsueh 1986, Ericson et al. 1989), as have the highly complex interactions of IGFs and their binding proteins on the modulation of gonadotropin action on follicular development (Lunenfeld and Insler 1993, Lunenfeld 1994, Costrici et al. 1994, Nakatani et al. 1991). These findings may have a significant impact on the understanding of ovulatory disorders such as the polycystic ovarian syndrome, or on ovulation-inducing therapy and its main complication, the ovarian hyperstimulation syndrome. Publications by

Homburg et al. (1988b) and Volpe et al. (1989) presented the claim that GH added to hMG protocols significantly reduced the hMG dose necessary for follicular stimulation.

However, Ronnberg et al. (1990) were unable to confirm these findings in a study of ovulatory patients undergoing a randomized stimulation protocol for in vitro fertilization. Based on our past and present studies, we believe that we can reconcile the discrepancy between these publications. We have shown that some patients with decreased levels of GH (Blumenfeld and Lunenfeld 1989) or anovulatory, normoprolactinemic, non-PCOD patients who are "poor responders" to gonadotropin stimulation and have a decreased level of GH reserve (Menashe et al. 1990a,b) may benefit from the addition of GH to gonadotropin stimulation protocols. The results of a prospective study on ovulation induction demonstrated that patients who responded to clonidine or to arginine with elevation of GH also responded normally to hMG therapy with a mean effective dose of 1.5 ampules/day (11.6 mean total dose), and patients who did not respond to clonidine with elevation of GH either needed excessive amounts of gonadotropins (mean effective dose of 3 ampules/day or a mean total dose of 36.5 ampules) to obtain an acceptable response or, despite higher doses of hMG, responded inadequately as expressed by either low serum estradiol levels or lack of sufficient follicular development, or both. The combined administration of GH and hMG to clonidine-negative patients resulted in a good ovarian response despite a significantly lower dose of hMG. In patients who responded to clonidine, arginine, or insulin with an elevation of GH (positive growth hormone reserve), the addition of GH had no significant effect on response or hMG dosage. This study also demonstrated that growth hormone reserve might be a preliminary differentiating indicator of the relative sensitivity of patients to hMG. We think that it will help to select patients who might benefit from the concomitant GH-hMG therapy. One fact should not be disregarded, however – namely the connection between patients' body weight and their response to clonidine. Lean women have normal GH pulsatility and growth hormone rise following the administration of clonidine. Obese patients and most patients with PCOD syndrome may show negligible GH pulses and lack of response to clonidine, probably due to an excess of GH-binding protein (Insler et al. 1993). Since IGF-1 may not be mandatory for normal ovarian response, the usefulness of GH or GRF as adjunctive therapy with gonadotropins must not be overestimated.

It has been shown (Laron et al. 1968, Dor et al. 1992) that a Laron-type dwarf (one with an autosomal recessive syndrome characterized by elevated GH levels concomitant with negligible serum IGF-1 levels) can spontaneously ovulate, conceive, and deliver. Due to secondary infertility, such a patient underwent superovulation with gonadotropins for in vitro fertilization, which permitted us to investigate her ovarian response in detail (Dor et al. 1992). Despite undetectable GH-binding protein, negligible IGF-1, and elevated IGF-BP levels in her serum and follicular fluid, fertilizable eggs were obtained. Together with IVF, this patient – who in effect provided an experiment of nature – permitted us to conclude that IGF-1 is not obligatory for ovarian response but seems to play a permissive modulating role in ovarian physiology. Whatever the exact role of GH and different growth factors in the normal ovulation process, GH may serve as an important addition to the clinical armamentarium employed in treating a specific but small group of patients with anovulation and infertility.

Monitoring of Gonadotropin Therapy

Proper monitoring is crucial for the results of gonadotropin therapy, i.e., to achieve a high rate of conceptions while avoiding hyperstimulation and reducing the incidence of multiple pregnancy to an acceptable minimum. Monitoring of the ovarian response to stimulation has four objectives:
1. To determine the effective daily dose of gonadotropins
2. To determine the length of gonadotropin administration
3. To determine the timing of administration of the ovulatory dose of hCG
4. To determine the occurrence and time of ovulation and to evaluate corpus luteum function.

Three types of parameters are used to monitor gonadotropin therapy: (a) clinical, (b) hormonal, and (c) ultrasonographic. Clinical parameters include vaginal examination, basal body temperature (BBT) records, and cervical mucus evaluation expressed as a semiquantitative cervical score (Insler et al. 1972). Hormonal assays required for monitoring of gonadotropin treatment consist of estrogen and progesterone estimations. The ultrasound examinations are aimed at determining the number and size of ovarian follicles and, if possible, also at observing their postovulatory transformation into corpora lutea (Hackeloer 1984, Cabau and Bessis 1981, Ritchie 1985). Ultrasonographic examination also permits assessment of endometrial quality (height and pattern), and combined with color Doppler sonography it may make it possible to evaluate the vascular pattern. These parameters may provide effective information to appraise whether the endometrium is ready for the implanting embryo.

The latent phase of gonadotropin therapy is "mute" to hormonal monitoring. During this time neither the clinical nor the hormonal parameters can give an objective measure of the ovarian response to stimulation. The role of monitoring at this stage is to establish the size of the effective daily dose of hMG. This is done empirically by successively increasing the daily dose of hMG (or FSH) by one ampule (or in some PCOD patients by half an ampule) every 5–7 days until a distinct ovarian response begins, as indicated by the initiation of steroidogenesis and by ultrasonically measurable follicular growth.

High-resolution vaginal sonography permits detection of small antral follicles with a diameter not exceeding 3–4 mm. It is speculated that in the near future it will be possible to recognize the initial recruitment of follicular cohort(s) relatively early in the latent phase of therapy. This may permit a more accurate and earlier tailoring of the gonadotropin dose required in each individual treatment course and consequently improve the final results of therapy.

The main monitoring effort is centered on the active phase of treatment. The number of follicles developing and their growth rhythm must be established, and the time when at least one follicle is ready to receive the ovulatory LH stimulus must be determined as accurately as possible.

The lessons learned from in vitro fertilization indicate that in order to carry out this complicated task it is best to use all three monitoring parameters: clinical, ultrasonographic, and hormonal. The number and diameter of follicles determined by ultrasound and the pattern of ascent of estrogen levels provide a good indication of the extent of follicular maturation. The clinical parameters (cervical score), in addition to being an indirect indicator of estrogen levels, reflect the functional state of the genital tract with regard to sperm transport.

It has been shown repeatedly that both plasma estradiol-17β and urinary total estrogen may be used for monitoring of gonadotropin therapy with equal efficiency (Brown 1986, Insler and Potashnik 1983, Lequin et al. 1986). A steady exponential rise of urinary or plasma estrogen is usually observed during the active phase of gonadotropin therapy. The ideal daily ascent rate is considered to be in the range of 40–100%. A slower ascent may reflect a suboptimal response, and a steeper daily increase is a warning sign of an exaggerated response, possibly heralding hyperstimulation.

For many years, the dominant follicle was considered to be the main source of estrogen, the contribution of smaller follicles being regarded as marginal. In vitro fertilization and ultrasound proved that this is true in monofollicular cycles only. In cycles with multifollicular development, peripheral estrogen levels reflect the sum total of steroidogenic activity of several leading follicles as well as of a number of "runner-up" follicles. Nitschke-Dabelstein et al. (1981) showed that an excellent correlation between the estradiol-17β levels and the number and size of follicles observed on ultrasound could be found in monofollicular but not in multifollicular cycles. On the other hand, the follicular size as measured by ultrasound is inadequate as a sole parameter of follicular maturation, the functional integrity of the follicle being probably better expressed by its steroidogenic activity. Moreover, the steroid production of the ovarian follicles is of primary importance in relation to the structural and functional changes of the endometrium. This is the main reason for combining hormonal and sonographic parameters in monitoring gonadotropin therapy. A steady daily rise of estrogen levels concomitant with a constant increase of follicular diameter and endometrial height on ultrasound are the best indicators of successful ovarian stimulation, as well as being reasonably good predictors of hyperstimulation.

In practice, gonadotropin treatment is monitored as follows: Patients are instructed to keep daily BBT records. Treatment is started between the third and fifth day of spontaneous or induced bleeding. If combined GnRH analogue/gonadotropin therapy is given, the treatment is started when complete pituitary-ovarian down-regulation has been obtained (see "Combined Therapy"). The initial FSH dose is usually one ampule per day in patients of group II (Fig. 7). In women of group I and in patients receiving the combined therapy, treatment is usually started with two ampules hMG per day. If the patient has received gonadotropin therapy in the past, treatment ordinarily commences at the level of the effective daily dose (EDD) of the previous course. Prior to initiation of every course of treatment an ultrasonographic scan of the pelvic region is performed in order

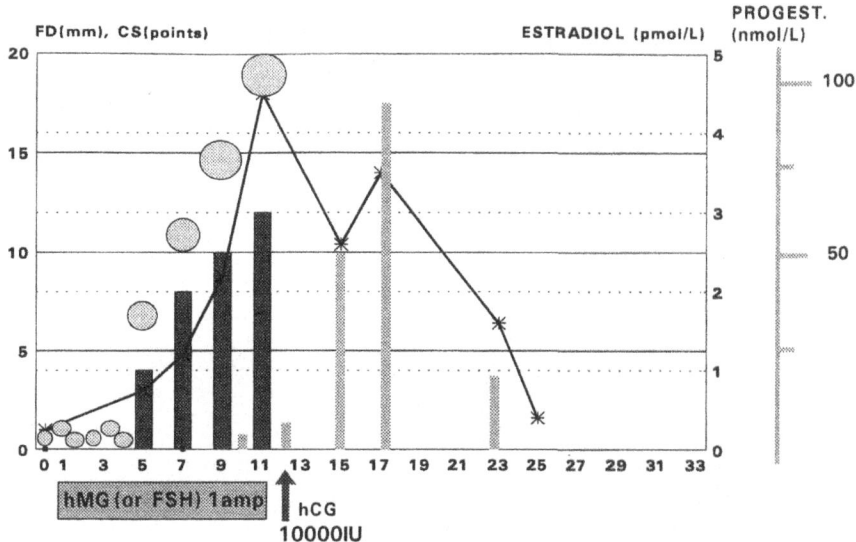

Fig. 7. Monitoring of gonadotropin therapy in a patient of group 2. *FD* diameter of the leading follicle (mm), *black bars* cervical score (*CS, points*), *solid line* estradiol (pm/l), *dotted bars* serum progesterone (nm/l)

to rule out the presence of abnormal follicular structures or cysts. Since such structures are associated with abnormal ovarian response to stimulation and/or with sonographic monitoring of treatment, either they should be punctured or the treatment should be delayed until they disappear spontaneously.

Patients are examined every 1–3 days. The examination includes palpation of the ovaries, estimation of cervical score, post-coital tests when indicated, and a short interview with the patient regarding her general well-being. The dose of gonadotropins is adjusted according to the patient's response as indicated by estrogens, ultrasonography, and clinical findings (Fig. 8).

If estrogens are low and not rising, the initial dose of gonadotropins is continued for 5–7 days and then increased by one ampule. This procedure is repeated until the EDD, i.e., the dose which causes a significant and steady estrogen rise, is achieved. In case of low endogenous estrogens at initiation of therapy, cervical score estimations may replace estrogen assays for the estimation of EDD, provided abnormal cervical response was previously excluded. From this day on the patient is examined daily or every 2 days. When estrogen levels reach or exceed 250 pg/ml (950 pmol/l), ultrasonography is performed. If estrogens increase too rapidly or the day-to-day difference exceeds the geometric rise, the dose is reduced by one ampule (75 IU FSH) and treatment is continued at this reduced dosage.

If the estrogen rise is steady and not excessive, the same dose is continued until an E2 level between 350 and 1200 pg/ml (1330–4500 pmol/l) is reached. Since the duration of the active phase is 4–6 days, this level should be reached within this time limit. At this stage of therapy the third sonographic scan is

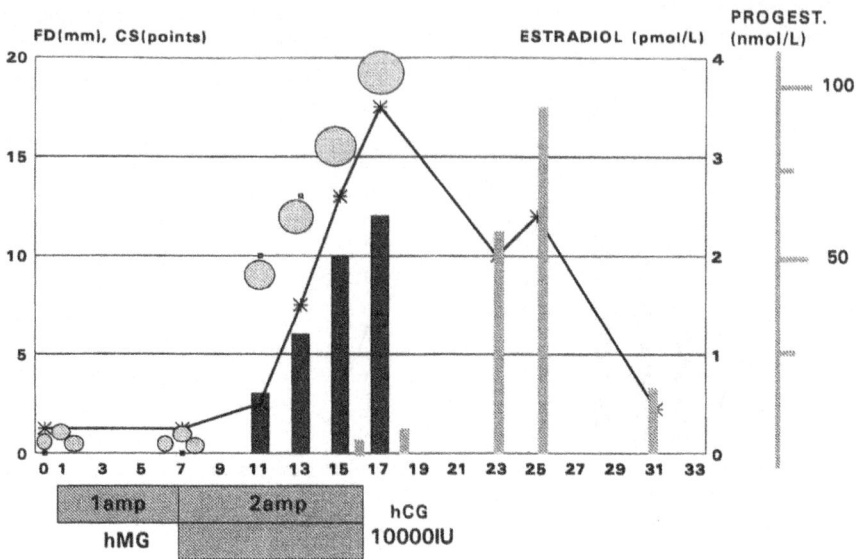

Fig. 8. Monitoring of gonadotropin therapy in a patient of group 1. *FD* diameter of the leading follicle (mm), *black bars* cervical score (*CS, points*), *solid line* estradiol (pm/l), *dotted bars* serum progesterone (nm/l)

performed. If, in both ovaries, the total number of measurable follicular structures does not exceed 10 and one to four follicles have a diameter exceeding 17 mm, the ovulatory dose of hCG (10000 IU) is administered. The patient is advised to have intercourse on three consecutive days, starting on the day of hCG administration. After induction of ovulation the patient is examined 3–5 and 7–9 days following the hCG injection. Special care is taken not to overlook possible ovarian enlargement, abdominal pains, tenderness or distention, and weight gain exceeding 3 kg. At least one blood sample is drawn and sent for progesterone assay. The patient is instructed to report back to the clinic if abdominal pains, nausea, vomiting, or diarrhea appear. If a sustained high phase of BBT lasts for more than 14 days, an hCG and progesterone assay should be performed to detect early pregnancy.

Clinical research and experience show that multifollicular and multiluteal cycles are a rule rather than an exception in gonadotropin therapy (Insler and Potashnik 1983). However, only a small proportion of the multiluteal cycles result also in multiple clinical pregnancies. Brown (1986) remarked that although multiple preovulatory follicles were seen by ultrasound in 50% of gonadotropin-induced cycles, the recorded multiple pregnancy rate was only 20%. O'Herlihy et al. (1981) showed that multiple preovulatory follicles were found in 71% of clomiphene cycles, but the incidence of multiple pregnancy was only 14%. It is thus probable that in hMG-induced conception cycles a number of ova are usually released and possibly fertilized, but only one or two of them are destined to produce a fetus.

The IVF programs are a very important contribution to the management of gonadotropin therapy, particularly when multiple follicles are stimulated. Some of the excessive follicles may be punctured under ultrasound control, thus reducing the E2 levels, leaving a smaller number of follicles to be luteinized by the hCG administration and possibly diminishing the chance of clinical hyperstimulation.

There is still no general agreement with regard to the integrity of corpus luteum function in stimulated cycles. Luteal insufficiency has been implicated as one of the major reasons for conception failure, nidation inadequacy, or early clinical abortion. The problem is too complicated to be explained by analysis of steroid levels and their ratios, or by examination of endometrial structure using light microscopy (and possibly also standard electron microscopy). In order to determine whether the luteal function in stimulated cycles is normal we must compare it with a gold standard, i.e., the corpus luteum function in spontaneous ovulatory cycles. Unfortunately, this standard is not made of "high-purity gold". Landgren et al. (1980) examined 68 meticulously selected spontaneously ovulating healthy women and found that the length of sustained high-phase BBT was 13 days or less in 20% of cases. On day 8 after LH peak the difference between lowest and highest levels of estradiol was fourfold, that of progesterone ninefold. Colston-Wentz (1980) examined 97 endometrial biopsies of presumably ovulating infertile women and reported that 33% of the samples showed an out-of-phase endometrium. Perez and co-workers (1981) examined the corpus luteum and its function in 50 presumably ovulating infertile patients. They used four parameters: laparoscopy, progesterone values, endometrial biopsy, and BBT. In 39 patients all four parameters were synchronized, indicating adequate luteal function. However, in three cases, despite the finding of an apparently normal corpus luteum on laparoscopy, the other parameters were abnormal. In eight other women, laparoscopy did not reveal the presence of a recent corpus luteum, but three of them had a secretory endometrium. It thus seems that accurate evaluation of corpus luteum function in normal ovulatory cycles is difficult, due to the following factors:

- There may be a large interindividual variation of hormone values.
- The high phase of BBT may be sustained by relatively low progesterone values.
- The timing of endometrial biopsy may be false.
- Standard histology of the endometrium may not accurately represent its functional capacity.

Since most of the stimulated cycles are multifollicular and probably multiluteal, the problem is even more complicated. However, Laufer et al. (1982) found that the estrogen and progesterone levels were significantly higher in stimulated, presumably ovulatory, cycles than in spontaneous ovulations, but in both groups steroid levels were similar in conceptional and nonconceptional cycles. Huang et al. (1986) reported that in IVF cycles the individual variation of progesterone levels during the luteal phase was large, but cycles with pregnancy did not significantly differ from those without pregnancy. Nylund et al. (1990)

studied 57 IVF cycles of which 15 resulted in clinical pregnancy and 42 in un-successful implantation. The values of estradiol, progesterone, testosterone, and sex hormone-binding globulin (SHBG) were not different in the two groups. The reports on endometrial structure in stimulated (or IVF) cycles are contro-versial. A review of the scientific literature of the past decade showed that some authors found frequent endometrial abnormalities (Garcia et al. 1981, Cohen et al. 1984, Sterzik et al. 1988, Paulson et al. 1990), while others reported that in stimulated and hyperstimulated cycles the endometrium was fully in phase, de-spite the high levels and/or abnormal ratios of sex steroids (Frydman et al. 1982, Dehou et al. 1987, Barash et al. 1992).

Considering the methodological and objective difficulties of assessing the corpus luteum function in stimulated cycles, which are usually multifollicular, it is obvious that no consensus has been reached with regard to exogenous hor-monal support of the corpus luteum function following induction of ovulation. Some authors advise supporting the corpus luteum by administering intramus-cular injections or vaginal suppositories of progesterone (Leeton et al. 1985, Yo-vich et al. 1985). Others suggest two or three booster injections of 2500–5000 IU of hCG on days 5 and 7 after ovulation induction (Buvat et al. 1990, Hutchinson-Williams et al. 1990, Yovich et al. 1991). A final conclusion as to the frequency and extent of corpus luteum insufficiency in stimulated cycles and the impact of this condition on the results of therapy cannot be established at this time. Consequently, luteal phase support is not considered an integral part of ovulation (or superovulation)-inducing therapy. It must be stressed, however, that luteal phase support is mandatory in the combined pituitary sup-pression/ovarian stimulation protocols, since in this type of therapy luteal insuf-ficiency is often part and parcel of treatment.

Results of Gonadotropin Therapy

Conception rates following gonadotropin therapy are dependent on the follow-ing factors (in order of importance):
1. Selection of patients
2. Type of monitoring
3. Treatment scheme.

In women with hypothalamic-pituitary failure (group I), substitution therapy with gonadotropins is very efficient in inducing ovulation and pregnancy. Go-nadotropin treatment applied as stimulation or regulation therapy in patients having some, albeit deranged, hypothalamic-pituitary-gonadal function (group II) is more complicated and less efficient by far (see also "Treatment Schemes").

While in patients of group I cumulative pregnancy rates of up to 82% were achieved, in group II conception rates varied between 20% and 35% (Lunenfeld and Insler 1978, Lunenfeld et al. 1981, 1985, Bettendorf et al. 1981, Australian Department of Health 1981, personal communication). The same discrepancy

Table 3. Conception rates following gonadotropin therapy

Reference	Patients (n)	Cycles (n)	Pregnancies		
			n	% cycles	% patients
Australian Dept. of Health (1981)[a]	1056	4008	552	13.8	52.3
Bettendorf et al. (1981)	756	1585	224	14.1	29.6
Butler (1970)	134	438	31	7.1	23.1
Caspi et al. (1974)	101	343	62	18.1	61.4
Ellis and Williamson (1975)	77	332	43	13.3	55.8
Gemzell (1970)	228	463	101	21.8	44.3
Goldfarb et al. (1982)	442	1098	118	10.7	26.7
Healy et al. (1980)	40	159	33	20.7	82.5
Kurachi et al. (1985)	2166	6096	523	8.6	24.2
Lunenfeld et al. (1985)	1107	3646	424	11.6	38.3
Insler et al. (1981)	364	?	157	–	32.4
Spadoni et al. (1974)	62	225	26	11.5	41.9
Thompson and Hansen (1970)	1190	2798	334	11.9	28.1
Tsapoulis et al. (1978)	320	?	163		50.9
Cumulative	8043	–	2791	–	43.0

[a] Personal communication.

was also seen when cumulative pregnancy rates were calculated using the life-table analysis method. In group I, after six cycles of therapy the cumulative pregnancy rate exceeded 90% among women less than 35 years old. In contrast, patients of group II required 12 cycles of therapy in order to reach a cumulative conception rate of less than 60%.

Age of the patient also influences the outcome of treatment markedly. Women over 35 years of age had a significantly reduced conception rate regardless of the type of diagnosis and treatment (Insler et al. 1981). The duration of amenorrhea, on the other hand, had no bearing on the results of gonadotropin therapy. The treatment was as efficient in women who had been amenorrheic for only 1 year as in those who had suffered from amenorrhea for 10 years or more.

Table 3 shows the results of gonadotropin therapy as reported by 18 different groups working independently on four continents. This list does not purport to include all data on gonadotropin therapy published so far. Nevertheless, it shows the overall dimension of this therapy and its importance in the therapeutic armamentarium of fertility clinics throughout the world. The list includes over 21000 treatment courses given to 8043 women and 2791 conceptions. Since the majority of entries deal with rather large groups of patients, this summary represents the results of gonadotropin treatment in unselected material typical for busy fertility clinics.

The pregnancy rates (per patients) varied between 23.1% and 82.5%, with an average of 43%. Pregnancy rates per cycle ranged from 7.1% to 21.8%. The intensity of treatment (the mean number of treatment courses per patient) fluctu-

Table 4. Conception rates following superovulation (controlled ovarian stimulation) gonadotropin therapy combined with IUI[a]

Reference	Patients (n)	Cycles (n)	Pregnancies		
			n	% cycles	% patients
Serhal et al. (1988)	48	77	5	6.5	15.6
Welner et al. (1988)	97	388	12	3.1	12.4
Chaffkin et al. (1991)	266	695	85	12.2	31.9
Chang et al. (1993)	343	467	72	15.6	–
Aboulghar et al. (1993)	268	463	93	20.1	34.7
Total	1022	2090	267	12.8	26.1

[a] Ovulatory women treated for unexplained or male infertility; hCG stimulation combined
with timed intercourse or IUI.

Table 5. Conception rates following superovulation (controlled ovarian hyperstimulation)
gonadotropin therapy for IVF, ICSI, and GIFT (ART World Report 1995, according to de-
Mouzon and Lancaster)

Treatment	No. of cycles started	Clinical pregnancies, n (%)	No. of live births n (%)
IVF	127 641	23 888 (18.7)	16 951 (13.3)
ICSI	19 318	4 067 (21.1)	2 756 (14.3)
GIFT	8 939	2 489 (27.7)	1 930 (21.6)
Cumulative	155 898	30 444 (19.5)	21 637 (13.9)

IVF in vitro fertilization, *ICSI* intracytoplasmic sperm injection, *GIFT* gamete intrafallopian
transfer

ated between 2.0 and 4.2. Using the pregnancy rate per cycle specific to each
clinic, one can easily calculate the overall prognosis and cost of this treatment.

During the past few years, gonadotropin stimulation has been used in spontaneously ovulating women with unexplained infertility or subfertility of the
male partner. In this group the ovarian stimulation (or controlled hyperstimulation) is usually combined with intrauterine insemination (IUI). The results
seem to be promising (Table 4). With a relatively low mean number of courses
per patient (2) 16.1% of women achieved conception. During the past decade
gonadotropin stimulation has been extensively used in spontaneously ovulating
women to achieve superovulation combined with ART procedures such as IVF-
ET, GIFT, TET, or micromanipulation.

In this setting ovarian stimulation by gonadotropins is only one component
of a complex clinical and laboratory process. Therefore, results achieved reflect
only in part the effectiveness of gonadotropin stimulation (Table 5).

Recombinant Versus Urinary FSH In ART

There are currently two recombinant human FSH preparations available: Gonal-F (Ares-Serono, Geneva, Switzerland) and Puregon(/Follistim: NV Organon, Oss, The Netherlands). The two r-hFSH molecules are structurally and biochemically almost indistinguishable, except for some minor differences in isoform profile. Furthermore, clinical data recently demonstrated that the two preparations, if administered on an equivalent IU basis, produce identical stimulation characteristics (Table 6) (Brinsden et al. 1998, Sargeant 1998). In view of their similar clinical effectiveness on an IU basis, data obtained on both preparations will be discussed together in the following paragraphs.

r-hFSH is approved for two main indications: anovulation in clomiphene-resistant (World Health Organization group II) patients and multiple follicular stimulation for normally ovulating women undergoing assisted reproduction techniques (ART).

The clinical effect of r-hFSH was first demonstrated in 1992, when case reports confirmed that r-hFSH used in combination with a gonadotropin-releasing hormone (GnRH) agonist successfully stimulated multiple follicular development and estradiol secretion in patients undergoing IVF and embryo transfer (Devroey et al. 1992, Germond et al. 1992). The retrieved oocytes were fertilized and pregnancies were achieved. Following these early case reports, the efficacy of r-hFSH in ART in combination with different GnRH agonists employed in a long protocol was investigated in a number of clinical trials. (Devroey et al. 1994, Reddy et al. 1996.)

As part of the clinical development program for both r-hFSH preparations, a number of key studies have been carried out to document the safety and efficacy of r-hFSH in ART compared with urine-derived FSH. Most have involved protocols that include pituitary desensitization [O'Dea et al. (personal communication), Hedon et al. 1995, Out et al. 1995, Recombinant Human FSH Study Group 1995, Bergh et al. 1997, Frydman et al. 1998] and will be discussed further in this chapter. Those studies designed with sufficient statistical power have clearly demonstrated that, with respect to units of hFSH used and days of

Table 6. Comparison of responses (mean ± SD) to follitropin alpha (Gonal-F, Ares-Serono) and follitropin beta (Puregon, NV Organon) in women undergoing in vitro fertilization

	Follitropin alpha (Gonal-F)	Follitropin beta (Puregon)
Patients	22	22
Total follicles	13±7	15±10
Oocytes retrieved	12±8	12±8
Days of FSH	9±1	9±1
Ampoules of FSH used (75 IU equivalent)	17.8±4.1	17.8±4.5
Embryos transferred	2±1	2±1
Clinical pregnancy/cycle (%)	32	18
Patients with injection reactions (%)	36	57

Table 7. Selected parameters of studies comparing recombinant human follicle-stimulating hormone (r-hFSH) with urinary human follicle-stimulating hormone (u-hFSH)

Parameter	r-hFSH	u-hFSH	p-value
Number of patients			
r-hFSH Study Group 1995	60	63	
O'Dea et al. 1993	60	60	
Hedon et al. 1995	60	39	
Out et al. 1995	585	396	
Bergh et al. 1997	119	114	
Frydman et al. 1998	60	63	
Number of ampules (75 IU)			
r-hFSH Study Group 1995	30.3	27.9	
O'Dea et al. 1993	33.3	28.3	0.00
Hedon et al. 1995	30.2	29.5	0.75
Out et al. 1995	28.5	31.8	<0.000
Bergh et al. 1997	21.9	31.9	<0.0001
Frydman et al. 1998	27.6	40.7	<0.0001
Total IU			
r-hFSH Study Group 1995	2270±714	2095±591	
O'Dea et al. 1993	2498	2123	0.00
Hedon et al. 1995	2265	2213	0.75
Out et al. 1995	2138	2385	<0.000
Bergh et al. 1997	1642.5	2392.5	<0.0001
Frydman et al. 1998	2070	3052.5	<0.0001
Days of treatment			
r-hFSH Study Group 1995	9.9±2.3	9.4±1.8	
O'Dea et al. 1993	10.0	9.0	0.00
Hedon et al. 1995	10.2	10.3	0.83
Out et al. 1995	10.7	11.3	<0.000
Bergh et al. 1997	11.0	13.5	<0.001
Frydman et al. 1998	11.7	14.5	<0.001
Number of embryos			
r-hFSH Study Group 1995	5.0±3.0	6.1±3.4	
O'Dea et al. 1993	5.6	6.4	0.36
Hedon et al. 1995	3.7	4.0	0.69
Out et al. 1995	3.1	2.6	<0.00
Bergh et al. 1997	8.1	4.7	<0.0001
Frydman et al. 1998	5.0	3.5	<0.0002

stimulation required, recombinant FSH is more effective than urinary gonadotropins in promoting the process of follicular development (Table 7).

The few studies which have investigated the safety and efficacy of r-hFSH in non-down-regulated cycles in ART will not be considered here. However, they too confirm the superior effectiveness of the recombinant product compared with urinary extracts.

In 1995, the results of the first multicenter, prospective, randomized clinical trial comparing r-hFSH and u-hFSH in women undergoing IVF-ET were published (Recombinant Human FSH Study Group 1995). In this small study, 60 patients were treated with r-hFSH (given s.c.) and 63 with u-hFSH (i.m.) follow-

Table 8. Comparison of the efficacy and tolerability of recombinant human follicle-stimulating hormone (r-hFSH) and urinary human follicle-stimulating hormone (u-hFSH) in a large, prospective, randomized, multicenter study

	r-hFSH	u-hFSH
Number of patients	615	412
Number of ampules (75 IU FSH)	28.5	31.8
Days of treatment	10.7	11.3
Total dose (IU)	2138	2385
Daily dose (ampules)	2.6	2.8
Estradiol (day of hCG; nm/l)	5.9	4.9
Number of follicles ≥15 mm	7.5	6.7
Number of follicles ≥17 mm	4.6	4.4
Total number of oocytes	10.8	8.9
Number of mature oocytes	8.6	6.5
Number of embryos	3.1	2.6
Number of cryopreserved embryos	2.6	1.2
Pregnancy/attempt (%)	22.4	18
Pregnancy rate/patient (including cryopreserved embryos; %)	25.4	20.4
Incidence of OHSS (%)	3.2	2.0

ing down-regulation with intranasal buserelin in a long protocol. The results confirmed r-hFSH to be as safe and effective as u-hFSH in stimulating ovarian follicular development.

Another prospective and very large, multicenter study (Table 8) compared r-hFSH with u-hFSH in an IVF-ET program. (Out et al. 1995). A total of 981 patients who received intranasal buserelin were randomized to treatment with r-hFSH or u-hFSH given i.m. Among patients receiving the recombinant product (n=585), a significantly higher number of oocytes (10.8 vs 8.9, adjusted for center effect; $p < 0.0001$) were retrieved with a lower total dose of FSH [2138 vs 2385 IU (28.5 vs 31.8 ampules of 75 IU FSH) $p < 0.0001$] over a shorter treatment period (10.7 vs 11.3 days; $p < 0.0001$) compared with u-hFSH. The number of high-quality embryos was also significantly higher among those receiving r-hFSH (3.1 vs 2.6 for u-hFSH; $p = 0.003$), but there were no differences between the two groups in implantation rates or clinical pregnancy rates per attempt and per transfer. However, more embryos were cryopreserved in the group receiving r-hFSH (mean 2.6 compared with 1.2 among the u-hFSH patients), reflecting the high number of mature oocytes and high-quality embryos obtained from these patients. When frozen embryo cycles were included in the analysis, ongoing pregnancy rates were significantly different in favor of r-hFSH (25.5% with r-hFSH vs 20.4% with u-hFSH; $p < 0.05$). The incidence of ovarian hyperstimulation syndrome (OHSS) was similar in the two treatment groups (3.2% with r-hFSH and 2.0% with u-hFSH) and no anti-FSH antibodies were detected in patients receiving the recombinant product.

In a further comparison of r-hFSH with u-hFSH in IFV-ET, down-regulation was accomplished with triptorelin given daily by s.c. injection (Brinsden et al. 1998). A total of 99 women were included in this prospective, assessor-blind, multicenter study and were randomized in a ratio of 3:2 to receive r-hFSH ($n = 60$) or u-hFSH ($n = 39$) given i.m. Although the differences between the r-hFSH and the u-hFSH group in this study were not statistically significant, there was a trend towards a higher number of retrieved oocytes (9.7 vs 8.9), higher serum estradiol levels (7551 vs 5514 pmol/l), and higher ongoing pregnancy rates per cycle (30.2% vs 17.4%) and per transfer (34% vs 18.8%) among those treated with the r-hFSH. Three patients (5%) who received r-hFSH were hospitalized for OHSS, but there was no OHSS in the u-FSH group.

These studies all confirmed the earlier observation that r-hFSH alone can successfully induce multiple follicular growth (Devroey et al. 1994) even in pituitary down-regulated cycles with very low endogenous LH activity. Furthermore, they indicated that r-hFSH was more effective than u-hFSH in inducing multiple ovulation for IVF-ET. Although the findings of these studies do not all show significant differences, it seems likely that this is a reflection of their statistical power to detect small differences (Mc Donough 1997).

That controlled ovarian stimulation with r-hFSH leads to statistically significant higher ongoing pregnancy rates compared with urinary FSH and hMG was further substantiated by a meta-analysis of three prospective multicenter, randomized comparative trials (Out et al. 1997). Such analyses are particularly useful when the results from several studies lack statistical significance yet appear to show effects with similar trends (D'Agostinho and Weintraub 1995). This meta-analysis found that the ongoing pregnancy rate at least 12 weeks after embryo transfer per started cycle was 22.9% for r-hFSH and 17.9% for urinary gonadotropins. The 5% treatment difference was statistically significant in favor of r-hFSH ($p = 0.044$). Furthermore, when the replacement of cryopreserved embryos was also taken into account, the treatment difference increased to 6.4% ($p = 0.011$) in favor of r-hFSH.

Comparison of Recombinant with Highly Purified Urinary FSH

The next question to be answered was: Is the recombinant product any more effective in inducing multiple follicular development for ART than highly purified urinary FSH, a product with a specific activity that approaches r-hFSH and that can also be injected s.c.?

The results of a prospective, randomized, assessor-blind, two-center study showing that r-hFSH (Gonal F) is more effective than highly purified urinary FSH (Metrodin HP; u-hFSH HP) in inducing multiple follicular development in women undergoing ovarian stimulation for IVF (including ICSI) were published in the latter half of 1997 (Table 9) (Bergh et al. 1997). Patients were down-regulated with intranasal buserelin in a long protocol and were then randomized to receive r-hFSH ($n = 119$) or u-hFSH HP ($n = 114$), both given s.c.

The mean number of oocytes retrieved, the primary end point of the study, was significantly higher among those given r-hFSH than among those who received u-hFSH HP. Furthermore, the number of FSH treatment days and the number of 75 IU ampules used were significantly less with r-hFSH than with

Table 9. Gonal-F vs. Metrodin HP

	Gonal-F	Metrodin	p-value
Ampules (75 IU)	21.9±5.1	31.9±13.4	<0.0001
FSH (days)	11.0±1.6	13.5±3.7	<0.0001
Oocytes retrieved	12.2±5.5	7.6±4.4	<0.0001
Embryos cleaved	8.1±4.2	4.7±3.5	<0.0001
Embryos transferred	2.0±02	1.9±0.4	ns
Pregnancy/cycle (%)	53/119 (45)	42/114 (37)	ns
Miscarriages (%)	13 (25)	6 (14)	ns
Twin pregnancies (%)	17 (32)	9 (21)	ns
Ongoing pregnancies/cycle (%)	40/119 (34)	36/114 (32)	ns
Implantation rate, %	32	31	ns

u-hFSH HP. Among patients treated using ICSI (63 in each group) no difference in oocyte maturation was observed between the two groups. However, the mean number of embryos obtained was higher among patients receiving r-hFSH. However, there were no significant differences between the r-hFSH and u-hFSH groups in the pregnancy rate per cycle (45% and 37%, respectively).The authors of this study commented that differences in the pregnancy rate may become apparent after the addition of cryopreserved embryo transfer cycles. The number of cryopreserved embryos was significantly higher in the r-hFSH group than in the u-hFSH HP group (3.2 versus 1.7; $p<0.0001$), giving a potentially higher chance of conceiving from a single stimulation cycle. Both treatments were well tolerated, and the incidence of OHSS was 5.1% and 1.7%, respectively, in the r-hFSH and u-hFSH HP groups.

The preliminary results of the first double-blind randomized comparison of r-HFSH (Gonal-F) and u-hFSH HP (Metrodin HP) administered s.c. in women undergoing ART were recently published (Frydman et al. 1998). This study included 246 pituitary down-regulated patients and found that, among those treated with r-hFSH, there was a significantly higher mean number of oocytes recovered and embryos obtained. Furthermore, the treatment duration was significantly shorter and the number of 75 IU ampules required significantly less in the r-hFSH group than in the u-hFSH HP group. The study power was not sufficient to detect a difference in ongoing clinical pregnancy rates. The incidence of severe OHSS was <1% in both groups (Table 10).

Although all these studies differ in their design and in the regimens used, the overall conclusion has to be that, compared with u-hFSH and u-hFSH HP, the use of r-hFSH to induce superovulation in women undergoing ART is associated with more embryos being obtained following the administration of a lower total FSH dose.

Furthermore, recent data demonstrate what has been suspected for many years: the number of embryos in culture is a major determinant of pregnancy outcome. An analysis of data entered in the Human Embryology and Fertilisation Authority database (Human Fertilisation and Embryology Authority Sixth

Table 10. Results of the first double-blind randomized comparison of r-hFSH and u-hFSH in women undergoing ART; values are means ±SD (from Frydman et al. 1998)

Parameter	r-hFSH ($n=130$)	u-hFSH HP ($n=116$)	p-value
Oocytes retrieved	11.0±5.9	8.8±4.8	0.0001
Ampules (75 IU) FSH	27.6±10.2	40.7±13.6	0.0001
FSH (days)	11.7±1.9	14.5±3.3	0.001
Embryos (day 2)	5.0±3.7	3.5±2.9	0.0002
Ongoing pregnancy rate/cycle (%)	20	20	ns
Multiple clinical pregnancy	41	28	ns

Annual Report 1997) has revealed that women who had more than four embryos in culture had a significantly higher chance of achieving a pregnancy than those with four embryos or less. This was true for all age-groups treated. Furthermore, among the women with more than four embryos in culture who subsequently had two or three embryos transferred (24.4% versus 23.4%) the incidence of pregnancy was similar irrespective of the number of embryos transferred. However, the chance of a multiple pregnancy increased from 6.6% with the replacement of two embryos to 9.2% with the replacement of three (Human Fertilisation and Embryology Authority Sixth Annual Report 1997). Thus, among women with multiple embryos, perhaps fewer embryos should be replaced in order to reduce the incidence of multiple pregnancies.

Another line of evidence clearly demonstrates the importance of having a large number (greater than 4) of gametes available for fertilization. Scholtes and Zeilmaker (1998), who replaced blastocysts in 265 sequential transfers, found that the chance of having at least one blastocyst to transfer was significantly increased if the woman had more than four oocytes collected. If the woman had 10–15 oocytes (the current 'ideal' number), the chance of blastocyst transfer was 80%.

If, as is apparent from this review, the use of r-hFSH to stimulate superovulation results in a higher number of embryos than obtained with urinary FSH products, the embryos that are not needed for immediate transfer can be cryopreserved. For couples who have cryopreserved embryos available, the potential for subsequent pregnancy is only slightly less than that obtained after the transfer of fresh embryos (Bachelot et al. 1996, Human Fertilisation and Embryology Authority Sixth Annual Report 1997, Society for Assisted Reproductive Technology 1998). This is a significant benefit for the couple, providing them with an additional boost in their pregnancy potential per stimulated cycle.

Comparison of the efficacy of recombinant and urinary FSH in 2227 IVF cycles demonstrated that the recombinant preparations yielded more embryos and a higher pregnancy rate with lesser amount (units) and shorter treatment (Table 7). Moreover, since in response to recombinant FSH more oocytes and consequently more embryos are produced, superfluous embryos may be frozen and replaced at an additional attempt, thus further increasing the chance for pregnancy. Recombinant FSH also produced high ovulation and pregnancy rates in anovulatory, clomiphene-resistant women (WHO group II).

In patients with hypogonadotropic hypogonadism (WHO group I) recombinant FSH alone was sufficient to stimulate follicular growth but was inadequate to induce competent follicular function. However, recombinant FSH combined with recombinant LH was able to produce follicular development and, following administration of hCG, ovulation and pregnancy (Kousta et al. 1996). It seems that the LH dose ensuring follicular development and function in hypogonadotropic women is in the range of 75–225 IU/day (European rec. LH study group 1998, personal communication).

The first birth following infertility treatment of a hypopituitary-hypogonadotropic woman (WHO group I) with recombinant FSH and recombinant LH to stimulate follicular growth and recombinant hCG to induce ovulation was reported by Agrawal et al. 1997. The highly potent, safe, and pure pharmaceutical-grade gonadotropin with full batch-to-batch consistency and with the additional convenience of s.c. self-administration, will hopefully shortly replace all urinary preparations.

New developments in the area of drug research will have a significant impact on the future of reproductive medicine. With recombinant DNA technology and highly defined cell culture techniques, genetically engineered gonadotropins are now being prepared on an industrial scale and are already on the market in many countries around the globe.

What would currently require 70 million liters of urine per year will ultimately be produced by genetically engineered cells in chemically defined culture medium comprising only a small fraction of that volume. When such recombinant gonadotropin preparations reach all the world markets, hMG and urinary FSH will have served their purpose and will become history (Fig. 9). Very soon we will be able to thank the thousands of women who have donated their urine over the past 30 years, permitting hMG to become history with the start of the new era of recombinant gonadotropins.

Outcome of Pregnancies

The course of gestation following induction of ovulation with gonadotropins appeared to be normal. Analysis of the mode of delivery showed a high incidence of interventions, breech extraction, vacuum extraction, forceps delivery, and cesarean sections. The high incidence of obstetrical intervention may be explained by an elevated multiple pregnancy rate, primiparity ratios, relatively high maternal age, and psychological factors involved in delivering a "premium child" in patients with long-standing infertility.

Our study (Ben-Rafael et al. 1986) showed that the sex ratio (M/F) of the single births was 1.06 (54% boys) and of the twins 0.72 (42% boys). The numbers of triplets were too small to analyze. In 1976 Caspi reported 32 males and 50 females among the single births (39%) with a twin M/F ratio of 0.78 (Caspi et al. 1976). In the series reported by Bettendorf et al. (1981) the incidence of male

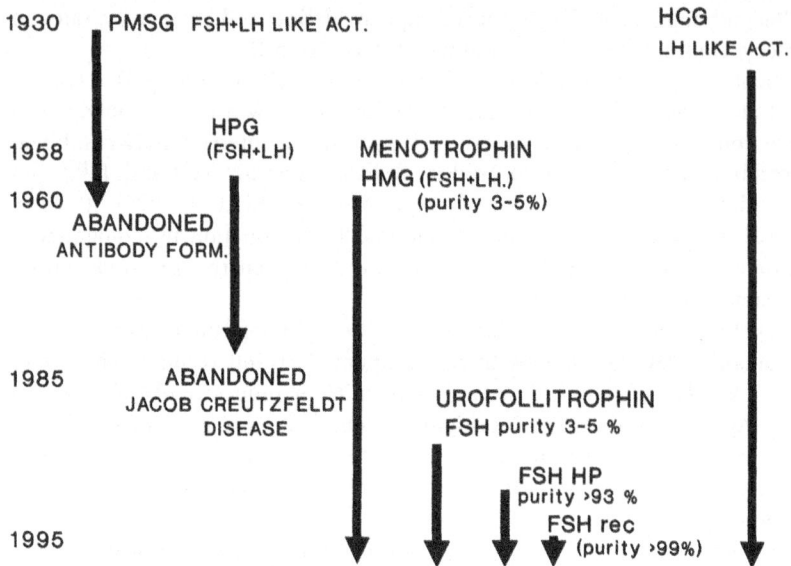

Fig. 9. History of gonadotropic preparations

children in single pregnancies was 51.8%. However, in their series the incidence of males among twins and triplets was 53.8% and 66.7%, respectively. The normal secondary sex ratio at 28 weeks is considered to be 106 boys to 100 girls (Tricomi et al. 1960, Serr and Ismajovich 1963). The sex ratio (M/F) was found by Nichols (1952) to be 1043 for twins, 1007 for triplets, and 0940 for quadruplets. The high incidence of girls in our twin series and the high incidence of male children among twins and triplets in the series of Bettendorf et al. (1981) are probably due to the rather small numbers involved. By combining all the three series, one approaches the expected sex ratios, indicating clearly the importance of sufficiently large numbers in order to estimate similarities or divergence in sex ratio.

Congenital Malformations

Table 11 shows the rate of congenital malformations found in a combined series of 941 babies born after induction of ovulation with hMG/hCG. The incidence of minor and major malformations was 22.3/1000 and 19.1/1000, respectively. The incidence of congenital malformations in normal populations has been reported to be 12.7/1000 after 28 weeks of gestation, with a range of 3.1 to 22.5 (McKeown 1960, Stevenson et al. 1966). There is a further rise to 23.1/1000 by the age of 5 years. Hendricks (1966) reported a rate of 3% in the neonatal period, with twice as many malformations in twin births, mostly monozygotic twins. Shoham et al. (1991) reviewed a large number of reports dealing with

Table 11. Congenital malformations after ovulation induction with human gonadotropins

Reference	n	Major	Minor
Kurachi et al. (1985)	509	9	1
Hack and Lunenfeld (1978)	209	4	4
Caspi et al. (1976b)	157	4	11
Harlap (1976)	66	1	5
Total	941	18 (1.91%)	21 (2.23%)
Normal population		(1.27%) (0.31–2.25%)	(7.24%)

congenital malformations in children born after induction of ovulation and concluded that clomiphene citrate, hMG/hCG, or the association of these drugs with IVF-ET and GIFT procedures do not carry an increased risk for congenital malformations as a whole, nor is there any specific malformation that has an increased incidence which is related in any way to the use of those drugs. It can thus be summarized that, at present, the clinical evidence does not indicate that babies born after hMG/hCG ovulation induction are at any greater risk of malformation than the general population.

Complications of Gonadotropin Therapy

All complications of gonadotropin treatment are due essentially to ovarian stimulation, follicular development, and luteinization or ovulation. To the best of our knowledge, direct side effects of the drug itself have not been reported. The main complications of gonadotropin treatment are:
1. Ovarian hyperstimulation syndrome
2. High incidence of multiple pregnancy
3. Abortion rate higher than in spontaneous conceptions.

Multiple Pregnancy

Multiple pregnancy is rather frequent following gonadotropin therapy. Brown (1986) reviewed 1712 pregnancies resulting from ovulation induction by human pituitary or menopausal gonadotropins and found that the average multiple pregnancy rate was 24.4%, fluctuating between 21% and 33%. As expected, small series showed a lower incidence of multiple gestations than large series. The causes of multiple conceptions following induced cycles are very similar to those causing ovarian hyperstimulation, i.e., the pharmacological stimulation of multifollicular development. Thus, the risk factors and the possibilities of avoiding (or at least reducing the incidence) of both complications are similar (see chapter on Ovarian Hyperstimulation). Insler and Potashnik (1983) reported that in 26% of gonadotropin-induced cycles three or more functional corpora

Table 12. Multiple births following IVF

Source	No. of cycles	No. of embryos transferred	Live births/ transfer	Multiple births (%)
French ART Registry (FIVNAT, 1995)	31 391 [a]	2.6	16.0	27.9 [b]
German ART Registry (1996)	36 727	2.3	15.4	24.1
UK ART Registry (April 1, 1995–March 31, 1996)	30 216	2 or 3 [c]	18.3	30.5
USA ART Registry (1996)	49 584	4.0	24.3	32.5

[a] Number of transfers.
[b] Mean for years 1991–1995.
[c] Mainly two, and not more than three, embryos transferred in the UK.

lutea were produced and that mean plateau progesterone levels were higher in the conceptional than in the nonconceptional cycles. Further analysis of the above data indicated that in hMG treatment cycles conception occurs in most cases in the presence of more than one corpus luteum and in one quarter of cases in the presence of three or more functioning corpora lutea. Since only around 25% of gonadotropin-induced pregnancies result in twins and only 5% produce three or more fetuses, and since the mean plateau progesterone levels are similar in single and multiple hMG-induced pregnancies, it could be speculated that in the majority of hMG conceptions a number of ova are released and fertilized but only one of them is destined to produce a living fetus. The others perish before reaching the uterine cavity or are absorbed or extruded prior to implantation (Table 12).

If, however, a quadruplet, quintuplet, etc. pregnancy reaches the gestational age of 7–8 weeks, its further development may represent a severe danger to the fetuses because of a very high probability of extreme prematurity, considerable medical complications for the mother, and a pronounced psychological, social, and financial burden for the family. The technique of fetal reduction under sonographic control has been developed. Breckwoldt et al. (1988) reported a case of gonadotropin-induced pregnancy with nine gestational sacks present in the uterus. Six of the fetuses were eliminated under sonographic guidance. This technique, although medically simple and logical, is still controversial for ethical, legal, and religious reasons.

Abortions

The abortion rate in conceptions following gonadotropin therapy is around 21%. Brown (1986) compiled and reviewed a series of 1712 pregnancies and found that the combined abortion and perinatal deaths rates fluctuated between 10% and 28% in different reports.

There was no significant difference in the abortion rate in relation to diagnostic groups. The rate was 26% in patients of group I and 32.6% in women of group II, respectively (Blankstein et al. 1986). However, the abortion rate was significantly higher in the first conception cycle (28.8%) than in the second or third gestation (12.8%). The main reasons for increased abortion rates in conceptions resulting from induction of ovulation have been presumed to be: (a) structural and functional inadequacy of the endometrium to ensure proper and timely nidation of the embryo; (b) functional incompetence of the corpus luteum, preventing it from reacting properly to the pregnancy signal, i.e., the initial increase of hCG produced by the trophoblast; (c) multiple pregnancy; (d) emotional factors. An in-depth analysis of the literature seems, however, to indicate that the dominant cause for early pregnancy wastage in conceptions resulting from ovarian stimulation is the quality of the ova, which in turn, depends on the nature of follicular environment during follicular maturation. This conclusion is also strongly supported by analysis of the fate of spontaneous pregnancies. According to Chard (1991), only 30% of natural conceptions produce a term pregnancy.

Long-term Safety

Nulliparity has been a consistently reported risk factor for carcinoma of the breast and endometrium (Kelsey 1979, Brinton et al. 1983, LaVecchia et al. 1984, Ron et al. 1987, Kelsey et al. 1991). A strong relation between age at first birth and breast cancer has been demonstrated. Although part of the association appears to be due to involuntary infertility, the biologic mechanism involved in the etiology of female reproductive cancers remains unclear. While results from case-control studies have consistently shown that multiparty and oral contraceptive use are associated with a reduced risk of ovarian cancer, excessive unopposed estrogen secretion has been linked to endometrial and breast carcinoma.

In the past decades, a multitude of epidemiological studies have been published on the association of ovarian cancer with environmental factors, with hereditary factors, and with factors related to reproductive history. However, conclusive etiologic studies are scarce, for the following reasons:

1. All examined associations appeared to be weak.
2. The etiology of ovarian cancer appeared to be multifactorial (this implies that considerable numbers of patients are needed to reach the threshold of statistical significance).
3. Based on the prevalence of ovarian carcinoma in the general population, it is difficult to find enough cases to undertake an epidemiological study.

Several authors have identified infertility as an independent risk factor on top of the nulliparity effect. Whittemore et al. (1989) called it "the ability to conceive" and found a significant correlation between the number of years of unprotected intercourse and the risk of ovarian cancer. Like Nasca et al. (1984), Joly et al. (1974) calculated the pregnancy rates per 1000 person-years at risk of pregnancy. They found significantly higher rates in controls than in the cases of ovarian cancer.

Hartge et al. (1989) showed that infertile nulliparous women with a history of infertility had a 2.8 times higher risk than nulliparous women without such a history, and Harlow et al. (1988) estimated this figure to be much higher, a factor of 6. Booth et al. (1989) concluded that the risk for ovarian cancer in nulligravid women with more than 10 years of unprotected intercourse is 6.5 times higher than in nulligravid women with less than 5 years of unprotected intercourse. Whittemore et al. (1989) found a relative risk of 1.8 for the same risk factor in all women, regardless of parity.

The above findings are confirmed by the observations of Lais et al. (1988), who found six ovarian malignancies in 571 consecutive patients who underwent microsurgery for infertility. Five of the six patients were nulligravid. Of the five patients who had undergone laparoscopy some months previously, three had been negative and in two, small "trivial" lesions had been reported. This prevalence figure is roughly ten times higher than that observed in general abdominal surgery or in pregnancy (Thornton and Wells 1987).

Among 296 cases and 343 controls, Hartge et al. (1989) found a clear difference in cancer risk between nonmarried nulliparous women (no risk increase) and married nulliparous women (70% risk increase). When they considered specifically nulliparous women who tried but failed to conceive, the risk ratio was 2.8. The authors thus demonstrated that infertility by itself is associated with an increased risk, in addition to the effect of nulliparity.

Among 215 cases and 215 controls, Cramer et al. (1983) did not find an effect of infertility alone. They found a 2.5 times higher risk in nulliparous women. They also found an increased risk associated with postmenopausal estrogen replacement therapy.

Concerning 403 cases and 806 controls, Nasca et al. (1984) concentrated on the infertility factor. They calculated the ratio of total pregnancies to the number of contraceptive-free years of marriage for each group. This ratio they found to be significantly lower in cancer patients (indicating an increasing risk with decreasing fertility). Their figures closely matched the findings of McGowan et al. (1979). Nasca's group concluded that infertility played an important role in the relationship between gravidity/parity and ovarian cancer risk. Fertility drugs were not mentioned in this paper.

Joly et al. (1974) did a case-control study on ovarian carcinoma. The authors found a consistent risk increase linked with infertility. Their data had been collected between 1957 and 1965, i.e., prior to the current use of fertility drugs.

Using a large combined data set derived from case-control studies in the United States, Whittemore et al. (1993) interpreted their findings in a recent publication to show that an increased risk of ovarian cancer associated with infertility may be due in part to the use of fertility drugs. The global study population of the three studies used by Whittemore et al. (1993) in their analysis was 2278 women, of whom only 1723 were included in the analysis. The data related to infertility drugs were calculated from 20 ever-married patients with invasive epithelial ovarian cancer treated with infertility drugs and 11 controls.

This very small number of cases is responsible for the extremely wide 95% confidence interval of 2.3–315.6 with a mean risk of 27.0 for women who did not conceive despite their receiving fertility drugs. Conception reduced this risk to levels of fertile controls. The study also found an increased relative risk for epithelial ovarian cancer of low malignant potential among women who had used fertility drugs. The mean relative risk for this group was 4.0 with 95% confidence limits of 1.1–13.9, based on four cases and nine controls.

If one translates the estimates of Whittemore et al. (1993) into absolute figures, then the added risk of cancer possibility being attributable to fertility drugs would be approximately 8.3/100 000 (1 in 12 000/year) at age 30–34 and 21.1/100 000 (1 in 5 000) for ages 40–44. This absolute risk would have to be balanced, however, against the benefit of achieving a birth.

The data of Whittemore et al. (1993) were in contrast to our results (Ron et al. 1987, Lunenfeld et al. 1986, 1987). Our studies indicated that hMG/hCG therapy does not increase the risk for cancer. Because the number of women receiving each specific treatment was small, and the majority of patients had not yet reached the age of maximal cancer risk, the statistical power to detect minor effects of treatment was low. We therefore reinvestigated our data again 10 years later (Modan et al. 1998). The results showed a similar trend, even though the mean age of the women reached 52.6 years and the follow-up period was prolonged to more than 22 years and presented over 53 000 women years.

Concluding Remarks

During the past two decades, human gonadotropins have become an integral part of the therapy of functional infertility. Introduced as a substitution therapy for hypogonadotropic hypogonadism, the indications for this modality have been gradually expanded to other types of fertility disturbances such as anovulation, oligo-ovulation, and PCOD. Finally, the concept of achieving superovulation by controlled ovarian hyperstimulation (COH) in spontaneous ovulators has been instigated. This, in combination with IVF, GIFT, IUI, and other ARTs, demanded the use of gonadotropins in treatment of mechanical, male, and unexplained infertility. The number of patients treated has grown to such proportions over the years that supply shortages of the drug have become imminent. Production of human FSH and LH by genetic engineering techniques seems to be within reach and will probably make it possible to cover the growing demand in the near future.

References

Aboulghar MA, Mansour RT, Serour GI, Amin Y, Abas AM, Salah IM (1993) Ovarian superstimulation and intrauterine insemination for the treatment of unexplained infertility. Fertil Steril 60:303–306

Adashi EY, Carol H, Resnick A, D'Ercole J, Svoboda EM, Van Wyk JJ (1985a) Insulin-like growth factors as intraovarian regulators of granulosa cell growth and function. Endocrinol Rev 6:400–410

Adashi EY, Resnick A, Svoboda EM, Van Wyk JJ (1985b) Somatomedin C synergizes with FSH in the acquisition of projection biosynthetic capacity by cultured rat granulosa cells. Endocrinology 116:2135–2142

Adashi EY, Resnick A, Svoboda EM, Van Wyk JJ (1985c) Somatomedin C enhances induction of LH receptors by FSH in cultured rat granulosa cells. Endocrinology 116:2369–2375

Adashi EY, Resnick CE, Hernandez ER et al (1990) The ovarian IGF-1 system as a paradigm for putative intra-ovarian regulators. In: Yen SSC, Vale WW (eds) Neuroendocrine regulation of reproduction, Serono Symposia. Norwell, Mass., pp 185–194

Agrawal R, West C, Conway GS, Page ML, Jacobs HS (1997) Pregnancy after treatment with three recombinant gonadotropins. Lancet 349:29–30

Anderson RE, Cragun JM, Chang RJ, Stancyk FZ, Lobo RA (1989) A pharmacodynamic comparison of human urinary stimulating hormone and human menopausal gonadotropins in normal women and polycystic ovary syndrome. Fertil Steril 52:216–220

Bachelot A, Rossin-Amar B et al (1996) Bilan FIVNAT 1995. Contracept Fertil Sex 24:694–699

Baird DT (1987) A model for follicular selection and ovulation: lessons from superovulation. J Steroid Biochem 27:15–23

Barash A, Czernobilsky B, Insler V, Borenstein R, Rosenberg M, Fink A (1992) Endometrial morphology and hormonal profiles in in vitro fertilization patients. Eur J Obstet Gynecol Reprod Biol 44:117–121

Ben-Nun I, Lunenfeld B, Ben-Aderet N (1984) Prevention de la luteinisation prematuree du follicle par hyperprolactinemie iatrogene volontaire au cours des traitements par HMG. Hormones 5:54–57

Ben-Rafael Z, Matalon A, Blankstein J, Serr DM, Lunenfeld B, Mashiach S (1986) Male to female ratio after gonadotropin-induced ovulation. Fertil Steril 45:36–40

Bergh C, Howles CM, Borg K, Hamberger L, Josefsson B, Nilsson L, Wikland M (1997) Recombinant human follicle-stimulating hormone (r-hFSH; Gonal-F) versus highly purified urinary FSH (Metrodin HP): results of a randomized comparative study in women undergoing assisted reproductive techniques. Hum Reprod 12:2133–2139

Bettendorf G (1963) Human hypophyseal gonadotropin in hypophysectomized women. Int J Fertil 8:799

Bettendorf G, Apostolakis M, Voigt KD (1961) Darstellung hochaktiver Gonadotropin Fraktionen aus menschlichen Hypophysen und deren Anwendung beim Menschen. Proc Int Fed Gynecol Obstet 1:76 (abstract)

Bettendorf G, Braendle W, Sprotte CH, Weise CH, Zimmerman R (1981) Overall results of gonadotropin therapy. In: Insler V, Bettendorf G (eds) Advances in diagnosis and treatment of infertility. Elsevier/North Holland, New York, pp 21–26

Blankstein J, Mashiah S, Lunenfeld B (1986) Ovulation induction and in vitro fertilization. Year Book, Chicago, p 148

Blumenfeld Z, Lunenfeld B (1989) The potential effect of growth hormone on follicle stimulation with human menopausal gonadotropin in a panhypopituitary patient. Fertil Steril 52:328–331

Blumenfeld Z, Nahhas F (1988) Luteal dysfunction in induction of ovulation: the role of repetitive human chorionic gonadotropin supplementation during luteal phase. Fertil Steril 50:403–407

Boime I, Keene J, Galway AB, Fares FA, Hsue AJW (1990) Regulation of secretion and molecular mechanisms of action. Springer, Berlin Heidelberg New York, pp 120–128

Booth M, Beral V, Smith P (1989) Risk factors for ovarian cancer: a case-control study. Br J Cancer 60:59208

Borth R, Lunenfeld B, de Watteville H (1954) Activite gonadotrope d'un extrait d'urines de femmes en menopause. Experientia 10:266–270

Borth R, Lunenfeld B, Riotton G, de Watteville H (1957) Activite gonadotrope d'un extrait d'urines de femmes en menopause (2me communication). Experientia 13:115–121

Breckwoldt M, Neulen J, Wieacker P, Schillinger H (1988) Induction of ovulation by combined GnRH-A/hMG/hCG treatment. In: Lunenfeld B (ed) Symposium on GnRH analogues in cancer and human reproduction. Parthenon Press, Casterton Hall, p 58

Brinsden P, Akagbosu F, Gibons L et al (1998) Gonal-F vs Puregon: results of a randomized assessor-blind, comparative study in women undergoing ART. 14th annual meeting of the European Society of Human Reproduction and Embryology. Gothenburg (abstract)

Brinton LA, Hoover R, Fraumeni JF jr (1983) Reproductive factors in the aetiology of breast cancer. Br J Cancer 47:757–762

Brown JB (1986) Gonadotropins. In: Insler V Lunenfeld B (eds) Infertility: male and female. Churchill Livingstone, London, pp 359–396

Butler JK (1970) Oestrone response patterns and clinical results following various Pergonal dosage schedules. In: Butler JK (ed) Developments in the pharmacology and clinical uses of human gonadotrophins. GD Searle & Co., High Wycombe, UK, pp 42–46

Butt WR, Kennedy JF (1971) Structure-activity relationships of protein and polypeptide hormones. In: Margoulis M, Greenwood PC (eds) Protein and polypeptide hormones. Excerpta Medica, Amsterdam, p 115

Buvat J, Marcolin G, Guittard C, Herbaut JC, Louvet AL, Dehaene JL (1990) Luteal support after luteinizing hormone-releasing hormone agonist for in vitro fertilization: superiority of human chorionic gonadotropin over oral progesterone. Fertil Steril 53:490

Cabau A, Bessis R (1981) Monitoring of ovulation induction with human menopausal gonadotropin and human chorionic gonadotropin by ultrasound. Fertil Steril 36:178

Caspi E, Levin S, Bukovsky J, Weintraub Z (1974) Induction of pregnancy with human gonadotropins after clomiphene failure in menstruating ovulatory infertility patients. Isr J Med Sci 10:249

Caspi E, Ronen J, Schreyer P, Goldberg MD (1976) The outcome of pregnancy after gonadotropin therapy. Br J Obstet Gynaecol 83:967–973

Chaffkin LM, Nulsen JC, Luciano AA, Metzger DA (1991) A comparative analysis of the cycle fecundity rates associated with combined human menopausal gonadotropin (hMG) and intrauterine insemination (IUI) versus either hMG or IUI alone. Fertil Steril 55:252–257

Chang MY, Huang HY, Lee CL, Lai YM, Chang SY, Swong YK (1993) Treatment of infertility using controlled ovarian hyperstimulation with intrauterine insemination: the experience of 343 cases. J Formos Med Assoc 92:341–348

Chard T (1991) Frequency of implantation and early pregnancy loss in natural cycles. Baillieres Clin Obstet Gynaecol 5:179–189

Cochius JI Mack K Burns RJ (1990) Creutzfeldt-Jakob disease in a recipient of human pituitary-derived gonadotropin. Aust N Z J Med 20:592

Cohen JJ, Debache C, Pigeau F, Mandelbaum J, Plachot M, de-Brux J (1984) Sequential use of clomiphene citrate, human menopausal gonadotropin, and human chorionic gonadotropin in human in vitro fertilization. II. Study of luteal phase adequacy following aspiration of the preovulatory follicles. Fertil Steril 42:360–365

Cohen J, DeMouzon J, Lancaster P (1993) World Collaborative Report 1991. VII World Congress on In Vitro Fertilization and Alternate Assisted Reproduction, Kyoto, September

Colston-Wentz A (1980) Endometrial biopsy in the evaluation of infertility. Fertil Steril 33:121–124

Cook AS, Webster BW, Terranova PF, Keel BA (1988) Variation in the biologic and biochemical characteristics of human menopausal gonadotropin. Fertil Steril 49:704–712

Costrici N, Lunenfeld B, Pariente C, Dor J, Rabinovici J, Kanety H, Karasik A (1994) Induction of aromatase in human granulosa cells by both follicle-stimulating hormone and insulin-like growth factor-I involves tyrosine phosphorylation. Gynecol Endocrinol 8:183–189

Cramer DW, Hutchison GB, Welch WR, Scully RE, Ryan KJ (1983) Determinants of ovarian cancer risk. I. Reproductive experiences and family history. J Natl Cancer Inst 71:711–716

Crawley WF, Comite F, Vale W, Rivier J, Loriaux DL, Cutler GB (1982) Inhibition of serum androgen levels by chronic intranasal and subcutaneous administration of a potent luteinizing hormone-releasing hormone (LH-RH) agonist in adult men. Fertil Steril 27:1240

Crooke AC (1970) Comparison of the effects of Pergonal and pituitary follicle-stimulating hormone. In: Butler JK (ed) Developments in the pharmacology and clinical uses of human gonadotrophins. GD Searle & Co, High Wycombe, UK, pp 36–41

D'Agostinho RB, Weintraub M (1995) Meta-analysis: a method for synthesizing research. Clin Pharmacol Ther 58:605–616

Davoren JB, Hsueh AJW (1986) Growth hormone increased ovarian levels of immunoreactive somatomedin C/insulin-like growth factor I in vivo. Endocrinology 118:888–890

Dehou MF, Lejeune B, Arijs C, Leroy F (1987) Endometrial morphology in stimulated in vitro fertilization cycles and after steroid replacement therapy in cases of primary ovarian failure. Fertil Steril 48:995

De la Llosa P, Jutisz M (1969) Protein and polypeptide hormones. In: Margoulis M (ed) Protein and polypeptide hormones. Exerpta Medica, Amsterdam, p 229

Devroey P, Van Steirteghem A, Mannaerts B, Coelingh Bennink K (1992) Successful in vitro fertilization and embryo transfer after treatment with recombinant human FSH. Lancet 339:1171

Devroey P, Mannaerts B, Smitz J, Coelingh Bennink K, Van Steirteghem A (1994) Clinical outcome of a pilot efficacy study on recombinant human follicle-stimulating hormone (org 32489) combined with various gonadotropin-releasing hormone agonist regimens. Hum Reprod 9:1064–1069

Diczfalusy E, Harlin J (1988) Clinical-pharmacological studies on human menopausal gonadotropin. Hum Reprod 3:21–27

Diedrich K, Felberbaum R (1998) New approaches to ovarian stimulation. Hum Reprod 13 [Suppl 3]:1–13

Dor J, Ben-Shlomo I, Lunenfeld B, Pariente C, Levran D, Seppala M (1992) Is insulin-like growth factor-1 essential for the human graafian follicle development: observation in a Laron-type dwarf during in vitro fertilization. J Clin Endocrinol Metab 74:539–542

Dumble LD, Klein RD (1992) Creutzfeldt-Jakob disease legacy for Australian women treated with human pituitary gonadotropins. Lancet 340:848

Ellis JD, Williamson JG (1975) Factors influencing the pregnancy and complication rates with human menopausal gonadotropin therapy. Br J Obstet Gynaecol 82:52

Ericson GF, Garzo VG, Magoffin DA (1989) Insulin-like growth factor-I regulates aromatase activity in human granulosa and granulosa luteal cells. J Clin Endocrinol Metab 69:716–724

Fares FAM, Suganuma N, Nishimori K, LaPolt P, Hsue AJW, Boime I (1992) Design of long-acting follitropin agonist by fusing the C terminal sequence of chorionic gonadotropin beta subunit to the follitropin beta subunit. Proc Natl Acad Sci USA 89:4304–4308

Fiddes JC, Goodman HM (1979) Isolation, cloning and sequence analysis of the cDNA for the alpha-subunit of human chorionic gonadotropin. Nature 281:351

Flack MR, Valove FM, Finch C, Froelich J, Anasti JN, Nisula BC (1994) Follicle-stimulating hormone signal transduction is distinct from receptor binding and each requires a different site on the hormone. Front Ovarian Res 1:20 (abstract)

Fleming R, Coutts JRT (1990) The use of exogenous gonadotrophins and GnRH analogues for ovulation induction in PCO syndrome. Res Clin Forums 11:77–85

Fleming R, Haxton MJ, Hamilton R (1985) Successful treatment of infertile women with oligomenorrhea using a combination of an LHRH agonist and exogenous gonadotropins. Br J Obstet Gynaecol 92:369–373

Frydman R, Testart J, Giacomini P, Imbert MC, Martin E, Nahoul K (1982) Hormonal and histological study of the luteal phase in women following aspiration of the preovulatory follicle. Fertil Steril 38:312–317

Frydman R, Avril C, Camier B et al (1998) A double-blind, randomised study comparing the efficacy of recombinant human follicle stimulating hormone (r-hFSH/Gonal-F) and highly purified urinary FSH (u-hFSH HP/Metrodin HP) in inducing superovulation in women undergoing assisted reproductive techniques (ART). 14th Annual Meeting of the European Society for Human Reproduction and Embryology, Gothenburg (abstract)

Garcia J, Jones GS, Acosta AA, Wright GL (1981) Corpus luteum function after follicle aspiration for oocyte retrieval. Fertil Steril 36:565–572

Garcia JE, Jones GS, Acosta AA, Wright G (1983) Human menopausal gonadotropin/human chorionic gonadotropin in follicular maturation for oocyte aspiration. Phase I. Fertil Steril 39:167–173

Gemzell CA (1964) Treatment of infertility after partial hypophysectomy with human pituitary gonadotropins. Lancet 1:644

Gemzell CA (1970) Recent results of human gonadotropin therapy. In: Bettendorf G, Insler V (eds) Clinical application of human gonadotropins. Thieme, Stuttgart, pp 6–20

Gemzell CA, Diczfalusy E, Tillinger G (1958) Clinical effect of human pituitary follicle-stimulating hormone. J Clin Endocrinol Metab 18:138–148

Gemzell CA, Diczfalusy E, Tillinger G (1960) Human pituitary follicle-stimulating hormone. 1. Clinical effect of a partly purified preparation. Ciba Found Colloquia Endocrinol 13:191

Germond M, Dessole S, Senn A, Loumaye E, Howles C, Beltrami V (1992) Successful in vitro fertilization and embryo transfer after treatment with recombinant human FSH. Lancet 339:1170–1171

Goldfarb AF, Schlaff S, Mansi ML (1982) A life-table analysis of pregnancy yield in fixed low-dose menotropin therapy for patients in whom clomiphene citrate failed to induce ovulation. Fertil Steril 37:629

Goodman AL, Nixon WE, Johnson DL, Hodgen GD (1977) Regulation of folliculogenesis in the rhesus monkey: selection of the dominant follicle. Endocrinology 100:155–161

Gougeon A (1986) Dynamics of follicular growth in the human: a model from preliminary results. Hum Reprod 1:81–87

Hackeloer BJ (1984) The role of ultrasound in female infertility management. Ultrasound Med Biol 10:35

Harlow BL, Weiss NS, Roth GJ et al (1988) Case-control study of borderline tumors: reproductive history and exposure to exogenous female hormones. Cancer Res 48:5849–5852

Hartge P, Schiffman MH, Hoover R, McGowan L, Lesher L, Norris HJ (1989) A case-control study of epithelial ovarian cancer. Am J Obstet Gynecol 161:10–16

Healy DL, Burger HG (1983) Serum FSH, LH and PRL during the induction of ovulation with exogenous gonadotropins. J Clin Endocrinol Metab 56:474–478

Healy DL, Kovacs GT, Pepperell RJ, Burger HG (1980) A normal cumulative conception rate after human pituitary gonadotropin. Fertil Steril 34:341

Hedon B, Out HJ, Hughes JN et al (1995) Efficacy and safety of recombinant FSH (Puregon) in infertile women pituitary-suppressed with triptorelin undergoing in vitro fertilisation: a prospective, randomised, assessor-blind, multicentre trial. Hum Reprod 10:3102–3106

Hendricks CH (1966) Twinning in relation to birth weight mortality and congenital malformations. Obstet Gynecol 27:47

Hodgen G (1983) The dominant follicle. Fertil Steril 38:81–300

Homburg R, Armar NA, Eshel A, Adams J, Jacobs HS (1988a) Influence of serum luteinising hormone concentration on ovulation, conception and early pregnancy loss in polycystic ovary syndrome. Br Med J 297:1024–1026

Homburg R, Eshel A, Abdallah HI, Jacobs HS (1988b) Growth hormone facilitates ovulation induction by gonadotropins. Clin Endocrinol 29:113–117

Homburg J, Balasch M, Birkhauser M et al (1994) Efficacy of recombinant human follicle-stimulating hormone Gonal F for inducing ovulation in WHO Group II anovulatory patients. Preliminary results of a comparative, multicenter study. In: Mori T, Aono T, Tominaga T, Hiroi M (eds) Frontiers in endocrinology: perspectives of assisted reproduction. Ares Serono Symposia, Rome, pp 463–668

Howles CM, Macnamee MC, Edwards RG, Goswamy R, Steptoe PC (1986) Effect of high tonic levels of luteinising hormone on outcome of in vitro fertilisation. Lancet II (8505):521–522

Huang KE, Muechler EK, Schwarz KR, Goggin M, Graham MC (1986) Serum progesterone levels in women treated with human menopausal gonadotropin and human chorionic gonadotropin for in vitro fertilization. Fertil Steril 46:903

Human Fertilisation and Embryology Authority (1997) Sixth annual report. Paxton House, 30 Artillery Lane, London E1 7LS

Hussa RO (1980) Biosynthesis of human chorionic gonadotropin. Endocr Rev 1:268–285

Hutchinson-Williams KA, DeCherney AH, Lavy G, Diamond MP, Naftolin F, Lunenfeld B (1990) Luteal rescue in in vitro fertilization-embryo transfer. Fertil Steril 53:495

Insler V, Lunenfeld B (1974) Application of human gonadotropins for induction of ovulation. In: Campos da Paz A, Hasegava T, Notake Y Hayashi M (eds) Human reproduction. Igaku Shoin, Tokyo, pp 25–38

Insler V, Lunenfeld B (1977) Human gonadotropins. In: Philip E, Barnes J, Newton M (eds) Scientific foundations of obstetrics and gynaecology. Heineman, London, p 629

Insler V, Potashnik G (1983) Monitoring of follicular development in gonadotropin-stimulated cycles. In: Beier HM, Lindner HM (eds) Fertilization of the human egg in vitro. Springer, Berlin Heidelberg New York, pp 111–122

Insler V, Melmed H, Mashiah S, Monselise M, Lunenfeld B, Rabau E (1968) Functional classification of patients selected for gonadotropin therapy. Obstet Gynecol 32:620–625

Insler V, Melmed H, Eichenbrenner I, Serr DM, Lunenfeld B (1972) The cervical score – a simple semiquantitative method for monitoring the menstrual cycle. Int J Obstet Gynecol 10:223–228

Insler V, Potashnik G, Glassner M (1981) Some epidemiological aspects of fertility evaluation. In: Insler V, Bettendorf G, Geissler KH (eds) Advances in diagnosis and treatment of infertility. Elsevier/North Holland, New York, pp 165–178

Insler V, Potashnik G, Lunenfeld E, Meizner I, Levy J (1989) The combined suppression/stimulation therapy in IVF-ET programmes: expectations and facts. Gynecol Endocrinol 4 [Suppl]:47–51

Insler V, Kleinman D, Sod-Moriah U (1990) Role of midcycle FSH surge in follicular development. Gynecol Obstet Invest 30:228–233

Insler V, Shoham Z, Barash A, Koistinen R, Seppala M, Hen M, Lunenfeld B, Zadik Z (1993) Polycystic ovaries in non-obese and obese patients: possible pathophysiological mechanism based on new interpretation of facts and findings. Hum Reprod 8:379–384

Jia XC, Kalmijin J, Hsueh AJW (1986) Growth hormone enhances FSH-induced differentiation of cultured rat granulosa cells. Endocrinology 118:1401–1409

Johnson P, Pearce JM (1990) Recurrent spontaneous abortion and polycystic ovarian disease: comparison of two regimens to induce ovulation. Br Med J 300:154–155

Joly DJ, Lilienfeld AM, Diamond EL, Bross ID (1974) An epidemiologic study of reproductive experience to cancer of the ovary. Am J Epidemiol 99:190–207

Kelsey JL (1979) A review of the epidemiology of human breast cancer. Epidemiol Rev 74–109

Kelsey JL, Gammon MD (1991) The epidemiology of breast cancer. Cancer J Clin 41:146–165

Kemmann E, Brandeis VT, Shelden RM, Nosher JL (1983) The initial experience with the use of a portable infusion pump in the delivery of human menopausal gonadotropins. Fertil Steril 40:448–453

Kousta E, White DM, Piazzi A, Loumay E, Franks S (1996) Successful induction of ovulation and completed pregnancy using recombinant human luteinising hormone and follicle-stimulating hormone in a woman with Kallman syndrome. Hum Reprod 11:70–71

Kurachi K, Aono T, Suzuki M, Hirano M, Kobayashi T, Kaibara M (1985) Results of HMG (Humegon)-HCG therapy in 6906 treatment cycles of 2166 women with anovulatory infertility. Eur J Obstet Gynecol Reprod Biol 19(1):43–45

Lais CW, Williams TJ, Gaffey TA (1988) Prevalence of ovarian cancer found at the time of infertility microsurgery. Fertil Steril 49:551–553

Landgren BM, Unden AL, Diczfalusy E (1980) Hormonal profile of the cycle in 68 normally menstruating women. Acta Endocrinol 94:89–98

Laron Z, Pertzelan A, Karp M (1968) Pituitary dwarfism with high serum levels of growth hormone. Isr J Med Sci 4:883–900

Laufer N, Navot D, Schenker JG (1982) The pattern of luteal phase plasma progesterone and estradiol in fertile cycles. Am J Obstet Gynecol 143:808–813

LaVecchia C, Franceschi S, Decarli A, Gallus G, Tognoni G (1984) Risk factors for endometrial cancer at different ages. J Natl Cancer Inst 3:667–671

Leethem JH, Rakoff AE (1948) Studies on antihormone specificity with particular reference to gonadotropic therapy in the female. J Clin Endocrinol Metab 8:262

Leeton J, Trounson A, Jessup D (1985) Support of the luteal phase in in vitro fertilization programs: results of a controlled trial with intramuscular Proluton. J In Vitro Fertiliz Embryo Transfer 2:166

Lequin L, Mendels E, Trimbos-Kemper G et al (1986) Oestrogens in urine or plasma to monitor ovarian response to exogenous gonadotropins. Serono Symposium on the control of follicular development, ovarian and luteal function: lessons from in vitro fertilization. (abstract)

Lopata A, Gronow MJ, Johnston WIH, McBain JC, Speirs AL, Leung PS (1986) In vitro fertilization and embryo implantation. In: Insler V, Lunenfeld B (eds) Infertility: male and female, Churchill Livingstone, Edinburgh, p 496

Loumaye E, Alvarez S, Barlow D et al. (1994) Efficacy of r-hFSH (Gonal-F) for stimulating multiple follicular development in assisted reproductive technologies. In: Mori T, Aono T, Tominaga T, Hiroi M (eds) Frontiers in endocrinology: perspectives on assisted reproduction. Ares-Serono Symposia Publications, Rome, pp 469–474

Lunenfeld B (1963) Treatment of anovulation by human gonadotropins. Int J Obstet Gynecol 1:153

Lunenfeld B (1994) The ovary – control from above and within. Aust N Z J Obstet Gynaecol 34:265–268

Lunenfeld B, Insler V (1978) Diagnosis and treatment of functional infertility. Grosse, Berlin

Lunenfeld B, Insler V (1993) Follicular development and its control. Gynecol Endocrinol 7:285–292

Lunenfeld B, Menzi A, Volet B (1960) Clinical effects of human post menopausal gonadotropins. Acta Endocrinol (Copenh) [Suppl] 51:587

Lunenfeld B, Serr DM, Mashiah S et al (1981) Therapy with gonadotropins: Where are we today. In: Insler V, Bettendorf G, Geissler KH (eds) Advances in diagnosis and treatment of infertility. Elsevier/North Holland, New York, p 27

Lunenfeld B, Mashiah S, Blankstein J (1985) Induction of ovulation with human gonadotropins. In: Shearman R (ed) Clinical reproductive endocrinology. Churchill Livingstone, London, p 523

Lunenfeld B, Blankenstein J et al (1986) Drugs used in ovulation induction. Safety of patient and offspring. Hum Reprod 1:435–439

Lunenfeld B, Blankenstein J, Ron E et al (1987) Short- and long-term survey of patients treated with HMG/HCG and follow-up of offspring. In: Genazziani AR, Volpe A, Facchinettie F (eds) Proc 1st International Congress on Gynecological Endocrinology, p 459

McDonough PG (1997) The coming of wonders (editorial comment). Fertil Steril 67:412–413

McFaul PB, Traub AI, Thompson W (1989) Premature luteinization and ovulation induction using human menopausal gonadotropins or pure follicle-stimulating hormone in patients with polycystic ovary syndrome. Acta Eur Fertil 20:157–162

McGowan L et al (1979) The woman at risk for developing ovarian cancer. Gynecol Oncol 7:325–344

McKeown J (1960) Malformations in a population observed for five years. In: Ciba Found Colloquia Congenital Malformations. J A Churchill, London, p 2

Macnamee MC (1990) The role of in vitro fertilization in polycystic ovarian disease. Res Clin Forums 11:89–95

Marshall JR, Jacobson A (1970) A technique of dose selection in ovulation induction with HMG. In: Butler JK (ed) Developments in the pharmacology and clinical uses of human gonadotrophins. GD Searle & Co., High Wycombe, UK, pp 141–150

Meldrum DR, Chang RJ, Lu J, Vale W, Rivier J, Judd HL (1982) Medical oophorectomy using a long-acting GnRH agonist – a possible new approach to treatment of endometriosis. J Clin Endocrinol Metab 54:1081–1083

Menashe Y, Lunenfeld B, Pariente C, Frenkel Y, Mashiach M (1990a) Can growth hormone increase, following clonidine administration, predict the dose of human menopausal hormone needed for induction of ovulation? Fertil Steril 53:432–435

Menashe Y, Lunenfeld B, Pariente C, Mashiach M (1990b) Effect of growth hormone on ovarian responsiveness. Gynecol Endocrinol 4:6

Milgrom E (1993) International Symposium on ovarian function, Jerusalem. Symposium on Ovarian Function 1:123 (abstract)

Modan B, Ron E, Lerner-Geva L, Blumstein T, Menczer J, Rabinovici J, Oelsner G, Freedman L, Mashiach S, Lunenfeld B (1998) Cancer incidence in a cohort of infertile women. Am J Epidemiol 147:1038–1042

Nakatani A, Shimasaki S, Erickson GS, Ling N (1991) Tissue-specific expression of four insulin-like growth factor binding proteins [1,2,3 and 4). J Endocrinol 129:1521-1529

Nasca PC, Greenwald P, Chorost S, Richart R, Caputo T (1984) An epidemiologic case-control study of ovarian cancer and reproductive factors. Am J Epidemiol 119:705-713

Nichols JB (1952) Statistics of births in the USA, 1915-1948. Am J Obstet Gynecol 64:376

Nitschke-Dabelstein S, Sturm G, Prinz H, Buchholz R (1981) Plasma 17 β-estradiol and plasma progesterone as indicators of cyclic changes in the follicle-bearing ovary. In: Insler V, Bettendorf G (eds) Advances in diagnosis and treatment of infertility. Elsevier/North Holland, New York, pp 57-64

Nylund L, Beskow C, Carstrom K et al (1990) The luteal phase in successful and unsuccessful implantation after IVF-ET. Hum Reprod 5:40

O'Herlihy C, Pepperell RJ, Brown JB, Smith MA, Sandri L, McBain JC (1981) Incremental clomiphene therapy: a new method for treating persistent anovulation. Obstet Gynecol 58:535

Oliviennes F, Bouchard P, Frydman R (1997) The use of a new GnRH antagonist (cetrorelix) with a single-dose protocol in IVF. J Assist Reprod Genet 14 [Suppl]:15S

Out HJ, Mannaerts BMJL, Driessen SGAJ et al (1995) A prospective, randomized, assessor-blind, multicentre study comparing recombinant and urinary follicle-stimulating hormone (Puregon versus Metrodin) in in vitro fertilization. Hum Reprod 10:2534-2540

Out HJ, Driessen SGAJ, Mannaerts BMJL, Coelingh Bennick HJT (1997) Recombinant follicle-stimulating hormone (follitropin beta, Puregon) yields higher pregnancy rates in in vitro fertilization than urinary gonadotrophins. Fertil Steril 68:138-142

Paulson RJ, Sauer MV, Lobo RA (1990) Embryo implantation after human in vitro fertilization: importance of endometrial receptivity. Fertil Steril 53:870

Perez RJ, Plurad AV, Palladino VS (1981) The relationship of the corpus luteum and the endometrium in infertile patients. Fertil Steril 35:423-427

Punnonen R, Ashorn R, Vilja P, Heinonen PK, Kunjansuu E, Tuohimaa P (1988) Spontaneous luteinizing hormone surge and cleavage of in vitro fertilized embryos. Fertil Steril 49:479-481

Quigley MM (1985) Selection of agents for enhanced follicular recruitment in an in vitro fertilization and embryo replacement treatment program. Ann N Y Acad Sci 442:96-111

Rabau E, Lunenfeld B, Insler V (1971) The treatment of fertility disturbances with special reference to the use of human gonadotropins. In: Joel CH (ed) Fertility disturbances in men and women. Karger, Basel, p 508

Recombinant Human FSH Study Group (1995) Clinical assessment of recombinant human follicle-stimulating hormone in stimulating ovarian follicular development before in vitro fertilization. Fertil Steril 63:77-86

Reddy R, Al-Oum M, Ledger W et al (1996) An alternate day step-down regimen using Gonal-F(r-hFSH) in IVF: a UK multicenter study. Hum Reprod 11:130-131

Ritchie WGM (1985) Ultrasound in the evaluation of normal and induced ovulation. Fertil Steril 43:167

Ron E, Lunenfeld B, Menczer J, Serr D, Katz L (1987) Cancer incidence in a cohort of infertile women. Am J Epidemiol 125:780-790

Ronnberg L, Martikainen H, Tapanainen J (1990) Is there any benefit to use growth hormone in ovarian hyperstimulation? Gynecol Endocrinol 4:7-27

Roux C, Elefant E, Biour B, Schatz B (1993) Follow-up of pregnancies after casual exposure to a GnRH analogue (Triptorelin). Gynecol Endocrinol 7:[Suppl 2] 137 (abstract)

Sargeant SD (1998) A study to evaluate the ease of use and tolerability by patients of gonadotrophins old and new. British Fertility Society, annual meeting, Sheffield (abstract F9)

Scholtes MCW, Zeilmaker GH (1998) Blastocyst transfer in day-5 embryo transfer depends primarily on number of oocytes retrieved and not on age. Fertil Steril 69:78-83

Seegar-Jones GEA-A, Garcia JE, Rosenwaks Z (1985) Specific effects of FSH and LH on follicular development and oocyte retrieved as determined by a program for in vitro fertilization. Ann N Y Acad Sci 442:119

Serhal PF, Katz M, Little V, Woronowski H (1988) Unexplained infertility - the value of Pergonal superovulation combined with intrauterine insemination. Fertil Steril 49:602-606

Serr DM, Ismajovich B (1963) Determination of the primary sex ratio for human abortions. Am J Obstet Gynecol 87:63

Shadmi AL, Lunenfeld B, Bahari C, Kokia E, Pariente C, Blankstein J (1987) Abolishment of the positive feedback mechanism: a criterion for temporary medical hypophysectomy by LHRH agonist. Gynecol Endocrinol 1:1–11

Shoham Z, Borenstein R, Lunenfeld B, Pariente C (1990) Hormonal profiles following CC therapy in conception and nonconception cycles. Clin Endocrinol 33:271–278

Shoham Z, Zosner A, Insler V (1991) Early miscarriage and fetal malformations after induction of ovulation by clomiphene citrate and/or human menopausal gonadotropins in in vitro fertilization, and gamete interfallopian transfer. Fertil Steril 55:1–10

Smith PE (1926) Hastening of development of female genital system by daily hemoplastic pituitary transplants. Proc Soc Exp Biol Med 24:131

Smith PE, Engle ET (1927) Experimental evidence of the role of anterior pituitary in development and regulation of gonads. Am J Anat 40:159

Society for Assisted Reproductive Technology and American Society for Reproductive Medicine (1998) Assisted reproductive technology in the US and Canada. Fertil Steril 69:389–398

Sopelak VM, Hodgen GD (1984) Blockade of the estrogen-induced luteinizing hormone surge in monkeys a nonsteroidal antigenic factor in porcine follicular fluid. Fertil Steril 41:108–113

Spadoni LR, Cox DW, Smith DC (1974) Use of human menopausal gonadotropin for the induction of ovulation. Am J Obstet Gynecol 120:988

Stanger JD, Yovitch JL (1985) Reduced in vitro fertilization of human oocytes from patients with raised basal luteinizing hormone levels during the follicular phase. Br J Obstet Gynaecol 92:385–390

Sterzik K, Dallenbach C, Schneider V, Sasse V, Dallenbach-Hellweg G (1988) In vitro fertilization: the degree of endometrial insufficiency varies with the type of stimulation. Fertil Steril 50:457

Stevenson AC, Johnson HA, Stewart PMI (1966) Congenital malformations: a report of a study of a series of consecutive births in two centers. Bull World Health Organ 34:9

Talmadge K, Boorstein WR, Fiddes JC (1983) The human genome contains seven genes for the beta subunit of chorionic gonadotropin but only one gene for the beta subunit of luteinizing hormone. DNA 2:281–289

Thompson LR, Hansen LM (1970) Pergonal (menotropin): a summary of clinical experience in the induction of ovulation and pregnancy. Fertil Steril 21:844

Thornton JG, Wells M (1987) Ovarian cysts in pregnancy: does ultrasound make traditional management inappropriate? Obstet Gynecol 69:717

Tricomi V, Serr DM, Solish G (1960) The ratio of male and female embryos as determined by sex chromatin. Am J Obstet Gynecol 75:504

Tsapoulis AD, Zourlaz PA, Comninos AC (1978) Observations on 320 infertile patients treated with human gonadotropins (human menopausal gonadotropin/human chorionic gonadotropin). Fertil Steril 29:492

Ulloa-Aguirre A, Espinoza R, Damian-Matsumura P, Chappel SC (1988) Immunological and biological potencies of the different molecular species of gonadotrophins. Hum Reprod 3:491–501

Volpe A, Coukos G, Barreca A et al (1989) Ovarian response to combined growth hormone gonadotropin treatment in patients resistant to induction of superovulation. Gynecol Endocrinol 3:125–133

Welner S, DeCherney AH, Polan ML (1988) Human menopausal gonadotropins: a justifiable therapy in ovulatory women with long-standing infertility. Am J Obstet Gynecol 158:111–117

Whittemore AS et al (1989) Epithelial ovarian cancer and the ability to conceive. Cancer Res 49:4047–4052

Whittemore AS, Harris, R, Itnyre J (1993) Characteristics relating to ovarian cancer risk: collaborative analysis of twelve US case-control studies. II. Invasive epithelial ovarian cancers in white women. Am J Epidemiol 136:1184–1203

World Health Organization (1976) WHO Technical Report Series, no 514

Wu C (1977) Plasma hormones in human gonadotropin-induced ovulation. Obstet Gynecol 49:308–313

Yen SSC (1983) Clinical applications of gonadotropin-releasing hormone and gonadotropin-releasing hormone analogs. Fertil Steril 39:257–266

Yovich JL, McColm SC, Yovich JM, Tuvik S (1985) Early luteal serum progesterone concentrations are higher in conception cycles. Fertil Steril 44:185

Yovich JL, Edirisinghe WR, Cummins JM (1991) Evaluation of luteal support therapy in a randomized controlled study within a gamete intrafallopian transfer program. Fertil Steril 55:31–139

Zondek B (1926) Über die Funktion des Ovariums. Z Geburtshilfe Gynakol 90:327

Zondek B, Aschheim S (1927) Das Hormon des Hypophysenvorderlappens; Testobject zum Nachweis des Hormons. Klin Wochenschr 6:248

Zondek B, Sulman F (1942) The antigonadotropic factor, with consideration of the anti-hormone problem. Williams and Wilkins, Baltimore, pp 1–185

Gonadotropin-Releasing Hormone: Agonists and Antagonists

R. Felberbaum, T. Rabe, K. Diedrich

Introduction

In adult women the cyclic function of the ovaries is embedded in the hypothalamic, pituitary, and ovarian feedback mechanisms [1]. The hypothalamus is
the superordinate organ releasing gonadotropin-releasing hormone (GnRH) in a
pulsatile manner. GnRH is secreted by the neural cells of the nucleus arcuatus
in the mediobasal portion of the hypothalamus. The axons in these neurons are
in close contact with the vessels of the hypothalamic-pituitary portal vein system. The pulsatile release of GnRH by the hypothalamic neurons causes the gonadotropic cells of the adenopituitary, which make up about 10% of its cell
mass, to release the gonadotropins follicle-stimulating hormone (FSH) and luteinizing hormone (LH), also in pulses. FSH and LH in turn control follicular
maturation and gonadal sexual steroid biosynthesis. The spontaneous activity
of the hypothalamic pulse generator is modulated by a number of neurotransmitters (norepinephrine, γ-aminobutyric acid, dopamine, serotonin), neuropeptides (neuropeptide Y, proenkephalin, prodynorphin, proopiomelanocortin, cor-
ticotropin-releasing hormone), endogenous opioids (β-endorphin), and steroids
(estradiol, progesterone, and testosterone). For example, an oversupply of endogenous opioids as seen in anorexia nervosa can slow the pulse generator and
cause hypothalamically induced hypogonadotropic amenorrhea. This has been
successfully treated and an ovulatory cycle established by using an opiate antagonist [2].

The Physiology of the Menstrual Cycle

The interval between two GnRH pulses is about 70–90 min [3]. When serum
FSH exceeds a certain level, which varies from individual to individual, a "follicular cohort" is recruited in both ovaries as they reach follicular maturation.
In the normal biphasic cycle, the FSH surge begins in the late luteal phase and
continues into the early follicular phase of the following cycle. The recruitment
of the follicular cohort is completed by day 3 of the cycle. The dominant follicle then appears; i.e., one follicle matures faster and earlier than the others. The
exact selection mechanism is not known, but the relationship between the androgens produced in the theca cells and the capacity of the granulosa cells to

aromatize them to become estrogens seems to be one of several intraovarian mechanisms [4]. While FSH binds to the granulosa cells to induce estrogen synthesis, LH binds to the theca cells, which form the precursors needed for estradiol synthesis. Follicles accumulating insufficient quantities of FSH are exposed to excessive concentrations of nonaromatized androgens and are degraded [5]. The selection of the dominant follicle is completed by day 7 of the cycle. The dominant follicle phase is characterized by an exponential rise in serum estradiol. The negative feedback causes a fall in the concentrations of FSH and LH. When a maximum estradiol concentration of 150–500 pg/ml is reached immediately before ovulation, the positive feedback triggers a massive release of LH from the pituitary. The LH peak induces ovulation, which occurs about 10–12 h afterwards [6]. It also causes the formation of the corpus luteum, which is reflected in a rise in progesterone. The corpus luteum continues to produce progesterone for 14 days, initiating the hyperthermic phase of the cycle due to its thermogenetic effect. Afterwards the progesterone level falls, menstruation starts, the FSH and LH levels rise slightly, a new follicular cohort is recruited, and a new cycle begins.

Gonadotropin-Releasing Hormone

The GnRH molecule is a chain of ten amino acids (decapeptide) first isolated and characterized in 1971 by two independent groups that had competed against each other for 10 years. Schally and Guillemin were awarded the Nobel prize for their pioneering work in 1977 [7, 8]. Figure 1 shows the amino acid sequence of native GnRH. It has a half-life of only 2–5 min. It is quickly inactivated enzymatically by the corresponding peptidases, especially in position 6. The consequence is that the single GnRH pulses released by the hypothalamus can act individually on the adenopituitary gland. It was only in 1978 that the crucial relevance of this for the maintenance of ovarian function was recognized, when it was shown that continuous administration of GnRH causes a decline in the secretion of FSH/LH [9]. This means that while position 6 is important for the inactivation of the decapeptide, the amino acids in positions 2 and 3 are needed for gonadotropin release and those in positions 1, 6, and 10 for maintaining the spatial structure and for binding [10]. The GnRH molecule binds to specific receptors on the membranes of the gonadotropic cells of the adenopituitary. A gonadotropic cell is capable of secreting both FSH and LH, but these functions seem to change cyclically. The synthesis and the release of FSH and LH are regulated by GnRH.

1	2	3	4	5	6	7	8	9	10

pGlu - His - Trp - Ser - Tyr - Gly - Leu - Arg - Pro - Gly-NH2

Fig. 1. Amino acids in native GnRH

GnRH Receptor Binding

When the GnRH receptor is occupied, complexes are formed by microaggregation of the GnRH receptors. These complexes seem to be the basis for the action of GnRH. Evidence of their importance can be derived from the fact that researchers have managed to convert a GnRH antagonist into a potent agonist using "double-linked" antibodies [11]. In addition to microaggregation, binding to the GnRH receptor on the surface of a gonadotropic cell leads to a change in the conformation of the receptor itself. These changes induce the calcium-dependent release of gonadotropins, a process involving many other "second messengers" such as phospholipids, diacyl glycerol, protein kinase C, inositol phosphates, arachidonic acid, leukotrienes, and cyclic adenosine monophosphate (cAMP) [12] (Fig. 2).

Natural GnRH has a binding affinity to the pituitary of about 1 nM^{-1}. It appears to bind to two sites: those of high affinity, which represent the actual receptors for GnRH, and those of low affinity, probably endopeptidases. The number of GnRH receptors on the gonadotropic cell is subject to physiological variations. It is reduced in elderly women and during lactation but increased by ovariectomy [10].

After the GnRH molecule has bound to its receptor, the whole receptor complex is incorporated into the cell; this is followed by its degradation. The GnRH receptor complex does not have to be incorporated for the gonadotropins to be released, but incorporation does play a major role in the mechanism of action of agonistic GnRH analogues.

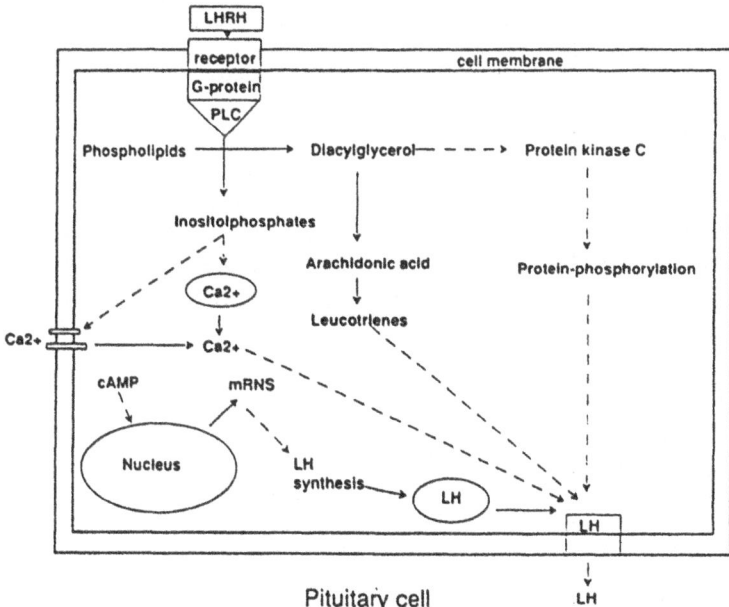

Fig. 2. Binding of GnRH at the gonadotropic cell of the anterior pituitary gland. (From [12])

Agonistic GnRH Analogues

Attempts have been made to modify the GnRH molecule to increase its resistance to enzymatic degradation and its affinity to the GnRH receptor. Agonistic GnRH analogues have been developed. Most structural modifications concern positions 6 and 10, and the modification of both sites has a cumulative effect [13]. Table 1 shows the available preparations and their amino acid sequences. These GnRH agonists have 100–200 times the affinity of native GnRH to GnRH receptors [12]. They were originally synthesized for a stronger and longer-lasting effect on the pituitary, and they cause an increased initial release of the FSH and LH stores and a short-term rise in the membrane-based receptors of the gonadotropic cell (up-regulation). When administered for a longer period, they simulate a chronic infusion of GnRH, and the pulsatile effect is neutralized. The agonist receptor complexes are incorporated, and the number of receptors falls. This process is commonly called down-regulation. The internalized agonist-receptor complexes are degraded by intracellular lysosomal enzymes, and the synthesis of new receptors is insufficient to cope with the loss of receptors. At the same time, postreceptor mechanisms are inhibited, and the synthesis of FSH and LH in the gonadotropic cell is reduced. The pituitary becomes refractory to the stimulating effect of native GnRH. The levels of FSH and LH in serum decline, their biological activity is depressed, and follicular maturation comes to a halt. Estradiol concentrations drop to the postmenopausal level (Fig. 3). The blockage of the pituitary function persists during therapy but is reversible afterwards. Follicular maturation can be suppressed chronically by daily intranasal or subcutaneous or monthly depot administration of the GnRH agonist. After therapy is discontinued, the cycle normalizes within an average of 6 weeks [14].

The "Flare-Up Effect"

It is important to note that the inhibitory effect of the GnRH agonists always occurs after an initial stimulatory effect. This flare-up triggers a fivefold increase in FSH concentration and a nearly tenfold rise in serum LH levels after 12 h. At the same time, estradiol levels rise briefly to about four times the base-

Table 1. GnRH and agonistic analogues

	1	2	3	4	5	6	7	8	9	10
GnRH	pGlu	His	Trp	Ser	Tyr	Gly	Leu	Arg	Pro	Gly-NH$_2$
Buserelin	1	2	3	4	5	D-Ser	7	8	9	Ethylamide
Goserelin	1	2	3	4	5	D-Ser	7	8	9	Az-Gly
Leuprorelin	1	2	3	4	5	D-Leu	7	8	9	Ethylamide
Triptorelin	1	2	3	4	5	D-Trp	7	8	9	Gly-NH$_2$
Nafarelin	1	2	3	4	5	D-Nal(2)	7	8	9	Gly-NH$_2$

Fig. 3. Pharmacological action of agonistic GnRH analogues. (From [12])

concentration of LHRH-receptors of the adeno hypophysis

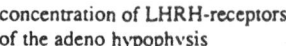
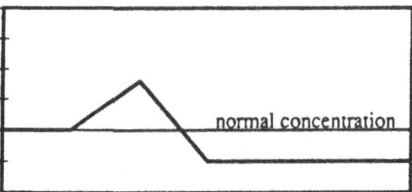

serum LH concentration

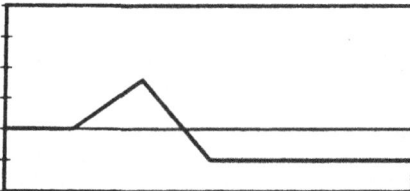

serum oestradiol

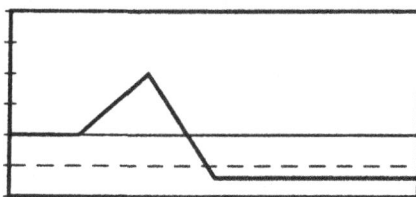

- - - - postmenopausal

line [15]. After the flare-up the levels decline continually, with FSH falling faster than LH. Postmenopausal estradiol levels are reached after an average of 21 days. Despite this flare-up, which is undesirable in nearly all cases, GnRH agonists have become common therapeutic agents when reversible medical castration is desired. They are used for endometriosis, uterus myomatosus, estrogen receptor-positive mammary cancer, prostate cancer, pubertas praecox, and infertility. Prior to the advent of GnRH agonists about 15–20% of stimulated cycles were lost due to a premature LH rise. The introduction of pretreatment by down-regulation reduced this rate to below 2% and increased the effectiveness of therapy, i.e., the rate of conception and pregnancy [16].

The fact that the negative effect of the flare-up is anything but negligible can be illustrated by the example of prostate cancer. The tumor flare syndrome is observed when bony metastases have formed, involving a deterioration in subjective complaints. For this reason the GnRH agonist is initially combined with the androgen antagonist cyproterone acetate before the desired suppression can start [17]. No similar observations have been made for gynecological indications, but a negative influence on these sexual steroid-dependent diseases can-

Table 2. Agonistic GnRH analogues (available preparations)

Substance	Pharmacology (half-life)	Preparation (manufacturer)	Formulation	Dosage
Buserelin	GnRH agonist, 120 times as potent as LH–RH (70–80 min)	Suprefact (Hoechst)	Nasal spray	1200 µg/day as a nasal spray; depending on indication, 600–900 µg is adequate
Buserelin acetate	GnRH agonist, 100 times as potent as LH–RH	Suprecur (Hoechst)	Nasal spray	900 µg daily as a nasal spray; 3 × 300 µg/day
Leuprorelin 'acetate	GnRH agonist, 50–80 times as potent as LH–RH (3 h)	Enantone Gyn Depot (Takeda)	Depot injection with 3.75 mg (prepacked)	1 amp/month
		Enantone uno (Takeda)	Injection solution with 1 µg/0.2 ml	Depending on indication
Goserelin	GnRH agonist; 100 times as potent as LH–RH (12 h)	Zoladex Gyn (Zeneca)	Implant 13 × 1.2 mm, 3.6 mg Goserelin s.c. prepacked	Every 28 days
Triptorelin	GnRH agonist D-Trp-6-LH–RH	Decapeptyl (Ferring)	Depot injection 3.75 mg (prepacked)	1 amp/month; daily release rate 100 µg for 21–30 days
		Decapeptyl 0.5 mg/0.1 mg (Ferring)	Prepacked injection with 0.5 mg/ 0.1 mg/ml	Depending on indication
Nafarelin 'acetate	GnRH agonist, 200 times as potent as LH–RH (2–4 h)	Synarella (Syntex)	Nasal spray	400–800 µg/day nasal spray

not be ruled out completely. In any event, about 3 weeks of therapeutic effect is lost. Table 2 lists the preparations currently available for clinical use, including their pharmacology, formulation, and dosage.

Use of GnRH Agonists for Controlled Ovarian Stimulation

The use of GnRH agonists for the purposes of ovarian stimulation marks the beginning of the "modern management" of assisted reproduction. The premature LH surge is responsible for the reduced effectiveness of ovarian stimulation by human menopausal gonadotropin (hMG) in an in vitro fertilization (IVF) program. At the same time, it negatively affects oocyte and embryo quality and the pregnancy rate [18, 19]. The introduction of agonist treatment has remedied most of these difficulties and drawbacks, and the rate of stimulated cycles which must be terminated has been brought down to 2% [16]. Ovulation induction has become planable, so that the psychological pressure on patients and physicians has been eased to some extent. Suppression of endogenous hormone production by GnRH analogues followed by hMG stimulation has developed from second-line into first-line therapy.

The Short and Ultrashort Protocols

Both the short and the ultrashort protocol try to harness the initial increase in gonadotropin secretion (flare-up) for follicular stimulation [20, 21]. Under the short protocol the GnRH agonist is given subcutaneously (e.g., buserelin 600 mg/day) or intranasally (e.g., 2 × 2 puffs of 200 mg nafarelin/day) from day 1 of the cycle to the induction of ovulation with human chorionic gonadotropin (hCG) [22]. hMG stimulation starts 2–3 days after the first agonist dose (Fig. 4).

Under the ultrashort protocol the GnRH agonist is administered subcutaneously or intranasally only on days 2–4 of the cycle. hMG stimulation starts on day 2, and ovulation induction with hCG begins when the well-known criteria are fulfilled (dominant follicle about 20 mm and estradiol about 400 pg/ml per follicle > 15 mm; Fig. 5).

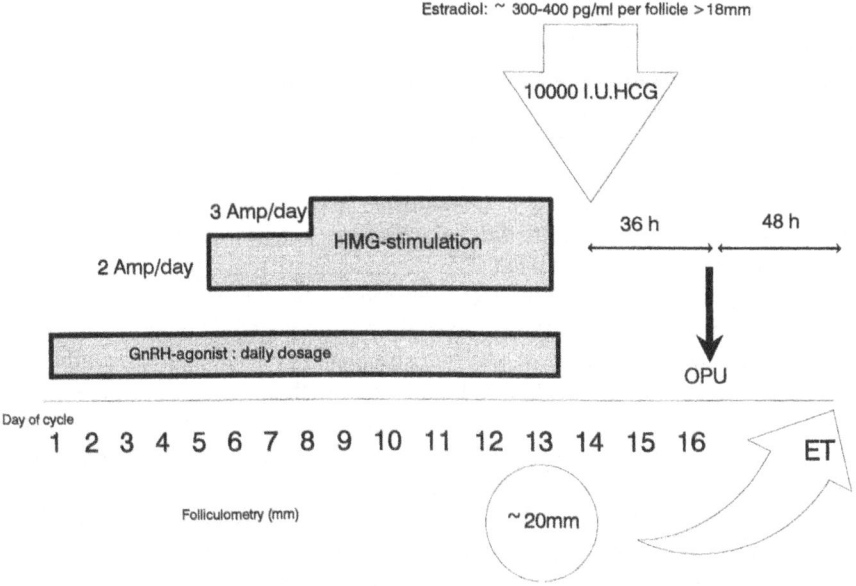

Fig. 4. Ovarian stimulation with hMG after pretreatment with GnRH agonists: the "short protocol"

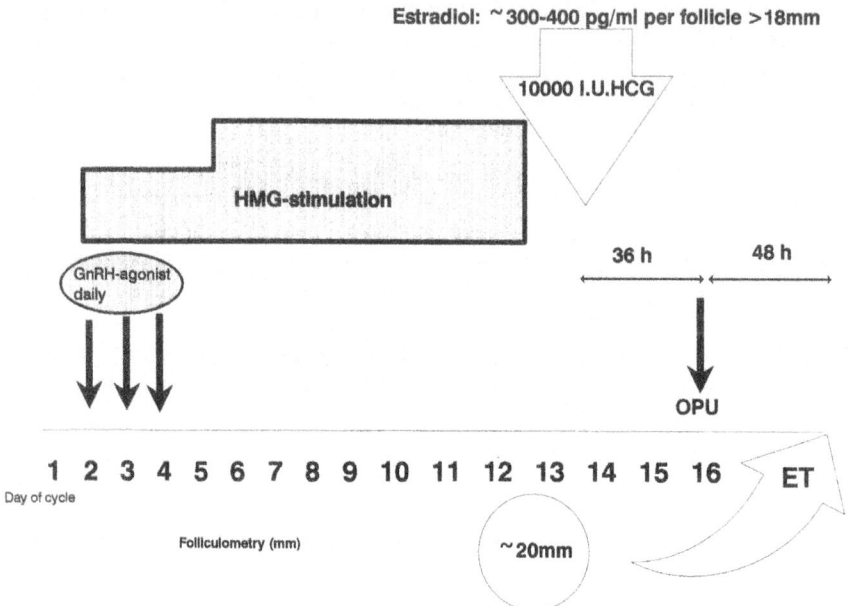

Fig. 5. Ovarian stimulation with hMG after pretreatment with GnRH agonists: the "ultrashort protocol"

Patient Monitoring in the Short and Ultrashort Protocols

The patient is monitored daily by measuring serum estradiol and LH combined with vaginal ultrasound to assess follicular growth, starting on day 5 of the cycle. On day 1, a baseline ultrasound is required before stimulation begins so as to exclude any functional ovarian cysts (>15 mm) or cystic adnexae caused by other factors.

If such factors are present, a spontaneous cycle or gestagen-induced menstruation should be awaited. If the cystic finding persists, it should be investigated before stimulation is started.

Both protocols are reliable ways of preventing a premature LH rise. Their advantage is that they prolong the stimulated cycle only slightly, if at all. At a consumption of about 27 ampules of hMG per stimulated cycle, both are cost-efficient, and consumption is only negligibly higher than with no analogue pretreatment [23]. One disadvantage is the increased LH concentration in the early follicular phase due to increased secretion of endogenous gonadotropin, which can affect follicular maturation adversely [24, 25]. In terms of the number of oocytes retrieved and embryos transferred, the long protocol has proven superior in prospective comparative studies [23]. Retrospective studies show that the long-term protocol yields significantly better pregnancy rates irrespective of the analogue used [26], and in prospective studies they were also higher under the long than under the short protocol (25.7% vs. 16.6%), but the difference was not significant [27].

The Long Protocol

The long protocol has become the standard method at most major centers. It aims at desensitizing the pituitary before hMG stimulation commences. For this purpose, the GnRH agonist is administered either daily subcutaneously or transnasally or in the form of a subcutaneous (e.g., 3.6 mg goserelin) or intramuscular (e.g., 3.2 mg triptorelin) depot preparation from the midluteal (day 22) or early follicular phase (day 1). The advantage of starting medication in the midluteal phase is that the flare-up coincides with the physiological rise in gonadotropin. The drawback is that therapy may accidentally clash with an existing pregnancy at a very early stage. However, no teratogenic effects of GnRH analogues are known [28]. No statistically significant advantages of one regimen over the other have so far emerged [29].

Patient Monitoring in the Long Protocol

Fourteen days after the start of GnRH agonist medication, it can be assumed that the hypothalamic-pituitary-ovarian axis has essentially been decoupled. The baseline hormone status is now assessed. hMG stimulation may start at LH levels below 10 mIU/ml and estradiol below 50 pg/ml, but the patient is first examined by vaginal ultrasound to exclude functional ovarian cysts. Such cysts occur in about 13–25% of the stimulated cycles, mainly under the first long protocol [30, 31]. In most cases, they are follicular cysts caused by the stimulatory flare-up acting on an already-growing follicle. Due to the subsequent pituitary blockade, however, these follicles do not ovulate and remain at the stage of functional cysts. Since this can cause an increase in the consumption of hMG and an enlargement of the ovaries, they should be treated prior to stimulation [32]. We recommend a transvaginal puncture. Alternatively, under the long protocol, regression of the cysts can be awaited as the administration of agonists continues. Regression seems to occur earlier when agonist administration has started in the midluteal phase [33].

Stimulation begins with two ampules of hMG daily on days 1, 2, and 3. On days 4–7, the patient receives three ampules of hMG daily, and from day 8, regular measurements of estradiol and LH are taken along with transvaginal ultrasound folliculometry to determine the subsequent dosage of hMG. When the patient has entered the active phase with continuously rising estradiol levels, the dose can be maintained. Until this phase is reached, the dose can be slowly increased by one ampule at a time at 2-day intervals. If the stimulated cycle proves unsuccessful after IVF and embryo transfer, the dose can be increased faster in the next cycle until the individual threshold is reached.

As soon as one or preferably several follicles measuring about 20 mm are identified by folliculometry and estradiol increases to a level of about 300–400 pg/ml per follicle larger than 17 mm, 10 000 IU hCG is administered i.m. in the evening (patient consent required). Follicular puncture monitored by transvaginal ultrasound is performed 36 h later under mild sedation or general anesthetic, as desired by the patient (Fig. 6). The timing of puncture has become

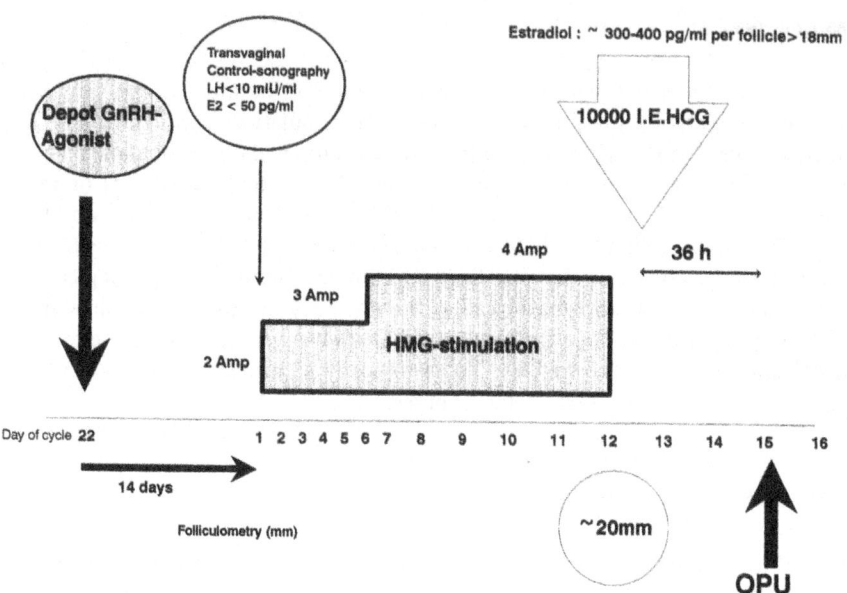

Fig. 6. Ovarian stimulation with hMG after pretreatment with GnRH agonists: the "long protocol"

fully calculable under this regimen and can be set to suit the requirements of both the center and the couple. It is no problem to postpone ovulation induction by 24 or 48 h for any reason, since some working groups have achieved even better results if the follicles were left to grow to an average diameter of 23 mm than under the standard regimen described above [34].

The long protocol synchronizes follicle maturation and makes it possible to select a larger number of follicles or oocytes for IVF than with the other protocols. A disadvantage is the high consumption of hMG, which averages 45 ampules per stimulated cycle [35]. This makes the therapy much more expensive.

The Effect of GnRH Agonist Medication on the Luteal Phase

An inadequate luteal phase after ovarian stimulation with hMG preceded by pituitary down-regulation by the GnRH agonist (long protocol) was first described by Smitz et al. in 1987 [36]. Eight days after the administration of hCG the serum levels of both progesterone and estradiol drop sharply. Pituitary LH secretion remains blocked until the end of the luteal phase and leads to premature luteolysis, thereby removing the stimulus necessary for the large number of corpora lutea [37]. Endometrial biopsies have shown a delay of secretory conversion in more than 50% of the stimulated cycles [38]. The GnRH agonists enter the growing follicles and bind to the GnRH receptors of the granulosa cells [39]. This could be the cause of reduced progesterone synthesis, as has been suggested by in vitro studies [40].

Luteal Support

Ovarian stimulation under the long protocol requires support in the luteal phase. Support may be provided in the form of further doses of hCG (5000 IU i.m. on days 2 and 5 after follicle puncture). This ensures a timely development of the endometrium and a corresponding increase in pregnancy rates [41]. However, this treatment may also cause or aggravate an ovarian hyperstimulation syndrome (OHSS) if multiple follicles are luteinized [42]. A now common alternative is to administer natural progesterone intravaginally over 14 days (3 × 2 Utrogestan vaginal tablets = 3 × 200 mg micronized progesterone daily) as an effective and safe method [43].

Luteal Phase Support as a Function of Response

The choice of medication must therefore be based on the response of the individual patient. We recommend the following approach:
- Estradiol levels below 2000 pg/ml at the time of follicular puncture: the patient is given 5000 IU hCG i.m. on the day of embryo transfer and again on day 5 after follicle puncture.
- Estradiol levels between 2000 and 5000 pg/ml at the time of follicular puncture and more than 15 follicles: 3 × 2 tablets of Utrogestan are administered daily for 14 days from the day of puncture. Additionally, 5000 IU hCG is given i.m. on the day of embryo transfer.
- Estradiol levels above 5000 pg/ml at the time of follicular puncture and/or more than 15 follicles: 2 × 2 tablets of Utrogestan are administered over 14 days from the day of puncture. No additional hCG is given. The same approach is taken if the patient has been diagnosed to suffer from polycystic ovary syndrome (PCO) with a hyperandrogenemic hormone status [44].

Agonistic GnRH Analogues for Uterus Myomatosus, Endometriosis, and Sexual Steroid-Dependent Malignomas

Although the flare-up effect is nearly always undesirable, GnRH agonists have become the therapy of choice wherever a temporary chemical castration is sought. This applies to the therapy of endometriosis, uterus myomatosus, estrogen receptor-positive mammary cancer, prostatic cancer, and pubertas praecox.

Patients with large myomas scheduled for a fertility-preserving operation, those with hemoglobin-reducing hypermenorrhea, and those scheduled for hysteroscopic ablation of myomas are commonly treated preoperatively with GnRH agonists. These therapies are rather effective; on average, myomas shrink by about 50% within 3–6 months. In the case of endometriosis GnRH analogues have become established alongside danazol as part of a three-step concept (primary surgery, follow-up drug treatment, second-look operation). All clinical symptoms of endometriosis are relieved markedly by GnRH agonists [45].

Antagonistic GnRH Analogues

In parallel with the development of agonists, other substances have been synthe-sized which also bind to the pituitary receptor for the GnRH molecule but do not trigger the secretion of gonadotropin. Several hundred of these so-called GnRH antagonists, which cause an immediate and sustained blockage of the pi-tuitary against native GnRH, have been synthesized since its discovery, by changing the amino acid sequence at positions 1, 2, 3, 6, and 10.

Histamine Release

The first generation of these GnRH antagonists proved to be effective only in vitro. At a higher dose they also produced an effect in vivo. Within hours the level of gonadotropins and sexual steroids dropped [13]. However, allergic side effects of varying degree occurred because of the histamine-releasing action of these agents. Localized reddening and induration as well as generalized edemas and anaphylactoid reactions made clinical application impossible. The localized and systemic histamine-releasing effect seems to be due to the presence of GnRH receptors on histamine-storing mast cells. When they are occupied by the GnRH antagonists, the histamine deposits degranulate [12]. Native GnRH can also release histamine, but in much smaller amounts (ED_{50} for native GnRH = 186 mg/ml; ED_{50} = molar concentration of a peptide releasing 50% of all the histamine to be released from rat peritoneum). On the molecular level, this effect seems to be due to a combination of the amino acid D-arginine in position 6 with hydrophobic amino acids at the N-terminal end. The hydropho-bic nature of the GnRH antagonists is the reason why the substances tend to jell after administration.

On account of these side effects antagonists initially appeared less likely to be used in therapy than agonists. The ideal GnRH antagonist was expected to have a potent and sustained effect with no histamine release and no jelling.

Modern GnRH Antagonists

When the second and especially the third generation of GnRH antagonists were developed, this goal came within reach. Figure 7 shows the structural formulas of the more recent GnRH antagonists Nal-Glu, Antide, and Cetrorelix, for which the largest body of clinical data is available. Cetrorelix seems to be the only sub-stance to have reached market maturity. In four studies covering more than 100 subjects no patient had to be excluded because of allergic side effects [46–49]. Compared with other antagonists, Cetrorelix is clearly the most potent per unit of weight.

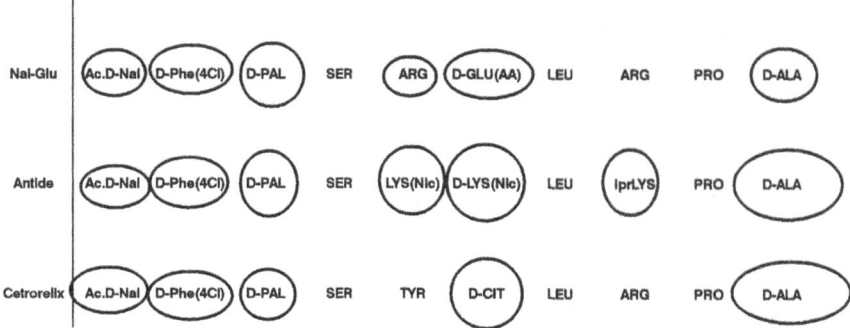

Fig. 7. Modern GnRH antagonists: Nal-Glu, Antide, Cetrorelix

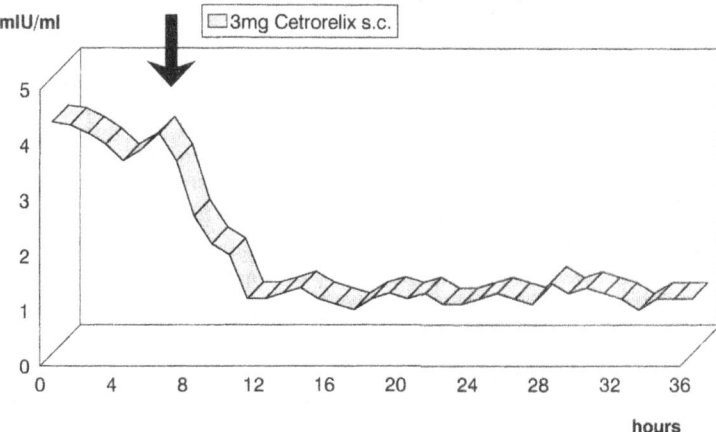

Fig. 8. Mean serum concentrations of LH (mIU/ml) after subcutaneous administration of 3 mg Cetrorelix in 30 healthy women with normal cycles. (From [46])

Mechanism of Action of GnRH Antagonists

The effect of GnRH antagonists is based on a completely different mechanism from that of the agonists. While agonists desensitize the gonadotropic cells by down-regulating the GnRH receptors, GnRH antagonists compete with native GnRH for binding to the receptors on the cell membranes, prevent their micro-aggregation, and block the postreceptor mechanism. Antagonists are devoid of any intrinsic activity and lead to a classic competitive inhibition at the GnRH receptor based on the law of mass action; therefore, their effect depends much more on dose than that of the agonists does. The antagonistic action on the pituitary is direct, i.e., without any intermediate stimulation.

Figure 8 shows the mean serum LH levels over time after subcutaneous administration of 3 mg in 30 healthy women ovulating regularly. Within 8 h LH levels start to fall, and sharply reduced levels are reached after 16 h [46]. In

1991, Dittkoff et al. showed that a GnRH antagonist applied for a short period is capable of suppressing the ovulation-inducing midcycle LH peak [50]. They administered 50 mg of Nal-Glu per kg body wt. and day for 4 days. The LH peak failed to occur, estradiol production came to a halt, and follicular growth was interrupted. After the antagonists were discontinued, gonadal function normalized within days, whereas this period may be as long as 6 weeks after down-regulation by agonists. Apparently, antagonists neither deplete the FSH and LH stores of gonadotropic cells nor inhibit gonadotropin synthesis.

Maintenance of Pituitary Response under GnRH Antagonists

Because of competitive inhibition it is possible to fine-tune the antigonadotropic effect by selecting the dose of the antagonist, either maintaining a residual secretion of estradiol or suppressing it completely, depending on the indication for therapy. This could help to avoid such typical side effects as hot flushes, sweating, and vaginal dryness. [51].

The pituitary remains susceptible to stimulation by GnRH and continues to react adequately. The maintenance of the pituitary response was demonstrated convincingly by a GnRH test in 20 patients treated with Cetrorelix at the start of an IVF program [52]. All patients were stimulated with hMG from day 2 of their cycles. Fifteen patients additionally received 3 mg Cetrorelix daily s.c. and five patients were given 1 mg Cetrorelix daily s.c., starting on day 7. Three hours prior to ovulation induction all patients received 25 mg GnRH. LH levels were measured before and 30 or 180 min after GnRH administration. LH levels were greatly suppressed in both groups by the antagonist. In the case of pretreatment with 3 mg Cetrorelix, LH levels reached an average of 10 mIU/ml 30 min after GnRH administration, while 32.5 mIU/ml on average were attained after pretreatment with 1 mg Cetrorelix (Fig. 9). It is also possible to restore the ovulatory cycle during an antagonist-induced suppressed phase with pulsatile GnRH [53]. This is the treatment regimen for infertile patients with hypothalamic dysfunction (WHO I), in whom ovulatory cycles can be induced with a GnRH pump (Zyklomat, Ferring) in more than 90% of cases [54].

GnRH Antagonists in Infertility Treatment

There has been a debate about the merits of the long protocol, aiming at complete pituitary desensitization before the start of hMG stimulation, compared with the short and ultrashort protocols, exploiting the flare-up. The long protocol as the most effective method has won the argument. However, its disadvantage is its long duration and high cost because large amounts of hMG are required. For this reason GnRH antagonists have a place in IVF programs.

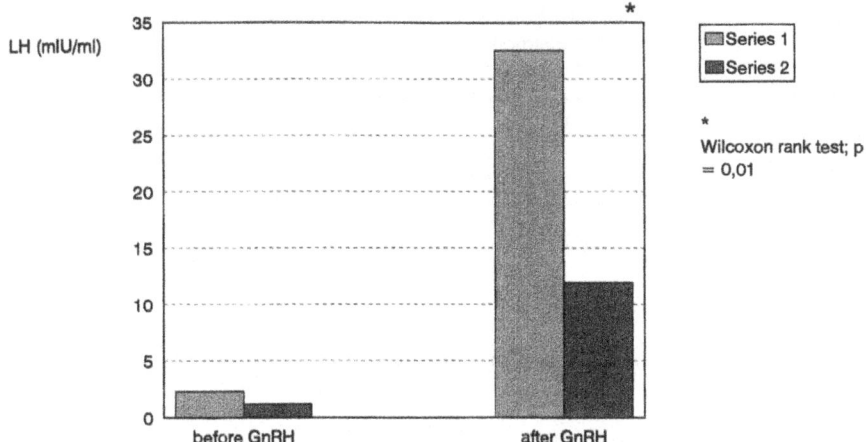

Fig. 9. Serum LH levels (mIU/ml) 30 min after GnRH; pretreatment with 3 mg (series 2: *n*=15) and 1 mg Cetrorelix (series 1: *n* = 5) daily

The Lübeck Protocol

Diedrich et al. used the regimen described in Fig. 10 to stimulate 15 patients, some of whom had shown a premature LH rise in preceding cycles. Five other patients received 1 mg instead of 3 mg/day Cetrorelix s.c. from day 7 to the day of ovulation induction [48]. Figures 11 and 12 show estradiol, progesterone, FSH, and LH concentrations over time. In no case did a premature LH surge occur. A total of 144 oocytes were retrieved, an average of 8.1 per patient. The fertilization rate was 61.5%; 42% of the embryos available for transfer were of excellent quality. The average number of hMG ampules used per cycle was 27. Under the long protocol the usual consumption per cycle is 40–50 ampules. This means that the amount of Cetrorelix required is within the range of the ultrashort protocol, which used to be considered cheapest [55]. Diedrich et al. supported the luteal phase with 5000 IU hCG on days 2 and 5 after follicular puncture, applying their experience with the agonist protocol to the antagonists. Whether this is really necessary remains to be determined in further studies. After Nal-Glu administration over 4 days at midcycle, ovulation occurred spontaneously, and the luteal phase was normal [50].

Ovarian Stimulation with hMG and Concomitant GnRH Antagonists at Different Doses

Thirty-five patients with tubal infertility and no other infertility factors to be observed were stimulated with hMG from the second day of the cycle. From day 7 up to ovulation induction with hCG 12 patients received the antagonist Cetrorelix at a dose of 3 mg/day subcutaneously, 12 patients received 1 mg, and a further 11 were treated with a dose of 0.5 mg. On day 5 the dose of hMG was

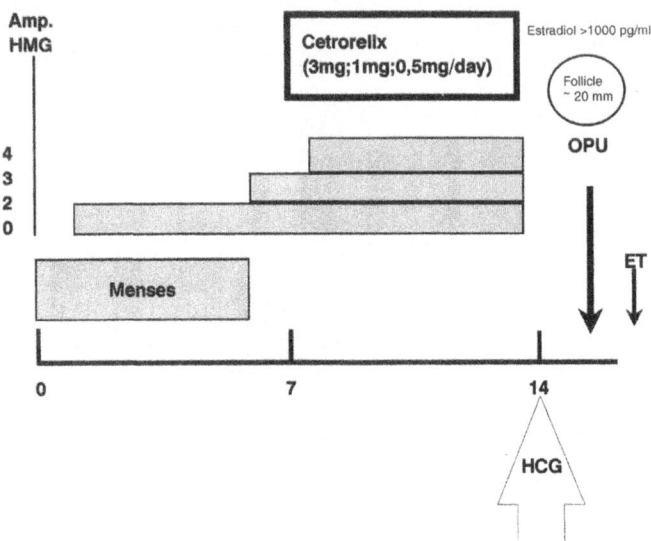

Fig. 10. Controlled ovarian hyperstimulation with hMG and concomitant GnRH antagonist administration (Cetrorelix): the Lübeck protocol

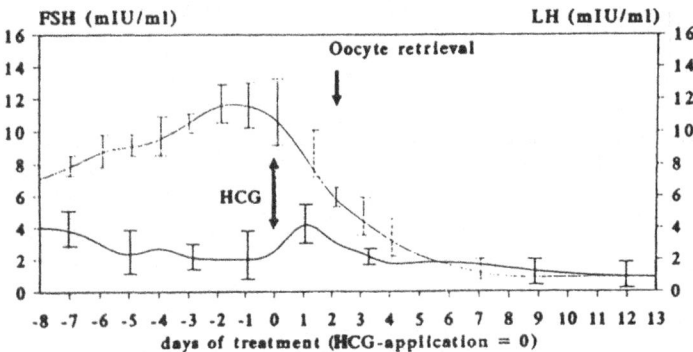

Fig. 11. Serum LH and FSH levels (mIU/ml) under controlled ovarian hyperstimulation with hMG and concomitant GnRH antagonist administration (Cetrorelix; mean ± SEM)

adjusted to the individual patient depending on ultrasound findings and estradiol levels. Treatment continued with 10 000 IU hCG up to ovulation if the dominant follicle was 18–20 mm in size and the estradiol levels indicated adequate follicular maturation. Transvaginal follicular puncture, IVF, and embryo transfer followed as usual in our IVF program. To support the luteal phase, patients received 5000 IU hCG i.m. on days 2 and 5 after follicular puncture. During the stimulated cycle, blood samples were collected daily to determine FSH, LH, estradiol, and progesterone. Figures 13 and 14 show the mean concentrations of FSH and LH over time. The levels of LH were below 2 mIU/ml from

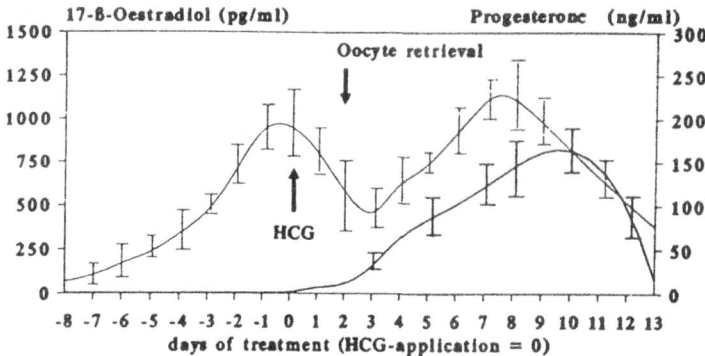

Fig. 12. Serum estradiol (pg/ml) and progesterone levels (ng/ml) under controlled ovarian hyperstimulation with hMG and concomitant GnRH antagonist administration (Cetrorelix; mean ± SEM)

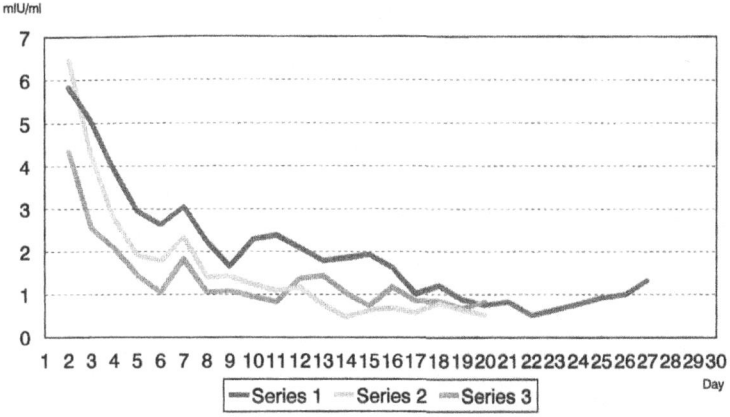

Fig. 13. Mean serum concentrations of FSH (mIU/ml) under controlled ovarian hyperstimulation with hMG and concomitant Cetrorelix administration at various dosages (series 1: 3 mg; series 2: 1 mg; series 3: 0.5 mg)

day 12 onwards. No premature endogenous LH rise was observed, and in no case die treatment have to be discontinued for this reason.

A continuous dose-dependent rise in estradiol concentrations was observed at all three doses. The rise between days 7 and 11 was much steeper in the 0.5-mg group than in the other two groups (Fig. 15). On day 10 maximum levels of 2164±2102 pg/ml were reached in the 0.5-mg group, compared with 852±325 pg/ml in the 3-mg group and 1022±602 pg/ml in the group receiving 1 mg Cetrorelix. The considerable standard deviation under 0.5 mg/ml can be attributed to one low responder in this group. Ovulation was not induced in this patient, but her hormone profile was included in the statistical analysis. In a matched-pair comparison of the rise in concentration on days 7–11 between

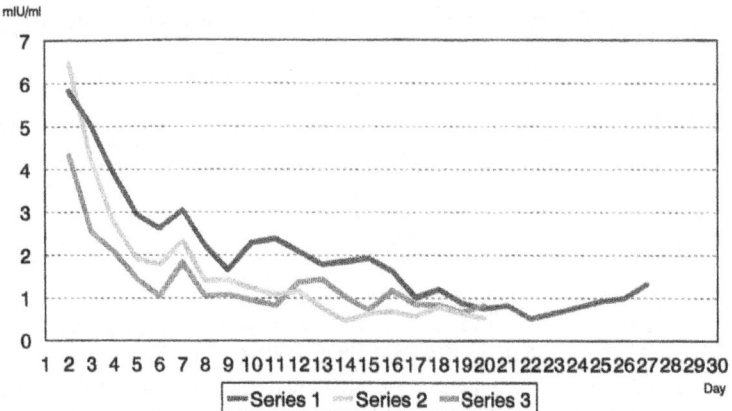

Fig. 14. Mean serum concentrations of LH (mIU/ml) under controlled ovarian hyperstimulation with hMG and concomitant Cetrorelix administration at various dosages (series 1: 3 mg; series 2: 1 mg; series 3: 0.5 mg)

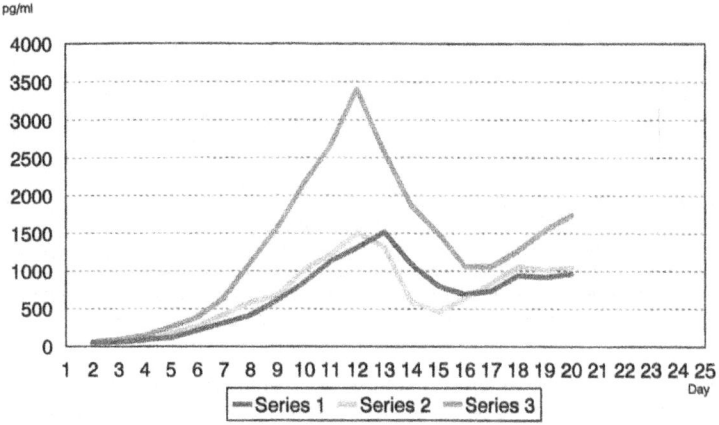

Fig. 15. Mean serum concentrations of estradiol (pg/ml) under controlled ovarian hyperstimulation with hMG and concomitant Cetrorelix administration at various dosages (series 1: 3 mg; series 2: 1 mg; series 3: 0.5 mg)

the patients treated with 0.5 mg and those treated with 1 mg, the Wilcoxon rank sum test suggested a difference in the gradient of the curve. Of course, due to the retrospective approach, this statistical analysis is of a merely explorative nature.

As expected, progesterone levels rose after day 12 of the cycle. No progesterone rise was observed during the follicular phase. hCG was administered for ovulation induction between days 10 and 14 (Fig. 16). The fertilization rate of the oocytes retrieved by follicular puncture was 45.3% in the 3-mg group, 53.2% in the 1-mg group, and 67.7% in the 0.5-mg group. In the 3-mg group

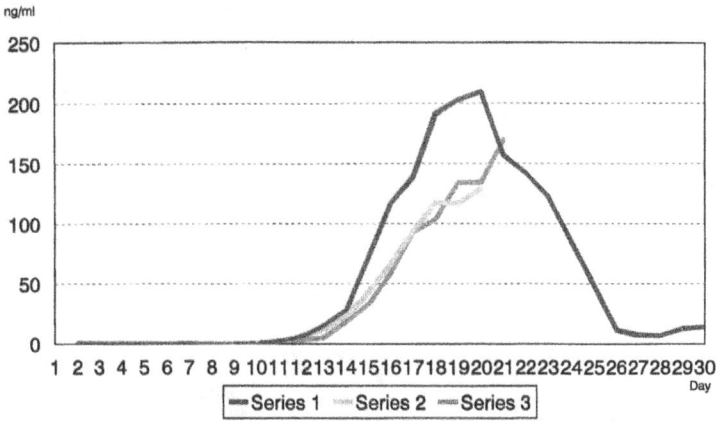

Fig. 16. Mean serum concentrations of progesterone (ng/ml) under controlled ovarian hyperstimulation with hMG and concomitant Cetrorelix administration at various dosages (series 1: 3 mg; series 2: 1 mg; series 3: 0.5 mg)

106 oocytes were retrieved and 30 embryos replaced after IVF. Of these, 36.7% were considered "excellent" by microscopic-morphological criteria [56]. In the 1-mg group 94 oocytes were retrieved, 28 embryos replaced, and 53.6% of them judged "excellent". In the 0.5-mg group 27 of 127 retrieved oocytes were replaced as embryos, of which 37% were "excellent". We cannot specify the cleavage rate after successful fertilization since, under the German Embryo Protection Act, the decision regarding which embryos are to be replaced must be made as early as in the pronuclear stage [57] (Table 3).

The average consumption of hMG per stimulated cycle was 30 ampules in the 3-mg group, 27 in the 1-mg group, and 26 in the 0.5-mg group. These differences are not statistically significant. The administration of 0.5 mg/day Cetrorelix s.c. from day 7 until the induction of ovulation is sufficient for the reliable prevention of an endogenous premature LH surge. This puts the stimulation protocol described above (Lübeck protocol) in the same league as the mode of administration published by Olivennes et al. [58]. They administered a single dose of Cetrorelix when serum estradiol levels reached between 150 and 200 pg/ml. A second injection was given 48 h later if ovulation had failed to occur in the meantime. The single dose was 5 mg (Fig. 17). No premature LH surge has been seen so far among 17 women treated under this protocol either [58].

As is the case with long agonist treatment, the luteal phase was supported in both study protocols. Under the Lübeck protocol natural hCG was used, while Olivennes et al. chose natural progesterone, administered intravaginally. Whether this is really necessary remains to be determined in other studies, since no luteal phase defect was found in the study by Dittkoff et al. after the GnRH antagonist Nal-Glu given at midcycle had been discontinued [50].

Judged by the gradients of estradiol rise, the ovaries were more sensitive to hMG stimulation in the 0.5-mg group than in the groups receiving higher doses. Because of the small number of subjects and the retrospective evaluation

Table 3. Controlled ovarian hyperstimulation with hMG and concomitant Cetrorelix at 3, 1, and 0.5 mg

	3 mg	1 mg	0.5 mg
No. of oocytes	106	94	127
Fertilization rate (%)	45.3	53.2	67.7
No. of embryos	30	28	27
Proportion of 'excellent' embryos (%)	36.7	53.6	37

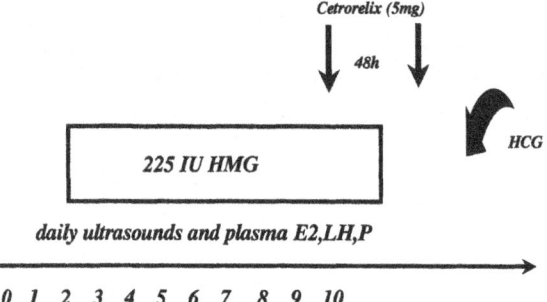

Fig. 17. Single or dual administration of Cetrorelix in IVF with embryo transfer. (From [58])

method, however, this is a mere observation rather than a statistically confirmed conclusion. Furthermore, there is no consistent explanation for this finding, since gonadotropin levels do not match it. At the moment it would be pure speculation to look for possible explanations on a paracrine-ovarian level, as has been discussed for GnRH agonists [55, 59].

Judging by the rate of fertilization of the oocytes retrieved after IVF, the lowest Cetrorelix dose of 0.5 mg/day was the most successful. At 28 ampules hMG per stimulated cycle for all three doses taken together, mean consumption was within the range of the short agonist protocol, which aims to integrate the flare-up of the gonadotropins into the stimulation but yields far lower fertilization rates. The average amount of hMG in the long agonist protocol, which attempts to reach complete desensitization of the pituitary before the onset of stimulation, is 40 ampules. The advantages of GnRH antagonists used in IVF are shorter stimulation, reduced hMG consumption, and lower costs.

Polycystic Ovary Syndrome

GnRH agonists have now been used for about 10 years to treat patients with polycystic ovary syndrome (PCO) [60]. It has become clear that the long-term administration of an agonist reduces the secretion of estradiol and ovarian androgens. The latter effect seems to be caused by reduced bioactive LH levels. Suppressing the pathological gonadotropin secretion (increase in the LH/FSH ratio) corrects the disruptive effect on the ovaries. After reaching suppression FSH/LH or FSH alone can normalize follicular maturation and synchronize the growth of the follicles. Unfortunately, pretreatment with GnRH agonists does not prevent hyperstimulation syndromes [61]. On the contrary, it has been shown that hMG stimulation following down-regulation results in a higher rate of OHSS than hMG therapy alone. Half of these cases were considered severe [33]. This effect is attributed to the more readily achieved high estradiol levels, resulting from the synchronous and rapid maturation of many follicles. In high-risk patients hyperstimulation can be reliably prevented by refraining from ovulation induction. The way in which the luteal phase is supported also plays an important role. When progesterone is given (e.g., 3×2 50-mg vaginal suppositories daily), the complication rate is probably lower in these risk patients than under repeated doses of hCG [43]. We can conclude that a patient with PCO must be monitored closely and frequently during therapy. Compared with GnRH agonists, antagonists have the advantage of immediate gonadotropin suppression without an initial flare-up. Furthermore, the suppression of LH secretion by GnRH antagonists seems to be more effective than that of FSH; this could be beneficial in those cases of PCO characterized by an LH/FSH ratio shifted in favor of LH.

Ovarian Hyperstimulation Syndrome

In the course of ovarian stimulation with hMG ovulation is normally induced by hCG. This effect is based on the similarity in molecular structure and biological activity of LH and hCG [62]. hCG can imitate the midcycle LH peak typical for a spontaneous cycle. Despite the similarity, hCG does not provoke the same physiological reaction as endogenous LH. It has a longer half-life than LH and fails to produce the physiological FSH rise at midcycle [63]. The extent to which these mechanisms play a role in the genesis of hyperstimulation is unclear, but researchers agree that the syndrome constitutes a serious complication of ovulation induction after treatment with gonadotropins. OHSS is characterized by massively enlarged ovaries, hemoconcentration, electrolytic changes, ascites, and an increased risk of thromboembolism. Women who are under 35 years of age and have PCO, very high estradiol levels under stimulation (>5000 pg/ml), and multiple immature and intermediary follicles seem to be at a particular risk of developing OHSS after ovulation induction.

Subsequent dose-finding studies using 0.5 mg Cetrorelix/day as well as 0.25 mg Cetrorelix/day and 0.1 mg Cetrorelix/day proved the efficacy and safety of 0.25 mg Cetrorelix/day in avoiding premature LH surges, while under 0.1 mg Cetrorelix/day premature LH surges were observed [64, 65]. In these studies ICSI for treatment of male subfertility was allowed, leading to fertilization rates within the range to be expected after normal oocyte maturation. It is really essential to emphasize that stepping down with the dosage of Cetrorelix did not have any negative impact on treatment outcome. There were no significant differences regarding two-pronuclei fertilization rates, increase in estradiol values, cleavage rate, clinical pregnancy rate per ET, and implantation rate between the group treated with 0.5 mg Cetrorelix/day and those patients treated with only 0.25 mg/day. The clinical pregnancy rates per transfer were 30.7% in the 0.5 mg group and 29.6% in the 0.25 mg group.

The "French Protocol": Single-Shot Injection

In parallel to the multiple-dose administration, a certainly different protocol for administration of GnRH antagonists within COH was developed by the French investigators Bouchard, Frydman and Olivennes, in which the compound was used in a dosage of 2 mg or 3 mg as single or dual administration around day 9. In this protocol the antagonist was injected at the time when estradiol reaches 150–200 pg/ml and the follicle size is > 14 mm, which usually is the case on day 8 or 9 of the cycle [59, 66]. They have not observed premature LH rises in any of the cycles studied and published to date. Since it was demonstrated that 3 mg Cetrorelix is able to suppress LH values for as long as 96 h, acting like an intermediate depot preparation, the protocol was modified: 3 mg Cetrorelix is now injected at cycle day 8 as a "jour fixe". If within these 96 h the criteria for ovulation induction are not met, 0.25 mg Cetrorelix is administered as daily injections. The injection of 3 mg Cetrorelix was capable of preventing LH surges in the patients treated, introducing a very simple treatment protocol. Clinical pregnancy rates of over 30% per transfer are reported, which sound very promising.

Luteal Phase Support in COH with Gonadotropins and GnRH Antagonist

After having discontinued the midcycle administration of 50 µg Nal-Glu per kg body wt. per day in women with normal cycles, Dittkoff and colleagues reported spontaneous ovulation after a certain delay and a normal, noncompromised luteal phase afterwards [50]. Based on this observation, it seemed reasonable to question the necessity of luteal phase support in COH with gonadotropins and GnRH antagonists for ART. However, using 0.5 mg Cetrorelix per day according to the multiple-dose protocol without luteal phase support in five patients, the luteal phase appeared to be insufficient, with preterm bleeding in all of these patients [67]. For this reason, in all subsequent study patients luteal phase support was performed either by repeated injections of hCG or by transvaginal administration of micronized progesterone. To date, luteal phase support seems to be mandatory in the case of COH with gonadotropins and concomitant GnRH antagonist treatment.

Results of Phase-III Studies

Both protocols described have been used in prospective, randomized, open-label phase-III studies, comparing the results obtained in the GnRH antagonist groups with those of treatment according to the long agonistic protocol.

A total of 188 patients treated with Cetrorelix in its minimal effective dose of 0.25 mg/day according to the multiple-dose protocol were compared with 85 patients treated according to the long protocol, using Buserelin as a nasal spray for desensitization of the pituitary gland. While in 84% of the patients in the antagonist group it was possible to perform an embryo transfer, this was the case in only 79% of the agonist group, reflecting a lower cancellation rate using Cetrorelix. The clinical pregnancy rate (intrauterine pregnancies with documented heart activity of the embryo) was 27% per transfer in the antagonist group and 33% in the agonist group. However, this difference was not statistically significant. Also, no differences were to be found in the implantation rates, which were 15.3% after the antagonist was used and 16.7% after COH according to the long protocol. Concerning those patients treated with ICSI due to infertility of the male partner, there were no differences to be observed regarding either oocytes in the metaphase II or fertilization rates after ICSI. Interestingly, the percentage of excellent embryos to be transferred was clearly higher in the Cetrorelix group (45%) in comparison to the agonist group (27%), although it may be difficult to attribute this observation to the use of a GnRH antagonist. The distribution of follicles on the day of hCG injection for ovulation induction was practically the same in the two groups, with a certain tendency towards fewer small follicles in the group of patients who had been treated with Cetrorelix. Although this tendency did not reach statistical significance, it became very clear that the synchronization of follicular recruitment is not impaired by the use of a GnRH antagonist according to the multiple-dose protocol. Also, the estradiol profiles throughout the time of treatment showed no significant differences between the two groups. Only a certain tendency towards higher estradiol levels was observed at the day of hCG. However, the incidence of ovarian hyperstimulation syndrome (OHSS II–III) was significantly different in the two groups ($p=0.03$). While in the Cetrorelix group only three cases (1.7%) were seen, all of them grade II, the incidence in the Buserelin group was 6.5%, with one case of severe OHSS that required hospitalization. The tendency towards higher estradiol levels in the late stimulatory phase in the agonist group, as well as the fewer small follicles at the day of hCG in the Cetrorelix group, may be of causal importance for this lower incidence with use of the antagonist [68].

One hundred and fifteen patients were treated according to the French single-shot protocol using 3 mg Cetrorelix to be injected on day 8 of the cycle. Their results were compared with those of 36 patients treated with Triptorelin as a depot preparation according to the long protocol. No significant statistical differences were observed between the two groups regarding stimulation length (9.4 days in the Cetrorelix group and 10.7 days in the Triptorelin group), estradiol levels on the day of hCG (1786 pg/ml and 2549 pg/ml, respectively), and

Table 4. Cumulus oocyte complexes (COCs), fertilization rates, embryos, quality of embryos, implantation rates, pregnancy rates, and abortion rate

	IVF	ICSI[a]	Overall
Patients (n)	149	173	322
COC	1279	1692	2971
Mature oocytes (IVF) (n)	811		
(% of COC)[c]	63.0±35.6		
Metaphase II oocytes (ICSI) (n)	1252		
(% of COC)[c]	74.7±25.0		
Fertilization rate (%)[b, c]	60.4±26.3	58.2±24.5	59.2±25.3
Embryos	605	647	1252
Excellent, n (% of all)	211 (34.9)	219 (33.8)	430 (34.3)
Good, n (% of all)	281 (46.4)	298 (46.1)	579 (46.2)
Fair, n (% of all)	113 (18.7)	130 (20.1)	243 (19.4)
Patients with embryo transfer	134	163	297
Clinical pregnancies (treatment cycle)	30	40	70
Pregnancy rate/ET (%)	22.4	24.5	23.6
Babies born after ET	33	45	78
Babies born/replaced embryos (%)	9.3	10.2	9.8
Miscarriages, n (%)	6 (20.0)	6 (15.0)	12 (17.1)

[a] IVF and ICSI were performed in 11 patients.
[b] Only patients with total number of obtained oocytes >0 are included.
[c] Patient-based ratios.

fertilization rates (50.5% and 54.7%, respectively). As in the case of the multiple-dose protocol, the pregnancy rate proved to be a little more favorable in the agonist group (27.3% per embryo transfer, ET) than in the Cetrorelix group (21.2% per ET). However, these differences were again not statistically significant. Again the incidence of OHSS (II–III) was remarkably lower among the patients who had been treated with Cetrorelix (3.5%) than in those who had been stimulated according to the long protocol using Triptorelin (11.1%). It is interesting that in all of those patients who had shown a starting rise in LH on day 8, when Cetrorelix was to be administered, the LH rise was reduced by the administration of the antagonist. None of these cycles had to be canceled, and pregnancies occurred as well [69].

In a prospective, open, nonrandomized study, also using 0.25 mg Cetrorelix according to the multiple-dose "Lübeck" protocol, 346 patients were treated at several European centers. By replacing a mean of 2.66 embryos per cycle a clinical ongoing pregnancy rate of 24% per transfer was obtained. The abortion rate was 17%. The median exposure time to Cetrorelix was 5 days, the mean time of stimulation with gonadotropins was 10.4 days per cycle, and the median number of ampules of hMG used per cycle was 23. The incidence of premature luteinization in this largest study to date using Cetrorelix for COH was as low as 0.89% after the commencement of antagonist administration (Table 4) [68].

Alternative Methods of Ovulation Induction

OHSS can always be avoided by refraining from using hCG. Alternatively, there have been successful attempts at inducing ovulation in PCO patients with 0.5 mg decapeptyl s.c. in hMG-stimulated cycles without preliminary agonist treatment. No case of severe OHSS has occurred [70]. Since pituitary reactivity is maintained, this approach seems to be practicable for antagonist treatment as well. It is also possible to trigger ovulation by pulsatile administration of GnRH under antagonist medication [53]. It is conceivable that downstream processes occur without any support for the luteal phase in the same way as in patients with WHO-I infertility. However, it remains to be seen whether the rate of OHSS is really lower with this therapy, or whether the syndrome is simply less acute.

Uterus Myomatosus, Endometriosis, and Sexual Steroid Sensitive Malignomas

Myomas are the most frequent benign tumor in women of reproductive age. Among women entering menopause after the age of 50 years, 40% develop myomas. Internationally, uterus myomatosus is the most frequent indication for gynecological surgery. In the United States an average of 6000 hysterectomies are performed daily because of uterus myomatosus [71]. Patients with larger myomas scheduled for a fertility-preserving operation, those with hemoglobin-reducing hypermenorrhea, and those requiring a hysteroscopic ablation of their myomas have become standard candidates for preoperative GnRH agonist therapy. Therapy is efficient and reduces the size of the myomas by about 50% in 3–6 months. Whether this very expensive therapy is reasonable in all cases is another question. The first results of daily GnRH antagonist treatment with Nal-Glu published by Kettel in 1993 show that the same shrinkage rate is reached within 1 month. Further shrinkage after this period has not been observed [72].

In a feasibility study performed in the department of obstetrics and gynecology at the Medical university of Lübeck a depot-preparation of the third-generation gonadotropin-releasing hormone antagonist Cetrorelix (SB-75) was used for preoperative treatment in 20 premenopausal patients with symptomatic uterine fibroids. In a prospective, open, randomized setting 60 mg Cetrorelix-pamoate salt was administered intramuscularly on cycle day 2. Patients were randomized for a second dose of 30 mg or 60 mg of Cetrorelix-depot, which was administered according to the degree of estradiol suppression (< 50 pg/ml) at treatment day 21 or 28. Surgery was done after 6 or 8 weeks of treatment, depending on second dose administration. Weekly transvaginal sonography (TVS) and magnetic resonance imaging (MRI) were performed before and after treatment to assess fibroid volume. Sixteen patients showed satisfactory suppression of gonadotropins and sexual steroid secretion, avoiding any initial flare-up effect, while four patients had an insufficient response to the medication. In those patients responding well to the depot antagonist preparation, according

mean and SEM in %

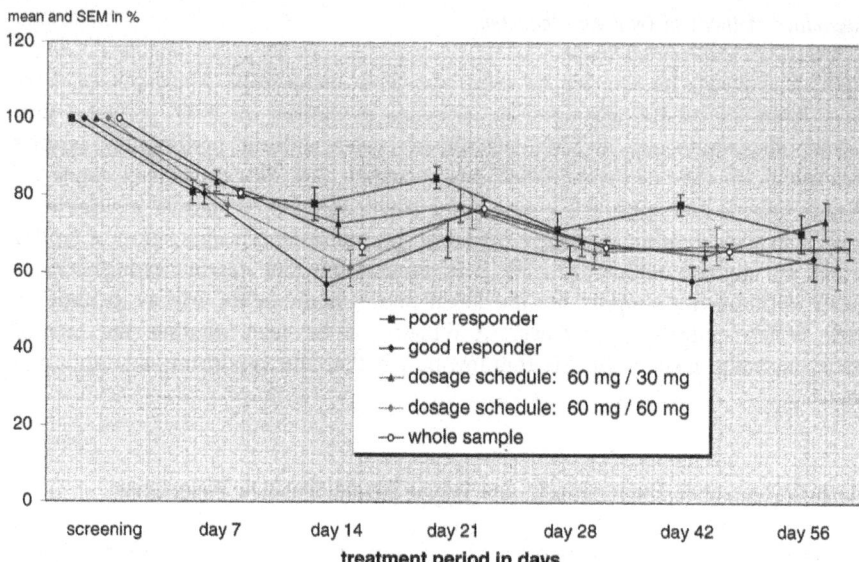

Fig. 18. Mean reduction in volume of largest fibroids as percentage of pretreatment value at screening (transvaginal ultrasound) following two doses of depot Cetrorelix

to TVS a mean shrinkage rate of leading fibroid volume of 33.5% at the end of treatment was observed, while the mean shrinkage rate obtained after 14 days of treatment was 31.3%. In good responders (shrinkage >20%) leading fibroid volume at day 14 was about 56.7% of the baseline assessment (Fig. 18). Although MRI showed shrinkage rates about 10% less than those seen with TVS, these differences were not statistically significant. The avoidance of any initial flare-up in gonadotropin secretion may explain this extremely fast reduction in fibroid size. We see the advantages of this protocol in the short treatment time with fast restoration of ovarian function. The rate of poor responders may be reducible using another galenic preparation [73].

Side Effects of GnRH Agonist Therapy

On the other hand, the side effects of long-term GnRH agonist therapy must not be neglected. Hot flushes occur in 81%, headaches in 30%, nausea and dizziness in 21%, and the patient suffers from loss of libido and a depressive mood. Furthermore, especially younger women are at risk of osteoporosis. Depending on the author, loss of bone mass is reported to be 3.4–7.4% after 6 months of continuous therapy, for example, in cases of severe endometriosis [74, 75].

GnRH Antagonists: An Alternative to the "Add-Back" Therapy?

However, in cases of uterus myomatosus and endometriosis, there seems to be a threshold concentration of estradiol at which no disease is induced but the symptoms of estrogen deprivation are prevented. Although this threshold has not yet been precisely defined, these observations are the basis for the so-called add-back therapy. As early as 1991, Maheux et al. administered 0.3 mg conjugated estrogens daily on days 1–25 after 3 months of Zoladex and managed to maintain the estradiol concentration at about 25 pg/ml. Zoladex administration continued, but no regrowth of the myomas was seen. Instead, subjective symptoms improved markedly [76]. Because of the specific mechanism of action of GnRH antagonists determined by the law of mass action, it is possible in principle to adjust the dose to maintain this threshold amount. It may be difficult to find the ideal dose of the depot preparation in view of interindividual and intraindividual fluctuations, but the mere possibility seems tempting. This would mean the end of time limits for therapy.

GnRH Antagonists and Sexual Steroid-Sensitive Malignomas

In the long run, GnRH antagonists will replace agonists for the therapy of hormone receptor-positive mammary cancer. Initial in vitro studies on endometrial cancer have suggested that antagonists inhibit proliferation and have a cytotoxic effect [77]. The situation is different for ovarian cancer. The administration of GnRH agonists as part of the so-called decapeptyl study has produced no therapeutic benefit. However, GnRH antagonists seem to interfere with the receptors for epidermal growth factor and insulin-like growth factor I. In nude mice transplanted with human ovarian cancer cells this led to an 85% reduction in the initial tumor volume, an effect which Triptorelin, administered in the control group, failed to achieve [78].

GnRH Antagonists and New Opportunities for Contraception

Contraceptive methods play a key role in gynecology. GnRH analogues could have a potential for male contraception. The results so far are promising, but a breakthrough still seems to be far away [79]. On the other hand, a combination of antigestagens such as RU 486, which have not been licensed in Germany, with oral GnRH antagonists, which remain to be developed, could lead to a completely new form of oral contraceptive for women [80].

References

1. Bettendorf G (1989) Diagnostik und Therapie der gestörten Ovarialfunktion. In: Schirren C, Bettendorf G, Leidenberger F, Frick-Bruder V (eds) Unerfüllter Kinderwunsch. Deutscher Ärzte-Verlag, Köln, pp 49–95
2. Wildt L, Leyendecker G (1987) Induction of ovulation by the chronic administration of naltrexone in hypothalamic amenorrhea. J Clin Endocrinol Metab 64:1334
3. Wildt L (1990) Die endokrine Kontrolle der Ovarialfunktion und die Pathophysiologie endokriner Ovarialfunktionsstörungen. In: Diedrich K (ed) Neue Wege in Diagnostik und Therapie der Sterilität. Enke, Stuttgart, pp 1–25
4. Hillier SG (1994) Current concepts of the role of FSH and LH in folliculogenesis. Hum Reprod 9:188–191
5. Erickson GF, Magolfin DA, Dyer CA, Hofeditz C (1985) The ovarian androgen production cells. A review of structure/function relationships. Endocr Rev 6:371
6. Diedrich K, Al-Hasani S, Van der Ven H, Diedrich C, Krebs D (1990) In vitro Fertilisation und Embryotransfer. In: Diedrich K (ed) Neue Wege in Diagnostik und Therapie der Sterilität. Enke, Stuttgart, pp 169–195
7. Burgus R, Butcher M, Ling N, Monahan M, Rivier J, Fellows R, Amoss M, Vale WW, Guillemin R (1971) Structure moléculaire du facteur hypothalamique (LFR) d'origine ovine contrôlant la sécretion de l'hormone gonadotrope hypophysaire de lutéinisation (LH). CR Acad Sci (D) 273:1611
8. Matsuo H, Baba Y, Nair RMG, Arimura A, Schally AV(1971) Structure of porcine LH and FSH releasing factor. I. The proposed amino acid sequence. Biochem Biophys Res Commun 43:1334–1339
9. Knobil E (1980) On the control of gonadotropin secretion in the rhesus monkey. Recent Prog Horm Res 30:53–88
10. Clayton RN, Catt KJ (1981) Gonadotropin-releasing hormone receptors: characterization, physiological regulation and relationship to reproductive function. Endocr Rev 2:186–209
11. Blum JJ, Conn PM (1982) Gonadotropin-releasing hormone stimulation of luteinizing hormone release: a ligand-receptor-effector model. Proc Natl Acad Sci USA 79:7307–7311
12. Kiesel L, Runnebaum B (1992) Gonadotropin-releasing-Hormon und Analoga – Physiologie und Pharmakologie. Gynakol Geburtshilfliche Rundsch 32:22–30
13. Coy DH, Horvath A, Nekola MV, Coy EJ, Ercheigyi J, Schally AV (1982) Peptide antagonists of LH-RH: large increases in antiovulatory activities produced by basic D-amino acids in the six position. Endocrinology 110:1445–1447
14. Gordon K, Hodgen GD (1993) Evolving role of gonadotrophin-releasing hormone antagonists. Trends Endocrinol Metab 3:259–263
15. Lemay A, Maheux R, Faure N, Jean C, Fazekas ATA (1984) Reversible hypogonadism induced by a luteinizing hormone-releasing hormone (LH-RH) agonist (Buserelin) as a new therapeutic approach for endometriosis. Fertil Steril 41:863–871
16. Schmutzler RK, Diedrich K (1990) Basic and clinical aspects of GnRH-agonists in reproduction. Int J Gynecol Obstet 32:311–324
17. Tunn UW, Goldschmidt AJW, Schweikert HU (1994) Tumor flare and treatment of prostate cancer with LH-RH agonists: prevention by simultaneous antiandrogenic treatment? In: Klingmüller D, Wildt L (eds) GnRH analogues in therapy. Thieme, Stuttgart, pp 67–82
18. Loumaye E (1990) The control of endogenous secretion of LH by gonadotrophin-releasing hormone agonists during ovarian hyperstimulation for in vitro fertilization and embryo transfer. Hum Reprod 5:357–376
19. Stanger JD, Yovich JL (1985) Reduced in vitro fertilization of human oocytes from patients with raised basal luteinizing hormone levels during the follicular phase. Br J Obstet Gynecol 92:385–393
20. Macnamee MC, Howles CM, Edwards RG, Taylor PJ, Elder KT (1989) Short-term luteinizing hormone-releasing hormone agonist treatment: prospective trial of a novel ovarian stimulation regimen for in vitro fertilization. Fertil Steril 52:264–269

21. Loumaye E, de Cooman S, Anoma M, Psalti I, Depreester S, Schmit M, Thomas K (1988) Short-term utilization of a gonadotropin releasing hormone agonist (Buserelin) for induction of ovulation in an in-vitro fertilization program. Ann NY Acad Sci 541:96–102
22. Insler V, Lunenfeld B (1993) Application of GnRH analogues in the treatment of female infertility. In: Lunenfeld B, Insler V (eds) GnRH analogues – the state of the art 1993. Parthenon, New York, pp 37–48
23. Pados G, Tarlatzis BC, Bontis J, Lagos S, Papadimas J, Spanos E, Mantalenakis S (1991) Ovarian stimulation with buserelin/HMG/HCG: prospective study of short vs long protocol. In abstract book of the 7th Annual meeting of the ESHRE, Paris, June 28–30, Hum Reprod 6:364–365
24. Howles CM, Macnamee MC, Edwards RG, Goswamy R, Steptoe PC (1986) Effect of high tonic levels of luteinizing hormone on outcome of in-vitro fertilization. Lancet 2:521–522
25. Regan L, Owen EJ, Jacobs HS (1990) Hypersecretion of luteinising hormone, infertility and miscarriage. Lancet 2:1141–1144
26. de Mouzon J, Belaisch-Allart J, Cohen J, Dubuisson JB, Guichard A, Parinaud J, Bachelot A, Chalais JJ (1988) Dossier FIVNAT, analyse des resultats 1987. Stimulations. Contracept Fertil Sexual 16:599–615
27. Tan SL, Kingsland C, Campbell S (1990) The use of buserelin in in vitro fertilization – a comparison between the long and short protocols of administration. Gynecol Endocrinol 4: abstract no 107
28. Ron-El R, Golan A, Herman A, Raziel A, Soffer Y, Caspi E (1990) Midluteal gonadotropin-releasing hormone analog administration in early pregnancy. Fertil Steril 572–574
29. Meldrum DR, Wisotn A, Hamilton F, Gutlay AL, Huynh D, Kempton W (1988) Timing of initiation and dose schedule of leuprolide influence the time course of ovarian suppression. Fertil Steril 50:400–402
30. Feldberg D, Ashkenazi J, Dicker D, Yeshaya Y, Goldman GA (1987) Ovarian cyst formation: a complication of gonadotrophin-releasing hormone analog agonist therapy. Fertil Steril 51:42–45
31. Ron-El R, Herman A, Golan A, Raziel A, Soffer Y, Caspi E (1990) Follicle cyst formation following long-acting gonadotropin-releasing hormone analog administration. Fertil Steril 52:1063–1066
32. Tummon IS, Henig I, Radwanska E, Binor Z, Rawlins R, Dmowski WP (1988) Persistent ovarian cyst following administration of human menopausal and chorionic gonadotrophins: an attenuated form of ovarian hyperstimulation syndrome. Fertil Steril 49:244–248
33. Smitz J, Ron-El R, Tarlatzis BC (1992) The use of gonadotrophin releasing hormone agonists for in vitro fertilization and other assisted procreation techniques: experience from three centres. Hum Reprod 7:49–66
34. Ron-El R, Raziel A, Nachum H, Strassburger D, Soffer Y, Bukovsky I, Herman A (1994) Immature oocyte production after ovulation induction. Hum Reprod 9 [Suppl 4]:85
35. Chetkowski RJ, Kruse LR, Nass TE (1989) Improved pregnancy outcome with the addition of leuproline acetate to gonadotrophins for in vitro fertilization. Fertil Steril 52:250–255
36. Smitz J, Devroey P, Braeckmans P, Camus M, Khan I, Staessen C, VanWasberghe L, Wisanto A, Van Steirteghem AC (1987) Management of failed cycles in an IVF/GIFT programme with the combination of a GnRH analog and hMG. Hum Reprod 2:309–314
37. Smitz J, Devroey P, Camus M, Deschacht J, Khan I, Staessen C, VanWasberghe L, Wisanto A, Van Steirteghem AC (1988) The luteal phase and early pregnancy after combined GnRH-agonist/HMG treatment for superovulation in IVF or GIFT. Hum Reprod 3:585–590
38. Smitz J, Camus M, Devroey P, Erard P, Wisanto A, Van Steirteghem AC (1990) Incidence of severe ovarian hyperstimulation syndrome after GnRH agonist/hMG superovulation for in vitro fertilization. Hum Reprod 5:933–937

39. Latouche J, Crumeyrolle-Arias M, Jordan D, Kopp N, Augende-Ferrante B, Cedard L, Haour F (1989) GnRH receptors in human granulosa cells: anatomical localization and characterization by autoradiographic study. Endocrinology 125:1739-1741
40. Pellicer A, Miro F (1990) Steroidogenesis in vitro of human granulosa luteal cells pretreated in vivo with gonadotropin-releasing hormone analogs. Fertil Steril 54:590-596
41. Smitz J, Devroey P, Bourgain C, Camus M, VanWasberghe L, Wisanto A, Van Steiteghem AC (1988) Luteal supplementation regimes after combined GnRH-agonist/HMG superovulation. J Reprod Fertil Abstr Ser 2:18
42. Herman A, Ron-El R, Golan A, Nachum H, Soffer Y, Caspi E (1990) Follicle cyst after menstrual versus midluteal administration of gonadotropin-releasing hormone analog in in vitro fertilization. Fertil Steril 53:854-858
43. Smitz J, Devroey P, Faguer B, Bourgain C, Camus M, Van Steirteghem AC (1992) A prospective randomized comparison of intramuscular or intravaginal natural progesterone as a luteal phase and early pregnancy supplement. Hum Reprod 7:168-175
44. Felberbaum R, Diedrich K (1995) Die ovarielle Stimulation in der asssistierten Reproduktion-Empfehlungen für ein modernes Management. In: Fischl FH (ed) Kinderwunsch. Krause und Pachernegg Verlag für Medizin und Wirtschaft, Vienna, pp 77-98
45. Schindler AE (1994) Treatment of endometriosis with GnRH agonists. In: Klingmüller D, Wildt L (eds) GnRH analogues in therapy. Thieme, Stuttgart, pp 36-52
46. Klingmüller D, Diedrich K, Sommer L (1993) Effects of the GnRH antagonist Cetrorelix in normal women. Gynecol Endocrinol 7:2
47. Klingmüller D, Schepke M, Enzweiler C, Bidlingmaier F (1993) Hormonal response to the new potent GnRH-antagonist Cetrorelix. Acta Endocrinol 128:15-18
48. Diedrich K, Diedrich C, Santos E, Zoll C, Al-Hasani S, Reissmann T, Krebs D, Klingmüller D (1994) Suppression of the endogenous luteinizing hormone surge by the gonadotrophin-releasing hormone antagonist Cetrorelix during ovarian stimulation. Hum Reprod 9:788-791
49. Felberbaum R, Reissmann T, Diedrich K (1995) Entwicklung und Anwendungsmöglichkeiten der GnRH-Antagonisten im Rahmen der Sterilitätstherapie - Eine Übersicht. Fertilitat 11:11-21
50. Dittkoff EC, Cassidenti DL, Paulson RJ, Sauer MV, Wellington LP, Rivier J, Yen SSC, Lobo RA (1991) The gonadotropin-releasing hormone antagonist (Nal-Glu) acutely blocks the luteinizing hormone surge but allows for resumption of folliculogenesis in normal women. Am J Obstet Gynecol 165:1811-1817
51. Bouchard P, Caraty A, Medalie D (1990) Mechanism of action and clinical uses of GnRH antagonists in women. In: Bouchard P, Haour F, Franchimont P, Schatz B (eds) Recent progress on GnRH and gonadal peptides. Elsevier, Paris, pp 209-219
52. Felberbaum R, Bauer O, Küpker W, Al-Hasani S, Zoll C, Germer U, Diedrich C, Diedrich K (1994) Hormone profiles and pituitary response under ovarian stimulation with HMG and GnRH-Antagonists (Cetrorelix). Hum Reprod 9 [Suppl 4]:13
53. Gordon K, Williams RF, Danforth DR, Hodgen GD (1990) A novel regime of gonadotrophin-releasing-hormone (GnRH)-antagonists plus pulsatile GnRH: controlled restoration of gonadotropin secretion and ovulation induction. Fertil Steril 54:1140-1145
54. Leyendecker G, Wildt L, Hansmann M (1980) Pregnancies following chronic intermittent (pulsatile) administration of GnRH by means of a portable pump ("Zyklomat") - a new approach to the treatment of infertility in hypothalamic amenorrhoea. J Clin Endocrinol Metab 51:1214-1216
55. Latouche J, Crmeyrolle-Arias M, Jordan D, Kopp N, Augende-Ferrante B, Cedard L, Haour F (1989) GnRH receptors in human granulosa cells: anatomical localization and characterization by autoradiographic study. Endocrinology 125:1739-1741
56. Stassen C, Camus M, Khan I, Smitz J, Van Waesberghe L, Wisanto A, Devroey P, Van Steirtheghem AC (1989) A 19-month survey of infertility treatment by in vitro fertilization, gamete and zygote intrafallopian transfer and replacement of frozen-thawed embryos. J In Vitro Fertil Embryo Transfer 6:22-29
57. Keller R, Günther HL, Kaiser P (1992) Embryonenschutzgesetz. Kohlhammer, Stuttgart

58. Olivennes F, Fanchin R, Bouchard P, DeZiegler D, Taieb J, Selva J, Frydman R (1994) The single or dual administration of the gonadotropin-releasing-hormone-antagonist Cetrorelix in an in vitro fertilization-embryo transfer program. Fertil Steril 62:468–476

59. Pellicer A, Miro F (1990) Steroidogenesis in vitro of human granulosa luteal cells pretreated in vivo with gonadotropin-releasing hormone analogs. Fertil Steril 54:590–596

60. Lamberts SWJ (1982) Testosterone secretion by cultured arrhenoblastoma cells: suppression by luteinizing-hormone agonist. J Clin Endocrinol Metab 54:450

61. Golan A, Ron-El R, Herman A, Weintraub Z, Soffer Y, Caspi E (1988) Ovarian hyperstimulation syndrome following D-Trp-6-luteinizing hormone-releasing hormone microcapsules and menotropins for in vitro fertilization. Fertil Steril 50:912–916

62. Dufau HL, Catt RJ, Tsuruhara T (1971) Retention of in vitro biological activities by desialated human luteinizing hormone and chorionic gonadotropin. Biochem Biophys Res Commun 44:1022–1029

63. Hoff YD, Quigley ME, Yen SCC (1983) Hormonal dynamics at midcycle: a reevaluation. J Clin Endocrinol Metab 57:892–896

64. Albano C, Smitz J, Camus M et al (1996) Hormonal profile during the follicular phase in cycles stimulated with a combination of human menopausal gonadotrophin and gonadotrophin-releasing hormone antagonist (Cetrorelix). Hum Reprod 11:2114–2118

65. Albano C, Smitz J, Camus M et al (1997) Comparison of different doses of gonadotrophin-releasing hormone antagonist cetrorelix during controlled ovarian hyperstimulation. Fertil Steril 67:917–922

66. Olivennes F, Fanchin R, Bouchard P et al (1995) Scheduled administration of a gonadotrophin-releasing hormone antagonist (cetrorelix) on day 8 of in vitro fertilization cycles: a pilot study. Hum Reprod 10:1382–1386

67. Albano C, Grimbizis G, Smitz J et al (1998) The luteal phase of nonsupplemented cycles after ovarian superovulation with the human menopausal gonadotrophin and the gonadotrophin-releasing hormone antagonist cetrorelix. Fertil Steril 70:357–359

68. Felberbaum RE (1999) Cetrorelix in controlled ovarian stimulation for ART. Results of phase III, multiple dose treatment. Gynecol Endocrinol 13 [Suppl 1]:14

69. Olivennes F, Belaisch-Allart J, Emperaire JC et al (1999) Comparison in a prospective multicentric randomized study in IVF-ET of a single dose of GnRH-antagonist (Cetrorelix) to a GnRh agonist long protocol (Triptorelin in depot formula). Gynecol Endocrinol 13 [Suppl 1]:14

70. Shalev E, Geslevich Y, Ben-Ami M (1994) Induction of pre-ovulatory luteinizing hormone surge by gonadotrophin-releasing hormone agonist for women at risk for developing the ovarian hyperstimulation syndrome. Hum Reprod 9:417–419

71. Wildt L, Jäger W (1994) Medical treatment of myomata uteri with decapeptyl-SR, a long acting agonistic analogue of GnRH. In: Klingmüller D, Wildt L (eds) GnRH analogues in therapy, Thieme, Stuttgart, pp 17–35

72. Kettel M, Murphy AA, Morales AJ, Rivier J, Vale WW, Yen SSC (1993) Rapid regression of uterine leiomyomas in response to daily administration of gonadotropin-releasing hormone antagonist. Fertil Steril 60:642–646

73. Felberbaum RE, Germer U, Ludwig M, Riethmüller-Winzen H, Heise S, Buttge I, Bauer O, Reissmann T, Engel J, Diedrich K (1998) Treatment of uterine fibroids with a slow-release formulation of the gonadotrophin-releasing hormone antagonist Cetrorelix. Hum Reprod 13:1660–1668

74. Uemura T, Mohri J, Osada H, Suzuki N, Katagiri N, Minaguchi H (1994) Effect of gonadotropin-releasing hormone agonist on the bone mineral density of patients with endometriosis. Fertil Steril 62:246–250

75. Matta WH, Shaw RW, Hesp R, Evans R (1988) Reversible trabecular bone density loss following induced hypo-estrogenism with GnRH analogue Buserelin in premenopausal women. Clin Endocrinol 29:45–51

76. Maheux R, Lemay A, Blanchet P, Friede J, Pratt X (1991) Maintained reduction of uterine leiomyoma following addition of hormonal replacement therapy to a monthly luteinizing hormone-releasing hormone agonist implant: a pilot study. Hum Reprod 6(4):500–505

77. Emons G, Schröder B, Ortmann O, Westphalen S, Schulz KD, Schally AV (1993) High-affinity binding and direct antiproliferative effects of LHRH analogues in human endometrial cancer cell lines. J Clin Endocrinol Metab 77:1458–1464
78. Yano T, Pinski J, Halmos G, Szepeshazi K, Groot K, Schally AV (1994) Inhibition of growth of OV-1063 human epithelial ovarian cancer xenografts in nude mice by treatment with luteinizing hormone-releasing hormone antagonist SB-75. Proc Natl Acad Sci USA 91:7090–7094
79. Pavlou SN, Sharp SC (1993) Clinical applications of GnRH antagonists in men. In: Bouchard P, Caraty A, Coelingh Bennink HJT, Pavlou SN (eds) GnRH, GnRH analogs, gonadotropins and gonadal peptides. Parthenon, London, pp 285–292
80. Spitz IM, Croxatto HB, Lähteenmäki P, Heikinheimo O, Bardin CW (1994) Effect of mifepriston on inhibition of ovulation and induction of luteolysis. In: Beier HM, Spitz IM (eds) Progesterone antagonists in reproductive medicine and oncology. Hum Reprod 9 [Suppl 1]:69–76

Ovarian Stimulation for In Vitro Fertilization: Past and Present

J. Urbancsek, T. Rabe, T. Strowitzki

Initially, "test tube babies" were born from pregnancies conceived by in vitro fertilization (IVF) of oocytes obtained from spontaneous, nonstimulated cycles (Steptoe and Edwards 1978; Lopata et al. 1980). Subsequently, the pioneers of IVF enhanced the efficacy of this procedure by developing methods for the hormonal stimulation of the ovaries. This treatment made the simultaneous development and fertilization of several oocytes possible, with the ultimate goal of transferring more than one embryo (Fishel et al. 1985). Thus, instead of the selection and development of a single dominant follicle, as seen in the spontaneous menstrual cycle, the primary objective of ovarian stimulation for IVF treatment has been, and still is, to promote the selection and simultaneous development of several dominant follicles during the same menstrual cycle.

The Mechanism of Ovarian Stimulation

According to Baird's theory (1987), the selection of the dominant follicle during a spontaneous cycle takes place as follows. Several antral follicles begin to grow simultaneously. Nevertheless, only one follicle can achieve dominance, provided it has developed to a certain size and maturation level before the rise of serum follicle stimulating hormone (FSH) levels occurs in the early follicular phase. This period, characterized by elevated FSH levels, is designated as the "FSH gate" in Baird's theory. Only the most advanced antral follicle will be able to "enter" the FSH gate and develop further as the single dominant follicle (Fig. 1a). Accordingly, there are two options for circumventing this process of follicular selection and ensure simultaneous dominance and development of several follicles (Fig. 1b,c). In theory, the number of small antral follicles (2–4 mm in diameter) growing simultaneously could be increased. However, the number of follicles entering the antral phase of development is genetically determined in humans, which rules out this method. Alternatively, the period characterized by increased serum FSH levels can be extended. According to Baird's pictorial analogy, this means that the FSH gate can be "widened". This enables several antral follicles to grow simultaneously to a size and develop to a level required for entrance through the widened FSH gate.

Consequently, multiple follicle growth can be achieved in humans by maintaining elevated serum FSH levels for an extended period. This can be achieved by stimulation of endogenous FSH release or administration of FSH. Figure 2 summarizes the therapeutic options for increasing serum FSH levels by influencing the hypothalamo-pituitary-ovarian axis at different levels to induce multiple follicular development.

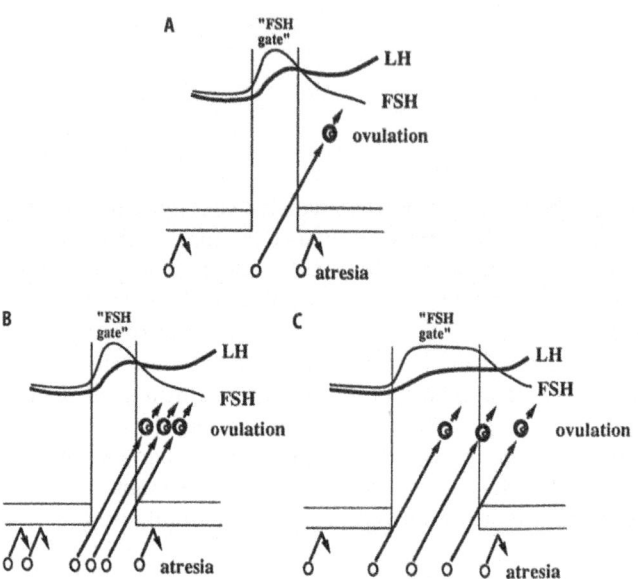

Fig. 1 A–C. Selection of the dominant follicle in a spontaneous cycle: only one follicle can enter the "FSH gate" (**A**). To increase the number of dominant follicles one can increase the number of antral follicles entering the "FSH gate" (**B**) or widen the "FSH gate" (**C**). (From Baird 1987)

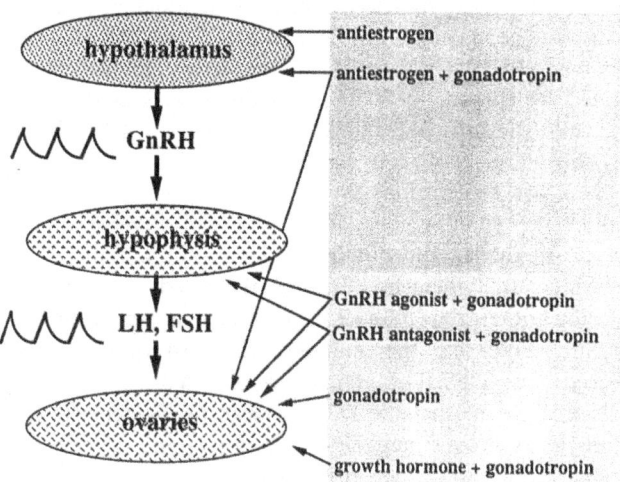

Fig. 2. Summary of different possibilities for ovarian stimulation for in vitro fertilization

Stimulation with Antiestrogens

Clomiphene citrate is the most established and widely used agent for inducing ovulation (Kistner 1965). It is administered from day 3 to day 7 or from day 5 to day 9 of the cycle in doses of 50–150 mg/day (Marrs et al. 1984). Essentially, its mechanism of action includes binding to hypothalamic estrogen receptors, resulting in the inhibition of the negative feedback regulation induced by serum estrogen (Adashi 1984). Inhibition of the negative feedback regulation stimulates GnRH release, which is followed by the elevation of FSH levels. Clomiphene citrate was first used by Lopata et al. (1978) to induce multiple follicular growth for subsequent in vitro fertilization. Similarly, these authors demonstrated for the first time the lower efficacy of clomiphene stimulation compared with that of human menopausal gonadotropin (hMG), as evidenced by the smaller number of follicles undergoing simultaneous maturation. The dose-dependent antiestrogenic effect of clomiphene citrate impairs both endometrial (Rogers et al. 1986) and luteal (Lamb et al. 1972) development. These effects, as well as lower oocyte yield, may explain the relatively low implantation and gestation rates observed during IVF (Table 1). Accordingly, clomiphene citrate is no longer used for IVF therapy by itself, although its discussed drawbacks can be eliminated by the combined use of clomiphene and gonadotropins.

Stimulation with Gonadotropins

Gonadotropins have been used for ovarian stimulation in infertile women for more than 30 years (Gemzell et al. 1958). The first successful stimulation that led to pregnancy was reported by Lunenfeld et al. (1960). The efforts of the Norfolk-based research team facilitated the incorporation of gonadotropins into the therapeutic arsenal of IVF (Jones et al. 1982). Similar to the administration of antiestrogens, the ultimate therapeutic goal of using gonadotropins is controlled hyperstimulation of ovarian function. Messinis and Templeton (1987) demonstrated that the administration of exogenous FSH (either as hMG or pure FSH) elevates serum FSH levels and induces multiple follicular development. Moreover, gonadotropin therapy during the follicular phase also enhances luteal function.

Since selection of the dominant follicle occurs between days 5 and 7 of the cycle (Hodgen 1982), treatment should be started early enough (i.e., on day 3) to establish the conditions necessary for the dominance and continuous growth of multiple follicles. The simultaneous persistence and development of several follicles to the time of ovulation is achieved by the FSH component of exogenous hMG. In the initial phase of follicular growth, exogenous FSH stimulates the estrogen production of granulosa cells. This prevents the enrichment of the hormonal environment with androgens, thereby precluding the degeneration of follicles that have started maturation at the beginning of the cycle. Moreover, FSH enhances the inhibin production of growing follicles; this is a safety mechanism that protects the system from excessive hyperstimulation. In addition, elevated serum inhibin levels observed during gonadotropin treatment may also moderate the LH surge occurring during the stimulated cycle (Urbancsek et al. 1992, 1993a,b).

It is widely known that different patients respond differently to hMG stimulation (García et al. 1983). Consequently, ovarian hyperstimulation should be performed flexibly, according to individualized protocols. Nevertheless, such interventions can be categorized into two essential groups. The Norfolk protocol involves "low dose, decreasing stimulation" (Jones et al. 1983) implemented by the administration of two ampules of hMG on days 3-6 of the cycle, followed by one or occasionally two ampules until the day before ovulation. The Bonn protocol applies "high dose, increasing stimulation" (Diedrich et al. 1988) by administering one ampule in the morning and at bedtime on days 3-6, followed by three ampules daily until the day before ovulation. As seen in Table 1, the number of oocytes retrieved is similar with both protocols.

In patients who respond poorly to stimulation with clomiphene and/or hMG as detailed above, superovulation can be induced by the administration of pure FSH (Diedrich et al. 1987). Multiple follicular growth can be achieved with pure FSH also in patients with polycystic ovary (PCO) syndrome (Raj et al. 1977) or abnormally high serum LH levels (Schoemaker et al. 1977). The optimized LH/FSH ratio and favorable estrogen/androgen ratio achieved by pure FSH create an environment that promotes the development of healthy oocytes suitable for subsequent fertilization (Jones et al. 1985). Two ampules containing 75 IU of FSH are administered on days 3-9 of the cycle; the daily dose can be increased to three ampules from day 10, depending on ovarian response (Diedrich et al. 1987). In PCO syndrome, a starting dose of one ampule daily seems reasonable, and this should be maintained over 2-3 weeks until a significant elevation of estradiol level occurs.

The active substance of conventional FSH (and hMG) preparations mentioned above is extracted from urine. Such preparations may cause occasional adverse reactions even if administered intramuscularly (Li and Hindle 1993). These untoward effects are attributed to the relatively high adjuvant protein content of these preparations (Howles et al. 1993). Recently, highly purified (HP) FSH preparations with a protein-specific activity over 9000 IU/mg have become available in addition to the "conventional" urinary FSH preparations (with a protein-specific activity of 150 IU/mg). Owing to its outstanding purity (95% compared with 3% for conventional FSH), the HP-FSH can be administered subcutaneously, which is more convenient for patients. Moreover, patients can administer subcutaneous injections themselves, which offers further advantages. In particular, this reduces the workload of medical personnel without decreasing the rate of successful pregnancies or the number of "take-home babies". Additionally, this method can be used without any increase in the number of ampules required for efficient stimulation or the risk of increased abortion rates. Furthermore, its use is not associated with a reduced oocyte yield or fertilization rate compared with the results of conventional FSH stimulation (Wikland et al. 1993).

Table 1. Success rates of in vitro fertilization after different protocols for ovarian stimulation

Stimulation protocol References	Oocyte retrievals (n)	Oocytes retrieved (n)	Pregnancy rate (%)		
			Per oocyte retrieval	Per embryo transfer	Per patient
Clomiphene citrate					
Lopata (1983)	155	2.3	10.9	15.1	–
McBain and Trounson (1984)	178	2.1	7.8	–	6.3
Speirs et al. (1984)	717	2.1	4.0	7.2	–
Kerin and Warnes (1986)	112	2.6	14.3	18.1	–
Diedrich et al. (1988)	98	2.4	22.0	31.0	22.0
Kemeter and Feichtinger (1989)	141	2.4	12.8	19.4	–
hMG treatment (low-dose, step-down dose regimen)					
Bernardus et al. (1985)	23	4.4	21.7	27.7	21.7
Jones et al. (1984)	560	–	18.8	24.5	32.9
Rosenwaks and Muasher (1986) (with FSH supplementation)	223	3.9	–	29.0	–
Leyendecker et al. (1990)	141	3.4	14.0	17.0	–
hMG treatment (high-dose, step-up dose regimen)					
Laufer et al. (1983)	55	3.2	16.3	17.3	14.2
Laufer et al. (1984)	106	4.0	15.0	16.1	13.0
Diedrich et al. (1988)	173	4.8	21.0	26.0	21.0
Urinary FSH treatment					
Rosenwaks and Muasher (1986)	78 (ET)	–	–	27.0	–
Diedrich et al. (1987)	38	5.4	18.4	–	–
Grillo et al. (1987)	40	6.4	25.0	31.3	18.9
Scoccia et al. (1987)	28	5.4	18.0	21.0	18.0
Clomiphene citrate+hMG treatment					
Lopata (1983)	217	6.1	17.5	23.6	–
Speirs et al. (1984)	155	4.6	14.0	19.7	–
Kerin and Warnes (1986)	293	3.9	17.0	21.2	–
Rainhorn et al. (1987)	240	–	17.0	24.8	13.8
Loumaye et al. (1988)	274	3.7	17.0	23.0	–
Rutherford et al. (1988)	225	5.5	21.3	30.1	14.6
Kemeter and Feichtinger (1989) (clomiphene citrate +hMG/FSH)	477	3.9	15.3	21.1	–
GnRH agonist+hMG treatment (long protocol)					
Daya et al. (1995)	332	–	15.5	16.5	–
Kondaveeti-Gordon U (1996) (starting on day 1 of the cycle)	36	10.3	25.0	25.7	–
Kondaveeti-Gordon (1996) (starting on day 21 of the cycle)	43	12.0	25.6	25.6	–
Fujii et al. (1997)	66	5.7	18.2	21.8	17.4
Jacob et al. (1998)	173	10.0	22.0	24.4	19.9

Table 1 (continued)

Stimulation protocol References	Oocyte retrievals (n)	Oocytes retrieved (n)	Pregnancy rate (%)		
			Per oocyte retrieval	Per embryo transfer	Per patient
GnRH agonist+hMG treatment (short protocol)					
Frydman et al. (1988)	40	6.0	20.0	23.5	–
Zorn et al. (1988)	136	3.7	18.0	25.0	–
Loumaye et al. (1988)	253	7.2	22.0	28.0	–
Abdalla et al. (1989)	116	2.7	24.1	-	–
Oyesanya et al. (1995)	71 (patients)	11.3	–	22.8	18.3
GnRH agonist+hMG treatment (ultra-short protocol)					
Howles et al. (1987)	7	4.4	42.0	42.0	–
Sharma et al. (1988)	14	2.7	20.0	22.0	–
Macnamee et al. (1989)	111	9.5	39.6	–	35.5
Ron-El et al. (1990)	80	7.7	–	19.0	–
Ron-El et al. (1998)	88	7.7	10.2	17.0	–
GnRH agonist+urinary FSH treatment (long protocol)					
Wikland et al. (1994)	230	10.4	–	45.6	–
Daya et al. (1995)	285	23.5	–	24.8	–
Out et al. (1995) (starting on day 1 of the cycle)	396 (patients)	9.0	–	30.5	–
Wikland et al. (1994) (highly purified FSH)	386	9.4	–	43.6	–
Bergh et al. (1997)	102	7.6	–	47.0	36.0
GnRH agonist+recombinant FSH treatment (long protocol)					
Recombinant Human FSH Study Group (1995)	55	9.3	21.8	24.0	20.0
Out et al. (1995) (starting on day 1 of the cycle)	585 (patients)	10.8	–	34.3	–
Bergh et al. (1997)	119	12.2	–	48.0	45.0
Vandervorst and Devroey (1998)	57	9.3	21.1	–	20.0
Jacob et al. (1998)	139	9.0	15.8	18.3	13.9
GnRH antagonist (cetrorelix) +hMG treatment (single-dose protocols)					
Olivennes et al. (1998) (2 mg cetrorelix on day 8)	31	8.4	25.8	25.8	25.0
Olivennes et al. (1998) (3 mg cetrorelix on day 8)	34	6.5	32.4	35.5	32.4
Rongieres-Bertrand et al. (1999) (0.5 or 1mg cetrorelix)	40	–	17.5	32.0	–
GnRH antagonist (cetrorelix) +hMG treatment (multiple-dose application)					
Albano et al. (1997) (0.5 mg cetrorelix daily from day 7 of the cycle)	32 (patients)	–	–	30.8	25.0

Table 1 (continued)

Stimulation protocol References	Oocyte retrievals (n)	Oocytes retrieved (n)	Pregnancy rate (%)		
			Per oocyte retrieval	Per embryo transfer	Per patient
Albano et al. (1997) (0.25 mg cetrorelix daily from day 7 of the cycle)	30 (patients)	–	–	29.6	26.7
Growth hormone (GH) +hMG treatment					
Homburg et al. (1988b)	12	7.4	–	–	–
Fixed protocols					
Rainhorn et al. (1987)	212	2.4	19.3	18.8	–
Kemeter and Feichtinger (1989)	277	4.5	21.3	25.7	–

The range of available gonadotropins is further expanded by recombinant FSH (rFSH) preparations. Recently, biotechnology has made available a recombinant preparation of FSH produced by inserting the genes encoding the alpha and beta subunits of FSH into expression vectors that are transfected into a Chinese hamster ovary cell line (Howles 1996). There are two rFSH preparations currently in clinical use: follitropin alpha and follitropin beta. Although both preparations were developed using the same technique, the post-translation glycosylation and purification processes are not identical (Olijve et al. 1996). The 100% purity of these preparations allows for the subcutaneous administration of the product with no marked differences in local tolerance symptoms and clinical efficacy compared with the intramuscular route (Out et al. 1997). Besides this, there are numerous obvious advantages of rFSH over its urinary predecessor: the product is more homogeneous with greatly reduced interbatch variability, resulting in more predictable and comparable reactions by the ovaries. The supply is practically unlimited, and shortages of urine should no longer bar their clinical use. There is no risk of infection or contamination as there is with products from a human source, and there have been no reported cases of seroconversion to anti-gonadotropin antibodies (Recombinant Human FSH Study Group 1995).

The first baby born from a pregnancy induced by IVF following ovarian stimulation with rFSH was reported in 1992 (Devroey et al. 1992). Studies performed with follitropin beta confirmed an increased potency of rFSH compared with uFSH and show that lower starting doses (100–200 IU) can safely and successfully be employed without jeopardizing the chance of pregnancy (Hoomans and Out 1999). Results from the first comprehensive study on stimulation with rFSH showed that the safety and efficacy of stimulation with rFSH for IVF treatment are comparable to those with urinary FSH (Recombinant Human FSH

Study Group 1995). Meanwhile, results from a prospective, randomized, multi-center trial of several hundred IVF cycles demonstrated that stimulation with rFSH requires the use of significantly fewer ampules and significantly shorter stimulation and yields significantly more oocytes than treatment with conventional urinary FSH (Out et al. 1995). Although a higher pregnancy rate has also been achieved with rFSH stimulation, this difference became statistically significant only after the inclusion of results from the transfer of cryopreserved-thawed embryos. This observation may suggest that the quality of oocytes obtained by ovarian rFSH stimulation is superior to that of oocytes retrieved after treatment with conventional urinary FSH. A clearer statement in favor of rFSH was made by Daya and Gunby (1999), who performed a meta-analysis of 12 selected randomized trials comparing the efficacy of urinary versus recombinant FSH preparations in infertility treatment cycles: the clinical pregnancy rate per cycle started is statistically significantly higher with rFSH. The total sample size on which this conclusion is based was 2875 (1556 allocated to rFSH and 1319 to uFSH). In this meta-analysis a marked difference was observed in favor of follitropin alpha, comparing the odds for clinical pregnancy in IVF stimulated with alpha or beta follitropin. This observation is supported by the results of Phillips et al. (1999) and von During et al. (1999), who found both the morphological quality of embryos and the numbers of good-quality embryos obtained significantly higher with follitropin alpha than with follitropin beta.

Combined Stimulation with Antiestrogens and Gonadotropins

The concomitant use of clomiphene citrate and gonadotropin (hMG) – once the most widely employed protocol for ovarian stimulation (Messinis 1989) – was first applied for in vitro fertilization by Trounson et al. (1981). Combined therapy increases serum FSH levels via the stimulatory effect of the antiestrogen component on endogenous FSH release, as well as owing to the exogenous FSH administered (Messinis 1986a). Patients receive 100 mg clomiphene citrate daily for 5 days (starting on day 2–5 of the cycle). According to the "simultaneous" combined protocol, this regimen is supplemented by administration of one to two ampules of hMG, first concomitantly, then by itself. When the "sequential" protocol is used, 5-day clomiphene administration is followed by gonadotropin treatment with one to two ampules of hMG. The latter method yields numbers of oocytes similar to those obtained after ovarian stimulation performed with gonadotropins only and ensures a significantly higher pregnancy rate than stimulation with clomiphene alone (see Table 1).

Evaluation of "Conventional" Stimulation Protocols

Unpredictability of the onset as well as the intensity of ovarian response is a common disadvantage of all "conventional" (clomiphene citrate and/or gonadotropins) methods for ovarian stimulation (García et al. 1983). Moreover, the number and maturity of growing follicles vary, and an LH surge may also occur prematurely (relative to the scheduled time of ovulation induction). The latter phenomenon can be attributed to the following: The cumulative quantity of estradiol produced by multiple growing follicles exceeds that usually synthesized by single dominant follicles during spontaneous cycles. As a result, the critical serum level of estradiol eliciting an LH surge by positive feedback is achieved significantly earlier (prematurely) than during normal cycles (Fig. 3b). However, individual follicles and oocytes are still immature for ovulation or follicular aspiration at this time. Moreover, a premature LH surge can induce endogenous luteinization – a threefold increase of serum progesterone levels may occur compared with the normal concentration seen during the follicular phase (0.5 ng/ml [1.59 nmol/l]; Fleming and Coutts 1986). The reduction of the oocyte yield as well as of fertilization and pregnancy rates have been demonstrated by several authors (Lejeune et al. 1986; Eibschitz et al. 1986; Stanger and Yovich 1985). These findings correspond to our experience regarding the unfavorable effect of the premature LH surge on the likelihood of a successful pregnancy. Accordingly, and similar to others, we have adopted a practice of recommending the cancellation of ovarian stimulation without retrieving oocytes in such cases (Urbancsek et al. 1990b).

Premature LH release and subsequent luteinization are common adverse endocrine reactions occurring during standard stimulation performed on patients with normal hypothalamo-pituitary-ovarian function. As observed by Zimmermann et al. (1982), the efficacy of gonadotropin therapy is superior in patients with hypothalamo-pituitary-ovarian dysfunction (WHO group I) compared with patients who have ovarian insufficiency and normal gonadotropin function (WHO group II). This observation prompted Fleming and his co-workers (1982) to induce hypogonadotropinism by selective inhibition of gonadotropin production before starting conventional ovarian stimulation with gonadotropins. The authors achieved pregnancy in three of five patients, and their unprecedented efforts led to the introduction of GnRH agonist–gonadotropin combinations to the therapy of female infertility.

Stimulation with the Combination of GnRH Agonists and Gonadotropins

The existence of a hypothesized neurohormonal substance, gonadotropin-releasing hormone (GnRH) was demonstrated by Schally and Guillemin only a decade prior to the pioneering work of Fleming (Schally et al. 1971; Burgus et al. 1971). Owing to its crucial importance, this discovery was rewarded with a Nobel prize.

The recognition of pulsatile GnRH release by Carmel et al. (1976) prompted Leyendecker et al. (1980) to apply GnRH clinically using an automatic infusor device. While the pulsatile administration of GnRH stimulates the pituitary synthesis and release of gonadotropins, its continuous administration to mammals and humans leads to reversible inhibition of gonadotropin secretion (LH primarily) and ovarian function after a temporary stimulatory effect (Belchetz et

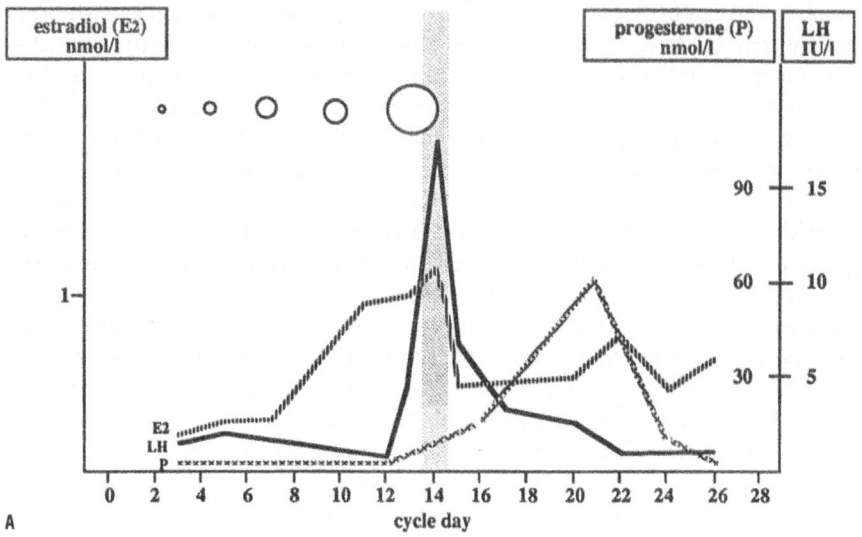

A

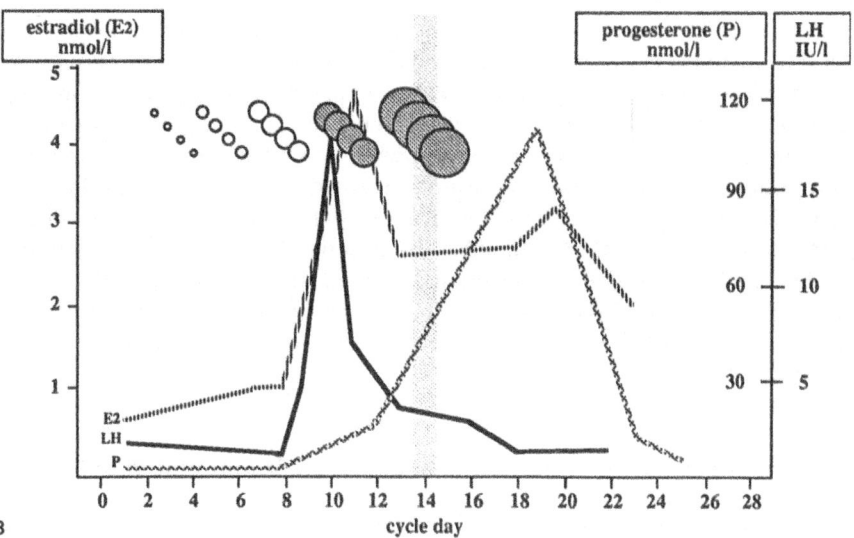

B

Fig. 3 A, B. Occurrence of premature LH surge and premature luteinization in a stimulated cycle: in stimulated cycles (B) rapidly increasing serum estradiol concentration reaches the value critical for induction of the LH surge in an earlier phase of the follicular phase than during the spontaneous cycle (A)

al. 1978). Initial hypersecretion is followed by the down-regulation of GnRH receptors, resulting in the inhibition of LH and FSH release. Consequently, the GnRH agonist exerts a paradoxical action; that is, it seems to act as a GnRH antagonist. Of course, this is not the case; this apparent effect results from the desensitization of hormone receptors by continuous exposure to the hormone

(Loumaye and Catt 1983). As a result, GnRH and its agonistic analogues are suitable for the treatment of hyperandrogenemia and estrogen-dependent diseases (such as endometriosis, uterine myoma, and breast cancer), as well as in combined hormone therapy for in vivo (Fleming et al. 1982; Fleming and Coutts 1986) and in vitro fertilization (Porter et al. 1984) of infertile women.

GnRH agonists are produced by the chemical modification of the native GnRH decapeptide (Fujino et al. 1972). Modification of the molecular structure increases the affinity of the compound for pituitary receptors (Loumaye et al. 1982) and enhances its resistance to enzymatic proteolysis responsible for the prompt inactivation of native GnRH (Swift and Crighton 1979). These properties increase the potency of GnRH agonists several-fold compared with the natural substance (Perrin et al. 1980) and explain their continuous effect on GnRH receptors despite discontinuous (four to six times daily) administration.

Inspired by the pioneering work of Fleming et al. (1982), the combination of GnRH agonists and gonadotropins was rapidly introduced also to in vitro fertilization (Porter et al. 1984). The most important indications for the use of this combination include premature LH surge associated with subsequent early luteinization (Wildt et al. 1986), elevated basal LH levels during the follicular phase (Macnamee and Howles 1987), polycystic ovary (PCO) syndrome (Salat-Baroux et al. 1988), and infertility unresponsive to conventional treatment (in "low-responders") (Neveu et al. 1987). Currently, most IVF teams use combined GnRH agonist–gonadotropin stimulation routinely. However, as Kingsland et al. (1992) demonstrated in their prospective, randomized trial, this is justified primarily by practical advantages rather than for medical reasons (see later). Nevertheless, GnRH agonist and gonadotropin combinations are extremely popular in in vitro fertilization programs: as many as as 78.8% of IVF stimulations worldwide are performed using this method (De Mouzon and Lancaster 1995).

Combined GnRH agonist–gonadotropin therapy is administered according to one of four regimens, i.e., ultra-short, short, long. and fast desensitizing protocols (see Fig. 4). Ultra-short and short protocols are based on the initial stimulatory effect of GnRH agonists on gonadotropin secretion ("flare-up effect"), which lasts 1–2 days and promotes the simultaneous maturation of several follicles. The GnRH agonist is administered from the first to the third day of the cycle (ultra-short protocol) or until the day of ovulation induction (short protocol). Gonadotropins are given from the third day of the cycle (Howles et al. 1987). When the long protocol is used, the GnRH agonist is administered for 10–14 days, from the first day of the cycle or the middle of the luteal phase, until a sufficient inhibition of gonadotropin release is achieved. Ovarian stimulation is then started with exogenous gonadotropins while GnRH agonist therapy is maintained (Wildt et al. 1986). In our experience, sufficient inhibition of pituitary function can be achieved earlier if GnRH agonist administration is started during the midluteal phase. This method also ensures higher fertilization and pregnancy rates than therapy started on the first day of the cycle (Urbancsek et al. 1991a; Urbancsek and Witthaus 1996). According to the results of prospective, randomized, comparative studies, the long protocol is probably more efficient than the short protocol in terms of follicular development and

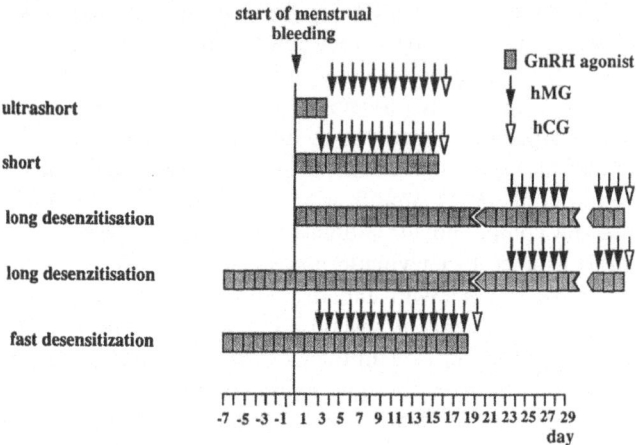

Fig. 4. Combined GnRH agonist and gonadotropin stimulation for in vitro fertilization: ultrashort, short, long-, and fast-desensitization protocols

fertilization rates, as well as of the number of embryos suitable for transfer (Tan et al. 1992). The fast desensitization protocol involves GnRH agonist administration from the middle of the luteal phase of a cycle; this treatment is supplemented by gonadotropins from the third day of the next cycle. This regimen combines the advantages of short and long desensitization protocols. In particular, the GnRH agonist started in the midluteal phase promptly inhibits pituitary gonadotropin secretion. Moreover, although the GnRH agonist is administered over a relatively brief period only, this method also precludes the initial increase of gonadotropin secretion at the beginning of the follicular phase (Loumaye et al. 1989).

The advantages and shortcomings of combined GnRH agonist–gonadotropin therapy can be summarized as follows: The occurrence of a premature LH surge can be prevented almost completely (Schmutzler et al. 1988), or at least its incidence can be reduced significantly (Urbancsek et al. 1990b). Basal serum LH levels also decrease considerably (Urbancsek et al. 1990a), and the number of canceled cycles can be reduced (Testart et al. 1989). The date of oocyte retrieval can be postponed and follicular punctures can thus be avoided on weekends (Abdalla et al. 1989). In patients with previous failures, pregnancy rates achieved by combined GnRH agonist + hMG treatment are similar to those observed with hMG or clomiphene + hMG treatment of women without previous unsuccessful ovarian stimulation (Urbancsek et al. 1991b). Drawbacks include luteal insufficiency resulting from the luteolytic effect of GnRH agonists (see last section) and a higher incidence of ovarian hyperstimulation syndrome (Forman et al. 1990). Multiple pregnancy occurs more frequently than after hMG and/or clomiphene stimulation. Moreover, GnRH agonists are very expensive.

Stimulation with Combination of GnRH Antagonists and Gonadotropins

A major problem with GnRH agonists is that LH secretion is stimulated at the initiation of treatment. In some women, prolonged daily use of a GnRH agonist may cause a small increase in LH secretion directly after the daily administration of the GnRH agonist. In turn, residual pituitary LH secretion stimulates ovarian androgen production, which may have detrimental effects on follicular development and endometrial function (Barbieri and Hornstein 1999). Synthetic GnRH antagonists inhibit endogenous LH and FSH release almost immediately (within a few hours), without the occurrence of the initial flare-up effect inherent to GnRH agonists (Chillik et al. 1987). Due to the immediate suppressive action, antagonists require analogue administration for a shorter period and the lower state of pituitary suppression may result in a smaller amount of FSH being required. Accordingly, the application of combined GnRH antagonist and gonadotropin therapy significantly reduces the duration of IVF therapy compared with the usual duration of combined GnRH agonist and gonadotropin treatment (Marshall et al. 1991). Furthermore, the potential for immediate recovery of the suppression of endogenous LH secretion may lead to less impairment of the luteal function (see last section). The immediate reversibility of pituitary suppression after withdrawal of the antagonist provides an opportunity for other stimulation strategies with reduced risk of ovarian hyperstimulation syndrome (OHSS): The final stage of follicular maturation can be triggered by a GnRH agonist instead of the commonly used hCG (Olivennes et al. 1996), which may reduce the risk of OHSS. The risk will even be minimal if the antagonist is used in natural or minimally stimulated cycles (Rongieres-Bertrand et al. 1999). Felberbaum et al. (1998) propose a so-called soft protocol, whereby the old-fashioned clomiphene citrate and hMG stimulation would be given under the cover of mid-cycle GnRH antagonist administration. This treatment would allow the retrieval of three to five mature oocytes which could be treated by ICSI, and the one to two developing embryos could be transferred in the blastocyst stage. This protocol could reduce the risk of OHSS to almost zero.

While GnRH agonists under chronic administration act on the gonadotropic pituitary cells by down-regulation of the GnRH receptors, the antagonists' pharmacological mode of action is based on a classic competitive receptor blockade. The GnRH antagonists suppress LH secretion in a dose-dependent manner: at small doses the suppression of LH is minimal, while at large doses near-complete suppression of LH can be achieved. Mannaerts et al. (1998) showed in a multicenter dose-finding study that larger doses of the antagonist were associated with markedly reduced pregnancy rates in IVF cycles.

Clinically safe GnRH agonists were developed relatively simply by just changing one or two amino acids. However, almost 30 years of trials with replacement of three or more amino acids were required (see Fig. 5) in order to obtain an antagonist with an acceptable pharmacokinetic, safety, and commercial profile. Unfortunately, first- and second-generation GnRH antagonists induce an intense histamine release as an adverse effect, which precludes their use in clinical practice. Third-generation preparations are almost devoid of this unfavorable effect and

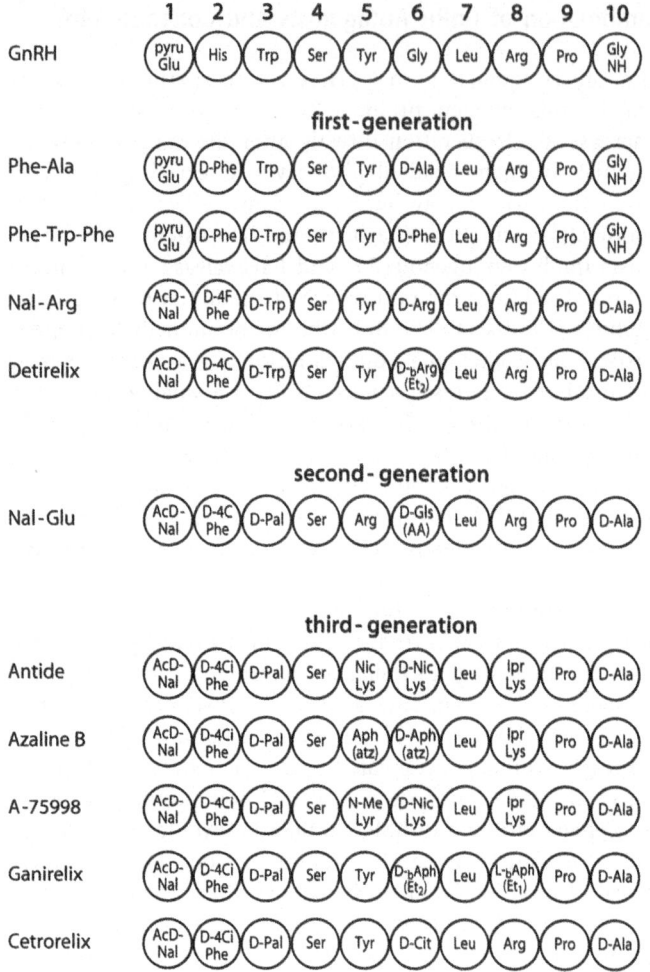

Fig. 5. Amino-acid sequence of the natural GnRH and its first-, second-, and third-generation antagonists

have been tested in clinical trials (Gordon et al. 1990). The two antagonists most commonly used in clinical studies are cetrorelix and ganirelix. Both are well tolerated, and all protocols were safe, effective, and convenient treatment regimens. The first pregnancies achieved by using GnRH antagonists for IVF in combination with gonadotropins were reported in 1994 for cetrorelix (Diedrich et al. 1994; Olivennes et al. 1994) and in 1998 for ganirelix (Itskovitz-Eldor et al. 1998).

The GnRH antagonists have been used either as small daily doses ("Lübeck protocol": cetrorelix, 0.25 mg daily s.c. injection from stimulation day 5 or 6 onwards until ovulation induction) (Diedrich et al. 1994) or as a single dose ("French protocol": cetrorelix, 3 mg s.c. on stimulation day 7) (Olivennes et al. 1994).

The interim analysis of the largest (531 patients) known prospective, multi-center study of a GnRH antagonist for controlled ovarian hyperstimulation in combination with gonadotropins for IVF showed that cetrorelix ("Lübeck proto-col") reliably prevents premature LH surges, is effective in terms of clinical pregnancy rate per started cycle and per ET (22% and 27%), and is safe in terms of a low incidence of patients hospitalized due to ovarian hyperstimula-tion syndrome grade II/III (Devroey 1999). Results of further smaller studies with the GnRH antagonists are given in Table 1.

Fixed Stimulation Protocols

Fixed stimulatory protocols were initially introduced for research purposes, to retrieve oocytes from volunteers at specific times (Braude et al. 1984). Subse-quently, these methods were applied also for clinical IVF (Rainhorn et al. 1987), and they gained remarkable popularity following improvement by Kemeter and Feichtinger (1989).

The fixed protocol consists of administering an oral contraceptive from the first day of the cycle for at least 18 days. This treatment is stopped on a Tues-day, and menstruation is expected within 2–7 days. Nevertheless, 100 mg/day clomiphene is started on the following Sunday, along with two ampules of hMG administered every other day and continued until the next Thursday. The pa-tient should present at the IVF center for the first follow-up visit on the next Sunday, that is, on day 8 of stimulation. Subsequently, treatment is adjusted to the individual response of the patient. The fixed protocol has the advantage that it can be adjusted to the time schedule of the IVF team, and a gynecologist not involved in IVF can also initiate it (Kemeter and Feichtinger 1989).

Stimulation in "Poor Responders"

The ideal approach for patients who respond poorly to standard controlled ovarian hyperstimulation regimens remains one of the major challenges for IVF. This condition, affecting 9–24% of patients undergoing IVF treatment (Keay et al. 1997), can be approached in either of two ways. Apart from exclud-ing these patients from IVF cycles, which may serve only to protect a program's success rates, the only ethical choice appears to be to attempt to improve their fertility chances by maximizing outcomes in IVF cycles.

Originally, the definition of poor response to ovarian stimulation was based on low peak estradiol levels (< 300 pg/ml) alone in cycles stimulated with hMG (García et al. 1983). Patients falling into this category produced fewer follicles and had fewer oocytes retrieved, fertilized, and transferred, and a lower preg-nancy rate compared with normal responders. With stimulation protocols be-coming more aggressive, this definition has also evolved. Although there is no universally accepted definition of poor responders, several programs use this term for patients with peak estradiol concentrations < 500 pg/ml, and three or fewer recruited dominant follicles or collected oocytes. However, some authors include patients whose cycle was canceled because of a spontaneous LH surge or who require a large dose of gonadotropins (Karande and Gleicher 1999; Hugues and Cédrin-Durnerin 1998). Other terms used to describe this condition include low responder, bad responder, and nonresponder.

Poor ovarian response can be explained, at least in part, by ovarian aging, i.e., diminishing ovarian reserve. Ovaries of women with a poor functional reserve contain fewer follicles, which are in a hypoxic environment and consist of fewer granulosa cells, with possibly impaired function. The decrease of the follicle pool brings about a reduction in inhibin levels (Seifer et al. 1996). The pituitary reacts by increasing FSH secretion, which in turn leads to an increase in basal estradiol levels (Klein et al. 1996). This situation leads to a greater risk of premature LH surge and ovulation and early luteinization, adversely affecting oocyte quality and the overall outcome of IVF treatment (Barri et al. 1998).

Since the decrease in ovarian reserve progresses with time, patient age has been found to be a risk factor for low ovarian response. Several studies have shown that cycle cancellation rates increase, the numbers of oocytes and embryos fall, and the pregnancy rates worsen as age rises, despite similar fertilization rates (Hull et al. 1996; Templeton et al. 1996). Furthermore, it has been observed that although poor response can also occur in young patients, pregnancy rates are still higher in younger women (Hanoch et al. 1998).

Several tests have been proposed to predict poor response to ovarian stimulation. These include simple serum measurements, as well as dynamic challenge tests and ultrasonographic assessment of the ovaries.

High basal FSH levels, measured in the early follicular phase (days 3–5) are considered to be reliable predictors of low response (Magarelli et al. 1996), and the value of this test is further increased by the observation that basal FSH levels do not vary significantly during a period of 1 year (Brown et al. 1995).

Recently, low (< 3 mIU/ml) basal LH levels have also been found to be predictive of a poor response (Noci et al. 1998). High basal estradiol (Smotrich et al. 1995) and low inhibin-B levels (Seifer et al. 1997) are associated with a worse response and higher cancellation rates. The clomiphene citrate challenge test has been proposed for the measurement of ovarian functional reserve, based on a higher rise of FSH concentrations after administration of clomiphene in case of low inhibin levels (Loumaye et al. 1990).

The use of high-frequency transvaginal transducers has made it possible to determine the number of small follicles after desensitization of the ovaries, just before starting ovarian stimulation. This number was found to correlate with the number of retrieved oocytes, thus predicting ovarian response (Tomás et al. 1997).

Another quick and cost-effective method for assessing the prognosis of stimulation is to measure ovarian volume before starting the administration of gonadotropins, as demonstrated by Lass et al. (1997). Although Tomás et al. (1997) found that the number of follicles gives a more accurate prognosis than ovarian volume, the latter method seems to be of great value in cases in which obesity or a distant localization of the ovaries perturbs the image quality.

In spite of the proven validity of these tests, there are still patients with normal endocrinological and ultrasound characteristics who will respond poorly to stimulation. Thus, a poor response may not be predicted until failure has occurred with standard stimulation protocols.

Several attempts have been made to improve cycle characteristics and IVF outcome for poor responders. One of these approaches includes increasing the doses of gonadotropins. However, a larger amount of gonadotropins produces only a slight improvement in serum estradiol levels or number of oocytes and does not increase the pregnancy rate because the fertilization rate is unchanged or even reduced (Land et al. 1996; Hugues and Cédrin-Durnerin 1998).

Currently, most IVF cycles are carried out following a long desensitization protocol. However, it has been established that GnRH agonists themselves may contribute to low ovarian response (Cédrin-Durnerin 1999). This has led to several approaches in which the dose and timing of GnRH agonist administration was adjusted so as to improve success rates in low responders. With reduction of the GnRH dosage at the end of the desensitization period ("mini-dose" protocol), a significant improvement in follicular as well as hormonal ovarian response was observed – i.e., lower cancellation rate, higher peak estradiol levels, smaller amounts of gonadotropins, shorter length of stimulation, increased numbers of retrieved oocytes and embryos transferred, and increased fertilization rates – in patients with a high basal FSH (Ben-Rafael and Feldberg 1993; Feldberg et al. 1994). The reduced amount of GnRH agonists was found to be still sufficient for maintaining pituitary suppression and preventing a premature LH surge.

Based on the protocol outlined above, the Norfolk group (Faber et al. 1998) developed a treatment regimen under which administration of the GnRH agonist leuprolide is terminated with the onset of menses ("stop-GnRH agonist" protocol), and high-dose gonadotropin therapy is applied thereafter. The authors reported an improved response to stimulation as well as higher pregnancy rates. Importantly, only one case of premature LH surge was observed among the 80 cycles, despite total withholding of the GnRH agonist.

Administration of GnRH agonists according to the short or "flare" protocol takes advantage of the initial stimulatory effect of GnRH agonists on endogenous secretion of FSH and LH. This treatment regimen, proposed by García et al. (1990) for poor responders, has met with limited success (Karande et al. 1997). However, "micro-doses" of GnRH agonists can trigger significant endogenous release of gonadotropins while providing adequate suppression of the pituitary and avoiding any premature LH surge. Several groups have reported improved ovarian response with this protocol, in which 20–40 µg leuprolide acetate is administered twice daily starting on cycle day 2, along with gonadotropins, and continuing until the administration of hCG (Scott and Navot 1994; Surrey et al. 1998). In order to avoid corpus luteum rescue, patients are pretreated with oral contraceptives through a cycle.

Homburg et al. (1988a) introduced combined ovarian stimulation with growth hormone (GH) and gonadotropins for the treatment of poor responders. The mode of action of GH as a component of this combination has not yet been clarified completely. Nevertheless, the favorable effects of GH are probably due to the stimulation of IGF-I (insulin-like growth factor I) production by granulosa cells (Homburg et al. 1988b) and/or hepatocytes (Homburg et al. 1991). IGF-I enhances the differentiation and FSH-dependent aromatase activity of granulosa cells (Carson et al. 1989). Combined therapy consists of supplementing continuous gonadotropin treatment with the administration of 20–24 IU synthetic growth hormone every other day for 1–2 weeks. A randomized, placebo-controlled study was conducted which did not show any significant improvement in response to GH preparations (Dor et al. 1995). More recent attempts with adjuvant administration of growth hormone-releasing factor have not proven effective in poor responders either (Howles et al. 1999).

Despite the wide range of possibilities made available by recent improvements to standard stimulation protocols, there are still patients who respond poorly to any treatment regimen. The only way to overcome this "oocyte factor" infertility is by oocyte donation.

Indications for Ovarian Stimulation for IVF

Although controlled ovarian hyperstimulation performed to induce multiple follicular growth is a major prerequisite to the success of IVF, pregnancy rates are probably influenced by other factors, too (Edwards 1984). Moreover, it is not yet understood whether relatively low (20%–30%) pregnancy rates result from the direct, unfavorable effects of stimulatory agents on oocyte maturation or are induced by changes in the hormonal milieu of the oocyte (Messinis 1989). It is currently believed that the efficacy of IVF can be improved by selecting an appropriate protocol as well as by individualizing treatment according to the needs of each patient. This can be accomplished by routine combined application of GnRH agonists and gonadotropins. Hughes et al. (1992) also recommend the use of combined GnRH agonist and gonadotropin stimulation in IVF programs, because their meta-analysis of ten clinical trials demonstrated significantly higher pregnancy rates per treatment cycle or embryo transfer with this approach. In addition, the number of canceled stimulation cycles was also considerably lower than during monotherapy with gonadotropins alone.

Several decades of experience with gonadotropin preparations demonstrate that both hMG and pure FSH are appropriate for inducing multiple follicular growth. Nevertheless, a review of the mechanisms of follicular growth and the selection of the dominant follicle (see first section, above) leads to the conclusion that FSH is the key factor in these processes, while the role of LH is almost negligible. A minimal increase in LH levels is sufficient to induce follicular development, and excessive elevation of serum LH reduces the likelihood of fertilization (see earlier in this chapter). Consequently, the administration of LH can exert unfavorable effects or even prove detrimental during ovarian stimulation. In a meta-analysis of eight randomized clinical studies, Daya et al. (1995) compared the efficacy of hMG stimulation and treatment with pure FSH by reviewing pregnancy rates achieved during IVF and GIFT treatment. The authors concluded that stimulation with pure FSH yields significantly higher pregnancy rates as evidenced by the number of stimulated cycles as well as of performed oocyte retrievals and embryo transfers. Higher therapeutic efficacy was unrelated to the use of GnRH agonists. However, the difference in pregnancy rates achieved by stimulation with FSH or hMG was substantially reduced when these were used in combination with GnRH agonists; this observation is in agreement with the known deleterious effect of elevated LH levels on clinical pregnancy rates. In another meta-analysis of ten randomized trials, Daya (1998) also proved a higher pregnancy rate with FSH, regardless of the type of GnRH agonist protocol used. Although no major differences in oocyte quality were observed in this analysis, complete fertilization failure was more likely with hMG use, and the cells obtained from FSH-primed follicles had greater steroidogenic activity. The advantages of stimulation with pure FSH have been demonstrated also by others (Wikland et al. 1994). Benefits included increases in clinical pregnancy rates and "take-home baby" rates, as well as a lower incidence of spontaneous abortions. All these observations led to the conclusion that stimulation with pure FSH reduces the number of canceled cycles (see two sections below), i.e., the interruption of treatment before or after oocyte retrieval. Presumably, this is attributable to the improved biological properties of oocytes retrieved following pure FSH stimulation as well as to the higher conception rates achieved with such oocytes.

In summary, the routine use of combined GnRH agonist and gonadotropin stimulation seems currently to be the method of choice for IVF treatment, especially when pure FSH is the gonadotropin component of the combination. Conventional FSH preparations extracted from urine are gradually being superseded by highly purified urinary FSH derivatives and, lately, by recombinant FSH preparations.

Regarding the use of GnRH antagonists in stimulation protocols for IVF, many questions need to be answered comparing the agonists with the antagonists. Concerning clinical results of IVF treatments with antagonists, unbiased comparison of the two analogues can only be ensured by double-blinding of trials. So far, only open trials comparing agonists and antagonists have been conducted. Hopefully, future results of larger, double-blind studies with extended follow-up will help us to decide what choice to make. A likely scenario for the future is a differentiated use of agonists and antagonists with optimal adjustment to need in the various IVF stimulation protocols (Huirme et al. 1999).

Ovulation Induction

There are two feasible methods for setting the time of oocyte retrieval during controlled ovarian hyperstimulation performed for the induction of multiple follicular development. In particular, either the time of the endogenous LH surge should be determined, or ovulation should be induced by hCG administration. The time of the LH surge is determined by measuring urinary or serum LH levels. Oocyte retrieval should be performed 24 or 36 h after detecting the LH surge in urine or serum (Yussman and Taymor 1970). Scheduling direct follicular puncture at the time of the LH surge yields lower pregnancy rates than oocyte retrieval performed after hCG administration (Lejeune et al. 1986). Moreover, the former method hardly conforms to the prevailing organizational principles of IVF programs: scheduling based on the time of LH surge requires IVF services to be available around the clock. Furthermore, accurate determination of the time of the LH surge is hindered by the pulsatile nature of pituitary LH release (Yen et al. 1972) and the short duration (approximately 29 h) of peak LH levels that are often lower in stimulated cycles (Messinis et al. 1986b). As a result, scheduling oocyte retrieval by ovulation induction with hCG administration has become almost universal practice in assisted reproduction. The structure and actions of human chorionic gonadotropin, the "pregnancy hormone", are very similar to those of LH (Daughaday 1981), which makes this hormone suitable for inducing ovulation at a desired time. Ovulation follows the intramuscular administration of hCG at 37 h. Accordingly, follicular puncture is performed earlier, i.e., 32–34 h (Edwards et al. 1980) or 35 h (Nader and Berkovitz 1990) after hCG administration. The usual dose of hCG for ovulation induction is 10,000 IU, administered 36 h before the scheduled time of oocyte retrieval. Ovulation induction can be performed if controlled ovarian hyperstimulation has resulted in the development of a 16- to 18-mm follicle as well as two to three additional follicles 15–16 mm in diameter, as seen on ultrasound examination. Moreover, a serum estradiol level of 200–300 pg/ml (0.73–1.1 nmol/l) per ≥15- to 16-mm follicles should be reached. Oocyte retrieval following the administration of a large hCG dose is associated with the additional benefit of supporting the luteal phase favorably through the induction of progesterone synthesis. However, hCG may cause ovarian hyperstimulation syndrome. This complication can be avoided by monitoring the patient closely.

Cycle Cancellation

Cancellation of an IVF cycle can be defined as the discontinuation of ovarian stimulation prematurely without oocyte retrieval (Acosta et al. 1989). The withdrawal of treatment may become necessary for several reasons, medical and nonmedical. Medical causes include delayed follicular development, the occurrence of a premature LH surge or luteinization, and the risk of ovarian hyperstimulation, whereas organizational issues constitute the majority of other factors. Most IVF teams agree that the number of canceled cycles can be reduced significantly by combined stimulation with a GnRH agonist and a gonadotropin (Schmutzler et al. 1988; Smitz et al. 1988; Urbancsek et al. 1991b). In our opinion, therapy should be abandoned when:
1. Follicular growth is delayed (ovarian stimulation over 10 days results in the development of fewer than three follicles ≥16 mm diameter and the serum estradiol level is less than 600 pg/ml [2.2 mmol/l])
2. Basal serum LH level is elevated (LH > 10 IU/l) or a premature LH surge occurs
3. Elevated serum progesterone (> 1.5 ng/ml [4.77 mmol/l]) is detected prior to ovulation induction

4. Ovarian hyperstimulation is suspected (ovary size exceeds 80 mm, both ovaries contain more than ten follicles < 16 mm diameter, and serum estradiol level is ≥ 3500 pg/ml).

Luteal Phase Support in Patients Undergoing Ovarian Stimulation for In Vitro Fertilization

Despite the high (70–80%) fertilization rates achieved with IVF treatment, pregnancy is established in only 15–20% of embryo transfers (Edwards 1984). This comparative failure is generally attributed to relative luteal insufficiency during stimulated cycles (Vaughan et al. 1985). There is much controversy surrounding the role of follicular puncture and aspiration of follicular fluid with partial evacuation of granulosa cells in the etiology of luteal insufficiency (García et al. 1981; Feichtinger et al. 1982). However, the causative role of ovarian hyperstimulation has been demonstrated unequivocally. Martikainen et al. (1987) have shown that combined stimulation with clomiphene citrate and hMG adversely affects luteal function through its excessive influence on pituitary gonadotropin and prolactin release. Others (Vaughan et al. 1985) regard relative luteal insufficiency as a consequence of progesterone deficiency resulting from controlled ovarian hyperstimulation. Originally, Fleming suggested that GnRH agonists probably have no adverse effect on luteal function (Fleming and Coutts 1986). Nevertheless, clinical studies performed in the meantime have demonstrated that GnRH agonists do impair luteal function and emphasized the need for hormone support of the luteal phase during combined treatment with GnRH agonists and gonadotropins (Smitz et al. 1988). Presumably, the detrimental effect of GnRH agonists is not related to any direct action on the corpus luteum, because these compounds are rapidly eliminated from the circulation after withdrawal (Sandow 1983). Clayton and Catt (1981) have demonstrated that suppression of gonadotropin synthesis and release persists for a considerable period after long-term therapy with GnRH agonists. Schriock et al. (1985) suggested that GnRH agonists "switch" pituitary functions to a refractory state. The results of these two studies consistently demonstrate that GnRH agonists impair luteal function indirectly, i.e., through the inhibition of LH release. In their study conducted on patients receiving combined IVF treatment, Smitz et al. (1988) found low LH levels 12 days after the withdrawal of the GnRH agonist.

Luteal insufficiency can be corrected by direct intervention (i.e., progesterone substitution) or indirectly (by hCG administration), or by the combination of these methods. The objective of progesterone substitution is to correct progesterone deficiency caused by the decline of endogenous synthesis. Natural progesterone can be applied in vaginal suppositories (2 × 100 mg daily from the day of embryo transfer) or, more recently, administered as capsules containing micronized natural progesterone. Successful treatment with these capsules can be implemented both by the oral and the vaginal route (in doses of 3 × 100–200 mg daily). Smitz et al. (1992) demonstrated unequivocally that the efficacy of intravaginal micronized progesterone is significantly superior to that of intramuscular treatment, as evidenced by the increased implantation and reduced spontaneous abortion rates. Moreover, progesterone administration has a protective effect against excessive ovarian hyperstimulation, owing to the inhibition of pituitary LH release.

According to Daya (1988), progesterone supplementation during the luteal phase is not associated with increased pregnancy rates. In contrast to these findings, Blumenfeld and Nahhas (1988) reported significantly higher pregnancy rates as well as considerable reduction of abortion rates following hCG administration during the luteal phase. Along with the stimulation of progesterone synthesis in the corpus luteum, hCG also enhances the production of other factors (such as relaxin; Yen 1986) with a potential influence on the process of implantation and the subsequent occurrence of pregnancy. Smitz et al. (1988) recommend the administration of hCG to alleviate LH deficiency associated with combined GnRH agonist and gonadotropin stimulation. Nowadays, luteal phase support with hCG administration is a widely accepted principle in ovarian stimulation with GnRH agonist and gonadotropin combinations (Belaisch-Allart et al. 1990). Hormone support is provided by administering 2500 IU hCG on days 1, 4, and 7 following oocyte retrieval. The only risk associated with hCG support is the development of ovarian hyperstimulation syndrome. When this risk is high, hCG supplementation should be avoided and replaced by progesterone administration. Moreover, sonographic as well as endocrinological monitoring of the ovaries is recommended even in cases where the risk of ovarian hyperstimulation is considered low.

The potential for immediate recovery from the suppression of endogenous LH secretion by the GnRH antagonists may lead to less impairment of the luteal function using GnRH antagonists instead of agonists. However, some luteal support seems to be necessary also after combined GnRH antagonist and gonadotropin stimulation. From the data of Albano et al. (1998), it seems that there may be impaired corpus luteum function even when GnRH antagonists are used. However, there is a need to document these findings in large prospective studies. There are in vitro data suggesting that progesterone accumulation by cultured granulosa-luteal cells from IVF patients treated with GnRH antagonists who are on hCG is better than that seen in agonist controls (Lin et al. 1999).

References

Abdalla HI, Baber RJ, Leonard T, Kirkland A, Mitchell A, Power M, Owen E, Studd JWW (1989) Timed oocyte collection in an assisted conception programme using GnRH analogue. Hum Reprod 4:927–930

Acosta AA, Oehninger SJ, Muasher SJ, Valdes H, Jones D (1989) Treatment cycle cancellation in the Norfolk in vitro fertilization (IVF) program: critical analysis and prognostic significance. Abstracts of the 6th World Congress of In Vitro Fertilization and Alternate Assisted Reproduction in Jerusalem, April 2–7, 1989, p 6

Adashi EY (1984) Clomiphene citrate: mechanism(s) and site(s) of action – a hypothesis revisited. Fertil Steril 42:331–344

Albano C, Smitz C, Camus M, Riethmüller-Winzen H, Van Steirteghem A, Devroey P (1997) Comparison of different doses of gonadotropin-releasing hormone antagonist Cetrorelix during controlled ovarian hyperstimulation. Fertil Steril 67:917–922

Albano C, Grimbizis G, Smitz J, Riethmüller-Winzen H, Reissmann T, Van Steirteghem A, Devroey P (1998) The luteal phase of nonsupplemented cycles after ovarian superovulation with human menopausal gonadotropin and the gonadotropin-releasing hormone antagonist Cetrorelix. Fertil Steril 70:357–359

Baird DT (1987) A model for follicle selection and ovulation: lessons from superovulation. J Steroid Biochem 27:15–23

Barbieri RL, Hornstein MD (1999) Assisted reproduction – in vitro fertilization success is improved by ovarian stimulation with exogenous gonadotropins and pituitary suppression with gonadotropin-releasing hormone analogues. Endocr Rev 20:249–252

Barri PN, Martínez F, Coroleu B, Parera N, Veiga A (1998) Managing nonresponders. Fertility and reproductive medicine. Proceedings of the 16th World Congress on Fertility and Sterility. San Francisco, October 4–9, 1998, pp 127–137

Belaisch-Allart J, De Mouzon J, Lapouterle C, Mayer M (1990) The effect of HCG supplementation after combined GnRH agonist/HMG treatment in IVF programme. Hum Reprod 5:163–166

Belchetz PE, Plant TM, Nakai Y, Keogh EJ, Knobil E (1978) Hypophyseal responses to continuous and intermittent delivery of hypothalamic gonadotropin-releasing hormone. Science 202:631–632

Ben-Rafael Z, Feldberg D (1993) The poor-responder patient in an in vitro fertilization-embryo transfer program. J Assist Reprod Genet 10:118–120

Bergh C, Howles CM, Borg K, Hamberger L, Josefsson B, Nilsson L, Wikland M (1997) Recombinant human follicle-stimulating hormone (r-FSH; Gonal-F) versus highly purified urinary FSH (Metrodin HP): results of a randomized comparative study in women undergoing assisted reproductive techniques. Hum Reprod 12:2133–2139

Bernardus RE, Jones GS, Acosta AA, García JE, Liu HC (1985) The significance of the ratio in follicle-stimulating hormone and luteinizing hormone in induction of multiple follicular growth. Fertil Steril 43:373–378

Blumenfeld Z, Nahhas F (1988) Luteal dysfunction in ovulation induction: the role of repetitive human chorionic gonadotropin supplementation during the luteal phase. Fertil Steril 50:403–407

Braude PR, Bright MV, Douglas CP, Milton PJ, Robinson RE, Williamson JG, Hutchinson J (1984) A regimen for obtaining mature human oocytes from donors for research into human fertilization in vitro. Feril Steril 42:34–38

Brown JR, Liu HC, Sewitch KF, Rosenwaks Z, Berkeley AS (1995) Variability of day 3 FSH levels in eumenorrheic women. J Reprod Med 40:620–624

Burgus R, Butcher M, Ling N, Monahan M, Rivier J, Fellows R, Amoss M, Blackwell R, Vale W, Guillemin R (1971) Molecular structure of the hypothalamic factor (LRF) of ovine origin monitoring the secretion of pituitary gonadotropic hormone ofluteinization. C R Acad Sci Hebd Seances Acad Sci D 273:1611–1613

Carmel PW, Araki S, Ferin M (1976) Pituitary stalk portal blood collection in rhesus monkeys: evidence of pulsatile release of gonadotropin-releasing hormone (GnRH). Endocrinology 99:243–248

Carson RS, Zhang Z, Hutchinson LA, Herington AC, Findlay JK (1989) Growth factors in ovarian function. J Reprod Fertil 85:735–746

Chillik CF, Itskovitz J, Hahn DW, McGuire JL, Danforth DR, Hodgen GD (1987) Characterizing pituitary response to a gonadotropin-releasing hormone (GnRH) antagonist in monkeys: tonic follicle-stimulating hormone/luteinizing hormone secretion versus acute GnRH challenge tests before, during and after treatment. Fertil Steril 48:480–485

Clayton RN, Catt KJ (1981) Gonadotropin-releasing hormone receptors: characterisation, physiological regulation and relationship to reproductive function. Endocr Rev 2:186–209

Daughaday WH (1981) The adenohypophysis. In: Williams RH (ed) Textbook of endocrinology. Saunders, London, pp 80–86

Daya S (1988) Efficacy of progesterone support in the luteal phase following in-vitro fertilisation and embryo transfer: meta-analysis of clinical trials. Hum Reprod 3:731–734

Daya S (1998) hMG versus FSH: is there any difference? In: Filicori M, Flamigni C (eds) Ovulation induction: update '98. Parthenon, Carnforth, pp 183–192

Daya S, Gunby J (1999) Recombinant versus urinary follicle-stimulating hormone for ovarian stimulation in assisted reproduction. Hum Reprod 14:2207–2215

Daya MB, Gunby J, Hughes EG, Collins JA, Sagle MA (1995) Follicle-stimulating hormone versus human menopausal gonadotropin for in vitro fertilization cycles: a meta-analysis. Fertil Steril 64:347–354

De Mouzon J, Lancaster P (1995) World collaborative report 1993. 15th World Congress on Fertility and Sterility, Montpellier, September 17–22, 1995

Devroey P (1999) Cetrotide multidose protocol: results of the largest multinational study with an antagonist in ART. Abstracts of the Symposium "Cetrotide in daily clinical practice", First Congress on Controversies in Obstetrics and Gynecology and Infertility. Prague, October 29, 1999, pp 10–12

Devroey P, Van Steirteghem A, Mannaerts B, Coelingh Bennink H (1992) First singleton term birth after ovarian superovulation with rh-FSH. Lancet 340:1108–1109

Diedrich K, Diedrich C, Wildt L, Van Der Ven H, Al-Hasani S, Werner A, Krebs D (1987) Ovarielle Stimulation mit reinem FSH in einem In-vitro-Fertilisationsprogramm. Geburtsh Frauenheilkd 47:612–618

Diedrich K, Van Der Ven H, Al-Hasani S, Krebs D (1988) Ovarian stimulation for in-vitro fertilisation. Hum Reprod 3:39–44

Diedrich K, Diedrich C, Santos E, Zoll C, Al-Hasani S, Reissmann T, Krebs D, Klingmüller D (1994) Suppression of the endogenous luteinizing hormone surge by the gonadotropin-releasing hormone antagonist Cetrorelix during ovarian stimulation. Hum Reprod 9:788–791

Dor J, Seidman DS, Amudai E, Bider D, Levran D, Mashiach S (1995) Adjuvant growth hormone therapy in poor responders to in-vitro fertilization: a prospective randomized placebo-controlled double-blind study. Hum Reprod 10:40–43

Edwards RG (1984) Human conception in vitro: new opportunities in medicine and research. In: Trounson AO, Wood EC (eds) In vitro fertilization and embryo transfer. Churchill Livingstone, Edinburgh, pp 217–250

Edwards RG, Steptoe PC, Purdy JM (1980) Establishing full-term human pregnancies using cleaving embryos grown in vitro. Br J Obstet Gynaecol 87:737–756

Eibschitz I, Belaisch-Allart J, Frydman R (1986) In vitro fertilization management and results in stimulated cycles with spontaneous luteinizing hormone discharge. Fertil Steril 45:231–236

Faber BM, Mayer J, Cox B, Jones D, Toner JP, Oehninger S, Muasher SJ (1998) Cessation of gonadotropin-releasing hormone agonist therapy combined with high-dose gonadotropin stimulation yields favorable pregnancy results in low responders. Fertil Steril 60:826–830

Feichtinger W, Kemeter A, Szalay S, Back A, Janish H (1982) Could aspiration of the graafian follicle cause luteal phase deficiency? Fertil Steril 37:205–208

Feldberg D, Farhi J, Ashkenazi J, Dicker D, Shalev J, Ben-Rafael Z (1994) Minidose gonadotropin-releasing hormone agonist is the treatment of choice in poor responders with high follicle-stimulating hormone levels. Fertil Steril 62:343–346

Felberbaum RE, Ludwig M, Diedrich K (1998) Are we on the verge of a new era in ART? Hum Reprod 13:1778–1780

Fishel SB, Edwards RG, Purdy JM, Steptoe PC, Webster J, Walters E, Cohen J, Fehilly C, Hewitt J, Rowland G (1985) Implantation, abortion and birth after in vitro fertilization using the natural menstrual cycle or follicular stimulation with clomiphene citrate and human menopausal gonadotropin. J In Vitro Fert Embryo Transf 2:123–131

Fleming J, Coutts JRT (1986) Induction of multiple follicular growth in normally menstruating women with endogenous gonadotropin suppression. Fertil Steril 45:226–230

Fleming R, Adam AH, Barlow DH, Black WP, Macnaughton MC, Coutts JRT (1982) A new systematic treatment for infertile women with abnormal hormone profiles. Br J Obstet Gynaecol 89:80–83

Forman RG, Frydman R, Egan D, Ross C, Barlow D (1990) Severe ovarian hyperstimulation syndrome using agonists of gonadotropin-releasing hormone for in vitro fertilization: a European series and a proposal for prevention. Fertil Steril 53:502–509

Frydman R, Parneix I, Belaish-Allart JC, Forman R, Hazout A (1988) LHRH agonists in IVF: different methods of utilisation and comparison with previous ovulation stimulation treatments. Hum Reprod 3:559–561

Fujii S, Sagara M, Kudo H, Kagiya A, Sato S, Saito Y (1997) A prospective randomized comparison between long and discontinuous-long protocols of gonadotropin-releasing hormone agonist for in vitro fertilization. Fertil Steril 67:1166–1168

Fujino M, Kobayashi S, Obayashi M (1972) Structure-activity relationships in the C-terminal part of luteinising-hormone releasing hormone (LHRH). Biochem Biophys Res Commun 49:863–869

García JE, Jones GS, Wright GL jr (1981) Prediction of the time of ovulation. Fertil Steril 36:308–315

García JE, Jones GS, Acosta AA, Wright G (1983) Human menopausal gonadotropin/human chorionic gonadotropin follicular maturation for oocyte aspiration: phase I and II. Fertil Steril 39:167–179

García JE, Padilla SL, Bayati J, Baramki TA (1990) Follicular phase gonadotropin-releasing hormone agonist and human gonadotropins: a better alternative for ovulation induction in in vitro fertilization. Fertil Steril 53:302–305

Gemzell CA, Diczfalusy E, Tillinger G (1958) Clinical effect of human pituitary follicle-stimulating hormone (FSH). J Clin Endocrinol Metab 18:1333–1348

Gordon K, Williams RF, Danforth DR, Hodgen GD (1990) A novel regimen of gonadotropin-releasing hormone (GnRH) antagonist plus pulsatile GnRH: controlled restoration of gonadotropin secretion and ovulation induction. Fertil Steril 54:1140–1145

Grillo M, Buck S, Mettler L (1987) Ovulationsinduktion mit reinem urinären FSH bei Patientinnen eines In Vitro Fertilisationsprogrammes. Fertilitat 3:181–185

Hanoch J, Lavy Y, Holzer H, Hurwitz A, Simon A, Revel A, Laufer N (1998) Young low responders protected from the untoward effects of reduced ovarian response. Fertil Steril 69:1001–1004

Hodgen GD (1982) The dominant ovarian follicle. Fertil Steril 38:281–300

Homburg R, Armar NA, Eshel A, Adams J, Jacobs HS (1988a) Influence of serum luteinising hormone concentrations on ovulation, conception, and early pregnancy loss in polycystic ovary syndrome. Br Med J 297:1024–1026

Homburg R, Eshel A, Abdalla I, Jacobs HS (1988b) Growth hormone facilitates ovulation induction by gonadotropins. Clin Endocrinol 29:113–117

Homburg R, West C, Ostergaard H, Jacobs HS (1991) Combined growth hormone and gonadotropin treatment for ovulation induction in patients with nonresponsive ovaries. Gynecol Endocrinol 5:33–36

Hoomans E, Out HJ (1999) The use of recombinant FSH (Puregon) in controlled ovarian hyperstimulation: a move to milder stimulation. Abstracts of the symposium: Changing perspectives in assisted reproduction. 11th World Congress on In Vitro Fertilization and Human Reproductive Genetics. pp 5–7

Howles CM (1996) Genetic engineering of human FSH (Gonal-F). Hum Reprod Update 2:172–191

Howles CM, Macnamee MC, Edwards RG (1987) Short-term use of an LHRH agonist to treat poor responders entering an in-vitro fertilisation programme. Hum Reprod 2:655–656

Howles C, Barri P, Cittadini E, Diedrich K, Fioretti P, Flamigini C, Hazout A, Herbaut N, Nicollet B, Schoysman R, Siebzehnrubl E, Lancaster S, Giroud-Venderickx D, Loumaye E (1993) Metrodin HP: clinical experience with a new highly purified follicle-stimulating hormone preparation suitable for subcutaneous administration. In: Lunenfeld B (ed) FSH alone in ovulation induction. Parthenon, New York, pp 45–61

Howles CM, Loumaye E, Germond M, Yates R, Brinsden P, Healy D, Bonaventura LM, Strowitzki T (1999) Does growth hormone-releasing factor assist follicular development in poor responder patients undergoing ovarian stimulation for in-vitro fertilization? Hum Reprod 14:1939–1943

Hughes EG, Fedorkow DM, Daya S, Sagle MA, Van de Koppel P, Collins JA (1992) The routine use of GnRHa prior to IVF and GIFT: a meta-analysis of randomized controlled trials. Fertil Steril 58:888–896

Hugues JN, Cédrin-Durnerin I (1998) Revisiting gonadotrophin-releasing hormone agonist protocols and management of poor ovarian responses to gonadotrophins. Hum Reprod Update 4:83–101

Huirme JAF, Lambalk CB, Janssens R, Schoemaker J (1999) Agonist versus antagonist: where are we today? Abstracts of the Symposium "Cetrotide in daily clinical practice", First Congress on Controversies in Obstetrics and Gynecology and Infertility. Prague, October 29, 1999, pp 4–8

Hull MGR, Fleming CF, Hughes AO, McDermott A (1996) The age-related decline in female fecundity: a quantitative controlled study of implanting capacity and survival of individual embryos after IVF. Fertil Steril 65:783–790

Itskovitz-Eldor J, Kol S, Mannaerts B, Coelingh Bennink H (1998) First established pregnancy after controlled ovarian hyperstimulation with recombinant follicle stimulating hormone and the gonadotrophin-releasing hormone antagonist ganirelix (Org 37462) Hum Reprod 13:294–295

Jacob S, Drudy L, Conroy R, Harrison RF (1998) Outcome from consecutive in-vitro fertilization/intracytoplasmic sperm injection attempts in the final group treated with urinary gonadotrophins and the first group treated with recombinant follicle-stimulating hormone. Hum Reprod 13:1783–1787

Jones HW, Jones GS, Andrews MC, Acosta A, Bundren C, García J, Sandow B, Veeck L, Wilkes C, Witmyer J (1982) The program for in vitro fertilization at Norfolk. Fertil Steril 38:14–21

Jones HW, Acosta A, Andrews MC, García JE, Jones GS, Mantzawinos T, McDowell J, Sandow B, Veeck L, Whibley T (1983) The importance of follicular phase to success and failure in in vitro fertilization. Fertil Steril 40:317–321

Jones GS, García JE, Rosewaks Z (1984) The role of pituitary gonadotropins in follicular stimulation and oocyte maturation in the human. J Clin Endocrinol Metab 59:178–80

Jones GS, Acosta AA, García JE, Bernardus RE, Rosenwaks Z (1985) The effect of follicle-stimulating hormone without additional luteinizing hormone on follicular stimulation and oocyte development in normal ovulatory woman. Fertil Steril 43:696–702

Karande V, Gleicher N (1999) A rational approach to the management of low responders in in-vitro fertilization. Hum Reprod 14:1744–1748

Karande V, Morris R, Rinehart J, Miller C, Rao R, Gleicher N (1997) Limited success using the "flare" protocol in poor responders in cycles with low basal follicle-stimulating hormone levels during in vitro fertilization. Fertil Steril 67:900–903

Keay SD, Liversedge NH, Mathur RS, Jenkins JM (1997) Assisted conception following poor ovarian response to gonadotrophin stimulation. Br J Obstet Gynaecol 104:521–527

Kemeter P, Feichtinger W (1989) Erste Erfahrungen mit einem fixen Stimulationsschema für die In-vitro-Fertilisation (IVF) ohne Bluthormonbestimmungen. Fertilitat 5:14–21

Kerin JF, Warnes GM (1986) Monitoring of ovarian response to stimulation in in-vitro fertilization cycles. Clin Obstet Gynecol 29:158–170

Kingsland C, Tan SL, Bickerton L, Mason B, Campbell S (1992) The routine use of gonadotropin-releasing hormone agonists for all patients undergoing in vitro fertilization. Is there any medical advantage? A prospective randomised study. Fertil Steril 57:804–809

Kistner RW (1965) Induction of ovulation with clomiphene citrate (Clomid). Obstet Gynecol Surv 20:873–899

Klein NA, Battaglia DE, Fujimoto VY, Davis GS, Bremner WJ, Soules MR (1996) Reproductive aging: accelerated ovarian follivular development associated with a monotropic FSH rise in normal older women. J Clin Endocrinol Metab 81:1038–1045

Kondaveeti-Gordon U, Harrison RF, Barry-Kinsella C, Gordon AC, Drudy L, Cottell E (1996) A randomized prospective study of early follicular or midluteal initiation of long protocol gonadotropin-releasing hormone in an in vitro fertilization program. Fertil Steril 66:582–586

Lamb EJ, Colliflower WW, Williams JW (1972) Endometrial histology and conception rates after clomiphene citrate. Obstet Gynecol 39:389–396

Land JA, Yarmolinskaya MI, Dumoulin JCM, Evers JLH (1996) High-dose human menopausal gonadotropin stimulation in poor responders does not improve in vitro fertilization outcome. Fertil Steril 65:961–965

Lass A, Skull J, McVeigh E, Margara R, Winston RML (1997) Measurement of ovarian volume by transvaginal sonography before ovulation induction with human menopausal gonadotrophin for in-vitro fertilization can predict poor response. Hum Reprod 12:294–297

Laufer N, DeCherney AH, Haseltine FP, Polan ML, Merzer HC (1983) The use of high-dose human menopausal gonadotropin in an in vitro fertilization program. Fertil Steril 40:731–741

Laufer N, DeCherney AH, Haseltine FP, Polan ML, Tarlatzis BC (1984) Human in vitro fertilization employing individualized ovulation induction by human menopausal gonadotropin. J In Vitro Fert Embryo Transf 1:56–62

Lejeune B, Degueldre M, Camus M, Vekemans M, Opsomer L, Leroy F (1986) In vitro fertilization and embryo transfer as related to endogenous luteinizing hormone rise or human chorionic gonadotropin administration. Fertil Steril 45:377–383

Leyendecker G, Wildt L, Hansmann M (1980) Pregnancies following chronic-intermittent (pulsatile) administration of GnRH by means of a portable pump ("Zyklomat") – a new approach to the treatment of infertility of hypothalamic amenorrhoea. J Clin Endocrinol Metab 51:1214–1216

Leyendecker G, Bernart W, Bremen T, Beck H, Kunz G, Waibel S, Blum A, Stenger P, Kaplan-Reiterer H (1990) Influence of the duration of the oestradiol rise on the success rate in GnRH analogue/HMG-stimulated IVF cycles. Hum Reprod 5:52–55

Li T, Hindle J (1993) Adverse local reaction to intramuscular injections of urinary-derived gonadotrophins. Hum Reprod 8:1835–1836

Lin Y, Kahn JA, Hillensjö T (1999) Is there a difference in the function of granulosa luteal cells in patients undergoing in vitro fertilization either with gonadotropin-releasing hormone agonist or gonadotropin-releasing hormone antagonist? Hum Reprod 14:885–888

Lopata A (1983) Concepts in human in vitro fertilization and embryo transfer. Fertil Steril 40:289–301

Lopata A, Brown JB, Leeton JF, McTalbot J, Wood C (1978) In vitro fertilization of preovulatory oocytes and embryo transfer in infertile patients treated with clomiphene and human choronic gonadotropin. Fertil Steril 30:27–35

Lopata A, Johnston IWH, Hoult IJ, Speirs AI (1980) Pregnancy following intrauterine implantation of an embryo obtained by in vitro fertilization of a preovulatory egg. Fertil Steril 33:117–120

Loumaye E, Catt KJ (1983) Agonist-induced regulation of pituitary receptors for gonadotropin-releasing hormone. J Biol Chem 258:12002–12009

Loumaye E, Naor Z, Catt KJ (1982) Binding affinity and biological activity of gonadotrophin-releasing hormone agonists in isolated pituitary cells. Endocrinology 111:730–736

Loumaye E, de Coorman S, Sartanaer JG, Psalti I, Depreester S, Thomas K (1988) Resultats obtenus en fecondation in vitro par administration de Buserelin et HMG chez des patients ayant presentés un echec de stimulation par CC-HMG ou HMG. Fertil Contracept Sexual 2:29–32

Loumaye E, Vankrieken L, Depreester S, Psalti J, De Cooman S, Thomas K (1989) Hormonal changes induced by short-term administration of a gonadotropin-releasing hormone agonist during ovarian hyperstimulation for in vitro fertilization and their consequences for embryo development. Fertil Steril 51:105–111

Loumaye E, Billion JM, Mine JM, Psalti I, Pensis M, Thomas K (1990) Prediction of individual response to controlled ovarian hyperstimulation by means of a clomiphene citrate challenge test. Fertil Steril 53:295–301

Lunenfeld B, Menzi A, Volet B (1960) Clinical effects of human postmenopausal gonadotropin. Rass Clin Ter Sci Affini 59:213–217

Macnamee MC, Howles CM (1987) The occurrence, characteristics and management of the LH surge in IVF. Hum Reprod 2 [Suppl 1]:46

Macnamee MC, Howles CM, Edwards RG, Taylor PJ, Elder KT (1989) Short-term luteinizing hormone-releasing hormone agonist treatment: prospective trial of a novel ovarian stimulation regimen for in vitro fertilization. Fertil Steril 52:264–269

Magarelli PC, Pearlstone AC, Buyalos RP (1996) Discrimination between chronological and ovarian age in infertile women aged 35 years and older: predicting pregnancy using basal FSH, age and number of ovulation induction/intra-uterine insemination cycles. Hum Reprod 11:1214–1219

Mannaerts B, Devroey P, Åbyholm T, Diedrich K, Hedon B, Itskovitz-Eldor J, Kahn J, Naether O, Olivennes F, Tarlatzis B, Westergaard L, Vanderheiden B (1998) A double blind randomised dose finding study to the efficacy of the gonadotropin-releasing hormone antagonist ganirelix (Org 37462) to prevent premature luteinizing surges in women undergoing ovarian stimulation with recombinant follicle stimulating hormone (Puregon-R). Hum Reprod 13:3023–3031

Marrs RP, Vargyas JM, Shangold GM, Yee B (1984) The effect of time of the initiation of clomiphene citrate on the multiple follicle development for human in vitro fertilization and embryo replacement procedures. Fertil Steril 41:682–685

Marshall LA, Fluker MR, Jaffe RB, Monroe SE (1991) Inhibition of follicular development by a potent antagonistic analog of gonadotropin-relesing hormone (detirelix). J Clin Endocrinol Metab 72:927–933

Martikainen H, Rønnberg L, Ruokonen A, Kauppila A (1987) Anterior pituitary dysfunction during the luteal phase following ovarian hyperstimulation. Fertil Steril 47:446

McBain JC, Trounson A (1984) Patient management: treatment cycle. In: Wood EC, Trounson AO (eds) Clinical in vitro fertilization. Springer, Berlin Heidelberg New York Tokyo, pp 49–65

Messinis IE (1989) Drugs used in in vitro fertilisation procedures. Drugs 38:148–159

Messinis IE, Templeton AA (1987) Endocrine and follicle characteristics of cycles with and without endogenous luteinizing hormone surges during superovulation induction with pulsatile follicle stimulating hormone. Hum Reprod 1:11–16

Messinis IE, Templeton AA, Baird DT (1986a) Comparison between clomiphene plus pulsatile human menopausal gonadotrophin and clomiphene plus pulsatile follicle stimulating hormone in induction of multiple follicular development in woman. Hum Reprod 1:223–226

Messinis IE, Templeton AA, Baird DT (1986b) Endogenous luteinizing hormone surge in women during induction of multiple follicular development with pulsatile follicle stimulating hormone. Clin Endocrinol 24:193–201

Nader S, Berkovitz A (1990) Study of the pharmakokinetics of human chorionic gonadotropin and its relation to ovulation. J In Vitro Fert Embryo Transf 7:114–118

Neveu S, Hedon B, Bringer J, Chinchole JM, Arnal F, Humeau C, Cristol P, Viala JL (1987) Ovarian stimulation by a combination of a gonadotropin-releasing hormone agonist and gonadotropins for in vitro fertilization. Fertil Steril 47:639–643

Noci I, Biagiotti R, Maggi M, Ricci F, Cinotti A, Scarselli G (1998) Low day 3 luteinizing hormone values are predictive of reduced response to ovarian stimulation. Hum Reprod 11:1169–1172

Olijve W, DeBoer W, Mulders JWM (1996) Molecular biology and biochemistry of human recombinant follicle-stimulating hormone (Puregon). Mol Hum Reprod 2:371–382

Olivennes F, Fanchin R, Bouchard P, de Ziegler D, Taieb J, Selva J, Frydman R (1994) The single or dual administration of the gonadotropin-releasing hormone antagonist Cetrorelix in an in vitro fertilization-embryo transfer program. Fertil Steril 62:468–476

Olivennes F, Fanchin R, Bouchard P (1996) Triggering of ovulation by a gonadotropin hormone-releasing hormone (GnRH) agonist in patients pretreated with a GnRH antagonist. Fertil Steril 66:151–153

Olivennes F, Alvarez S, Bouchard P, Fanchin R, Salat-Baroux J, Frydman R (1998) The use of a GnRH antagonist (Cetrorelix) in a single dose protocol in IVF-embryo transfer: a dose finding study of 3 versus 2 mg. Hum Reprod 13:2411–2414

Out HJ, Mannaerts BMJL, Driessen SGAJ, Bennink HJTC (1995) A prospective, randomized, assessor-blind, multicentre study comparing recombinant and urinary follicle-stimulating hormone (Puregon versus Metrodin) in in-vitro fertilization. Hum Reprod 10:2534–2540

Out HJ, Reimitz PE, Coelingh Bennink HJT (1997) A prospective, randomized study to assess the tolerance and efficacy of intramuscular and subcutaneous administration of recombinant follicle-stimulating hormone (Puregon). Fertil Steril 67:278-283

Oyesanya OA, Teo SK, Quah E, Abdurazak N, Lee FY, Cheng WC (1995) Pituitary down-regulation prior to in-vitro fertilization and embryo transfer: a comparison between a single dose of Zoladex depot and multiple daily doses of Suprefact. Hum Reprod 10:1042-1044

Perrin MH, Rivier JE, Vale WW (1980) Radioligand assay for gonadotrophin-releasing hormone: relative potencies of agonists and antagonists. Endocrinology 106:1289-1296

Phillips E, Page M, Fleming SD (1999) A prospective comparison of two different recombinant FSH preparations. Abstract book of the 11th World Congress on In Vitro Fertilization and Human Reproductive Genetics, p 88

Porter RN, Smith W, Craft IL, Abdulwahid NA, Jacobs HS (1984) Induction of ovulation for in-vitro fertilisation using buserelin and gonadotrophins. Lancet 2:1284-1285

Rainhorn JD, Forman RG, Belaish-Allart J, Hazout A, Fries N, Tesstart J, Frydman R (1987) One year's experience with programmed oocyte retrieval for IVF. Hum Reprod 2:491-494

Raj SG, Berger MJ, Grimes EM, Taymor ML (1977) The use of gonadotropins for the induction of ovulation in women with polycystic ovarian disease. Fertil Steril 28:1280-1284

Recombinant Human FSH Study Group (1995) Clinical assessment of recombinant human follicle-stimulating hormone in stimulating ovarian follicular development before in vitro fertilization. Fertil Steril 63:77-86

Rogers P, Milne B, Trounson A (1986) A model to show uterine receptivity and embryo viability following ovarian stimulation for in vitro fertilization. J In Vitro Fert Embryo Transf 3:93-98

Ron-El R, Herman A, Golan A, Bahar R, Weinraub Z, Soffer Y, Caspi E (1990) Ultrashort luteinizing hormone-releasing hormone agonist protocol in ovarian hyperstimulation for IVF. Abstracts of the 2nd Joint ESCO-ESHRE Meeting, Milan 1990, 114-115

Ron-El, Raziel A, Friedler S, et al (1998) Characteristics of very short regimens. Ovulation Induction Update '98. Proceedings of 2nd World Conference on Ovulation Induction. Bologna, September 12-13, 1997, pp 91-95

Rongieres-Bertrand C, Olivennes F, Righini C, Fanchin R, Taïeb J, Hamamah S, Bouchard P, Frydman R (1999) Revival of the natural cycles in in-vitro fertilization with the use of a new gonadotrophin-releasing hormone antagonist (Cetrorelix): a pilot study with minimal stimulation. Hum Reprod 14:683-688

Rosenwaks Z, Muasher SJ (1986) Recruitment of fertilizable eggs. In: Jones GS, et al (eds) In vitro fertilization Norfolk. Williams and Wilkins, Baltimore, pp 30-51

Rutherford AJ, Subak-Sharpe RJ, Dawson KJ, Margara RA, Franks S (1988) Improvement on in vitro fertilisation after treatment with buserelin, an agonist of luteinizing hormone-releasing hormone. Br Med J 296:1965-1968

Salat-Baroux J, Alvarez S, Antoine JM, Tibi C, Cornet D, Mandelbaum J, Plachot M, Junca AM (1988) Comparison between long and short protocols of LHRH agonist in the treatment of polycystic ovary desease by in-vitro fertilization. Hum Reprod 3:535-539

Sandow J (1983) Clinical application of LHRH and its analogues. Clin Endocrinol 18:517-592

Schally AV, Arimura AA, Baba Y, Nair RMG, Matsuo H, Redding TW, Debeljuk L (1971) Isolation and properties of the FSH- and LH-releasing hormone. Biochem Biophys Res Commun 43:393-399

Schmutzler RK, Reichert C, Diedrich K, Wildt L, Diedrich C, Al-Hasani S, Van Der Ven H, Krebs D (1988) Combined GnRH-agonist/gonadotropin stimulation for in-vitro fertilisation. Hum Reprod 3 [Suppl 2]:29-33

Schoemaker J, Wentz A, Jones GS (1977) Induction of ovulation with pure FSH in patients with amenorrhea and elevated LH levels. Fertil Steril 28:295-298

Schriock ED, Monroe SE, Martin MC, Henzel MR, Jaffe RB (1985) Effect on corpus luteum function of luteal phase administration of a potent gonadotropin-releasing hormone analog (Nafarelin). Fertil Steril 43:844-850

Scoccia B, Blumenthal P, Wagner C, Prins G, Scommegna A, Marut EL (1987) Comparison of urinary human follicle-stimulating hormone and human menopausal gonadotropin for ovarian stimulation in an in vitro fertilization program. Fertil Steril 48:446–449

Scott RT, Navot D (1994) Enhancement of ovarian responsiveness with microdoses of gonadotropin-releasing hormone agonist during ovulation induction for in vitro fertilization. Fertil Steril 61:880–885

Seifer DB, Gardiner AC, Lambert-Messerlian G, Schweyer AL (1996) Differential secretion of dimeric inhibin in cultured luteinized granulosa cells as a function of ovarian reserve. J Clin Endocrinol Metab 81:736–739

Seifer DB, Lambert-Messercian G, Hogan JW, Gardiner AC, Blazar AS, Berk CA (1997) Day 3 serum inhibin-B is predictive of assisted reproductive technologies outcome. Fertil Steril 67:110–114

Sharma V, Williams J, Collins W, Riddle A, Mason B, Whitehead M (1988) The sequential use of a luteinizing hormone-releasing hormone (LH-RH) agonist and human menopausal gonadotropin to stimulate folliculogenesis in patients with resistant ovaries. J In Vitro Fert Embryo Transf 5:38–42

Smitz J, Devroey P, Camus M, Deschacht J, Khan I, Staessen C, Van Waesberghe L, Wisanto A, Van Steirteghem AC (1988) The luteal phase and early pregnancy after combined GnRH-agonist/HMG treatment for superovulation in IVF or GIFT. Hum Reprod 3:585–590

Smitz J, Devroey P, Faguer B, Bopurgain C, Camus M, Van Steirteghem (1992) A prospective randomized comparison of intramuscular or intravaginal natural progesterone as a luteal phase and early pregnancy supplement. Hum Reprod 7:168–175

Smotrich BB, Widra EA, Gindoff PR, Levy MJ, Hall JL, Stillman RJ (1995) Prognostic value of day 3 estradiol on in vitro fertilization outcome. Fertil Steril 64:1136–1140

Speirs A, Trounson A, Warmer GM, Yovich JL, Saunders DM (1984) Summary of results. In: Wood EC, Trounson AO (eds) Clinical in vitro fertilization. Springer, Berlin Heidelberg New York Tokyo, pp 157–163

Stanger JD, Yovich JL (1985) Reduced in-vitro fertilisation of human oocytes from patients with raised basal luteinising hormone levels during the follicular phase. Br J Obstet Gynaecol 92:385–393

Steptoe PC, Edwards RG (1978) Birth after the reimplantation of a human embryo. Lancet 2:366

Surrey ES, Bower JA, Hill DM, Ramsey J, Surrey MW (1998) Clinical and endocrine effects of a microdose GnRH agonist flare regimen administered to poor responders who are undergoing in vitro fertilization. Fertil Steril 69:419–424

Swift AD, Crighton DB (1979) Relative activity, plasma elimination and tissue degradation of synthetic luteinising hormone-releasing hormone and certain of its analogues. J Endocrinol 80:141–152

Tan SL, Kingsland C, Campbell S, Mills C, Bradfield J, Alexander N, Yovich J, Jacobs HS (1992) The long protocol of administration of gonadotropin-releasing hormone agonist is superior to the short protocol for ovarian stimulation for in vitro fertilization. Fertil Steril 57:810–814

Templeton A, Morris JK, Parslow W (1996) Factors that affect outcome of IVF treatment. Lancet 348:1402–1406

Testart J, Forman R, Belaisch-Allart J, Volante M, Hazout A, Strubb N, Frydman R (1989) Embryo quality and uterine receptivity in in-vitro fertilisation cycles with or without agonists of gonadotrophin-releasing hormone. Hum Reprod 4:198–201

Tom C, Nuojua-Huttunen S, Martikainen H (1997) Pretreatment transvaginal ultrasound examination predicts ovarian responsiveness to gonadotrophins in in-vitro fertilization. Hum Reprod 12:220–223

Trounson AO, Leeton JF, Wood EC, Webb J, Wood J (1981) Pregnancies in humans by fertilization in vitro and embryo transfer in the controlled ovulatory cycle. Science 212:681–682

Urbancsek J, Witthaus E (1996) The midluteal buserelin administration is superior to early follicular phase administration in combined GnRH-analogue and gonadotropin stimulation for controlled ovarian hyperstimulation. Fertil Steril 65:966–971

Urbancsek J, Rabe T, Grunwald K, Kiesel L, Runnebaum B (1990a) Analysis of hormonal changes during combined buserelin/hMG treatment. Hum Reprod 5:675–681

Urbancsek J, Rabe T, Grunwald K, Runnebaum B (1990b) Diagnose, Häufigkeit und klinische Bedeutung des vorzeitigen LH-Anstiegs-/Gipfels bei Patientinnen eines In-vitro-Fertilisierungs- und Gametentransfer-Programmes. Geburtsh Frauenheilkd 50:454–462

Urbancsek J, Rabe T, Gör Ü, Schulte B, Grunwald K, Papp Z, Runnebaum B (1991a) Wirkung des GnRH-Analogons Buserelin auf die Serum-Spiegel von Sexualhormonen in Abhängigkeit von Behandlungsbeginn und Behandlungsdauer. Geburtsh Frauenheilkd 51:617–625

Urbancsek J, Rabe T, Grunwald K, Thuro H, Runnebaum B (1991b) Kombinierte Behandlung mit einem GnRH-Analogon und Gonadotropinen bei IVF-ET/GIFT-Patientinnen nach vorangegangen erfolglosen reinen HMG-Stimulation. Zentralbl Gynakol 113:563–574

Urbancsek J, Rabe T, Grunwald K, Kiesel L, Klinga K, Papp Z, Runnebaum B (1992) Serum inhibin levels in gonadotropin stimulated in-vitro fertilization/gamete intra-fallopian transfer cycles. Hum Reprod 7:1195–1200

Urbancsek J, Rabe T, Grunwald K, Sztanyik L, Ibrahim M, Papp Z, Runnebaum B (1993a) Serum inhibin levels in gonadotropin-stimulated IVF/GIFT cycles. In: Rodriguez OA, Baumgartner W, Burgos L (eds) Fertility and sterility, progress in research and practice. Parthenon, Carnforth, pp 415–430

Urbancsek J, Rabe T, Grunwald K, Kiesel L, Sztanyik L, Papp Z, Runnebaum B (1993b) Elevated serum inhibin levels and suppressed luteinizing hormone surge in young patients stimulated with gonadotropins. Gynecol Endocrinol 7:23–31

Vandervorst M, Devroey P (1998) Recombinant FSH: results in assisted reproduction. Ovulation Induction Update '98. Proceedings 2nd World Conference on Ovulation Induction. Bologna, September 12–13, 1997, pp 137–146

Vaughan J, Safro E, Gidley-Baird A, Saunders DM, O'Neill C (1985) Luteal phase endocrine defects as a possible cause of failure of IVF and ET. Abstracts handbook of the 4th World Conference of In Vitro Fertilization, Melbourne, November 1985, p 211

Von During V, Kahn JA, Sunde A (1999) Results of a prospective, randomized study comparing two recombinant FSH preparations (Gonal-F, Puregon) in IVF and ICSI treatments. Abstract book of the 11th World Congress on In Vitro Fertilization and Human Reproductive Genetics, p 265

Wikland M, Borg K, Borg J, Forsberg AS, Hammar M, Jakobsson AH, Svalander P, Waldenström U (1993) Human chorionic gonadotrophin (hCG) administered by the subcutaneous route for induction of oocyte maturation in an IVF-embryo transfer program. Hum Reprod 8:S262

Wikland M, Borg J, Hamberger L, Svalender P (1994) Simplification of IVF: minimal monitoring and the use of subcutaneous highly purified FSH administration for ovulation induction. Hum Reprod 9:1430–1436

Wildt L, Diedrich K, Van Der Ven H, Al-Hasani S, Hübner H, Klasen R (1986) Ovarian hyperstimulation for in-vitro fertilisation controlled by GnRH agonist administered in combination with human menopausal gonadotrophins. Hum Reprod 1:15–19

Yen SSC (1986) The human menstrual cycle. In: Yen SSC, Jaffe RB (eds) Reproductive endocrinology, 2nd edn. Saunders, Philadelphia, p 213

Yen SSC, Tsai CC, Naftolin F, Vendenberg G, Ajabor L (1972) Pulsatile patterns of gonadotropin release in subjects with and without ovarian function. J Clin Endocrinol Metab 34:671–675

Yussman MA, Taymor ML (1970) Serum levels of follicle-stimulating hormone and luteinizing hormone and of plasma progesterone related to ovulation by corpus luteum biopsy. J Clin Endocrinol Metab 30:396–399

Zimmermann R, Soor B, Braendle W, Lehmann F, Weise HC, Bettendorf G (1982) Gonadotropin therapy of female infertility. Analysis of results in 416 cases. Gynecol Obstet Invest 14:1–18

Zorn JR, Barata M, Brami C, Epelboin S, Nathan C, Papageorgiou G, Quantin P, Rolet F, Savale M, Boyer P, et al (1988) Ovarian stimulation for in vitro fertilisation combining administration of gonadotropins and blockade of the pituitary with D-Trp6-LHRH microcapsules: pilot studies with two protocols. Hum Reprod 3:235–239

Ovarian Hyperstimulation Syndrome

V. Insler, E. Lunenfeld, B. Lunenfeld

Introduction

Almost all complications of gonadotropin treatment are due essentially to ovarian stimulation, multiple follicular development, and luteinization or ovulation of numerous follicles. The main complications are:
1. A high incidence of multiple pregnancy, which may result in serious gestational and perinatal complications such as increased abortion rate, prematurity, pathological lies and presentations, and high incidence of cesarean sections
2. Ovarian hyperstimulation syndrome (OHSS)

Modern treatment of infertility makes extensive use of ovulation-inducing drugs such as clomiphene citrate (CC), human menopausal gonadotropins (hMG), highly purified or recombinant follicle-stimulating hormone (FSH-HP, rFSH), synthetic native gonadotropin-releasing hormone (GnRH), and its numerous agonists (GnRHa). These drugs are applied as three different treatment modalities:
1. Substitution therapy – to replace lacking endogenous ovarian stimulation capacity
2. Regulation therapy – to override inappropriate endogenous signal transmission
3. Superovulation therapy – aimed at developing an oversized follicular cohort which will subsequently yield a high number of ova ready for natural or in vitro fertilization

All of the above types of ovarian stimulation, but particularly the latter variant, may result in the development of multiple follicles which, when luteinized, produce excessive quantities of steroids and peptides regulating the growth and permeability of blood vessels. The final effect of this sequence of events may be a massive fluid shift and recompartmentalization resulting in hypovolemia on the one hand and in edema, ascites, hydrothorax, or hydropericardium on the other hand; in consequence, this may lead to impaired function of the heart, kidneys, and liver, as well as to thromboembolic phenomena.

Any form of ovulation-induction therapy may result in OHSS. As early as 1977, Insler and Lunenfeld [1] stated: "To obtain a reasonable pregnancy rate in gonadotropin-induced ovulations one has to operate at a dose level very close to the hyperstimulation dose."

It has to be realized, and accepted, that OHSS is an iatrogenic disorder which cannot be entirely avoided at present, but its incidence may be significantly reduced by flexible planning and meticulous monitoring of ovarian stimulation, and its outcome may be dramatically improved by appropriate therapy.

Ovarian hyperstimulation has been observed after the administration of clomiphene citrate [2], gonadotropins [3], native gonadotropin-releasing hormone [4], and its agonists [5]. Of special interest is also the report of Ludwig et al. [6] describing a case of severe OHSS which occurred in a spontaneous pregnancy with triploidy and hydatidiform mole and persisted even after induced abortion. The abnormally high levels of hCG produced by molar pregnancy were probably the driving force for development and persistence of ovarian hyperstimulation.

Classification of Ovarian Hyperstimulation Syndrome

A comprehensive classification of hyperstimulation into six grades based on the severity of the symptoms, signs, and laboratory findings was originally proposed by our group in 1967 [7]. It was later modified into three grades [8] (Table 1). Grade I (mild hyperstimulation) is characterized by bilateral ovarian enlargement (multiple follicular and corpus luteum cysts measuring up to 5×5 cm). Laboratory findings in serum include E2 values greater than 1500 pg/ml (6000 pmol/l), progesterone levels greater than 30 ng/ml (115 nmol/l) in the early part of the luteal phase, or urinary estrogen levels above 150 µg/24 h and pregnanediol excretion above 10 mg/24 h.

Grade II (moderate hyperstimulation) is characterized by ovaries enlarged up to 12×12 cm accompanied by abdominal discomfort and gastrointestinal symptoms such as nausea, vomiting, and diarrhea. A sudden increase in weight above 3 kg may be an early sign of moderate hyperstimulation.

Table 1. Grading of OHSS

Signs and symptoms	Grade I	Grade II	Grade III
Excessive steroids	+	+	+
Ovary size	Enlarged	6–12 cm	>12 cm
Abdominal discomfort	?	+	+
Abdominal distention		+	+
Nausea		+	+
Vomiting		?	+
Diarrhea		?	+
Ascites		?	+
Hydrothorax			+
Hydropericardium			?
Oliguria			+
Severe hemoconcentra-tion			+
Thromboembolic phe-nomena			?

Grade III (severe hyperstimulation) is defined by the presence of large ovarian cysts, ascites, in some cases also pleural and/or pericardial effusion, electrolyte imbalance, hypovolemia, and even hypovolemic shock. In extreme cases there is severe hemoconcentration, increased blood viscosity, and thromboembolic phenomena.

The incidence of moderate and severe hyperstimulation compiled from more than 11 300 ovulation-induction cycles reported in the literature varied from 3.1% to 6% and from 0.25% to 1.8%, respectively [9]. Sonographic monitoring of ovulation induction raised hopes for reduction of the incidence of OHSS. On the other hand, advanced reproductive technologies (ART), all using aggressive ovarian stimulation, carried with them a forecast of increased risk of ovarian hyperstimulation. It seems, however, that neither the optimistic hopes nor the pessimistic forecasts for changes in the OHSS frequency were realized. In 1998, Grudzinskas and Egbase [10] still maintained that clinically relevant ovarian hyperstimulation occurs in up to 10% of cycles and may become a life-threatening complication in 0.5%–2.0% of these.

Tulandi et al. [11] found the pregnancy rate to be three times greater in hyperstimulated than in nonhyperstimulated cycles. It is generally agreed that mild hyperstimulation (multifollicular development) is associated with an increased pregnancy rate. This indicates that causing mild OHSS might be beneficial to increasing the pregnancy rate. However, it should be noted that in severe hyperstimulation the abortion rate is significantly increased.

Thus, induction of mild hyperstimulation renamed with a probably more correct term "superovulation" or "controlled ovarian hyperstimulation (COH)" is today generally used in IVF protocols, and, combined with IUI, in treatment of unexplained, cervical, and some forms of male infertility. It has been pointed out that aspiration of follicles may lower the chance of development of clinical hyperstimulation by reducing the mass of luteinized granulosa cells, although it may not and should not be considered a complete safeguard. This practice has also been suggested as a measure to prevent hyperstimulation due to ovulation induction in anovulatory patients. Hazout and Belaisch [12] reported that in treatment cycles in which more than three large follicles were present prior to the administration of hCG, follicular aspiration was performed 36 h after administration of the ovulatory dose of hCG, leaving only two follicles. The aspirated oocytes were fertilized in the laboratory and frozen. If the patient did not become pregnant these extra embryos were transferred in later cycles.

Pathogenesis

The primary basis of ovarian hyperstimulation is multifollicular development. In the spontaneous ovulatory cycle, delicate but efficient feedback mechanisms ensure recruitment of a limited number of early antral follicles into a functional cohort and full development of a single leading follicle capable of ovulating in response to the midcycle LH surge (Fig. 1). In gonadotropin-stimulated cycles, this fine endogenous control does not exist and cannot be fully replaced by

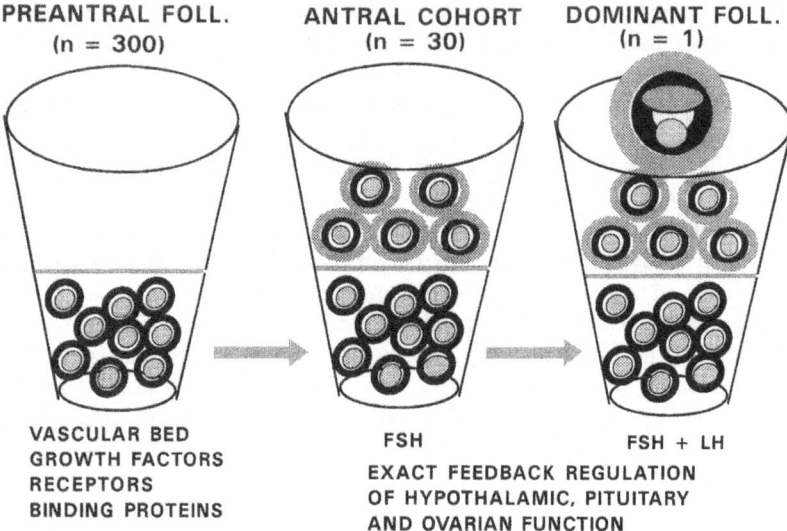

PREANTRAL FOLL.
(n = 300)

ANTRAL COHORT
(n = 30)

DOMINANT FOLL.
(n = 1)

VASCULAR BED
GROWTH FACTORS
RECEPTORS
BINDING PROTEINS

FSH

EXACT FEEDBACK REGULATION
OF HYPOTHALAMIC, PITUITARY
AND OVARIAN FUNCTION

FSH + LH

Fig. 1. Follicular development in a spontaneous cycle. Depending on their proximity to the ovarian vascular bed and the possible action of some yet undefined growth factors, approximately 300 primordial and preantral follicles start to develop, until several of them reach the early antral stage and acquire FSH receptors. These early antral follicles are then recruited into a cyclic cohort by rising levels of FSH. Continuous FSH stimulation permits the selection of one representative of an antral follicular cohort for further growth. The selected dominant follicle regulates the inhibin, FSH, and LH levels in a manner that ensures its further development, on the one hand, and atresia of all other follicles originating from the same cohort, on the other

even the most meticulous monitoring. A pharmacological dose of gonadotropins is administered in order to ensure successful therapy. This results in recruitment and maintenance of a number of antral follicles, several of them being sustained as leading follicles and capable of either luteinization or ovulation (Fig. 2).

Final maturation and luteinization of multiple follicles results in excessive production of vascular endothelial growth factor (VEGF). This peptide has been shown to exert a twofold action: it serves as a potent promoter of neovasculogenesis, on the one hand, and may increase the permeability of blood vessels walls, thus disrupting functional integrity of the vascular bed, on the other hand [13–15]. Thus, the appearance of OHSS may be perceived as an exaggeration of a physiological process. Its successive stages (Fig. 3), as described by Insler and Lunenfeld [16], consist of:

1. Recruitment of a large number of small antral follicles into a functional cohort
2. Development of numerous large antral follicles until ovulation (or luteinization)
3. Excessive production of VEGF by the developing large follicles
4. Exaggerated perifollicular neovascularization, with some of the new blood vessels exhibiting increased permeability

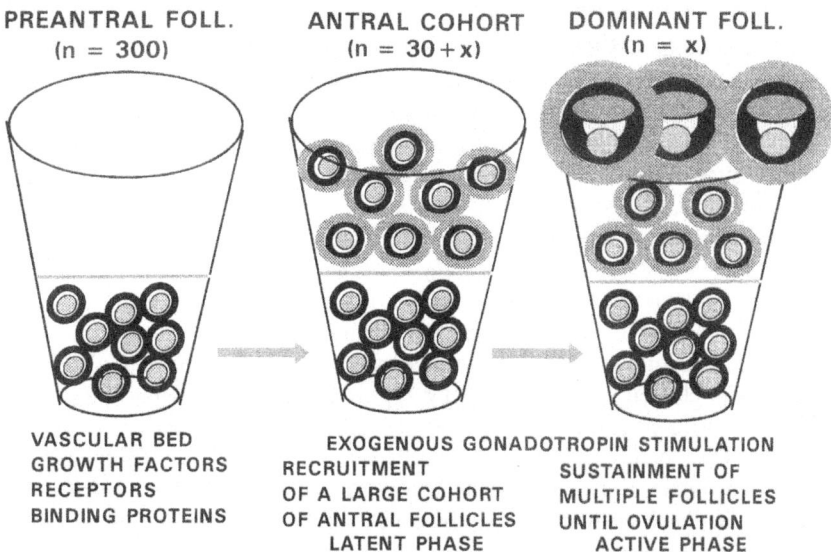

PREANTRAL FOLL.
(n = 300)

ANTRAL COHORT
(n = 30 + x)

DOMINANT FOLL.
(n = x)

VASCULAR BED
GROWTH FACTORS
RECEPTORS
BINDING PROTEINS

EXOGENOUS GONADOTROPIN STIMULATION
RECRUITMENT
OF A LARGE COHORT
OF ANTRAL FOLLICLES
LATENT PHASE

SUSTAINMENT OF
MULTIPLE FOLLICLES
UNTIL OVULATION
ACTIVE PHASE

Fig. 2. Follicular development stimulated by application of exogenous gonadotropins. Depending on their proximity to the ovarian vascular bed and the possible action of some yet undefined growth factors, approximately 300 primordial and preantral follicles start to develop, until several of them reach the early antral stage and acquire FSH receptors. Administration of a pharmacological dose of gonadotropins results in recruitment of a large cohort of early antral follicles (latent phase of therapy). Continuous administration of exogenous gonadotropins sustains the development of multiple follicles (active phase of therapy), several of them acting as dominant follicles and reaching pre-ovulatory stage

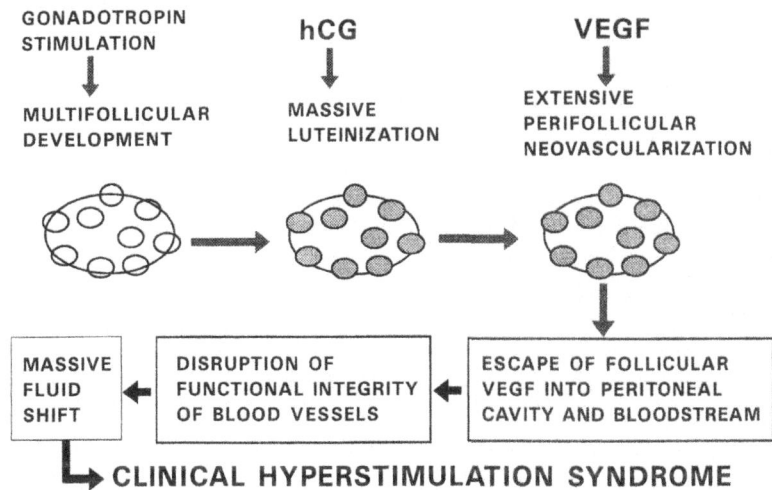

GONADOTROPIN
STIMULATION

hCG

VEGF

MULTIFOLLICULAR
DEVELOPMENT

MASSIVE
LUTEINIZATION

EXTENSIVE
PERIFOLLICULAR
NEOVASCULARIZATION

MASSIVE
FLUID
SHIFT

DISRUPTION OF
FUNCTIONAL INTEGRITY
OF BLOOD VESSELS

ESCAPE OF FOLLICULAR
VEGF INTO PERITONEAL
CAVITY AND BLOODSTREAM

CLINICAL HYPERSTIMULATION SYNDROME

Fig. 3. Pathophysiological mechanism of ovarian hyperstimulation syndrome (*hCG* human chorionic gonadotropin, *VEGF* vasculoendothelial growth factor)

5. Escape of follicular fluid and perifollicular blood vessels content including large amounts of VEGF into the peritoneal cavity and its subsequent absorption into the general vascular bed
6. Functional impairment of general vascular bed
7. Massive fluid shift from the intravascular into the third compartment
8. Intravascular hypovolemia, concomitant with development of edema, ascites, hydrothorax, and/or hydropericardium
9. Impairment of cardiac, renal, pulmonary, and liver function

Ovarian hyperstimulation occurs after massive follicular luteinization. It is therefore observed only following hCG administration or following a spontaneous LH peak induced by the elevated estrogen production of multifollicular growth. The clinical symptoms usually appear 5–10 days following the first dose of hCG. In women with a spontaneous LH surge hyperstimulation is rare. This might be due to intraovarian regulatory components such as inhibin, insulin-like growth factor-1 (IGF-1) and its binding proteins (IGF-BPs), and/or ovarian pituitary feedback regulation including also secretion of specific gonadotropin-secretion-attenuating factor (GnSAF).

With the increased use of "triphasic therapeutic regimens" consisting of hMG stimulation following desensitization of the pituitary gland by GnRH agonists, the estrogen-induced endogenous LH surge is practically eliminated. This therapeutic method will reduce hyperstimulation caused by a spontaneous LH surge, but it may increase the rate of hyperstimulation following hCG, because in combined pituitary suppression/ovarian stimulation therapy significantly larger doses of hMG are employed. As will be discussed later, preventing ovulation by withholding hCG is an effective method of avoiding hyperstimulation in overstimulated ovaries.

The fact that ovulation (luteinization) is necessary for the OHSS to occur suggests the involvement of intraovarian regulators in the pathogenesis of this syndrome. Polishuk and Schenker [17] found that high-dose hMG treatment caused no complications in male rabbits while all hyperstimulated female rabbits, including a group with extraperitonealized ovaries, displayed ovarian enlargement and ascites. They concluded that ovarian secretion is responsible for increased capillary permeability, causing an extraperitoneal fluid shift. In fact, high levels of ovarian hormones have been detected in severe cases of clinical hyperstimulation, including estradiol, estriol, progesterone, 17-OH-progesterone, pregnanediol, pregnanetriol, testosterone, 17-hydroxycorticosteroids, and 17-ketosteroids [18].

The exact factor(s) responsible for enhanced capillary permeability have been, until recently, the subject of lively debate. While Schenker and Polishuk [19] have proposed prostaglandins, others have implicated estrogens in this role. Schenker's hypothesis is supported by the fact that antiprostaglandins such as indomethacin alleviate ascites formation. However, Pride et al. [20] contested the above hypothesis. In their experiments with rabbits, ascites formation was not influenced despite good suppression of ovarian prostaglandins. Thus they suggest that prostaglandins are not obligatory mediators of the third space fluid shifting.

Other findings support a role of estrogen in increasing capillary permeability. Davis [21] found that injection of estradiol increased the rate of labeled albumin loss into the extravascular space. Cecil et al. [22] reported effects of estrogen upon the uterus, such as water imbibition, hyperemia, electrolyte changes, and vasodilation. The length of the effect was dose related, with permeability returning to normal after 48 h. However, findings of other authors question the estrogen hypothesis; for example, administration of large doses of exogenous estrogens does not cause the syndrome [23].

Regardless of its etiology, the increased capillary permeability results in massive ascites and hypovolemia, which Engel et al. [24] term the "cardinal events" in the pathogenesis of OHSS. Hypovolemia is associated with hemoconcentration, decreased central venous pressure, low blood pressure, and tachycardia. Severe hypovolemia also causes decreased renal perfusion, leading to increased reabsorption of sodium and water in the proximal tubule [17], which results in oliguria and low urinary sodium. Exchange of hydrogen and potassium for sodium in the distal tubule is reduced, resulting in an accumulation of H^+ and K^+ and causing hyperkalemia and a tendency to acidosis [24]. Additional factors leading to increased sodium retention in patients with OHSS include:

1. Increased renin production
2. Enhanced aldosterone secretion
3. Elevated androgens

Sims [25] proposed that increased progesterone in these patients might cause a natriuretic effect which could stimulate increased aldosterone secretion. This effect could be further compounded by elevated androgens, which might increase retention of water and Na^+ in human beings [26].

Cytokines such as interleukin-1 (IL-1) or interleukin-6 (Il-6) were also suggested as possible actors on the OHSS stage, since they have an effect on vascular permeability. Both serum and ascitic fluid from women with OHSS contained significantly higher levels of Il-6 than did control sera and peritoneal fluids [27]. An explicit cause-effect relationship between cytokines and the incidence or severity of OHSS has not yet been established. Several authors proposed that the sequence of events leading to clinical ovarian hyperstimulation is initiated by excessive activation of the angiotensin-renin system [28, 29] Navot et al. [30] reported that plasma renin activity has been significantly elevated in hyperstimulated cycles and correlated with severity of hyperstimulation. On the other hand, some signs and/or components of hyperstimulation syndrome such as ascites, hypovolemia, and enlarged ovaries may, by themselves, stimulate renin production [31–33]. As pointed out above, the preeminent theory is that VEGF of follicular origin is the main, although possibly not the sole, component responsible for development of OHSS. The idea that additional substances produced or concentrated by the hyperstimulated ovary may play a role in the development and/or progression of OHSS can certainly not be dismissed at this stage. The exact roles of IL-6, of renin-angiotensin cascade [34], and of kinin-kallikrein system [35] as promoters or abettors of ovarian hyperstimulation must be elucidated in detail.

The extensiveness of ascites is reflected in the patient's weight gain. Indeed, an initial gain of more than 3 kg following hCG administration should be considered a serious warning sign of developing OHSS, warranting close patient observation. Patients with severe OHSS can gain as much as 15–20 kg.

A quite dangerous but rare side effect of OHSS is the occurrence of thromboembolic phenomena. The connection between hMG/hCG treatment and clotting abnormalities was first described by our group [36]. While the cause of thromboembolic phenomena is still not fully established, they are probably related to hemoconcentration and associated with elevated estrogen levels. Phillips et al. [37] reported high levels of factor V, platelets, fibrinogen, profibrinolysin, and fibrinolytic inhibitors and increased thromboplastin generation in patients with OHSS. All these findings may be regarded as the result of hemoconcentration and the majority of them as a corollary to hyperestrogenicity.

Management

Recognition of Risk Factors in the Development of OHSS

Knowledge of the risk factors and close observation of clinical conditions are useful for preventing the occurrence, or at least reducing the incidence, of severe hyperstimulation. Factors which should be considered include:
- Patient risk (age, diagnosis)
- Estrogen levels prior to hCG administration
- Method of drug administration
- Results of ovarian ultrasonography
- FSH/LH ratio
- Probably, the level of growth hormone (GH) and/or IGF-1,which have been shown to modulate ovarian sensitivity to gonadotropic stimulation

Whereas young oligomenorrheic, anovulatory women are at greater risk for ovarian hyperstimulation, increased age is associated with a decrease in the risk of OHSS [38] but probably with a higher risk for thromboembolic complications and, obviously, with a much lower chance for success. The lower GH reserve in this age-group may be one of the factors explaining lower risk for OHSS. Amenorrheic patients who respond to progestational agents with withdrawal bleeding are at greater risk than hypoestrogenic amenorrheic women and should be treated more conservatively and monitored more closely. Tulandi et al. [11] found that when hyperstimulation occurs in hypoestrogenic amenorrheic patients it tends to occur in their first treatment cycle, because the response of this group of women to ovarian stimulation is relatively uniform in consecutive cycles. On the other hand, spontaneously menstruating patients are notoriously capricious in their reaction to gonadotropin therapy and it is extremely difficult to predict the hMG dose required for stimulation on the strength of previous treatment cycles.

The risk of PCOD patients with elevated LH levels for developing OHSS is high following clomiphene citrate and gonadotropin treatment. Since growth factors have a role in modulating ovarian sensitivity, and PCOD patients have decreased IGF-1 binding proteins (IGF-1BP), it can be speculated that the resulting excessive level of free IGF-1 increases ovarian sensitivity to gonadotropic stimulation and may increase the risk of hyperstimulation. Future management may involve monitoring of growth hormone (GH), IGF-1, and or IGF-1BP levels to reduce this risk.

Recently, Fulghesu et al. [39] reported the results of a clinical experiment carried out in 34 PCOD patients treated with urinary FSH/hCG for induction of ovulation. In the early follicular phase of the cycle preceding the treatment cycle, all women were subjected to a 75-g oral glucose tolerance test (OGTT). Twenty patients were classified as hyperinsulinemic and 14 as normoinsulinemic. The majority (70%) of the hyperinsulinemic women were also obese, while obesity was observed in only 21% of the normoinsulinemic subjects. The mean total FSH dose and the number of large (>16 mm) follicles were similar in both groups. The number of midsize follicles (12–16 mm) and mean serum estradiol levels were significantly higher in the hyperinsulinemic group. The incidence of OHSS was also higher in hyperinsulinemic as compared with normoinsulinemic PCO patients.

Hyperinsulinemia resulting from insulin resistance is a fairly typical feature in women with PCOD and is known to be considerably amplified by obesity [40, 41]. Insulin, either directly or indirectly through IGF-1, can act upon the ovary and exert some gonadotropin-like stimulatory function. It would be logical to presume that hyperinsulinemic women have an amplified ovarian response to stimulation and thus develop more follicles when treated with gonadotropins. If the report of Fulghesu and co-workers is confirmed by other research, measurement of insulin levels during a simple OGTT might prove to be useful for predicting increased risk of hyperstimulation in women with PCOD and/or obesity.

The Role of Treatment Schedule in Prevention of OHSS

Incidence or severity of OHSS is also related to the treatment schedule and to the dose of hMG or FSH and hCG. Administration of hMG or FSH according to an individually adjusted treatment scheme (with daily doses increasing or decreasing stepwise) is associated with a lower incidence of OHSS than when gonadotropins are administered according to other, particularly fixed, regimens. In addition, a lower incidence of OHSS is found in cycles in which hCG administration does not overlap with hMG treatment [42]. Polishuk and Schenker [17] found that increased doses of hMG are associated with increased OHSS severity, as indicated by ovarian size and severity of ascites and pleural effusion. The study by Tulandi et al. [11] of 27 anovulatory women who had experienced at least one episode of hyperstimulation during hMG/hCG therapy suggests that there is no such correlation. These authors found no significant difference in either the duration of treatment or the amount of hMG administered between nonhyperstimulated and hyperstimulated cycles. It seems that the variability of patient response is of greater significance than the variability of dosage. Modern monitoring techniques facilitate the establishment of proper dosage to stimulate a proper level of follicular development, but it is unlikely that it will be possible to entirely eliminate the occurrence of hyperstimulation.

Due to its prolonged biological half-life (30 h), administration of hCG creates an ovulatory surge of rather long duration. Following intramuscular or subcutaneous injection of a single dose of 10 000 IU hCG, high levels of the hormone were observed for 3 or 4 days and the substance was still detectable in serum after 8 days (Shoham et al., personal communication).

Recently, several authors proposed the creation of a more attenuated and shorter mid-cycle gonadotropin surge by stimulating secretion of endogenous LH with administration of GnRH agonists [43–46]. Indeed, the results published so far are encouraging. The GnRH agonists are capable of evoking an LH surge sufficient to induce ovulation but not prominent or long enough to provoke ovarian hyperstimulation. Although promising, this therapeutic variant should not be regarded as a foolproof insurance against ovarian hyperstimulation, since pharmacological ovarian stimulation will probably always carry some likelihood of triggering this complication. Indeed, van der Meer et al. [47] reported that moderate OHSS was observed in three of 48 cycles of ovarian stimulation with hMG followed by ovulation induction via nasal application of GnRHa. It is still not certain whether the corpus luteum function following ovulation induced by GnRHa is adequate to sustain nidation and continuation of pregnancy or whether pharmacological luteal support is mandatory [48]. Animal experiments indicate also that the GnRHa may have a direct effect on the developing follicle. It has been shown that GnRHa can induce ovulation in hypophysectomized rats by affecting the levels and function of ovarian tissue-type plasminogen activator (tPA). Hsueh et al. [49] showed that in PMSG-primed hypophysectomized rats GnRHa stimulated the induction of tPA and its specific mRNA in granulosa cells. Recombinant human LH (rhLH) is already available for clinical use. Since this preparation has a biological half-life of approximately 10 h, which is significantly shorter than that of hCG (30 h), this might enable treatment protocols creating a shorter and or lower LH peak than that created by standard hCG. Such protocols might reduce the incidence of OHSS.

The Role of Monitoring in Prevention of OHSS

The pattern of estrogen rise, reflecting follicular development, is a useful parameter for monitoring hMG treatment. A steep increase of estrogens, i.e., doubling of serum levels on consecutive days, should be regarded as an important warning sign. Serious consideration must be given to the timing and amount of hCG administration. It has been recommended that whenever urinary estrogen levels exceed 200 µg/24 h or plasma estrogens are above 1500 pg/ml (or, in SI units, >6000 pmol/l), the administration of hCG to induce ovulation should be withheld in that treatment cycle. We generally adhere to this rule; however, since strict adherence may be over-conservative and cause a fall in pregnancy rate, in special cases we have given hCG when urinary estrogen levels exceeded

200 µg/24 h or serum levels were higher than 1500 pg/ml, and this has usually not resulted in severe hyperstimulation.

Modern monitoring techniques have facilitated determination of the hMG dose appropriate to obtain optimal conditions for follicular development. The profile of estrogen response reflects follicular development and function and constitutes a useful parameter for the surveillance of hMG treatment. It furnishes a general index of follicular function but does not give any precise indication about number and size of the follicles present. Elevated estrogen levels may reflect the presence of one or two mature follicles or a large number of intermediate-size follicles.

Thus if estrogen levels are elevated, ultrasonographic visualization of the follicles makes it possible to interpret more precisely the meaning of estrogen level and facilitates decision-making. It is clear that OHSS appears generally in patients with high estrogen levels; however, it has also been observed in women in whom estrogens were not excessive and, conversely, some patients with high estrogen levels did not develop OHSS. This demonstrates that determination of the number and size of follicles probably is a more precise criterion for the prediction of OHSS. In our opinion, ultrasonography constitutes the best predictive parameter for assessing the risk of OHSS.

We have noted that induction of ovulation with hCG in the presence of more than five intermediate-size follicles (9–15 mm) significantly correlated with the appearance of OHSS. Tal et al. [50] came to a similar conclusion, showing that in cycles under gonadotropin therapy the administration of hCG in the presence of one dominant and fewer than four immature follicles never provoked OHSS. However, the presence of more than four follicles 14–16 mm in diameter significantly correlated with the occurrence of OHSS. They suggested that ovarian follicles 14–16 mm in diameter should cause concern and that the number of secondary follicles, rather than that of dominant follicles, are a valuable sign of possible development of OHSS.

Our own data [51] suggest that the number and size of different types of follicles correlate well with the appearance of OHSS. Patients without hyperstimulation had the lowest total number of follicles in the preovulatory period (fewer than six). In mild hyperstimulation, the number of preovulatory follicles increased by 38% and in moderate or severe hyperstimulation they increased by 76% (9.6 follicles). Furthermore, the distribution of the follicular categories small, intermediate, and large on the day of hCG administration characterized the severity of OHSS. Patients in whom hyperstimulation did not develop showed a near equal distribution of all three follicular groups. Mild OHSS was characterized by a significantly increased number of intermediate-size follicles (68.7%). In women who developed severe hyperstimulation, 54% of the follicles were less than 9 mm in diameter. Thus a decrease in the fraction of the mature follicles and an increase in the fraction of the small functioning follicles correlated with an augmented risk for the development of severe OHSS.

The measurement of estrogens, together with ultrasonography, may prevent hyperstimulation by contraindicating the administration of hCG. Thus it could be recommended that in gonadotropin-stimulated cycles combined with in vivo fertilization, the injection of hCG should be withheld in the presence of estradiol above 1500 pg/ml (or >6000 pmol/l) and the presence of more than two follicles greater than 17 mm together with more than four follicles of less than 17 mm. If estradiol is above 1500 pg/ml in the presence of more than two large follicles but fewer than four smaller follicles, hCG may be administered and follicular reduction [11] may be considered, as described above. In patients with estradiol levels of less than 1500 pg/ml in the presence of no more than two follicles above 17 mm and fewer than four smaller follicles, hCG may be administered, and it is unlikely that OHSS will occur.

Analysis of several large series comprising 11 342 treatment cycles showed that the incidence of moderate and severe hyperstimulation was 3.4% and 0.8%, respectively [9]. Only some of the women who received hCG despite inappropriate rise or excessive levels of estrogen developed ovarian hyperstimulation. It is certain, however, that most women who did develop the syndrome had abnormally high preovulatory estrogen levels. It should also be noted that these data were based on reports describing ovulation-inducing therapy instituted prior to the introduction of combined hormonal/sonographic monitoring.

Preventive Therapy

Tan et al. [52] injected women prone to develop severe hyperstimulation as indicated by high estrogen levels and multiple follicular cohort (more than 20 follicles observed on ultrasound) with 100 mg of hydrocortisone i.v. immediately after oocyte recovery; this was followed by oral prednisolone administration for 5 days. The hyperstimulation rates in treated patients and in the control group were very similar (41.2% and 42.9%, respectively). Asch and his co-workers [53] administered human albumin to patients prone to develop OHSS at the time of oocyte retrieval and immediately thereafter. Of the 36 women treated, none developed ovarian hyperstimulation. Another randomized placebo-controlled study of 31 women undergoing IVF-ET, all of them with multifollicular development accompanied by high serum estradiol levels (>7000 pmol/l), indicated that while none of patients treated with albumin developed OHSS, four women in the placebo group had to be hospitalized and treated for severe ovarian hyperstimulation [54]. Albumin is effective in correcting hemodynamic instability and balancing hypovolemia. It also has a remarkable absorption capacity and could possibly reduce the amount of VEGF circulating in the blood, thus removing the main factor disrupting blood vessel integrity.

Orvieto and Ben-Rafael [55] assembled from the literature six articles which claimed that albumin was efficient in preventing OHSS and six other studies asserting the opposite view. They concluded that albumin was ineffective in preventing late severe OHSS but might be a feasible utensil for secondary prevention and/or amelioration of its severity. As stated by the authors, the number of cases in all studies has been insufficient to draw unequivocal conclusions.

Fisher et al. [56] proposed to replace albumin with a 10% hydroxyethyl starch (HES) infusion, which is commercially available, cheaper, and free of the risk factors inherent in blood products. Recently, the efficacy of (HES) in prevention of OHSS was confirmed in a prospective, randomized, placebo-controlled study [57]. A total of 101 women in an IVF program were recruited. All had serum estradiol concentrations higher than 1500 pg/ml (in SI units more than 6000 pmol/l) and/or more than ten follicles on the day of hCG administration. Fifty-one women received 1000 ml of 6% (HES) as an intravenous infusion and 50 control patients received 1000 ml saline shortly after embryo transfer. In the HES group only one case of moderate OHSS was observed, while in the placebo group seven cases of moderate hyperstimulation occurred. Furthermore, serum estradiol, leukocyte count, increase in abdominal circumference, and weight gain 14 days after embryo transfer were significantly higher in the placebo group.

Treatment of Clinical OHSS

As ovarian hyperstimulation is a self-limiting disease, its treatment should be symptomatic and conservative, although the severity of its symptoms may demand radical, intensive care. Treatment is generally medical, with laparotomy reserved for cases of abdominal catastrophe (i.e., ovarian torsion or rupture and internal hemorrhage). The ovarian cysts are so large and brittle that surgical attempts as a palliative procedure usually result in oophorectomy.

Mild hyperstimulation can proceed to moderate and severe form, especially if conception ensues. Therefore, the patient should be observed until vaginal bleeding appears and, if not, for at least 2 weeks. Treatment of moderate hyperstimulation (Fig. 4a,b) consists of observation, bed rest, adequate fluid supply, and monitoring of cyst size by ultrasound. If the cysts regress, as evidenced by reduction in their size on two consecutive ultrasound scans, and clinical symptoms recede, it may be assumed that the disease has run its course and will not progress to the severe form. The most important feature of moderate OHSS management is early detection of the severe form of the syndrome. This may be heralded by continuous weight gain, increase in severity of existing symptoms, or appearance of additional symptoms such as vomiting, diarrhea, and dyspnea.

Medical treatment of severe hyperstimulation is aimed at: (a) maintaining blood volume while correcting the disturbed fluid and electrolyte balance, (b) relieving secondary complications of ascites and hydrothorax, and (c) preventing thromboembolic phenomena. Fluid balance should be accurately monitored by determination of net fluid flow (intake/output record), weight and girth measurements, and hematocrit examinations. In severe cases central venous pressure should be monitored.

Plasma expanders such as hemacell, dextran, human albumin, and plasma (500–1000 ml/24 h) supplemented with appropriate electrolytes should be administered early. The effect of this treatment may be complemented by reducing capillary permeability with indomethacin, a blocker of prostaglandin synthesis. However, pregnancy should be excluded before prescribing this drug, as it is possibly teratogenic. Diuretic agents are not recommended, since fluid in the

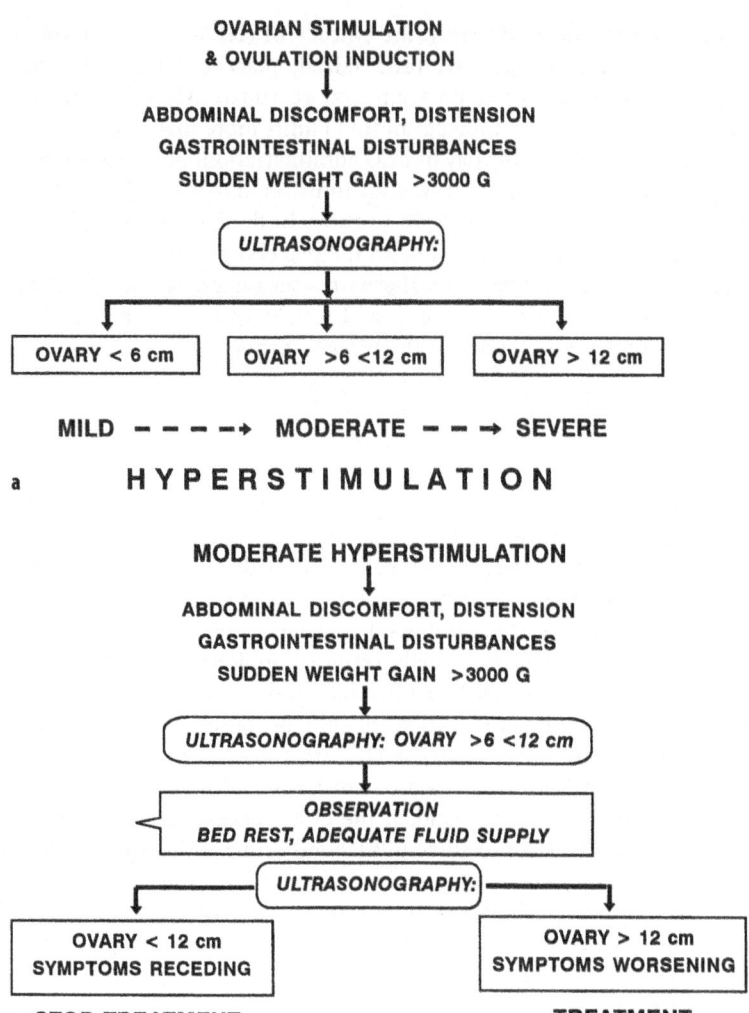

Fig. 4a, b. Treatment scheme for moderate ovarian hyperstimulation syndrome

third space is not affected by these drugs and most diuretics influence the distal tubule with minimal effect on the proximal tubule [24]. Thus the artificially induced diuresis may further diminish the intravascular volume but may be unable to cause reduction of the ascites or hydrothorax.

Another important goal of treatment is the relief of pulmonary and/or abdominal pressure symptoms. Pleural effusions should be drained, and Rabau et al. [2] proposed paracentesis to further alleviate breathing difficulty. Insler and Lunenfeld [58] have used paracentesis successfully in such patients.

Thaler et al. [59] reported a dramatic improvement of creatinine clearance and urine volume and a significant weight loss following abdominal paracentesis performed on a pregnant patient with severe OHSS. Schenker and Weinstein [60] stated that abdominal paracentesis for drainage of ascites should not be performed, as there was a danger of puncturing large ovarian cysts, which could result in intraperitoneal hemorrhage. Although theoretically correct, this danger has been significantly reduced by performing paracentesis under sonographic control. Indeed, in our experience, not a single case of intraperitoneal hemorrhage requiring surgical intervention was observed following drainage of ascites in severe hyperstimulation syndrome. Moreover, a marked improvement of renal function and blood osmolarity was achieved, most probably owing to increased venous return and reduction of hemoconcentration, and striking relief from dyspnea and abdominal discomfort was reported by the patients [61].

Aboulghar and his colleagues [62] reported on 42 cases of severe OHSS treated by transvaginal sonographically guided aspiration of ascites and intravenous fluid infusion. This treatment significantly relieved symptoms, improved hematocrit, renal clearance, and urine output, and shortened the duration of hospitalization. Some authors [63, 64] reinfused the withdrawn ascitic fluid (after microfiltration) and reported relief of symptoms and improvement of renal function.

Experimental animal studies have demonstrated that in the presence of OHSS, ascites formation is not effectively suppressed by indomethacin [42]. The poor clinical and experimental efficacy, as well as the theoretical hazard of indomethacin medication in early pregnancy [65, 66], make the use of this agent in cases of severe OHSS questionable. Thus, based on the retrospective experience, we would like to propose an algorithmic guideline for the therapeutic approach to OHSS (see Fig. 4). Anticoagulant therapy is usually unnecessary if the above-mentioned steps are taken promptly. However, because of the danger of disseminated intravascular clotting, the blood coagulation should be monitored.

Modern management of infertility is very efficient and successful but certainly holds inherent dangers of serious complications, one of them being the OHSS. This iatrogenic entity, although self-limited, may be exceptionally severe and requires prompt and extensive therapy. Since OHSS is an exaggeration of physiological processes taking place during ovarian stimulation, it is logical to assume that it must be accepted as part and parcel of ovulation induction. Resilient, individually adjusted treatment schemes using gonadotropic preparations tailor-made for specific groups of patients, meticulous monitoring, suitable preventive measures, and intelligent active therapy will certainly reduce the incidence and ameliorate the course of the ovarian hyperstimulation syndrome.

References

1. Insler V, Lunenfeld B (1977) Human gonadotrophins. In: Philipp EE, Barnes J, Newton M (eds) Scientific foundations of obstetrics and gynaecology, 2nd edn. Heinemann, London, pp 629–649
2. Rabau E, Serr DM, David A, Mashiach S, Lunenfeld B (1967) Human menopausal gonadotropins for anovulation and sterility. Am J Obstet Gynecol. 96:92
3. Southam AL, Janovski NA (1962) Massive ovarian hyperstimulation with clomiphene citrate. JAMA 181:443

4. Neuwirth RS, Turksoy RN, Vande Wiele RL (1965) Acute Meig's syndrome secondary to ovarian stimulation with menopausal gonadotropins. Am J Obstet Gynecol 91:977–981
5. Lunenfeld B, Insler V, Glezerman M (1993) Diagnosis and treatment of functional infertility, 3d edn. Blackwell Wissenschaft, Berlin, p 42, 98
6. Weissman A, Barash A, Shapiro H, Casper RF (1998) Ovarian hyperstimulation following the sole administration of agonistic analogues of gonadotrophin-releasing hormone. Hum Reprod 13:3421–3424
7. Ludwig M, Gembruch U, Bauer O, Diedrich K (1998) Case report. Ovarian hyperstimulation syndrome (OHSS) in a spontaneous pregnancy with fetal and placental triploidy: information about the general pathophysiology of OHSS. Hum Reprod 13:2082–2087
8. World Health Organization (1973) Agents stimulating gonadal function in humans. WHO Techn. Rep. Series, no 514
9. Lunenfeld B, Insler V, Glezerman M (1993) Diagnosis and treatment of functional infertility. Publ Blackwell Wissenschaft, Berlin (3rd revised edition) p 98
10. Grudzinskas JG, Egbase PE (1998) Prevention of ovarian hyperstimulation syndrome: novel strategies. Hum Reprod 13:2051
11. Tulandi T, McInnes RA, Arronet GH (1984) Ovarian hyperstimulation following ovulation induction with human menopausal gonadotropin. Int J Fertil 29:113
12. Hazout A, Belaisch-Allart J (1986) In: Buvat J, Bringer J (eds) Progres en gynecologie. Doin, Paris
13. Yan ZH, Weich HA, Bernart W, Breckwoldt M, Neulen J (1993) Vascular endothelial growth factor (VEGF) messenger ribonucleic acid (mRNA) expression in luteinized human granulosa cells in vitro. J Clin Endocrinol Metab, 77:1723–1725
14. McLure N, Healy DL, Rogers PA, Sullivan J, Beaton L, Haning RV, Connoly DT, Robertson DM (1994) Vascular endothelial growth factor as capillary permeability agent in ovarian hyperstimulation syndrome. Lancet 344:235–236
15. Shweiki D, Itin A, Neufeld G, Gitay-Goren H, Keshet E (1993) Patterns of expression of vascular endothelial growth factor (VEGF) and VEGF receptors in mice suggest a role in hormonally regulated angiogenesis. J Clin Invest 91:2235–2243
16. Insler V, Lunenfeld B (1997) Pathogenesis of ovarian hyperstimulation syndrome. In: Gomel V, Leung PCK (eds) In vitro fertilization and assisted reproduction. Monduzzi, Bologna, pp 433–439
17. Polishuk WZ, Schenker JG (1969) Ovarian overstimulation syndrome. Fertil Steril 20:443
18. Schenker JG, Schumert Z, Shifrin A, Spitz I (1977) Steroid pattern in experimental hyperstimulation syndrome and the response to indomethacin. Paper presented at 2nd Int. Congress of Human Reproduction, Tel Aviv, October
19. Schenker JG, Polishuk WZ (1976) The role of prostaglandins in ovarian hyperstimulation syndrome. Eur J Obstet Gynecol Reprod 6:47
20. Pride SM, Yuen BH, Young SM, Leung PCS (1986) Relationship of gonadotropin-releasing hormone, danazol and prostaglandin blockade to ovarian enlargement and ascites formation or the ovarian hyperstimulation syndrome in the rabbit. Am J Obstet Gynecol 154:1155
21. Davis JS (1960) Hormonal control of plasma and erythrocyte volume of rat uterus. Am J Physiol 199:841
22. Cecil HC, Hannun JA jr, Bitman J (1966) Quantitative characterization of uterine vascular permeability changes with estrogen. Am J Physiol 211:1099
23 Schenker JG, Polishuk WZ (1976) An experimental model of ovarian hyperstimulation syndrome. In: Tishner M, Pilch J (eds) Proceedings of the international congress on animal reproduction, vol 4. Drukarnia Naukowa, Krakow, p 635
24. Engel J, Jewelewicz R, Dyrenfurth I, Speroff L, VandeWiele RL (1972) Ovarian hyperstimulation syndrome. Report of a case with notes on pathogenesis and treatment. Am J Obstet Gynecol 112:1052
25. Sims EA (1967) Renal function in normal pregnancy. Clin Obstet Gynecol 11:961
26. Mudge GH, Welt LG (1975) Agents affecting volume and composition of body fluids. In: Goodman LS, Gilman A (eds) The pharmacological basis of therapeutics, 5th edn. Macmillan, New York, pp 733–781

27. Friedlander MA, Loret-de-Mola JR, Goldfarb JM (1993) Elevated levels of interleukin-6 in ascites and serum from women with ovarian hyperstimulation syndrome. Fertil Steril 60:826–833

28. Balasch J, Arroyo V, Carmona F, Llach J, Jimenez W, Pare JC, Vanrell JA (1991) Severe ovarian hyperstimulation syndrome: role of peripheral vasodilation. Fertil Steril 56:1077–1083

29. Ong AC, Eisen V, Rennie DP, Homburg R, Lachelin GC, Jacobs HS, Slater JD (1991) The pathogenesis of the ovarian hyperstimulation syndrome (OHS): a possible role for ovarian renin. Clin Endocrinol (Oxf) 34:43–49

30. Navot D, Margalioth EJ, Laufer N, Birkenfeld A, Relou A, Rosler A, Schenker JG (1987) Direct correlation between plasma renin activity and severity of the ovarian hyperstimulation syndrome. Fertil Steril 48:57–61

31. Dirks JH, Cirksena WJ, Berliner RW (1966) Micropuncture study of the effect of various diuretics on sodium reabsorption by the proximal tubules of the dog. J Clin Invest 45:1875–1878

32. Berliner RW, Kennedy TJJ, Hilton JG (1950) Renal clearance of ferranocyanide in dog. Am J Physiol 160:348–353

33. Landau RL, Lugibihl K (1958) Inhibition of the sodium-retaining influence of aldosterone by progesterone. J Clin Endocrinol Metab 18:1237–1242

34. Navot D, Bergh PA, Palermo R (1994) Pathophysiology and clinical management of ovarian hyperstimulation. In: Filicori M, Flamigni C (eds) Ovulation induction. Elsevier Science BV, Amsterdam, pp 319–329

35. Ujioka T, Matsuura K, Tanaka N, Okamura H (1998) Involvement of ovarian kinin-kallikrein system in the pathophysiology of ovarian hyperstimulation syndrome: studies in a rat model. Hum Reprod 13:3009–3015

36. Moses M, Bogowsky H, Anteby E, Lunenfeld B, Rabau E, Serr D, David A, Salomy M (1965) Thromboembolic phenomena after ovarian stimulation with human menopausal gonadotrophins. Lancet 2:1213

37. Phillips LL, Glanstone W, VandeWiele R (1975) Studies of the coagulation and fibrinolytic systems in hyperstimulation syndrome after administration of human gonadotrophins. J Reprod Med 14:138

38. Schenker JG, Weinstein D (1978) Ovarian hyperstimulation syndrome: a current survey. Fertil Steril 30:255

39. Fulghesu AM, Villa P, Pavone V, Guido M, Apa R, Caruso A, Lanzone A, Rossidivita A, Mancuso S (1997) The impact of insulin secretion on the ovarian response to exogenous gonadotropins in polycystic ovary syndrome. J Clin Endocrinol Metab 82:644–648

40. Dunaif A, Segal KA, Futterweit W, Dobrjansky A (1989) Profound peripheral insulin resistance, independent of obesity in polycystic ovary syndrome. Diabetes 38:1165–1174

41. Norman RJ, Masters SC, Hague W, Beng C, Pannal P, Wang JX (1995) Metabolic approaches to the subclassification of polycystic ovary syndrome. Fertil Steril 63:329–335

42. Haning RV jr, Strawn EY, Nolten WE (1985) Pathophysiology of the ovarian hyperstimulation syndrome. Obstet Gynecol 66:220

43. Gonen Y, Balakier H, Powell W, Casper RF (1990) Use of gonadotropin releasing hormone agonist to trigger follicular maturation for in vitro fertilization. J Clin Endocrinol Metab 71:918–922

44. Emperaire JC, Ruffie A (1991) Triggering ovulation with endogenous luteinizing hormone may prevent the ovarian hyperstimulation syndrome. Hum Reprod 6:506–510

45. Itskovitz J, Boldes R, Levron J, Erlik Y, Kahana L, Brandes JM (1991) Induction of preovulatory luteinizing hormone surge and prevention of ovarian hyperstimulation syndrome by gonadotropin-releasing hormone agonist. Fertil Steril 56:213–220

46. Corson SL, Batzer FR, Gocial B, Meislin G (1993) The luteal phase after ovulation induction with human menopausal gonadotropin and one versus two doses of gonadotropin-releasing hormone agonist. Fertil Steril 59:1251–1256

47. van der Meer S, Gerris J, Joostens M, Tas B (1993) Triggering of ovulation using a gonadotropin-releasing hormone agonist does not prevent ovarian hyperstimulation syndrome. Hum Reprod 8:1628

48. Lanzone A, Fulghesu AM, Villa P, Guida C, Guido M, Nicoletti MC, Caruso A, Mancuso S (1994) Gonadotropin-releasing hormone agonist versus human chorionic gonadotropin as a trigger of ovulation in polycystic ovarian disease gonadotropin hyperstimulated cycles. Fertil Steril 62:35–41

49. Hsueh AJ, Liu YX, Cajander S, Peng XR, Dahl K, Kristensen P, Ny T (1988) Gonadotropin-releasing hormone induces ovulation in hypophysectomized rats: studies on ovarian tissue-type plasminogen activator activity, messenger ribonucleic acid content and cellular localization. Endocrinology 122:1486–1495

50. Tal J, Paz B, Samberg I, Lazarov M, Sharf M (1985) Ultrasonographic and clinical correlates of menotropin versus sequential clomiphene citrate: menotropin therapy for induction of ovulation. Fertil Steril 44:342

51. Blankstein J, Shalef J, Saadon T, Kukia E, Rabinovich J, Pariente C, Lunenfeld B, Serr D, Mashiach S (1987) Prediction OHSS by preovulatory follicles. Fertil Steril 47:4

52 Tan SL, Balen A, Hussein E, Campbell S, Jacobs HS (1992) The administration of glucocorticosteroids for the prevention of ovarian hyperstimulation syndrome in in-vitro fertilization: a prospective randomized study. Fertil Steril 58:378–383

53. Asch RH, Ivery G, Goldman M, Frederick JL, Stone SC, Balmaceda JP (1993) The role of intravenous albumin in patients at high risk for severe ovarian hyperstimulation syndrome. Hum Reprod 8:1015–1020

54. Shoham Z, Weissman A, Barash A, Borenstein R, Schachter M, Insler V (1994) Intravenous albumin for the prevention of severe ovarian hyperstimulation syndrome in an in vitro fertilization program: a prospective, randomized, placebo-controlled study. Fertil Steril 62:137–142

55. Orvieto R, Ben-Rafael Z (1998) Role of intravenous albumin in the prevention of severe ovarian hyperstimulation syndrome. Hum Reprod 13:3306–3309

56. Fischer R, Baukohl V, Naether O, Nuckel M (1994) Human serum albumin and 10% hydroxyethyl starch infusion as a preventive treatment of severe ovarian hyperstimulation syndrome. Hum Reprod 9:123–124

57. Kynig E, Bussen S, Sutterlin M, Steck T (1998) Prophylactic intravenous hydroxyethyl starch solution prevents moderate-severe ovarian hyperstimulation in in-vitro fertilization patients: a prospective, randomized, double-blind and placebo-controlled study. Hum Reprod 13:2421–2424

58. Insler V, Lunenfeld B (1983) Diagnosis und Therapie endokriner Fertilitätsstörungen der Frau. Grosse Verlag, Berlin, p 96

59. Thaler I, Yoffe N, Kaftory JK, Brandes JM (1981) Treatment of ovarian hyperstimulation syndrome: the physiologic basis for a modified approach. Fertil Steril 36:110

60. Schenker JG, Weinstein D (1978) Ovarian hyperstimulation syndrome: a current survey. Fert Steril 30:255

61 Borenstein R, Elhalal U, Lunenfeld B, Schwartz ZS (1989) Severe ovarian hyperstimulation syndrome: a re-evaluated therapeutic approach. Fertil Steril 51:791–795

62. Aboulghar MA, Mansour RT, Serour GI, Sattar MA, Amin YM, Elattar I (1993) Management of severe ovarian hyperstimulation syndrome by ascitic fluid aspiration and intensive intravenous fluid therapy. Obstet Gynecol 81:108–111

63. Aboulghar MA, Mansour RT, Serour GI, Riad R, Ramzi AM (1992) Autotransfusion of the ascitic fluid in the treatment of severe ovarian hyperstimulation syndrome. Fertil Steril 58:1056–1059

64. Fukaya T, Chida S, Terada Y, Funayama Y, Yajima A (1994) Treatment of severe ovarian hyperstimulation syndrome by ultrafiltration and reinfusion of ascitic fluid. Fertil Steril 61:561–564

65. Physician Desk Reference (1986) 40th edn. INDOCIN 1187

66. Katz Z, Lancet M, Borenstein R, Chemke J (1984) Absence of teratogenicity of indomethacin in ovarian hyperstimulation syndrome. Int J Fertil 29:186

Luteal Phase: Physiology and Pharmacotherapy

H. W. Jones Jr., G. S. Jones

Corpus Luteum Physiology

The new corpus luteum of each cycle is formed from the ovulatory follicle or, in the case of assisted reproductive technology, from any follicle from which an egg is removed and is composed in part of granulosa cells which luteinize. As the corpus luteum forms, there is an infolding of the cell columns, and into these interstices come theca cells which themselves become luteinized. The latter carry with them an abundant vascular supply, in contrast to the granulosa cells which are very poorly vascularized. The two types of luteal cells have long been recognized in the human on a morphological basis, and the theca lutein cells are usually referred to as para-lutein cells. The differential function of these two cells in the human has been poorly addressed, and it is only animal studies that have indicated that there is a marked difference between the function of these two types of luteal cells.

The granulosa cell from being the fastest replicating cell in the body becomes fully differentiated and does not mitose after luteinization. Luteinizing hormone (LH) receptors have been induced late in the follicular phase, presumably by follicle-stimulating hormone (FSH) and estradiol stimulation, and differ from the endogenous LH receptors of the theca lutein cells in that the receptors of the granulosa lutein cells are fully occupied by the midcycle LH surge. The granulosa cell LH receptors do not internalize, i.e., are not replenished, and they continue to translate progesterone synthesis for only 10 days. They are responsible for the major progesterone production during the first ten days of the luteal phase, but they do not respond to an LH pulse or to human chorionic gonadotropin (hCG).

The luteinized theca cells respond to the luteal LH pulses, and also to hCG. Therefore, it is the theca lutein cells which are responsible for the pulsatile progesterone release and allows the corpus luteum rescue by trophoblastic hCG. They also provide the progesterone secretion during the last 4 days of the menstrual cycle.

The demise of the corpus luteum after 14 days of function has not been fully elucidated, although it may be related to a change of the gonadotropin-releasing hormone (GnRH) pulse at about this time, to a frequency and magnitude which characterizes the ensuing follicular phase. The central nervous system mechanism by which these changes occur remains to be clearly set forth.

Abnormal Luteal Function and Reproduction

Abnormal, i.e., decreased luteal function, has serious implications for reproduction. A luteal phase defect may be defined as a defect in the production of progesterone by the corpus luteum. Of course, this operates by inducing an abnormal endometrial response, with a cascade of events which results in failure of the reproductive process.

Luteal phase defects can be divided into (a) a corpus luteum with a normal 14-day span, but low progesterone production as judged by either a total measurement of progesterone production in that cycle, or more practically, by an examination of an adequately timed endometrial biopsy; (b) a short luteal phase usually about 10 days in length; and (c) a short luteal phase associated by a poor progesterone production during that 10-day span.

Luteal phase deficiencies are not common causes of infertility and repeated miscarriages, and etiologically they are associated with a variety of problems which cause central nervous system or pituitary malfunction. It is beyond the scope of this chapter to discuss these types of abnormal luteal function. Suffice it to say that in assisted reproductive technology, the controlled ovarian stimulation usually corrects inadequate progesterone production, but as is seen below, can of itself cause a short luteal function, i.e., a luteal function limited to only 10 days. The significance of these events in controlled ovarian stimulation is discussed.

Events in the Natural Cycle

In normal reproduction after ovulation the residual follicle is converted into a corpus luteum. If serum progesterone values are examined on a daily basis, the maximum progesterone secretion is reached on about the 6th or 7th day of the luteal phase, i.e., the 20th or 21st day of the cycle, considering day-14 as the day of ovulation or of aspiration. Several studies of progesterone secretion in the normal luteal phase have shown that there is usually a notch at about corpus luteum day 10 in progesterone secretion (Fig. 1). This notch may be interpreted as the transition between the corpus luteum function dependent primarily on the granulosa cells and the progesterone secretion by the thecal luteal cells, which as was mentioned above, are chiefly responsible for the progesterone output on days 10–14 of the normal menstrual cycle.

It has been shown that in the normal cycle the ovulated egg is fertilized in the ampullary portion of the fallopian tube and reaches the endometrial cavity at the morula stage on about day 18 or 19 of the menstrual cycle, when the peripheral serum progesterone level is around 15 ng/ml. A study of the endometrium during these days indicates that basal endometrial vacuole secretion is very prominent. It is thought that hatching occurs soon after this, and that the implantation process begins on about day 20, i.e., when the peripheral progesterone concentration is at its maximum. In a normal pregnancy implantation should be complete, i.e., the endometrium completely healed over the implanta-

Fig. 1. Estradiol and progesterone values in a natural cycle. Note that the progesterone peak is at about days 21–22

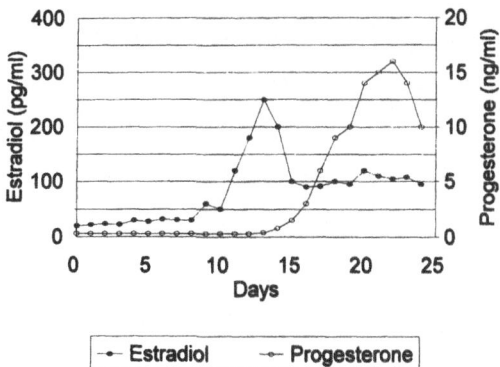

tion site by day 24 or 25, that is, at about the time of transition of the progesterone secretion from the granulosa cells to the theca lutein cells.

It is worth noting that, in natural cycle in vitro fertilization (IVF), which has proven to be inefficient, the transfer procedure usually takes place 48 h (cycle day 16) or 72 h (cycle day 17) after oocyte retrieval. Thus, there is a double asynchrony in that the preembryo is placed in the uterus 24–48 h before it would normally arrive there at a preembryonic developmental stage considerably earlier than would be if it arrived at its physiological time on day 18 or 19 of the cycle. It has been pointed out above that when the morula arrives physiologically, the endometrium has considerable secretory activity as expressed by basal vacuoles. On the other hand, in the artificial transfer situation the endometrium on day 16 or 17, when the four- to eight-cell conceptus arrives, is still in a proliferative stage. Whether these asynchronies are related to the inefficiency of the natural cycle for IVF is highly speculative, but it is entirely possible that these asynchronies are related to the poor results in natural cycle in vitro fertilization.

Alteration in Luteal Function by Controlled Ovarian Stimulation for IVF

The Controlled Stimulation Cycle

The use of controlled ovarian stimulation by the administration of exogenous gonadotropins was early noted to cause severe disruption in the events of the normal menstrual cycle. Numerous studies indicated that the midcycle spontaneous LH surge necessary for the initiation of ovulation and corpus luteum function is in fact inhibited in stimulated cycles. Ferraretti et al. [1] observed that estradiol levels in the stimulated cycles are often well above the trigger point for an LH surge release, but that no surge occurs. Furthermore, these investigators noted that there is a spectrum of estradiol response to a standard dose of exogenous gonadotropin stimulation so that patients can be divided into low responders, intermediate responders, and high responders. Intermediate and high responders have sustained estradiol values well above the trigger point, but no LH surge occurs (Fig. 2). Furthermore, it was also noted early on that in stimulated cycles the corpus luteum function cuts off at about the 10th day (Fig. 3). Early investigators attributed their failure with stimulated cycles to the short luteal phase, which is associated with the controlled stimulation. It was only some years later that an understanding of these abnormal events was possible. It has been shown that the follicular content of GnRH surge-inhibiting factor is greatly increased in the follicular fluid in stimulated cycles. This increased concentration of surge-inhibiting factor prevents the normal surge mechanism. Furthermore, this increased surge-inhibiting factor probably also inhibits the normal pulsation of the hypothalamus responsible for the pulsatile

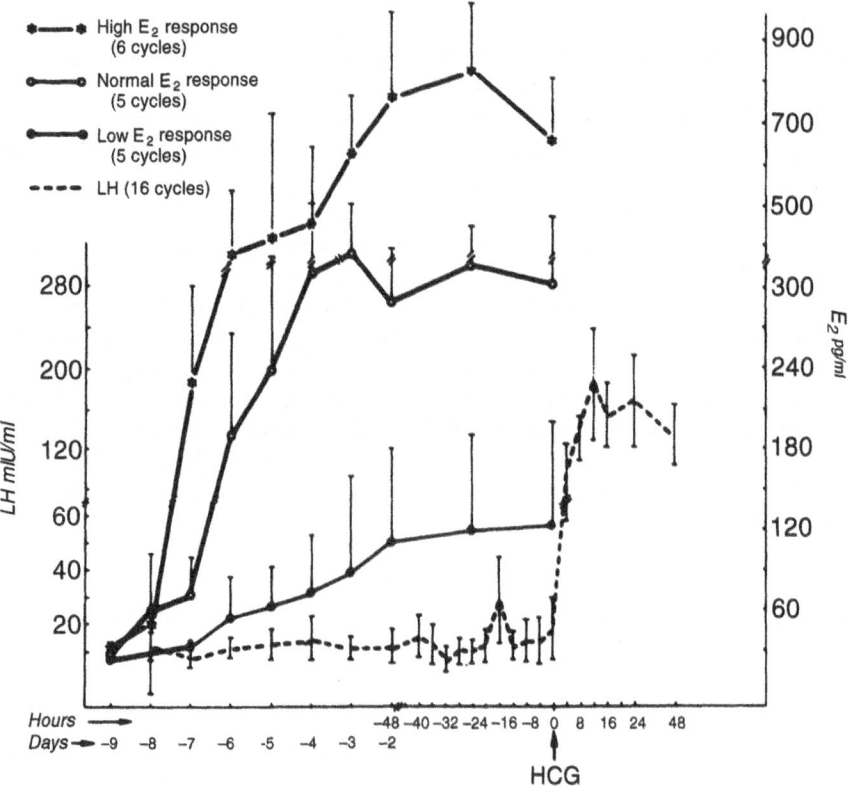

Fig. 2. Estradiol (E_2) values among 16 cycles in normal menstruating women, each receiving a standard dose of hMG. Note that there is a considerable variation in the estradiol response to this standard stimulation, so that the patients may be divided into low responders, intermediate responders, and high responders. Note likewise that there is no LH response among these patients until after the hCG is given. The assay used in this study cannot distinguish between LH and hCG. Note also that the estradiol values for the intermediate and high responders are well above the trigger point for an LH release in the normal cycle. It can be concluded that exogenous hMG in the normal menstruating woman inhibits the spontaneous LH surge

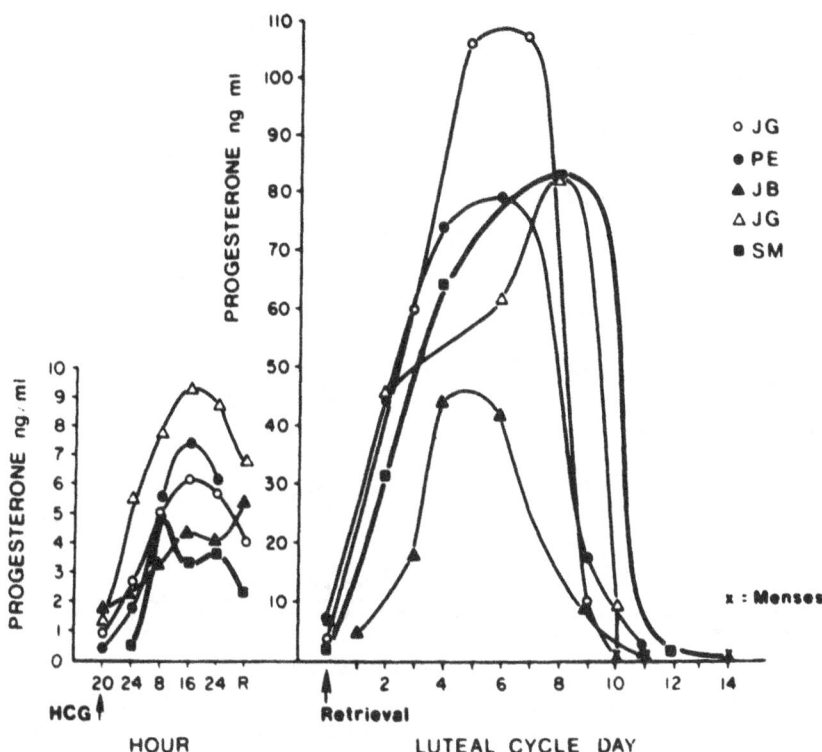

Fig. 3. Progesterone values in five patients who were stimulated with hMG. Note the very high progesterone values and note also that they cut off at about day 10. The reason for this is discussed in the text

release of LH from the theca cells of corpus luteum prolongs the luteal function from 10–14 days.

At one time it was thought that the GnRH surge-inhibiting factor might be a form of inhibin, but further studies have shown that this is a distinct protein hormone [2].

As noted above, in the event that pregnancy occurs, the corpus luteum is rescued (Fig. 4). This rescue is possible because the theca lutein cells respond to hCG by progesterone production, and the suppression of the LH pulse becomes irrelevant. Thus, the rescue of the corpus luteum is entirely due to the response of the theca lutein cells. The corpus luteum of pregnancy is composed essentially of theca lutein cells, the granulosa cells becoming degenerate and disappearing after about 10 days of the luteal phase.

The question arises as to the effect of the above endocrinological changes on the endometrium, and the relationship of the endometrial changes to the transfer and to the implantation window. In a study of endometrial biopsies at the time of transfer in cycles stimulated by hMG and/or hMG and FSH, it was shown on day-16 of the idealized cycle, when most transfers were occurring,

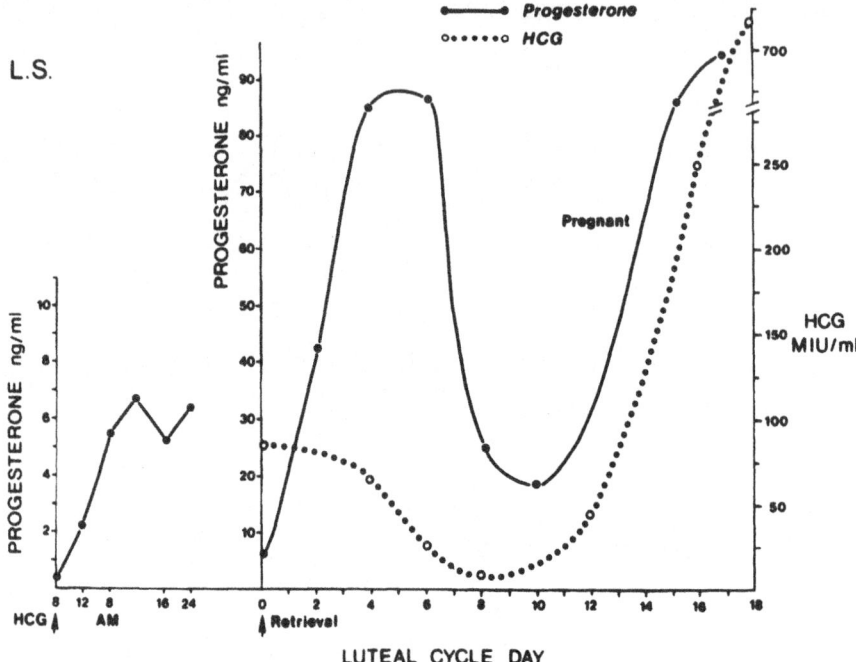

Fig. 4. The rescue of the corpus luteum by the pregnant patient. Note that in this patient who was stimulated by hMG without previous GnRH agonist exposure had a rapidly falling progesterone value which probably would have resulted in an early menstrual period, were it not for the fact that the endogenous hCG caused a rise in the progesterone value, noticeable as early as day 12. The elevated hCG values prior to day 8 are the result of the ovulatory dose of hCG to substitute for the LH surge which does not occur in stimulated patients

that the endometrium was advanced, i.e., showed patterns of day 17 or day 18 in many cases. This endometrial pattern therefore corresponded to the endometrial pattern that would normally be seen 24–48 h later in the unstimulated cycle [3]. It therefore seemed possible that the gonadotrophic-stimulated ovary with its excessive production of progesterone was a favorable development in providing receptive endometrium at the time of transfer. The status of the endometrium at some 48–72 h after this, i.e., at days 18–19 of the stimulated cycle, has not been adequately studied, and it is therefore completely unknown whether implantation in the stimulated cycle begins at the normal cycle time of day 20 or 21, or whether it begins earlier, i.e., day 18 or 19. If implantation is required for the appearance of hCG in the peripheral circulation, the evidence suggests that implantation in the stimulated cycles is not too different in terms of cycle day as compared with the normal cycle. This point is in need of further study; however, the current evidence seems to suggest that there is a longer interval between the transfer point and the beginning of implantation in the stimulated situation.

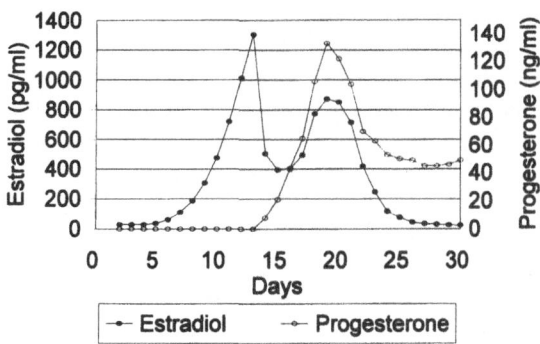

Fig. 5. Estradiol and progesterone values in a patient who were exposed to a GnRH agonist from the midluteal phase of the previous cycle. Note that the estradiol values and the progesterone values are substantially higher than in the luteal phase, and indeed, they may be substantially higher than in those patients stimulated without exposure to a GnRH agonist. Note that the scales in Figs. 1 and 5 are considerably different

The Use of GnRH agonist Followed by Exogenous Gonadotropin for Controlled Ovarian Stimulation

In the late 1980s the use of gonadotropin agonist became available and had become widely used as a method of downregulating the pituitary prior to the use of exogenous gonadotropins. This sequential use of drugs enables higher amounts of gonadotropins to be used and prevents the inadvertent spontaneous LH surges which sometimes occur, thereby interfering with the intended sequence of events.

The progesterone output and the estradiol output from the corpus luteum under this circumstance is substantially greater than the output when GnRH agonists are not used (Fig. 5).

Endometrial studies at the time of transfer and at the presumed time of implantation in patients so treated, but who were not transferred, indicate that at 48–72 h after aspiration the endometrium is likely to be at day 17±1 for biopsies taken on day 16 and at day 18±1 for biopsies taken on day 17. Thus, the endometrium is "advanced" under this circumstance, just as it was in the use of exogenous gonadotropins without GnRH agonists. On the other hand, studies of the endometrium at the expected implantation time indicate that there may be some disparity between glands and the stroma, but pinopodes which were found to occur in the stimulated cycle at about day 20 or 21 of the menstrual cycle, with the day of ovulation at 14, are therefore unchanged in time from that of the normal unstimulated cycle (unpublished data).

The Treatment of the Luteal Phase in IVF Cycles

The treatment of the luteal phase in IVF cycles with progesterone is highly problematic. It may not be necessary at all. Clearly, in stimulated cycles the amount of progesterone secreted by the corpus luteum is far in excess of the amount secreted in an unstimulated normal cycle. Thus, treatment cannot be justified on the basis of treatment for a luteal phase defect, i.e., inadequate progesterone production. Furthermore, treatment based on the hMG-induced cutoff at 10 days is not reasonable, as it has been amply demonstrated that if pregnancy occurs, the corpus luteum is rescued prior to its demise by the endogenous hCG generated by the developing conceptus. However, it is possible that exogenous progesterone can be useful. There are really no adequate controlled prospective studies that have been designed to elucidate the truth in this circumstance. There are theoretical reasons to believe that exogenous progesterone, even in the face of large amounts of endogenous progesterone, might be useful. The rationale for this revolves around the fact that, given the excessive amount of estrogen in the luteal phase, the endometrium does not seem to be converted in an adequate way to the secretory phase [4]. Presumably, this may be associated with the fact that large amounts of estrogen downregulate the progesterone receptors, and therefore that the endometrium does not "see" the progesterone. This situation could be overcome by larger amounts of progesterone to protect the progesterone receptors from the downregulation of the excessive estrogen. It would be on this theoretical basis that exogenous progesterone might prove to be helpful, and in many clinical situations it is empirically given on these grounds. If this is done, 50 mg a day by vaginal suppository or, at the most, 100 mg a day, or a corresponding amount by whatever route of administration is probably appropriate. It has been suggested that the continuation of progesterone after pregnancy is well established and can be justified by its use as a pharmacological agent to prevent miscarriage in these premium pregnancies. The use of long-acting progesterone in this circumstance is convenient.

References

1. Ferraretti AP, Garcia JE, Acosta AA, Jones GS (1983) Serum luteinizing hormone during ovulation induction with human menopausal gonadotrophin for in vitro fertilization in normally menstruating women. Fertil Steril 40: 742
2. Danforth DR, Cheng CY (1995) Purification of a candidate gonadotrophin surge inhibiting factor from porcine follicular fluid. Endocrinology 136: 1658–1665
3. Garcia JE, Acosta AA, Hsiu J-G, Jones HW Jr (1984) Advanced endometrial maturation after ovulation with human menopausal gonadotrophin/human chorionic gonadotrophin for in vitro fertilization. Fertil Steril 41: 31
4. Toner JP, Hassiakos DK, Muasher SJ, Hsiu JG, Jones HW Jr (1991) Endometrial receptivities after leuprolide suppression and gonadotrophin stimulation: histology steroid receptor concentrations and implantation rates. Ann NY Acad Sci 622: 220–229

An Andrological Approach to Assisted Reproduction

F.-M. Köhn, W.-B. Schill

Introduction

The World Health Organization (WHO) describes "reproductive health" as the ability of women and men to realize their reproductive wishes, to have intact sexual relations, and to maintain the health of the following generations [429]. Infertility is defined as lack of conception after 12 [431] or 24 [87] months of unprotected intercourse. The exact prevalence of involuntary infertility is not known. It is thought that 10–15 million couples in the United States have fertility problems; in Germany the estimated number of infertile couples in 1989 was 0.585 million [53]. A male factor is considered to be present in 40–50% of these cases. Therefore, medical evaluation of the male partner is a prerequisite in the treatment of couples with involuntary infertility. However, intracytoplasmic sperm injection has not only enlarged the spectrum of indications for assisted reproduction techniques (ART), but also questioned the position of andrology in reproductive medicine. Andrology has been criticized mainly because of the lack of convincing therapeutic approaches. Male factors are the indications in 16% of in vitro fertilization (IVF) cycles and 75% of intracytoplasmic sperm injections (ICSI).

The overall effectiveness of ART in the treatment of male infertility is generally accepted [259, 375]. The position of andrology has been strengthened again, since testicular sperm extraction (TESE) or microsurgical epididymal sperm aspiration (MESA) require andrological differential diagnosis (obstructive/nonobstructive azoospermia, congenital bilateral absence of the vas deferens) and at least testicular biopsies. Other pathological findings (e.g., testicular tumors) can be diagnosed only after physical examination of the male partner. The effect of treatment of varicoceles on spontaneous pregnancy rates is still a matter of discussion. However, Matthews et al. [266] demonstrated that spermatogenesis can be induced after microsurgical varicocelectomy in some men with azoospermia. Thereafter, at least ICSI with ejaculated spermatozoa would be possible. The medical history is important to identify risk factors (e.g., cryptorchidism, environmental hazards), which stresses the importance of an andrological evaluation. The financial factor is another argument for andrologists to diagnose treatable factors of infertility and to recommend therapeutic procedures where these seem more appropriate than ART. In the United States, for example, the costs per one successful delivery after in vitro fertilization (IVF) are approximately $100,000 [293]. In our experience, especially couples with a short history of infertility want to be assured that ART are recommended only if more "natural" ways of conception are not possible. Since in Germany health insurance pays for IVF but no longer covers the costs of ICSI, more patients are sent to andrologists in order to improve semen quality. Andrologists are also helpful for avoiding time- and money-consuming trials of intrauterine insemination or IVF when sperm functions (acrosin activity, acrosome reaction or zona binding) are impaired and ICSI is preferred [300]. Liu et al. [250] have demonstrated high fertilization and pregnancy rates after ICSI with spermatozoa from men with impaired sperm functions.

Quality management is a very important factor for andrological laboratories. Therefore, the new WHO laboratory manual [432] includes detailed instructions for quality controls of the standard semen analysis. The need for better standardization is emphasized by low interlaboratory consistency, especially for the evaluation of sperm motility and sperm morphology [199]. Feedback of results to the technicians of the laboratories participating in external quality control programs leads to the harmonization of results between different laboratories [84].

Andrological Medical History

Without knowledge of the medical history or physical examination, the results of semen analysis are not sufficient to recommend ART. Febrile infections or medical treatment occurring within 3 months of sperm collection may affect semen quality temporarily; in such cases, special andrological therapy is usually not required. Drugs that interfere with male infertility include [159]:
- Those that cause direct damage to spermatogenesis
    - Cytotoxic drugs
    - Colchicine
    - Sulfasalazine
    - Nitrofurantoin
    - Niridazole
    - Gossypol
    - Those that are toxic to the epididymis
    - Amiodarone
- Those that inhibit sperm motility
    - Propanolol, procaine
    - Chlorpromazine
    - Quinine
- Those that interfere with the hypothalamic-pituitary-testicular axis
    - High-dose corticosteroids
    - Androgens
    - Progestagens
    - Estrogens
    - LHRH agonists
    - Ketoconazole

- Those that interfere with the action of androgens at the testicle
  - Spironolactone
  - Cimetidine
  - Antiandrogens.

Taking of the medical history includes questions about children's diseases (especially epidemic parotitis after puberty), other bacterial or viral infections, metabolic diseases (diabetes mellitus), cardiac diseases, hepatopathy, neurological disorders, (testicular) neoplasm, genital or pelvic traumata, operations, and drug intake. The patient should also be asked about specific genital infections (orchitis, epididymitis, prostatitis, urethritis, sexually transmitted diseases), unilateral or bilateral undescended testes, testicular torsion, genital or pelvic operations of inguinal hernia, varicoceles, hydroceles, bladder neck, orchidopexy, and urogenital malformations (epispadia, hypospadia). In addition, information about nicotine and alcohol abuse, stress factors, and possible environmental hazards (pesticides, heat) is important. Decreased libido or reduced hair growth may be caused by endocrine disorders. Kartagener' syndrome may be indicated by recurrent respiratory infections, and Kallmann's syndrome by anosmia.

The medical history should address sexual habits, such as frequency of sexual intercourse or use of contraceptives and spermatotoxic lubricants. Erectile dysfunction or premature ejaculation are estimated to affect 5% of infertile men [143]. It is important to ask whether the patient has fathered children before. Primary male infertility is diagnosed if the man has never impregnated a woman, secondary male infertility if the man has impregnated a woman, irrespective of whether she is his present partner and irrespective of the outcome of pregnancy [159].

Infertile men attending andrological centers are a selective group who have already experienced diagnostic and therapeutic procedures; consequently, special details such as testicular biopsies or epididymal surgery and results of previous IUI, IVF, or ICSI must be considered. IVF cycles without fertilization of oocytes may indicate impaired sperm functions (acrosome reaction, acrosin activity, zona binding). In addition, it is advisable to reevaluate thin sections from earlier testicular biopsies, because single seminiferous tubules with spermatozoa may be present despite the reported diagnosis of Sertoli cell-only syndrome. In these cases, TESE can be recommended. Pregnancies can be achieved by MESA or TESE even with spermatozoa from men with infertility related to genetic disorders. It is particularly important to ask about cystic fibrosis or familial infertility.

Physical Examination

Inspection is the first step in the physical examination of andrological patients. Disproportions of the body (e.g., low ratio upper/lower segment height), gynecomastia, reduced body hair and lack of androgenetic alopecia may indicate genetic (Klinefelter's syndrome) or endocrine disorders. Epispadia, hypospadia, or grade-III varicoceles can also be diagnosed by inspection.

Thereafter, the position and size of the testicles are examined. Usually, they are both palpable in the lower scrotum of a standing man. Their consistency is comparable to that of rubber. Soft consistency is often found in combination with reduced spermatogenesis. Areas with hard consistency may indicate a testicular tumor. The volume (normal: >15 ml) is evaluated with a Prader or Hynie orchidometer, calipers, or hollow forms. Alternatively, ultrasonography can be used, because volumes determined by this method are highly correlated with actual testicular volumes and with the outcome of Prader orchidometer measurements [34, 124]. The advantage of ultrasonography is the testicular evaluation even in cases of large hydroceles or inguinal position. It also allows the diagnosis of testicular tumors, hydroceles, epididymal abnormalities, spermatoceles, intratesticular cysts, and hyper- or hypoechoic structures, which may not be detected by palpation [289]. Behre et al. [35] reported sonographic abnormalities in 50.4% of 1048 patients attending an andrological outpatient department.

Caput and corpus epididymidis are normally palpable as elongated structures attached to the upper part of the testis. Palpation of the epididymis usually causes no or only little discomfort. Pain or palpation of fibrotic structures may indicate inflammation. Solid round nodules are spermatoceles or other epididymal cysts and should also be examined by means of ultrasonography (Fig. 1). Enlargement of the epididymis in combination with missing vasa deferentia may result from dilatation of the epididymal duct system due to obstructive processes.

Both vasa deferentia are felt as lead- or wire-like structures. Especially in azoospermic men, absence of the vasa deferentia should be recorded for the diagnosis of congenital bilateral absence of the vas deferens (CBAVD).

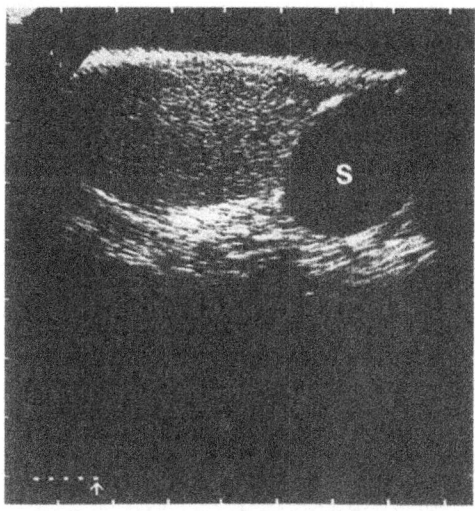

Fig. 1. Spermatocele (S)

Fig. 2. Prostate gland (*P*) with utriculus cyst (*U*)

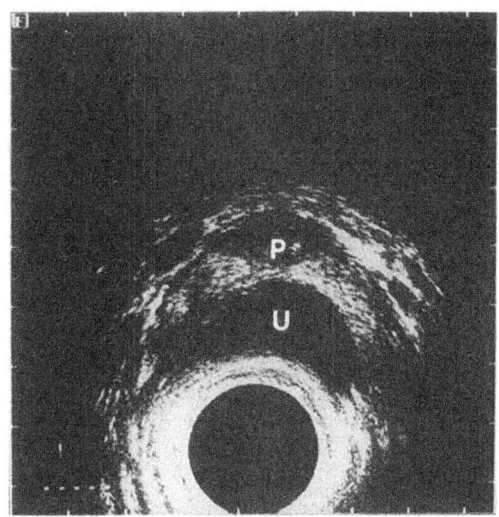

The pampiniform plexus is palpable in patients in the standing position. Four types of varicoceles are differentiated [159]: grade-III varicoceles are visible through the scrotal skin; in patients with grade-II varicocele the pampiniform plexus is palpable without being visible; grade-I varicoceles are palpable only during the Valsalva maneuver. Since subclinical varicoceles can be diagnosed only by Doppler ultrasonography, this technique or scrotal thermography of the pampiniform plexus on both sides is generally recommended.

Inspection and palpation of the penis before and after retraction of the foreskin reveal urogenital malformations, meatal strictures, phimosis, ulcerations (e.g., syphilis, genital herpes), condylomas, and plaques caused by Peyronie's disease.

The physical examination should conclude with a rectal examination of the prostate gland. Since most patients attending andrological outpatient departments are young, pathological findings during palpation are not likely. Nevertheless, transrectal ultrasound of the prostate gland is recommended in cases of severe oligozoospermia, azoospermia, or inflammatory signs. This allows detection of prostatic, utricle (Fig. 2), or ejaculatory duct cysts and calcifications of the prostatic glands. In addition, the seminal vesicles, which are not palpable, can be evaluated.

Semen Analysis, Biochemical Semen Parameters, and Sperm Function Tests

Semen analysis has been standardized by the WHO [432]. However, abnormal values do not necessarily indicate infertility [329, 376]. Bostofte et al. [47] considered a sperm concentration of 5×10^6/ml the clinical borderline of male fertility. Schill and Dasilva [352] found that 16% of samples from men who had impregnated their wives within 10 weeks before or after semen analysis showed sperm concentrations between 1 and 10×10^6/ml, and 13% had no progressive sperm motility. Rather than single semen parameters, a combination of these (volume, sperm count, motility, morphology) has been suggested to be a better diagnostic tool for discriminating between fertile and infertile men [31]. The limited value of standard semen parameters for fertility prognosis must be considered before recommending ART. Duleba et al. [105] have demonstrated that independent predictors of pregnancy are the duration of infertility and a history of pregnancy in the female partner. Therefore, the andrologist may advise ART in cases of long infertility even if semen parameters or functional semen tests are not pathological. On the other hand, pathological semen parameters do not automatically require ART when patients are young and the duration of infertility is short.

Sample Collection

Semen is collected by masturbation into a sterile plastic or glass container after 3–5 days of sexual abstinence. Longer periods of abstinence (10 days) after depletion of sperm reserves may be advantageous, depending on sperm numbers and motility [83].

The container should be tested for spermicidal effects (plasticizers) and labeled with the patient's name or identification code. Since psychological stress factors on the day of IUI, IVF, or ICSI keep some patients from producing ejaculates, special rooms should be available which guarantee a private atmosphere. Compared with the semen quality during pre-IVF workup, 4–8% of men show a severe deterioration on the day of IVF [161]. If the patient is not able to deliver his ejaculate, he may try it at home and transport the semen container at body temperature to the hospital within 30–60 min. Cryopreservation of semen samples before IVF or ICSI may be useful [320]. Kenntenich et al. [208] recommended sample collection in the presence of the patient's wife to reduce stress during the IVF procedure.

For cases of impaired semen quality (in particular, sperm concentration and motility), several modifications of sample collection have been established. One method is the separate collection of the first (two contractions) and second (remaining contractions) semen fractions (split ejaculate). The first fraction of split ejaculate usually contains more spermatozoa with better motility than the second fraction [257]. However, pregnancy rates after artificial insemination with the first portion of the husband's semen are not consistently better than those after use of the whole ejaculate [277]. In the case of male infertility, washed spermatozoa achieve significantly higher pregnancy rates than split ejaculates [140]. This is in agreement with Sokol et al. [382], who found no differences between spermatozoa from the first and second portions concerning penetration into zona-free hamster ova or bovine cervical mucus.

In contrast to split ejaculates, the total number of motile spermatozoa can be increased by pooled sequential ejaculates [153]. Patients are asked to produce two ejaculates within a period of 1–4 h. In normozoospermic men the total number of motile spermatozoa decreases significantly in the second ejaculate; oligozoospermic men show similar or even higher sperm counts in the second sample [150, 410]. The total number of motile spermatozoa is increased more than three times by pooling both ejaculates. Since at least 500,000 progressively motile spermatozoa should be available for successful IVF in couples with male infertility factors [101], sperm preparation is performed in both pool samples; thereafter, IVF or GIFT may be possible even in cases of severe oligoasthenozoospermia.

Barash et al. [27] demonstrated improved sperm motility and higher motile sperm counts after swim-up preparation of the second pool ejaculate. In addition, the fertilization rate was significantly higher after IVF with spermatozoa from the second ejaculate than that achieved using sperm cells from the first ejaculate (29.6% vs. 18.3%).

In patients with oligozoospermia due to functional semen transport disturbances [220] the sperm concentration may be increased by intravenous injection of 10–15 mg of the alpha-sympathomimetic midodrin 30 min prior to ejaculation.

Standard Semen Analysis

For standardization and better comparison of results obtained in different laboratories, standard semen analysis according to WHO [432] is recommended. Standard semen parameters include appearance (homogeneous, opalescent gray), time of liquefaction (< 60 min), volume, consistency, pH, presence of agglutinations, sperm concentration, total sperm count, motility, sperm viability, and morphology.

These standard semen parameters allow the differentiation of special andrological disorders. For example, reduced semen volume in combination with low pH and fructose levels indicates agenesis of the seminal vesicles or obstruction of their ducts. Azoospermia should be diagnosed only if no sperm cells can be found after centrifugation of the ejaculate.

In cases of extreme asthenozoospermia sperm viability must be determined by trypan blue, eosin Y, Hoechst 33258, or the hypo-osmotic swelling (HOS) test. This is important because viable, but not necessarily motile, spermatozoa are required for ICSI.

In 1984, Jeyendran et al. [192] introduced the HOS test to determine the functional integrity of human sperm membranes. The WHO recommends it only as an optional, additional vitality test.

Because of the variety of morphological malformations, sperm morphology is probably the least standardized parameter of semen analysis. The purpose of the WHO recommendations is to provide a compromise as a suitable classification for clinical practice. However, special morphological abnormalities of the flagellum have not been included. Kruger et al. [228] defined the "strict criteria" of sperm morphology and demonstrated low fertilization rates in IVF with spermatozoa showing normal morphology < 14%. Other classifications considered both the origin and the severity of tail defects [151, 152].

The standard semen analysis must be performed in at least two ejaculates produced within 6–12 weeks. This allows intraindividual variations in semen quality to be considered prior to ART. It may be advisable to cryopreserve semen samples as backups for use following ART. In addition, this procedure may help patients to reduce the psychological stress during semen donation on the day of ART.

Biochemical Semen Parameters

The use of biochemical markers in the diagnostic workup of male infertility provides specific information about anatomical and functional disturbances at the level of the accessory sex glands and the epididymis, the occurrence of acute and chronic male genital tract inflammation, and the fertilizing capacity of human spermatozoa. In contrast to bioassays, marker substances are advantageous in that they are objective methods subject to common conditions of laboratory methods, including quality control.

The following biochemical markers can be used in clinical andrology to determine and identify: (a) sperm fertilizing capability (aniline blue, acrosin, reactive oxygen species [ROS]); (b) male genital tract inflammation (elastase, C'3 complement component, ceruloplasmin, IgA, IgG); (c) accessory sex gland and epididymal dysfunction and obstruction (fructose, α-glucosidase, acid phosphatase, prostatic specific antigen [PSA]).

Acrosin Activity

Acrosin, a serine proteinase, is located within the acrosome. The enzyme is released during an exocytic process known as the acrosome reaction (AR). It is considered to be the major enzyme required for zona penetration through limited proteolysis of zona proteins. Another important function is its ability to bind to the zona pellucida. Acrosin is apparently also involved in capacitation and AR. In addition, it may act as a sperm-stimulating agent during intrauterine sperm migration, since it is able to liberate kinins from kininogen. Kinins have been demonstrated to enhance sperm metabolism and sperm motility in vitro [349]. No acrosin activity, or only traces, can be measured in men with round-headed spermatozoa [193, 343]. The acrosin activity is also reduced in semen samples from patients with polyzoospermia and severe teratozoospermia, including the syndrome of decapitated spermatozoa [347]. In most other sperm populations acrosin activity is normal. However, a wide overlap of the range of acrosin levels is seen in most andrological groups [349]. Factors that may affect acrosin activity are the duration of sexual abstinence [347] and varicoceles [108].

Several methods have been described for assessing acrosin activity in human spermatozoa [347]. A simple way is to measure the proteolytic potential of spermatozoa on gelatin plates [166]. Acrosin is released by hyperosmolaric rupture of the acrosome and leads to halo formation during incubation in a humid chamber at 37 °C. Halo formation is brought about predominantly by living spermatozoa; this method is supported by correlation with the eosin test ($r=0.619$). The more dead spermatozoa are identified, the lower is the halo formation rate. No acrosin is available in case of globozoospermia. The method of gelatinolysis is advantageous in that the equipment is simple and acrosin activity can be determined in individual spermatozoa. Its results show good correlation with the biochemical assay [345].

A more sophisticated method is the spectrophotometric determination of acrosin after acid extraction from the sperm acrosome, performed in the presence of synthetic acrosin inhibitors to avoid autoactivation from proacrosin. Proacrosin is the zymogen form predominating in epididymal and freshly ejaculated spermatozoa. This method allows the determination of active, nonzymogen acrosin, proacrosin, and total acrosin activity. In most sperm populations, acrosin activity shows normal values and a wide overlap in the range of acrosin levels. In contrast, significantly lower acrosin activity is observed in patients with severe teratozoospermia and polyzoospermia [347]. This supports the concept that acrosin may be a useful parameter for predicting the fertilizing potential of spermatozoa [349].

Aniline Blue Staining for Determination of Chromatin Condensation, Acridine Orange Staining

During spermiogenesis the sperm chromatin is condensed within the nucleus. Chromatin condensation is associated with the replacement of lysine-rich histones by protamines. This process is a prerequisite for subsequent decondensation to form a male pronucleus during oocyte fertilization. In cases of disturbed chromatin condensation, histones persist and can be identified by staining with acid aniline blue [399]. Since nuclear proteins play a significant role in chromatin condensation, this method uses nuclear maturity as a parameter for discriminating between fertile and infertile men.

The stability of sperm DNA and the degree of chromatin condensation can also be determined by acridine orange staining [451]. When acridine orange binds to double-stranded DNA, it shows green fluorescence, while red fluorescence indicates single-stranded DNA or RNA. Since ejaculated spermatozoa usually do not contain significant amounts of RNA, acridine orange staining provides information about the ratio of double-stranded to denatured single-stranded DNA.

Reactive Oxygen Species

The influence of reactive oxygen species (ROS) on human spermatozoa was first reported by McLeod [256]; oxidative stress is thought to be associated with male infertility [9, 12]. The two major sources of reactive species in ejaculates are leukocytes [10, 209] and spermatozoa [9, 190, 452]. Spermatozoa have a much higher content of polyunsaturated fatty acids in their membranes than somatic cells. Therefore, they are particularly susceptible to oxidation by ROS, which causes lipid peroxidation. In extreme cases this may result in dramatic damage to sperm function, for example, markedly reduced motility [282] and penetration in the zona-free hamster ovum penetration test [10, 12], reduced inducibility of AR [144], and impaired membrane integrity [126]. In addition, oxidative damage to spermatozoa is closely correlated with inflammatory processes in the genital tract and the occurrence of leukocytes, particularly granulocytes, which generate at least 100 times more ROS than spermatozoa themselves [117].

Several authors have reported that 30–40% of ejaculates from infertile men generate excessive levels of ROS [5, 190]. Especially oligozoospermic patients tend to have high ROS production by spermatozoa [13].

Biochemical Markers for Male Genital Tract Inflammation

From a clinical point of view it is mandatory to differentiate between chronic male genital tract inflammations and noninflammatory complaints such as vegetative urogenital syndrome and anogenital symptom complex. In contrast to autonomic nervous system complaints, chronic inflammatory processes require antibiotic-antiphlogistic therapy. More than 1×10^6/ml peroxidase-positive round cells (neutral granulocytes) indicate a reproductive tract infection. However, the absence of leukocytes does not exclude the possibility of an accessory sex gland infection. Therefore, biochemical markers have been suggested as sensitive indicators of an inflammatory reaction [435]. The determination of elastase in seminal plasma as a specific inflammatory parameter of polymorphonuclear granulocytes (PMN) enables the diagnosis of silent male genital tract inflammations [196]. In addition, sequential determinations allow the course of the disease to be followed during and after therapy. Granulocyte elastase is determined in cell-free seminal plasma by the method of Neumann and Jochum [292]. PMN elastase levels above 1000 ng/ml are diagnostic of leukocytospermia [435]. Clinically silent inflammations can be measured by PMN elastase in semen [436]. Recent investigations with an exact quantification of granulocyte elastase in 305 andrological patients have confirmed its high specificity and sensitivity in distinguishing inflammatory from noninflammatory male adnexal affections [330].

Apart from elastase measurements, a permeable blood-seminal plasma barrier indicates adnexal disturbance and provides information about accessory sex gland infections. Particularly helpful is the quantitative determination of complement component C'3 and ceruloplasmin. Normally, C'3 complement component is detectable only in traces, or not at all, in seminal plasma. During inflammatory reactions transudation from the blood is increased, and levels of both C'3 complement component and ceruloplasmin are significantly elevated in semen samples.

Determination of Accessory Sex Gland Secretory Function

The secretory capacity of seminal vesicles, the prostate, and the epididymis can be determined by means of various biochemical markers, for example fructose, PSA, and neutral a-glucosidase [432]. Low or missing secretory function due to an occlusion is reflected in a low total output of the specific markers; therefore, they may be used to assess both accessory sex gland secretory function and location of an obstruction.

Fructose in semen is determined, according to the WHO laboratory manual, by means of a colometric reaction with indole [432]. In cases of azoospermia caused by CBAVD low fructose levels indicate associated dysgenesis of the seminal vesicles. Fructose levels are also low in postinflammatory atrophy of the seminal vesicle epithelium or relative androgen deficiency.

Assessment of neutral a-glucosidase, which originates from the corpus and cauda epididymidis, has been found to provide more reliable and reproducible results than determination of l-carnitine. Since a-glucosidase is significantly decreased in seminal plasma from patients with distal ductal obstruction [147], it should be determined prior to invasive diagnostic procedures; in case of azoospermia in combination with low a-glucosidase values, reconstructive surgery or MESA/TESE may be suitable. Measurement of a-glucosidase also provides information about epididymal functions [148]. The activity of this enzyme is significantly reduced in ejaculates from men with epididymitis [82]. According to the WHO [432], values of 20 mU a-glucosidase or more per ejaculate are normal. Other authors suggest discriminatory levels of 10 mU/ml [227].

Marker substances for prostatic gland secretion include zinc, citric acid, and prostatic acid phosphatase [432]. Assessment of the specific prostatic marker PSA, a kallikrein-like protease, may provide information about inflammatory reactions and tumor cells in the prostate [213, 236]. PSA determination is used as a screening test to exclude prostatic cancer or chronic inflammatory processes within the prostatic tissue.

Nonbiochemical Sperm Function Tests

Sperm function tests include biochemical markers such as acrosin activity and staining of histones by aniline blue and the detection of ROS (see above). In addition, special functions of the plasma membrane and the acrosomal cap can be assessed. Bioassays (hamster ovum penetration test, hemizona assay) are useful in the evaluation of sperm/egg interactions [6, 244, 350, 451]. Two aspects demonstrate the diagnostic and clinical benefit of sperm function tests: (a) Since their results are correlated with those of IVF, they should be performed prior to ART. In cases of reduced AR, acrosin activity, or disturbed sperm/egg interaction, ICSI should be preferred. IVF could be performed only for diagnostic purposes; the chance of achieving a pregnancy would be significantly lower. (b) Therapeutic approaches to pathological sperm functions are not available in most cases; therefore, ART should be planned early, without useless treatment preceding it.

Acrosome Reaction

The AR is an exocytotic process including dispersal of the acrosomal content (see above) after fusion and fenestration of the plasma and outer acrosomal membrane [450]. After complete AR the inner acrosomal membrane is exposed, and spermatozoa are able to penetrate the oocyte. Various second-messenger systems are involved in regulating the AR [94, 95]. AR assays detect the ability of spermatozoa to undergo AR in response to a stimulus.

A variety of methods have been introduced to measure the AR. These use triple or double staining [93, 395], fluorescein isothiocyanate (FITC)-labeled *Pisum sativum* agglutinin [88], FITC-labeled Concanavalin A [179], *Arachis hypogaea* agglutinin [283], chlortetracycline [341], paramagnetic beads [301, 302, 304], and monoclonal antibodies [8, 115, 201, 280, 433]. Triple staining and assays based on fluorescent lectins are probably the most common techniques (Fig. 3). To differentiate between live and dead acrosome-reacted spermatozoa the majority of methods are used in combination with live/dead stainings.

Hemizona Assay

Prior to fusion with the oocyte, spermatozoa must bind to the zona pellucida. This first step of fertilization is evaluated by the hemizona assay [57]. The zona pellucida is used as a functional surface to measure the ability of spermatozoa to bind to the glycoprotein coat of the oocyte (Fig. 4). After the zona pellucida has been dissected into equal halves, one hemizona is incubated with the patient's spermatozoa and the other with spermatozoa from a fertile donor (con-

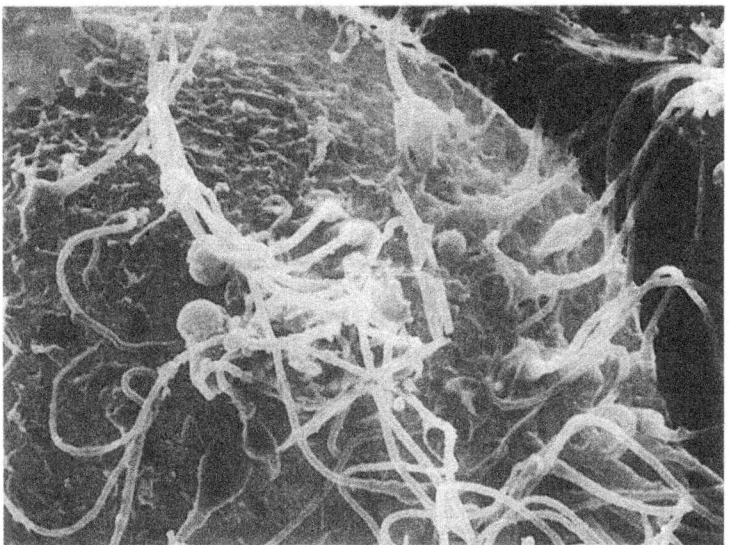

Fig. 3. Scanning electron microscopy of spermatozoa bound to the zona pellucida

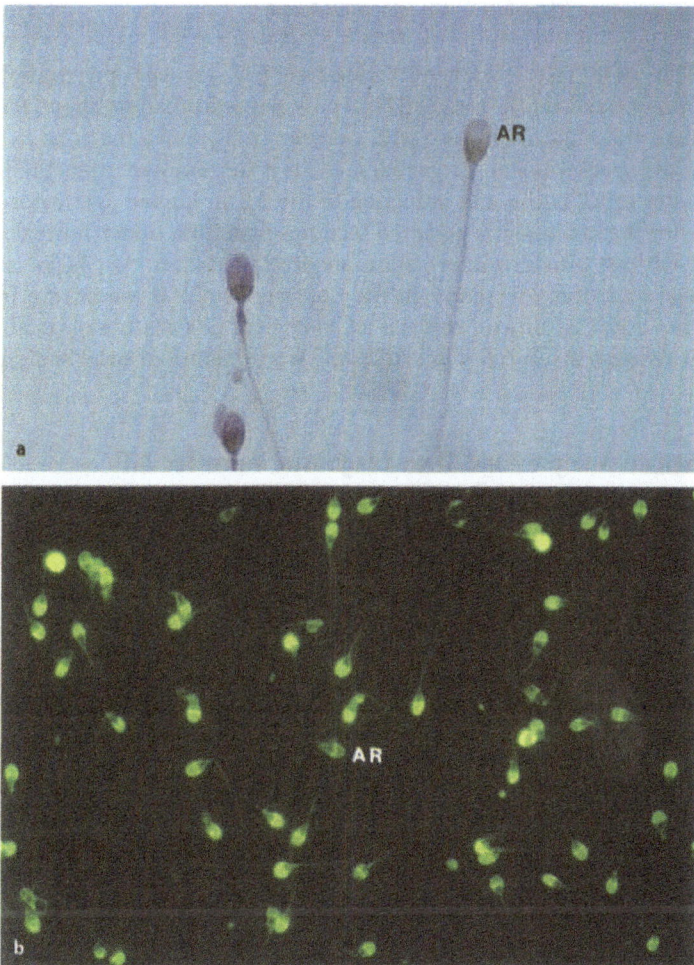

Fig. 4. a Human spermatozoa after staining with rose bengal and Bismarck brown (*AR* acrosome-reacted spermatozoon). **b** Human spermatozoa after staining with FITC-PSA (*AR* acrosome-reacted spermatozoon)

trol). The numbers of spermatozoa bound to the outer surface of each hemizona are determined and compared by calculating the hemizona assay index (number of patient's spermatozoa bound to the outer surface of each hemizona, divided by the number of donor's spermatozoa bound per hemizona, multiplied by 100). The hemizona assay index is correlated with IVF outcome [121]. Binding of human spermatozoa to the zona pellucida is also related to the immunohistochemical presence of proacrosin and acrosin in sperm cells [120]. Therefore, an important indication for this bioassay is failed fertilization in preceding IVF programs. In case of disturbed zona binding, ICSI should be recommended rather than further IVF trials.

Heterologous (Hamster) Ovum Penetration Test

The HOP test (synonyms: zona-free hamster egg penetration test [HEPT], sperm penetration assay [SPA]) provides information about the ability of human spermatozoa to fuse with oocytes [443]. Since the zona pellucida prevents cross-species fusion of gametes, it must be removed from the hamster oocyte. After capacitation and induction of the AR in human spermatozoa [432], fusion with the oolemma is achieved in more than 10% under normal conditions. The HOP test provides information about capacitation, AR, fusion with the oolemma, and decondensation in the ooplasm [142]. However, the interpretation of this assay is difficult because of biological and methodological variations, and it remains a subject of debate in the investigation of male subfertility.

Semen Analyses and Their Diagnostic Value for ART

Diagnostic criteria with predictive value must be developed in order to decide which form of ART should be recommended. The standard semen parameters and functional sperm tests have been studied most extensively. In addition, new assays or biochemical markers have been suggested, such as mannose receptor expression on sperm heads [40], sperm creatine phosphokinase M-isoform ratios [188], and hyaluronidase activity in human semen [2].

Standard Semen Analysis

Intrauterine Insemination

Several studies of IUI in couples with male infertility and after ovarian stimulation have reported pregnancy rates between 3.16% and 14.3% per cycle [18, 127, 174, 396]. Comhaire et al. [80] evaluated cumulative pregnancy rates in differently treated infertile men and demonstrated the favorable effect of IUI (average monthly pregnancy rate: 3.9%) compared with a control group (average monthly pregnancy rate: 1.1%). For successful IUI, the minimal cut-off values were 15×10^6/ml for sperm concentration, 9% for WHO (a)+(b) motility, and 8% for normal morphology. Other authors reported significantly lower pregnancy rates after use of ejaculates with sperm concentrations less than 5×10^6/ml [18], total sperm count less than 10×10^6/ml, progressive motility less than 30%, or a total motile sperm count less than 5×10^6/ml [102]. Since IUI is usually performed with prepared semen samples (swim-up, glass-wool filtration, Percoll), the total number of motile spermatozoa is an important discriminative factor. It is generally accepted that more than 1×10^6/ml motile spermatozoa should be available for successful IUI [19, 182]. The chance for conception is higher with increasing total motile sperm count [51], or more than 70% motile spermatozoa after swim-up [19, 267].

Reports about the predictive value of sperm morphology for the outcome of IUI are contradictory. Toner et al. [401] claimed that normal morphology as detected by strict criteria is the most significant predictor of pregnancy: when it was 14% or higher, the pregnancy rate was 15% per cycle, compared with 7% per cycle in case of normal morphology <14%. However, a cut-off value of 4% (strict criteria) does not discriminate between ejaculates that achieve pregnancies after IUI and those that do not [265]. Using WHO criteria to evaluate sperm morphology, Francavilla et al. [118] demonstrated that teratozoospermia (<50% normal morphology) is correlated with lower pregnancy rates after IUI.

In conclusion, IUI achieves better results in cases of reduced male fertility if certain criteria of semen quality are considered (sperm concentration in the native ejaculate $>5 \times 10^6$/ml, $>1 \times 10^6$/ml motile spermatozoa after sperm preparation). In patients showing extreme variations of semen quality, occasionally improved semen samples can be cryopreserved and later pooled with fresh samples for IUI [3]. IUI may also be successful in cases of male immunological infertility [232, 306], provided that not all spermatozoa are coated with antibodies [119].

In Vitro Fertilization, Gamete Intrafallopian Transfer

A variety of studies have examined the predictive value of standard semen parameters with regard to the IVF outcome. Biljan et al. [43] found a slight correlation between sperm concentrations in native ejaculates and fertilization rates ($r=0.28$). Similar results were reported by Duncan et al. [106] and Barlow et al. [29]. Significantly higher sperm concentrations have been demonstrated in patient groups achieving pregnancies after IVF [14]. Cut-off levels of $15-20 \times 10^6$/ml spermatozoa in the native sample have been suggested for successful IVF [80, 110]. However, the total motile sperm count after sperm preparation has a higher predictive value. Acceptance of male partners in IVF programs requires at least $0.4-3.0 \times 10^6$/ml progressively motile spermatozoa [69, 101, 110, 116, 171]. Fertilization rates after IVF are directly correlated with the total sperm number. Following use of ejaculates with 0.5×10^6 motile spermatozoa or fewer, the pregnancy rates after IVF were still 7.8% per retrieval [39]. However, spontaneous abortions were observed more frequently after IVF using spermatozoa from men with oligoasthenozoospermia [211]. Significant correlations between clinical pregnancy rates and sperm count, total sperm count, motile sperm count, and total motile sperm count were found in GIFT programs [335]. In contrast to Rodriguez-Rigau et al. [335], Nelson et al. [291] suggested the percentage of motile spermatozoa to be of predictive value for GIFT. GIFT is useful in cases of sperm concentrations $>20 \times 10^6$/ml [171]. Therefore, diagnostic semen preparation should always be performed prior to ART. This procedure is helpful in deciding whether a patient's ejaculate is suitable for IUI, IVF, GIFT, or ICSI.

The native sperm motility parameters according to the WHO are correlated with fertilization rates after IVF [29, 45, 103]. Fertilization is significantly reduced after use of ejaculates with <30% motile spermatozoa [146]. This is in agreement with Enginsu et al. [110], who studied 200 consecutive couples in an IVF program and defined 30% as the cut-off for progressive motility. In contrast, Biljan et al. [43] did not find significant correlations between motility and fertilization rates. However, a recent controlled study suggests that ICSI should be preferred in cases of low sperm motility, since fertilization rates were significantly lower after conventional IVF [416].

Data on the predictive value of motility parameters achieved by computer-aided sperm analysis (CASA) are contradictory. Maximum fertilization rates were achieved with sperm velocity >50 μm/s (CellSoft) and mean lateral head displacement (ALH) <2.89 μm [45]. Grunert et al. [146] also reported lower fertilization rates after IVF with spermatozoa showing average velocities (Cell-Soft) <50 μm/s. However, they considered conventional semen parameters such as sperm motility or morphology to be more predictive than values obtained by CASA. Since no differences in motility parameters were detectable in semen samples from patients achieving pregnancies after IVF and those who did not, CASA was not suggested to be helpful as a diagnostic tool before IVF [169]. Another problem of CASA is the limited availability of motile spermatozoa before IVF [29]. Hyperactivation after 3 or 6 h of capacitation has been shown to be correlated with fertilization rates [389, 422].

One of the best discriminants of the fertilization potential of human spermatozoa is sperm morphology. However, results and cut-off levels depend on the criteria for normal morphology. A variety of studies have used the WHO criteria to predict IVF outcome [29, 106, 146], whereas other authors were unable to confirm these results [43]. The clinical value of the WHO sperm morphology for in vivo fertility has been criticized [30].

The percentage of morphologically normal spermatozoa (according to WHO criteria) is significantly lower in semen samples achieving <50% fertilization rates in IVF programs [388]. Ejaculates with normal morphology (WHO) are associated with higher numbers of fertilized oocytes per couple [281]. However, the cut-off values for normal sperm morphology as recommended by the WHO were found to be too high. Hinting et al. [172] suggested a threshold value of 16% normal sperm morphology as a predictor of successful IVF. Spermatozoa showing normal morphology of less than 5% should not be used for IVF.

In 1986, Kruger et al. [228] introduced new criteria for normal sperm morphology and found high fertilization and pregnancy rates after IVF in patients with more than 14% normal spermatozoa. Later they reported a very low fertilization rate of 7.6% with fewer than 4% normal spermatozoa, whereas higher (63.9%) and even normal fertilization rates were achieved with samples containing 4–14% and more than 14% normal spermatozoa, respectively [229]. The value of strict criteria for prediction of IVF outcome was still obvious when slightly different cut-off levels were used: fertilization and pregnancy rates were significantly lower with semen samples showing less than 9% normal forms; no pregnancy was observed when normal sperm morphology was less than 5% [305]. In a structured literature review Coetzoe et al. [76] demonstrated that the overall fertilization rate was 59.3% for the <4% normal sperm morphology threshold, whereas it was 77.6% in patients with >4% normal sperm morphology. The clinically reliable cut-off limit for normal sperm morphology according to strict criteria was suggested to be 8% in post-swim-up spermatozoa [111]. The majority of studies have confirmed the predictive value of strict criteria [145, 218, 306, 445, 449], whereas Matorras et al. [265] did not find a correlation with pregnancy rates after IUI. However, severe sperm head abnormalities affect pregnancy rates more than fertilization after IVF [296]. Therefore, additional parameters such as normal acrosomal morphology are useful in the prediction of IVF outcome [264, 270].

The percentages of normal morphology according to other morphological classifications (Düsseldorf classification) are also correlated with fertilization and pregnancy rates after IVF [178].

A recent study about the frequency of cytoplasmic residues on sperm midpieces found an association between defective sperm functions and reduced fertilization rates after IVF [205].

Intracytoplasmic Sperm Injection

Since the first report about pregnancies after intracytoplasmic sperm injections appeared in 1992 [311], severe male infertility has become the major indication for ICSI. The outcome of ICSI is not correlated to any of the standard semen parameters [234], although fertilization rates are affected by the concentration of motile spermatozoa in the ejaculate and by the origin of samples (e.g., epididymis, ejaculate) [312]. Nagy et al. [285] demonstrated significantly lower fertilization rates when no spermatozoa had been found in the initial semen samples after checking the area of grids of the Makler or Neubauer counting chamber. However, the pregnancy rates did not differ significantly. In addition, the fertilization rate (2 pronuclear; % of intact oocytes) was significantly lower (10.9±12.1%) after ICSI with semen samples containing no motile spermatozoa. Morphology did not affect the outcome of microinjection [260, 299, 319]. However, implantation and ongoing pregnancy rates were lower after using spermatozoa with total teratozoospermia and abnormal head morphology [398]. Fertilization rates after use of spermatozoa from patients with male genital tract obstruction are better than those in cases of severe oligozoospermia, oligoasthenoteratozoospermia, or asthenoteratozoospermia [158].

Failure of previous IVF has no negative effect on the outcome of ICSI. Apparently more important for pregnancy rates are the egg number and the age of the female partner (<34 years: 48.9%; 35–39 years: 22.9%; ≥40 years: 5.9% clinical pregnancy per transfer) [299, 369]. In contrast, the paternal age has no influence on pregnancy outcome after ICSI [383].

Since only one living spermatozoon is required for microinjection, ICSI has also been performed in cases of extreme male infertility. Harari et al. [157] reported fertilization of four oocytes with spermatozoa from a patient with mosaic Klinefelter's syndrome; sperm concentration was less than 1000/ml. The authors suggested that in these cases spermatozoa may be used for ICSI without genetic risk. Pregnancies were also reported in patients with Klinefelter's syndrome after ICSI with testicular spermatozoa [338].

Fertilization and pregnancy with acrosomeless ("round-headed") spermatozoa or immotile spermatozoa presenting a "tail stump syndrome" or deficient dynein arms and disordered microtubular configuration are examples for the clinical benefit of ICSI in severe morphological disorders [204, 254, 384, 387]. Since sperm quality does not correlate with the outcome of ICSI, and even men with severe andrological disorders are able to have children, the genetic risk of this technique is a major concern [316].

Bonduelle et al. [44] found no differences in the pediatric follow-up of 130 ICSI children in comparison to 130 children born after conventional IVF. Generally, the present data do not suggest a significantly increased incidence of genetic-based diseases or male infertility [109]. This may also be due to the fact that selection mechanisms against genetic-based defects occur after fertilization of the oocyte. According to Engel et al. [109], inherited male infertility may be a problem of ICSI if mutations of X- or Y-chromosomal genes play a major role in male fertility disorders.

A set of genes located at the long (q) arm of the Y chromosome is required for spermatogenesis [334]. This region was described as "azoospermia factor" (AZF), since it was originally thought to harbor an azoospermia factor gene [60, 419]. The Y chromosome has been mapped into a series of deletion intervals. In infertile patients most deletions are observed in three regions within the deletion intervals 5 and 6. These regions were designated AZFa, AZFb, and AZFc. Each of these regions seems to be associated with a distinct testicular histology [420]. Two candidate AZF genes are RBM (RNA-binding motif) and DAZ (deleted in azoospermia). In patients with severe oligozoospermia ($<5 \times 10^6$/ml spermatozoa) the frequency of Y chromosome microdeletions ranges from 3% to 29% [334, 380]. Spermatozoa from men with microdeletions of the Y chromosome seem to be capable of undergoing capacitation and AR and of fertilizing during IVF [339]. The transmission of Y chromosomal deletions from fathers to sons through ICSI have been described recently [202, 310].

It is generally recommended that patients and their children born after ICSI undergo careful follow-up to clarify possible genetic risks of micromanipulation techniques [197, 273, 315]. Molecular analysis of Y-chromosomal microdeletions should also be performed in all men with sperm concentration $<5 \times 10^6$/ml [380].

Acrosin Activity

The predictive value of sperm acrosin activity has been examined in a variety of studies. Figure 5 compares fertilization rates and acrosin activity index calculated from halo diameter and halo formation rate in an IVF program (110 patients) [166]. Normal acrosin activity indices were observed in men with high fertilization rates, while the halo diameters and halo formation rates were smaller in most cases of poor fertilization ($<50\%$). Patients showing a normal acrosin activity index but low fertilization probably had defects other than im-

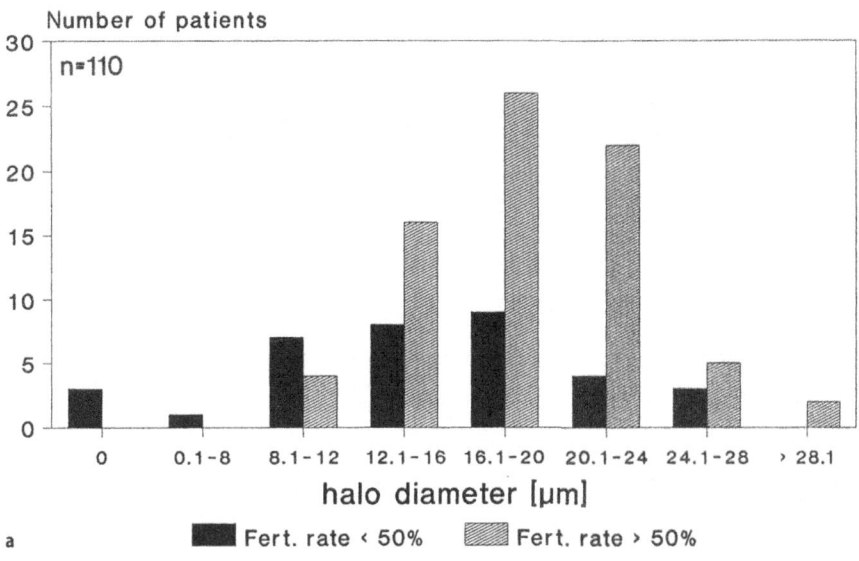

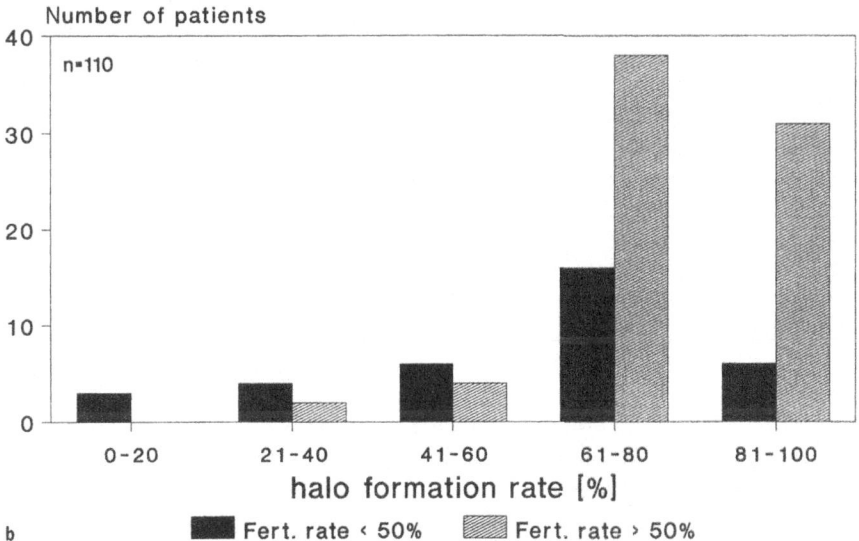

Fig. 5a, b. Correlation between fertilization rates after in vitro fertilization and halo diameter (a) and halo formation rate (b) detected by gelatinolysis (from Henkel et al. [166])

paired acrosin activity (e.g., impaired AR, impaired sperm-oolemma interaction, or disturbance of chromatin decondensation). This is also a reason why statistical calculations showed a low sensitivity (26%), while high specificity (98%) and a high predictive value (positive predictive value 90%, negative predictive value 74%) are observed for human IVF outcome [166]. These data confirm results reported by other groups [32, 96, 368], who have also found correlations between acrosin activity and fertilization rates in IVF programs. Acrosin activity is correlated with the proportion of mature oocytes that are transferred as cleaving embryos [408]. In contrast, Menkveld et al. [270] demonstrated only a low correlation between fertilization rates and acrosin activity. After the use of a polyclonal antibody against acrosin, spermatozoa from a patient group with no fertilization in IVF showed significantly less normal staining of the anterior head membranes than spermatozoa from a group in which fertilization was achieved [365]. Other studies have reported no significant differences in sperm acrosin activity between groups showing good or poor fertilization rates after IVF [230, 245, 444].

Only little information is available about the influence of acrosin on the outcome of other forms of ART. Total acrosin activity is correlated with the pregnancy rate after partial zona dissection [409].

Acrosome Reaction

A variety of artificial and physiological stimuli have been reported to induce the human sperm acrosome reaction in vitro [450]. The percentage of spermatozoa undergoing spontaneous AR during 9 h incubation was found to be negatively correlated with the outcome of IUI [263]. While the spontaneous acrosome reaction is not correlated with fertilization rates in IVF programs [321], the following are of prognostic value for sperm fertilization capacity: inducibility of AR (i.e., difference between induced and spontaneous AR) by calcium ionophore A 23187 [11, 90, 115, 314, 389, 448], human follicular fluid [58, 59], progesterone [226], phorbol 12-myristate 13-acetate 4-O-methyl ether [315], zona pellucida [246], pentoxifylline [397], N-acetylglucosamine-neoglycoprotein [49], and low-temperature [164] or incubation in capacitation medium [392, 422].

Henkel et al. [164] demonstrated that patients with fewer than 13% acrosome-reacted spermatozoa and less than 7.5% inducible AR have significantly lower fertilization rates in IVF programs (Fig. 6). Liu and Baker [247] observed reduced fertilization rates after IVF with spermatozoa showing normal morphology <15% and low response to induction of the AR by calcium ionophore.

In cases with <30% normal sperm morphology according to the WHO, the proportion of spermatozoa with normal intact acrosomes in the insemination medium (as detected by FITC-PSA) is related to the fertilization rates after IVF [242]. All studies on the inducibility of AR should consider the high degree of inter- and intrasubject variability of AR in both patients and fertile donors; the duration of sexual abstinence does not seem to have a significant effect [406].

As noted above, human sperm AR may be affected in spermatozoa with head malformations. Acrosome reaction and acrosin activity seem also to be impaired in polyzoospermic patients [402]. In addition, other factors such as smoking or environmental toxins may alter the AR [108, 221]. Hershlag et al. [168] described a case of male infertility in a patient treated with a calcium ion channel blocker. After discontinuation of this therapy, expression of mannose-specific lectin and AR normalized, and a pregnancy was achieved after IUI.

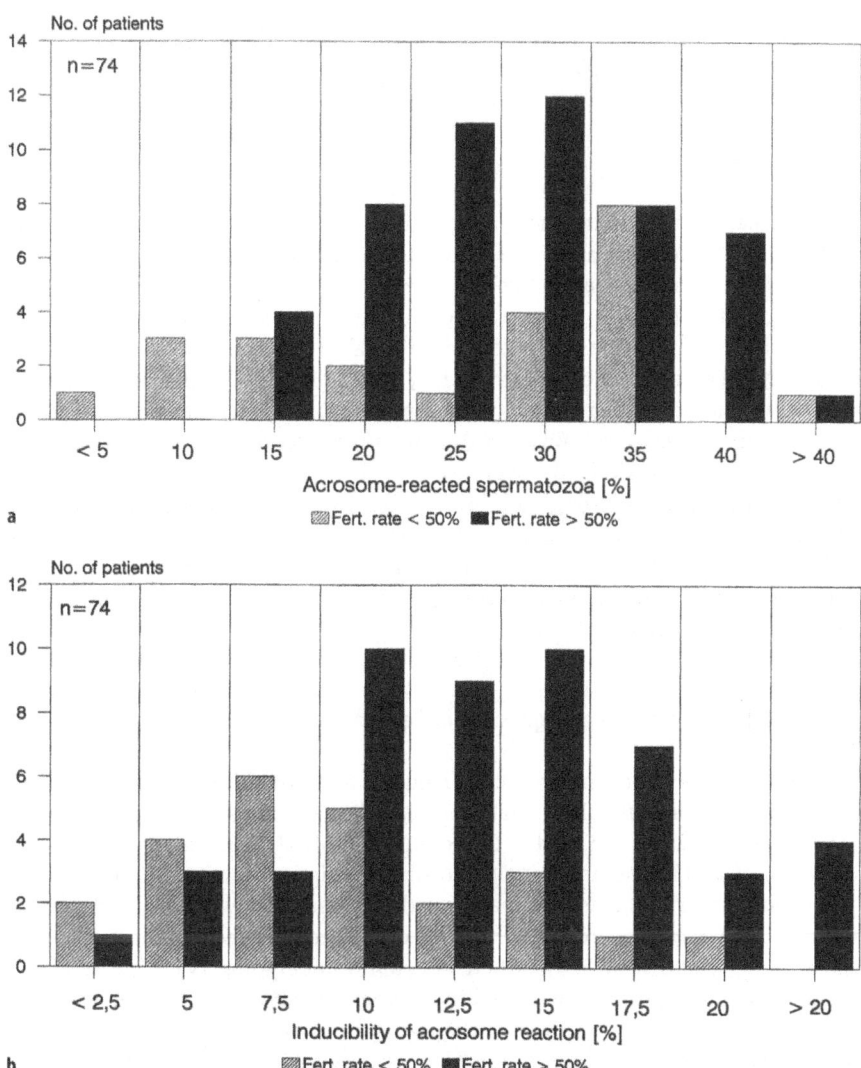

Fig. 6. Correlation between fertilization rates after in vitro fertilization and the percentage of acrosome-reacted spermatozoa (AR) and AR inducibility after cold induction (from Henkel et al. [164])

However, the acrosome reaction is not required for ICSI. Liu et al. [251] demonstrated that spermatozoa with impaired zona pellucida-induced AR achieve 50% or more normal fertilization and embryo development. Therefore, AR assays are useful for pre-IVF diagnostics. Insufficient AR may be improved by in vitro sperm treatment, for example, with pentoxifylline [400]. Otherwise, microinjection should be recommended for andrological reasons. Successful fertilizations with this method have been described even in severe cases of acrosomal dysfunction such as globozoospermia [252].

Hemizona Assay

Since normal sperm-egg interaction is required for all ART not based on microinjection, the hemizona assay has been developed as a biological test system with predictive value especially for IVF [57]. The positive predictive value for fertilization after IVF was initially reported to be 83%, with 83% sensitivity and 95% specificity [297]. The positive predictive value was confirmed in later studies with higher numbers of IVF trials [73, 122, 123, 125]. Therefore, the hemizona assay should be performed with spermatozoa from patients who fail to achieve fertilization in IVF programs or are suspected to have fertilization disorders [298]. Liu et al. [248] demonstrated a significant correlation between sperm-zona pellucida binding and fertilization during IVF programs in patients with less than 30% normal sperm morphology. They recommended HZA as a useful tool before IVF, especially in cases of poor sperm morphology. Low sperm binding to the zona pellucida is associated with sperm defects, rather than with oocyte defects [249].

Sperm Penetration Test (Heterologous Ovum Penetration Test)

Data from studies about the predictive value of SPA are contradictory. This may be due to technical difficulties which make it difficult to repeat the assay [451]. The results of SPA are not related to the outcome of IUI [233, 263].

Belkien et al. [38] reported a 95% positive predictive value of SPA for IVF in normozoospermic patients, compared with 0% in men with reduced semen quality. These results were confirmed by other groups who demonstrated the high specificity and sensitivity of SPA in couples undergoing IVF because of tubal infertility or unexplained infertility. Therefore, SPA is of limited value in cases of male subfertility [189, 261, 414]. In addition, a negative SPA ($\leq 10\%$ fusions) is associated with a high rate (65%) of false-negative results in IVF [74]. The results of SPA are also not correlated with the outcome of GIFT cycles [335]. However, Soffer et al. [381] found correlations between SPA and fertilization (IVF) after preincubation of spermatozoa with TEST-yolk buffer.

In conclusion, the sperm penetration assay has to be evaluated in combination with other semen or sperm function parameters (e.g., AR). It is of only limited use in cases of male infertility.

Hypo-osmotic Swelling Test

Despite the fact that the HOS test seems to be correlated with fertility in vivo [61, 62], many studies have failed to demonstrate significant correlations between hypo-osmotic sperm swelling and IVF outcome [23, 43, 75]. The WHO therefore recommended the HOS test as a marker of cell viability rather than fertilizing capacity. However, the percentage of sperm swelling has been shown to be higher in semen samples successfully used for IUI [276, 411]. In contrast, the hypo-osmotic swelling test score is significantly lower in samples from men whose partners have had unexplained recurrent spontaneous abortions [56].

Aniline Blue Staining, Acridine Orange Staining

As noted above, nuclear proteins play a significant role in chromatin condensation. Using nuclear maturity as a parameter, this method is an attempt to discriminate between fertile men and those suspected of being infertile [22, 175]. Disturbed chromatin condensation is often observed in combination with an increased number of acrosomal defects [177]. A protamine gene defect is thought to be involved in case of more than 50% aniline blue-positive spermatozoa. Results in 33 men showed a close correlation ($r=0.825$) between normal chromatin condensation and fertilization rate after IVF [150]. Liu and Baker [245] reported similar findings with aniline blue staining of spermatozoa from 91 men in an IVF program. Nucleus maturity was significantly correlated with fertilization rates when normal sperm morphology was 15% or more. Higher percentages of chromatin decondensation in spermatozoa that failed to fertilize human oocytes in vitro were also observed by electron microscopy [65]. This indicates that normal chromatin condensation is mandatory for induction of fertilization. Thus, aniline blue staining is highly predictive and may be used as an additional function test prior to ART. However, its value is apparently restricted to conventional IVF procedures, because in ejaculated or testicular spermatozoa used for ICSI, chromatin condensation was not a predictive factor for fertilization [155, 156, 413]. In this context it should be mentioned that glass-wool filtration showed a selective capacity to enrich the number of normal chromatin-condensed spermatozoa [165].

Fertilization rates after IVF are correlated not only with sperm nucleus maturity but also with intact DNA, as detected with acridine orange staining [247]. Claassens et al. [70] demonstrated a high positive predictive value of the acridine orange test, while the negative predictive value was low.

Reactive Oxygen Species

Especially oligozoospermic patients tend to have high ROS production by spermatozoa [13]. From a clinical point of view it is important to determine semen samples producing excessive amounts of ROS, and to separate leukocytes and damaged spermatozoa from sperm cells that do not show signs of lipid peroxidation. Because spermatozoa are sensitive to oxidative damage, sperm separation should be performed very carefully, preferably by means of density gradient centrifugation with Percoll or glass-wool filtration. Both methods maintain normal sperm function with regard to motility and penetration into zona-free hamster oocytes [12, 282, 327]. Compared with fertile controls, more ROS are produced by spermatozoa from patients who do not achieve pregnancies after IUI [91].

Krausz et al. [225] investigated ROS levels in semen samples that were used for IVF. Formylleucylphenylalanine and a phorbolester induced the generation of ROS from spermatozoa and leukocytes, respectively. ROS production was associated with reduced sperm motility. However, the fertilization rates were correlated only with ROS generation from leukocytes. This is in agreement with Sukcharoen et al. [388], who also found formylleucylphenylalanine-induced chemiluminescence to be one of the most informative predictive factors for fertilization after IVF. Measuring the antioxidant capacity of seminal plasma, Lewis et al. [241] observed higher levels in men whose partners had ongoing pregnancies after IVF than in infertile patients attending a subfertility clinic.

Male Urogenital Infection and ART

Acute inflammatory urogenital processes (e.g., epididymitis) are known to affect semen quality. Therefore, acute infections have to be cured before methods of assisted reproduction are indicated. In contrast, temporary inflammatory episodes do not have a significant effect on sperm quality [325]. However, Eliasson [107] reported that inflammation of the male accessory sex glands is often found in infertile men and recommended the routine examination of prostatic fluid. Comhaire et al. [79] defined the following indicators of male genital tract infections: growth of more than 1000/ml pathogenic bacteria; growth of more than 10,000 nonpathogenic bacteria in seminal plasma after 1:2 dilution; more than 1×10^6 leukocytes per milliliter ejaculate; pathological secretory function of the accessory sex glands.

The possible effect of chronic inflammation on fertility is still a matter of discussion. Chronic prostatitis may decrease sperm concentration and sperm motility. These parameters were improved after antibiotic treatment [133]. Leib et al. [237] confirmed that patients with chronic nonbacterial prostatitis have lower sperm quality than fertile men. Other groups have not found different sperm concentrations, motility, or morphology in control groups and patients with chronic bacterial prostatitis, nonbacterial prostatitis, or prostatodynia [424]. Although high numbers of bacteria do not necessarily affect semen quality [68, 97, 160, 423], some studies demonstrate that motility and viability are reduced in bacteriospermic men [272]. However, antibiotic treatment did not improve semen quality in comparison to a control group treated with placebo [271]. Thus, the clinical significance of asymptomatic bacteriospermia for male fertility remains to be clarified. When semen samples are used for ART, microbiological or serological examinations are recommended because micro-organisms may be transferred [42, 279]. In four of five women with positive peritoneal cultures, Stone et al. [386] found the same organisms that had also been cultured in semen samples. In cases of significant bacteriospermia (>104 bacteria per milliliter) antibiotic therapy should be performed. Sperm preparation techniques may also reduce the number of micro-organisms [437]. Nevertheless, transfer of bacteria after preparation techniques can never be excluded because some micro-organisms are able to penetrate spermatozoa and may be carried into the IVF medium or the female genital tract during ART. Repeated embryo degeneration caused by bacterial infection with *Escherichia coli* originating in the ejaculate has been reported. In these cases, TESE with ICSI may be successful [364]. Positive bacteriological results have been reported in 50–72% of semen samples used for IVF [332]. Aerobic or anaerobic bacteria were found in 44–88% of these ejaculates, and *Mycoplasma* was present in 6–33%. Concerning *Ureaplasma urealyticum*, similar percentages were reported by Montagut et al. [278], who demonstrated significantly reduced pregnancy rates after embryo transfer in these cases. In contrast, Riedel et al. [331] did not find correlations between bacteriospermia and fertilization rates. Similar data were reported by Kanakas et al. [203], who observed higher abortion rates after IVF with ejaculates containing *U. urealyticum*. The fertilization rates were not affected. *Chlamydia trachomatis* was detected in 14% of semen samples from men participating in an IVF program, but semen quality was not different from that of the noninfected group [284]. Data on the association of chlamydial antibodies in serum and fertilization in IVF programs are contradictory [255]. According to Torode et al. [403], these antibodies are not related to impaired semen quality or reduced fertilization rates after IVF. Thus, bacteriospermia requires antibiotic therapy because negative effects on implantation or embryonic development cannot be excluded.

Leukocytes as generators of ROS are associated with impaired sperm functions. White blood cells originate from the epididymis and the prostate gland [434]. They may interfere with fertilization in IVF programs [7, 77, 412]. Therefore, leukocytes or other markers of inflammation should be determined in seminal plasma prior to IVF.

Ejaculatory Disorders and ART

Male infertility is only rarely caused by ejaculatory disorders, including reduced volume of ejaculate, painful ejaculation, premature or delayed ejaculation, retrograde ejaculation, anejaculation, and anorgasmia [323]. With regard to ART, clinically important disorders are retrograde ejaculation and anejaculation. The ejaculation and emission processes may be affected by traumatic or surgical injury (prostatectomy, bilateral radical lymph node dissection, spinal cord injury), diabetic neuropathy, drugs, and congenital factors. Retrograde ejaculation can be diagnosed in 0.3–2.0% of infertile patients. However, the incidence is higher (18%) in azoospermic men [446]. Therefore, the postejaculatory urine sediment should always be examined in cases of azoospermia. Therapeutic approaches include conversion into antegrade ejaculation and collection of spermatozoa directly from the bladder for ART. Medical treatment of retrograde ejaculation includes α-adrenergic agents (phenylpropanalamine hydrochloride, synephrine, oxedrin, midodrin), anticholinergics (brompheniramine maleate), and imipramine [167, 446].

Since urine has a deleterious effect on sperm quality, recovery of spermatozoa from urine is only successful when pH (7.4) and osmolarity (320 mOsm/kg) are adjusted by oral intake of sodium bicarbonate and water [63]. Alternatively, medium can be injected into the bladder before ejaculation; nevertheless, urine may interfere with sperm functions [64]. Following these procedures, pregnancies have been reported after sexual intercourse [348], IUI [328, 340, 366, 391], direct intraperitoneal insemination [421], IVF [46], GIFT [417], pronuclear stage tubal transfer (PROST) [186], and ICSI [129, 294]. Pregnancies have also been reported after IUI or IVF with spermatozoa obtained from the vas deferens by microsurgical aspiration [37, 92, 183]. Retrograde ejaculated spermatozoa obtained from the patient's urine can be cryopreserved and later successfully used for ICSI [195].

In cases of anejaculation and intact sacral reflexes, penile vibratory stimulation (PVS) to the frenulum may be useful [33, 427]. PVS is not indicated for anejaculation due to lesions of the peripheral nerve fibers. Dahlberg et al. [92] reported 17 pregnancies following vibrator use and "home insemination", IUI, or IVF.

Rectal probe electroejaculation can be used to treat anemission irresponsive to conservative therapy or after unsuccessful vibratory stimulation. Electroejaculation has also been used in men with spinal cord injury. Since semen quality after electroejaculation is usually poor, better results are obtained with ART [66]. Pregnancies have been reported after IUI, IVF, and ICSI [52, 66, 67, 92, 154, 303]. Hulting et al. [187] achieved five IVF pregnancies and a fertilization rate of 54% in six couples with anejaculatory infertility after testicular spermatozoa had been obtained via electroejaculation. If conservative treatment, vibratory stimulation, and electroejaculation are not successful, MESA or TESE may be suitable to retrieve spermatozoa for ICSI.

Cryopreservation of Human Spermatozoa and ART

In 1973, Steinberger and Smith [385] reported similar conception rates after cryopreservation and insemination using ejaculates of very good quality (61%) or fresh semen samples (73%). However, the majority of ejaculates had been stored for less than 6 months. Insemination with frozen/thawed spermatozoa required 5.3 cycles for pregnancy to occur, whereas fresh spermatozoa induced pregnancies after 4.4 cycles. Minimal criteria for cryopreservation were developed before the new methods of assisted reproduction became available, (e.g., progressive motility $>10\%$, $>15 \times 10^6$/ml spermatozoa after thawing) [219]. Since only one living spermatozoon is necessary for ICSI, such cut-off values are no longer useful.

Two major indications for human sperm cryopreservation are: (a) IUI with donor semen [379] and (b) fertility insurance before surgery, radiation, or chemotherapy. In the age of AIDS, artificial donor insemination with cryopreserved semen is mandatory after exclusion of HIV infection in the donor [370]. Cryopreservation does not necessarily destroy micro-organisms present in the semen: *Streptococcus*, *Neisseria gonorrhoeae*, *Chlamydia*, mycoplasms, HIV, cytomegalovirus, hepatitis B virus, *Trichomonas vaginalis*, herpes simplex virus, and *Treponema pallidum* may survive freezing and thawing. "Fertility insurance" is an important indication for sperm cryopreservation. However, various studies have shown that only few patients want to use their ejaculates for later inseminations [180, 206, 219, 224]. Since modern ART were introduced in reproductive medicine, cryopreserved semen has been successfully used for IVF [112, 258, 346] and GIFT [16].

Another indication for cryopreservation is the storage of epididymal or testicular spermatozoa until they are to be used for ICSI [286, 342]. The fertilization rates after ICSI with fresh or frozen/thawed epididymal spermatozoa are comparable [286, 405]. Epididymal sperm cryopreservation is advantageous in that epididymal surgery and ICSI can be planned independently. In addition, cryopreserved spermatozoa may be used for further ICSI without second or third scrotal surgery [100]. The quality of microsurgically aspirated and cryopreserved spermatozoa can be improved with pentoxifylline [54].

Microsurgical Epididymal Sperm Aspiration, Testicular Sperm Extraction

Microsurgical Epididymal Sperm Aspiration

Nonobstructive azoospermia is classified into reparable and irreparable disorders. Obstructive azoospermia may be treated by surgical procedures on the epididymis, vas deferens, or ejaculatory duct [324, 426]. Partial epididymal and vasal obstruction in association with severe oligozoospermia has been corrected microsurgically [162]. Since ICSI was established as a new ART, an alternative therapeutic approach is available for men presenting with azoospermia.

MESA has replaced the alloplastic spermatocele in cases of surgically untreatable azoospermia. Obstructive azoospermia may be caused by congenital or acquired reproductive tract occlusion [137]. CBAVD, which occurs in 1–2% of infertile men [191], represents a mild form of cystic fibrosis (CF) [17]. The vasa deferentia are also absent in almost all men with CF. Therefore, the medical history (respiratory infections, known CF) and physical examination (impalpable scrotal vasa deferentia or corpus/cauda epididymidis) are important in all cases of azoospermia. However, obstructive azoospermia in combination with chronic suppurating respiratory disease may also be caused by a Young's syndrome which is not related to CF [238].

CBAVD is often associated with morphological abnormalities of the seminal vesicles [295], which can be detected by transrectal ultrasonography. While testicular size and function and caput epididymidis are usually normal, corpus or cauda epididymidis may be missing. Since patients with CBAVD but without clinical signs of CF may transmit CF mutations, genetic screening of both partners is mandatory before performing MESA and ICSI. The incidence of CF is

1:1600 in the general population, with a carrier frequency of 1:25 [295]. More than 300 mutations of the CF gene are known. The most frequent mutation is ΔF508, which is found on 70% of CF chromosomes. Screening for 12 mutations in the CF transmembrane regulator gene (CFTR), Patrizio et al. [317] found 64% of 63 patients positive. A higher incidence (77%) was reported by Le Lannou et al. [238]. If the common mutations are not present in the patient's spouse, and no cases of CF are reported in her family history, the CF carrier risk is reduced to 0.4% [295].

Patients with congenital unilateral absence of the vas deferens represent a clinically, anatomically, and genetically heterogeneous group. When the contralateral vas deferens is anatomically intact and patent, CF mutations are not found, whereas occlusions are associated with mutations [274].

Spermatozoa can be obtained by MESA or TESE from patients with CBAVD. Patrizio et al. [317] reported significantly lower fertilization and pregnancy rates following IVF with spermatozoa from men carrying the ΔF508 mutation; in contrast, men with CBAVD and no or other mutations showed better IVF outcomes. However, these differences were not observed after IVF procedures in combination with micromanipulations (partial zona dissection, subzonal sperm injection, ICSI) [358]. The IVF outcome is related to the length of the epididymis in men with CBAVD. Patients with an epididymal length greater than 4.0 cm show the highest fertilization and pregnancy rates [318]. Generally, ICSI should be preferred in cases of CBAVD because fertilization and pregnancy rates per cycle are significantly higher than after IVF [173, 377].

Several modified epididymal sperm retrieval techniques have been demonstrated. It is still a matter of discussion whether percutaneous epididymal aspiration (PESA) is an equivalent method. In 20% of cases, Tsirigotis and Craft [407] failed to obtain spermatozoa. In later studies the epididymal sperm retrieval rate was 83%. Retrieved spermatozoa were found to be motile in 67–100%. Differences between the clinical pregnancy rates after ICSI with ejaculated spermatozoa and those retrieved by PESA were not different [269]. However, most microsurgeons do not accept this method for fear of causing uncontrollable damage to the epididymal duct system. Moreover, MESA in combination with ICSI is superior to percutaneous aspiration procedures because of higher pregnancy rates, availability of spermatozoa for cryopreservation, lower frequency of blood contamination, lower risk of tissue damage, and higher numbers and better quality of spermatozoa [137, 371].

Yamamoto et al. [442] collected epididymal spermatozoa by micropuncture after stimulation of the spermatic nerve. Spermatozoa were obtained in all 15 patients included in their study. Three pregnancies were achieved after partial zona dissection or SUZI.

Kim and Han [212] detached epididymides surgically and extracted spermatozoa after mechanical dissection of epididymal tissue in IVF medium.

Testicular Sperm Extraction

The development of TESE has also changed the diagnostic procedure in andrology. Testicular biopsies are now performed for diagnostic and therapeutic reasons because testicular spermatozoa can be used for ICSI. TESE is suitable for patients suffering from CBAVD and obstructive or nonobstructive azoospermia [98, 360]. In patients with obstructive azoospermia, fertilization and pregnancy rates after ICSI with testicular spermatozoa are similar to those with epididymal or ejaculated sperm cells [135, 378]. In cases of nonobstructive azoospermia, fertilization and pregnancy rates with testicular spermatozoa are significantly lower than those achieved with epididymal spermatozoa from men with obstructive azoospermia [313]. Fertilization rates are significantly higher after injection of motile testicular spermatozoa, which can be more frequently retrieved in cases with normal spermatogenesis [288, 373]. Single seminiferous tubules with intact spermatogenesis may also be present in damaged testes [136, 447]; therefore, elevated follicle-stimulating hormone (FSH) levels or reduced testicular size are no longer contraindications for testicular biopsies. More than one biopsy may be necessary to find spermatozoa in cases of testicular failure [99, 163]. Spermatozoa can be extracted from testicular tissue in 50–60% of patients with elevated FSH levels [194]. In addition to the histological evaluation, a TESE test should be performed to determine whether spermatozoa from native or cryopreserved testicular tissue can be extracted. Various techniques have been developed for this purpose. Separation methods such as Percoll centrifugation are not practicable because of increased sperm loss [415]. Gentle enzymatic and mechanical disintegration of the testicular tissue preserves testicular sperm viability [342]. The presence of motile spermatozoa may indicate genital tract obstruction [200].

Similar to MESA, the retrieval of testicular spermatozoa has also been modified. Bourne et al. [48] reported two pregnancies in two couples after ICSI with living spermatozoa obtained by fine-needle biopsy of the testis. The men suffered from obstructive azoospermia. Hovatta et al. [185] confirmed the effectiveness of testicular needle biopsy in cases of obstructive azoospermia in a larger group of patients. However, it should be noted that in three of 17 patients no spermatozoa were found in the needle biopsy specimens, while they were present in the open biopsy samples. The spermatozoa recovery rate may be better after more than one biopsy by fine-needle aspiration [141]. Using percutaneous testicular sperm aspiration, Craft and Tsirigotis [86] retrieved spermatozoa from patients with nonobstructive azoospermia. A prospective study showed that spermatozoa were retrieved in only 14% of patients with nonobstructive azoospermia by fine-needle biopsies, whereas spermatozoa were extracted in 63% of men with open testicular biopsies [114]. Tournaye et al. [404] also demonstrated that more spermatozoa were recovered after open biopsy than after fine-needle aspiration. Fertilization, cleavage, ongoing pregnancy, and implantation rates after ICSI with these spermatozoa were comparable. Similar to percutaneous puncture of the epididymis, needle biopsy or aspiration of the testis are not generally accepted because they may damage testicular tissue and usually do not provide enough material for cryopreservation [137].

Recently, a new technique for microdissection of testicular tubules was introduced. Larger and more opaque seminiferous tubules containing developing germ cells were identified by optical magnification. Schlegel [357] thus increased the ability to find spermatozoa from 45% to 63% in patients with nonobstructive azoospermia.

Fertilization and pregnancy rates after ICSI with ejaculated, epididymal, or testicular spermatozoa are comparable. However, some groups reported reduced live birth rates after ICSI with spermatozoa from patients with nonobstructive azoospermia [131].

Since 1995, first pregnancies have been reported after ICSI with round spermatids (round spermatid injection, ROSI) and elongated spermatids (elongated spermatid injection, ELSI) [21]. However, fertilization and pregnancy rates after ICSI with round spermatids are significantly lower than those achieved with testicular spermatozoa [132].

Medical Therapy

Despite considerable basic research efforts, the therapeutic possibilities for improving impaired male fertility are still limited [351]. This is due partly to the fact that the cause of reduced fertility is unknown in most cases, and consequently no specific therapy is available. Another major problem concerns the objective assessment of the treatment response. Biological variations of semen parameters and the effects of endogenous or exogenous factors contribute to make this a difficult task. Nevertheless, medical therapy may be more appropriate than ART; it may also improve semen quality and the outcome of ART. Causal medical treatments in andrology include the treatment of sperm transport disturbances, endocrine insufficiency, male adnexitis and sperm autoantibodies [355].

A variety of therapeutic approaches have been developed to modify sperm functions in vitro [290]. Adjuvant male therapy during IVF procedures has been suggested by Acosta et al. [4], Abdelmassih et al. [1], and Comhaire et al. [81]. For example, administration of exogenous testosterone or systemic treatment with FSH may improve the fertilizing capacity of spermatozoa. Increased fertilization rates after IVF were observed following treatment of the male partner with FSH (150 units, three times a week for 3 months). Interestingly, endocrine profiles or semen quality did not change during treatment [4]. Concomitant treatment of the male by recombinant FSH has also been suggested [24]. Ashkenazi et al. [20] treated male partners of ICSI couples with pure FSH for more than 50 days prior to oocyte retrieval and observed significantly higher implantation rates.

Approaches to andrological therapy at different levels include stimulation of spermatogenesis, improvement of epididymal function or sperm transport within the male genital tract, and stimulation of sperm metabolism. All agents for improvement of spermatogenesis must be administered for at least 3 months before a significant increase in sperm count can be expected. Empirical administration of drugs may be discussed in individual cases. It is known that even a placebo may be an effective therapy in some patients, leading to improved semen parameters and/or pregnancy rates [25].

For a therapy to be considered effective the increase in sperm count should be greater than 50%. So far, no clinical studies have fulfilled these conditions [223]. There is only one exception: A "yes" or "no" response is expected during substitution therapy in case of azoospermia caused by hormonal insufficiency.

In the medical therapy of male fertility disturbances, specific and empirical treatment procedures have to be distinguished. Specific treatment is based on a pathophysiological concept and entails accurate patient selection; the therapeutic success is predictable. In contrast, empirical treatment involves no patient selection according to specific criteria, and the results are not predictable. Empirical treatment is performed regardless of whether the mechanism of action of the drug used is hypothetical, partially known, or well established.

Pentoxifylline

Pentoxifylline is a methylxanthine derivative, approved for treatment of various circulatory disturbances. Its effectiveness in andrological indications is thought to be based on increased intracellular ATP and cAMP concentrations by inhibition of phosphodiesterase [240]. However, the seminal plasma levels of the substance during therapy have been lower than those required for stimulation of sperm motility in vitro. Suggested andrological indications for pentoxifylline are asthenozoospermia, oligozoospermia, and decreased ejaculatory volume, as well as vascular erectile dysfunction. Treatment attempts and studies have been performed with daily oral administration of 3×400 mg or 3×600 mg pentoxifylline for 6–12 weeks. Only smaller control studies have reported on the effectiveness of pentoxifylline in male fertility disorders [361]. Randomized double-blind studies are lacking. Thus a positive effect of pentoxifylline on male fertility and especially on pregnancy rates during therapy has not been proven.

Tamoxifen

Tamoxifen is the *trans*-isomer of a triphenylethylene derivative with antiestrogenic action, approved for the adjuvant therapy of (metastatic) carcinoma of the breast. Its antiestrogenic action is based on the inhibition of estrogen binding of the genomic receptor, followed by reduced synthesis of estrogen receptors and growth factors. In andrological indications, its effectiveness is thought to result from competitive inhibition of estrogen binding to hypothalamic and pituitary receptors, which leads to increased production of gonadotropins and stimulation of spermatogenesis. Whether there is a direct effect of tamoxifen on the testis remains controversial. The incidence of endometrial carcinoma is increased during tamoxifen therapy. Animal experiments have shown a hepatocarcinogenic effect in rats, but not in mice. Suggested andrological indications for tamoxifen are oligozoospermia in normogonadotropic and hypergonadotropic patients, as well as (reportedly) partial androgen resistance. Treatment attempts and studies have been performed with daily doses of 5–40 mg tamoxifen. A dosage of 2×10 mg/day has been used most frequently. Rolf et al. [336] evaluated 29 studies on tamoxifen in andrological indications. Nearly all major studies revealed significantly elevated LH, FSH, and testosterone serum levels. While a significant increase in sperm concentration was observed in most open studies, this was not uniformly reported in randomized trials. At any rate, the largest randomized study comprising 239 men revealed increased sperm concentrations in about 50%, the number of spermatozoa being higher in patients with high-grade oligozoospermia. A positive effect on sperm motility was observed in only 20%, but the influence on pregnancy rates was not considered [222]. Thus, a positive effect of tamoxifen therapy on ejaculate quality is possible. However, improved pregnancy rates have not been documented so far.

Clomiphene

Clomiphene is a mixture of cis- and trans-isomers (zuclomiphene, enclomiphene), a nonsteroidal, synthetic substance. The cis-isomer is many times more effective than the trans-isomer. It has a moderate antiestrogenic action and a mild estrogenic effect. In andrological indications, clomiphene citrate is thought to be effective through competitive inhibition of estrogen binding to hypothalamic and pituitary estrogen receptors (see Tamoxifen). Liver and testicular carcinomas have occasionally been observed during therapy with clomiphene citrate, without a causal relation with the drug having been confirmed. Suggested andrological indications for clomiphene citrate are oligo- and asthenozoospermia at the following dosage: 25 mg clomiphene citrate per day for 3 months or 25 mg clomiphene citrate daily for 25 days, followed by a treatment pause of 5 days. By the early 1990s, about 20 open and controlled studies had demonstrated controversial results concerning the effectiveness of clomiphene citrate in andrological indications. Finally, the WHO [430] arranged for a double-blind, randomized, placebo-controlled study in 190 men with idiopathic oligo- or asthenozoospermia. No significant treatment effects on ejaculate quality or pregnancy rates were demonstrated. However, another study showed that alternate therapy with 25 mg chlomiphene citrate every other day was superior to daily administration of this dose [181]. Akin [15] reported a successful conversion from azoospermia to cryptozoospermia after treatment with clomiphene citrate in a patient with incomplete androgen resistance. The author suggested that medical treatment may be helpful in combination with micromanipulation techniques in this case. Thus, a positive effect of chlomiphene citrate on ejaculate quality or pregnancy rates has not yet been documented. Apart from studies, the use of this drug for andrological indications is therefore not recommended.

Mast Cell Blockers (Ketotifen, Tranilast)

Ketotifen is a tricyclic benzocycloheptathiophene, approved for prevention and therapy of allergic diseases of the respiratory tract. It has a stabilizing effect on the mast cell. Furthermore, Ketotifen blocks histamine (H1) receptors and inhibits the SRS-A (slow-reacting substance of anaphylaxis) as well as phosphodiesterase with increased cAMP concentrations. In andrological indications, Ketotifen is thought to be effective by inhibiting mast cells, which are sometimes increased in the testicular tissue of infertile men [36, 353]. Suggested andrological indications are oligozoospermia and asthenozoospermia. In these cases, the daily dosage is 2×1 mg. Significant positive effects on sperm concentration and motility were demonstrated in an open study comprising 17 oligospermic or asthenozoospermic men. However, the pregnancy rates during therapy were not different from the spontaneous conception rates [353]. On the other hand, a placebo-controlled, non-double-blind study using the mast cell blocker Tranilast (300 mg daily for 3 months) in 50 men with $< 5 \times 10^6$/ml spermatozoa achieved a pregnancy rate of 28.6% in the treatment group, as against 0% in the placebo group. Sperm concentration and motility were also significantly improved [441]. Thus, positive effects of mast cell blockers on ejaculate quality and pregnancy rates are possible. However, extended controlled studies are still lacking.

Testolactone

Testolactone is a synthetic testosterone derivative without significant androgenic action, approved for treatment of advanced female breast cancer. It inhibits aromatase and thus the production of estradiol. Its mechanism of action in the treatment of male fertility disturbances is explained by reduction of intra-testicular estradiol concentrations. Normogonadotropic oligozoospermia has been suggested as an andrological indication for testolactone. In these cases, the daily dosage is 2×500 mg testolactone. Open studies with small numbers of patients (9 and 13) over 3–6 months revealed a significant increase in sperm concentrations [104, 354]. However, the pregnancy rates were not higher than the expected spontaneous conception rates. A double-blind, placebo-controlled crossover study of 25 men with idiopathic oligozoospermia who were given 2 g testolactone daily for 8 months demonstrated endocrinologic effects with elevated free testosterone, LH, and FSH, but no effects on sperm concentration or pregnancy rates [71]. Thus, as long as major controlled studies are lacking, the use of testolactone for andrological indications cannot be recommended.

Vitamin E

Vitamin E (alpha-tocopherol) is a liposoluble vitamin, approved for treatment of decreased vitality and vitamin deficiency. In andrological indications, the action of vitamin E is explained by a protective effect on lipid peroxidation in sperm membranes through free oxygen radicals [390]. Suggested andrological indications for vitamin E are asthenozoospermia and sperm dysfunction. In these cases, the daily dosage is 300–600 mg alpha-tocopherol. In a double-blind, randomized, placebo-controlled study of 87 men who received 3×100 mg vitamin E daily for 6 months, Suleiman et al. [390] observed an increase in sperm motility. Furthermore, an open study demonstrated a positive effect on the fertilization rates in the IVF program after daily administration of 200 mg vitamin E for 4 weeks to men whose spermatozoa had shown low fertilization rates in IVF [130]. Improved sperm function was also achieved in a double-blind, placebo-controlled crossover study of 30 healthy men with increased concentrations of radical oxygen species in the seminal plasma, who were given daily doses of 600 mg vitamin E for 3 months. The sperm-zona pellucida binding capacity increased significantly during therapy with vitamin E, while other ejaculate parameters remained unaffected [210]. A recent double-blind, randomized, placebo-controlled study of 31 asthenozoospermic or oligozoospermic men failed to demonstrate improved ejaculate quality after treatment with 1000 mg vitamin C and 800 mg vitamin E [337]. Although major controlled studies are still lacking, because of its favorable spectrum of side effects, vitamin E can be recommended within the framework of an attempted cure, especially for men with increased concentrations of ROS in the seminal plasma.

Captopril

Captopril is an angiotensin-converting enzyme inhibitor, approved for treatment of hypertension and heart failure. In andrological indications it is thought to be effective by influencing the paracrine regulation of spermatogenesis [356]. Initially, asthenozoospermia was suggested as an andrological indication for captopril, because sperm motility was thought to be increased by elevated kinin concentrations after inhibition of kininase II. The daily dosage in this study was 2×25 mg captopril. During a 3-month double-blind, randomized, placebo-controlled study of 58 men with asthenozoospermia or oligozoospermia, Schill et al. [356] did not observe a significant improvement in sperm motility, but sperm concentrations were increased. However, there was no effect on the pregnancy rates. Major controlled studies are still lacking.

Alpha Receptor Blockers

Bunazosin is a selective alpha-1 adrenergic receptor blocker, approved for treatment of essential hypertension. In andrological indications its effect is explained by dilatation of stenotic sections of the seminiferous tubules through relaxation of myoid cells [439]. Oligozoospermia and azoospermia have been suggested as andrological indications for bunazosin. To date, there has been only one open, neither randomized nor placebo-controlled study in which bunazosin was used together with the beta-adrenoceptor agonist procaterol [439].

The daily dosage was 2 mg bunazosin plus 100 µg procaterol. The effect was investigated in 20 men with sperm concentrations $< 20 \times 10^6$/ml; six men had azoospermia. At the end of 5 months of therapy, the authors observed increased sperm concentration and volume in 16 of the 20 men. Spermatozoa were demonstrable again in five of the six azoospermic men. The pregnancy rate during the treatment period was 15%. Major controlled studies are still missing.

Zinc Salts

Zinc salts are approved for treatment of zinc deficiency, acne vulgaris, wound-healing impairment, potency disorders, immune activation, alopecia areata, diabetes mellitus, and for concomitant therapy with penicillamine. Zinc hydrogen aspartate and zinc sulfate are used in andrological indications. The effect of these zinc salts on spermatogenesis or cell functions is still unclear. Zinc therapy has been recommended in cases of increased exfoliation of spermatogenic cells and resultant testicular zinc loss, as well as for patients with secretory dysfunction of the prostate and seminal vesicles [351]. Only studies on zinc sulfate are available so far. Marmar et al. [262] treated 11 patients who had sperm concentrations $< 60 \times 10^6$/ml and reduced zinc concentrations in their seminal plasma with daily doses of 3×80 mg zinc sulfate for at least 6 months. In this open, neither randomized nor placebo-controlled study, significant improvements in sperm count, motility, and morphology were achieved. Three pregnancies occurred during the treatment period, while no pregnancy had been recorded in the preceding year. It appears that the positive effect on sperm motility is even enhanced when zinc sulfate is combined with an androgen [393]. In another open, neither randomized nor placebo-controlled study, 101 infertile men with low zinc levels in their seminal plasma were given 440 mg zinc sulfate daily for 2–24 months [394]. Kynaston et al. [231] observed significantly improved sperm motility in 33 patients with idiopathic asthenozoospermia and/or oligozoospermia after administration of 220 mg zinc sulfate twice daily for 3 months. However, double-blind studies to support this concept are missing. Thus, although controlled studies are still lacking, because of their low spectrum of side effects, zinc salts can be used for treatment attempts in andrological indications.

Growth Hormone

The biosynthetically produced polypeptide somatropin is therapeutically applied; its amino acid sequence is identical to that of growth hormone. Growth hormone deficiencies are the most frequent indication for somatropin therapy. In andrological indications, growth hormone has been used because secretion of the hormone seems to be disturbed in azoospermic, oligozoospermic and asthenozoospermic men [308, 372]. The effect of growth hormone on spermatogenesis is still unclear; indirect effects via "insulin-like growth factor I" and "insulin-like growth factor-binding proteins" are discussed [308]. The risk of leukemia associated with growth hormone therapy is a possibility but remains to be clarified. The therapeutic success with growth hormone has been investigated in oligozoospermic and asthenozoospermic patients. In a prospective, open, controlled pilot study, Lee et al. [235] treated 12 endocrinologically normal men with sperm concentrations $< 10 \times 10^6$/ml by daily subcutaneous injections of growth hormone for 5 months. No effect on sperm count was demonstrated. Another open, neither randomized nor placebo-controlled study of nine men each with oligozoospermia ($< 10 \times 10^6$/ml spermatozoa) and asthenozoospermia (motility < 30) who received daily subcutaneous injections of 2 IU (weeks 1–2), 4 IU (weeks 3–4), and 6 IU (weeks 5–12) growth hormone also failed to demonstrate altered sperm concentrations, although the number of motile spermatozoa was significantly increased [309]. In contrast to the study by Lee et al. [235], all patients showed suppressed response to the growth hormone stimulation test. Thus, growth hormone appears to have a positive effect on sperm motility under defined conditions. However, until double-blind, randomized and placebo-controlled studies are available, its use cannot be recommended, not even within the framework of an attempted cure.

L-Carnitine

While L-carnitine can be produced in various human tissues (liver, kidneys, testes) by lysin and methionine, most of the body's L-carnitine is of exogenous origin. After gastrointestinal absorption, it accumulates in the skeletal and cardiac muscles. The concentration of L-carnitine in the epididymal secretion is 2000 times higher than that in the serum. About half of total L-carnitine is present as acetyl-L-carnitine. In the epididymis it is secreted into the seminal plasma and can stimulate human sperm motility in vitro. Seminal plasma L-carnitine concentrations are reduced in oligoasthenozoospermic men [268]. From this observation it has been deduced that the substance may be of therapeutic benefit in patients with poor ejaculate quality. The motility enhancing action of L-carnitine is explained by effects on the mitochondrial energy metabolism. In the USA, L-carnitine and acetyl-L-carnitine are available as food additives without prescription for improvement of sperm quality. So far, the effectiveness of both substances has been documented only in uncontrolled studies. Vitali et al. [418] treated 47 patients with daily doses of 3 g L-carnitine. After 3 months, sperm concentration and motility were significantly increased. Similar results were obtained in a major multicenter but uncontrolled study [85]. A final judgement concerning L-carnitine and acetyl-L-carnitine is not yet possible. The substances offer the advantage of being free from side effects and contraindications. The results of a multicenter controlled study are expected to be available in the last 6 months of the year 2000.

Other Drugs

Apart from the aforementioned drugs, which are not approved for treatment of male fertility disorders, other substances have been tested for this indication, sometimes in a small number of patients. Barkay et al. [28] investigated the use of anti-inflammatory drugs such as indomethacin ($2-3 \times 25$ mg daily for 60 days) or ketoprofen (3×50 mg daily for 60 days) in a total of 100 patients with sperm concentrations between 1 and 30×10^6/ml. A significant increase in sperm count and motility was achieved with both drugs. The pregnancy rates during therapy with indomethacin and ketoprofen were significantly higher compared with those in the placebo-treated control group. The mechanism of action of these drugs in the study remained unclear. An effect on the prostaglandin metabolism was discussed. Declining seminal plasma prostaglandin concentrations were also observed during indomethacin therapy in a later study [217]. There was no change in the motility parameters. However, the men examined were healthy volunteers, and indomethacin was administered for only 14 days.

A more recent investigation searched for a positive effect of interferon alpha on sperm concentration. So far, only case experience has been reported with four patients who had markedly higher sperm concentrations and motility after injection of interferon alpha (3 million units daily, 5 days a week, for 8–12 weeks) [438].

Another open, neither randomized nor placebo-controlled study demonstrated a positive effect of glutathione on sperm motility [239]. However, only 11 men were treated with this substance (600 mg daily for 2 months), which is not approved for oral use in Germany. The effect was thought to result from protective action against damage by ROS. Glutathione and interferon alpha cannot be recommended for treatment of male infertility, not even within the framework of an attempted cure. Their use should be restricted to controlled studies.

Only a single report is available on the use of folic acid. However, this investigation was an uncontrolled study. Daily administration of 15 mg folic acid for 3 months resulted in improved sperm motility [41].

Antibiotics are used for the treatment of male adnexitis – as monotherapy of prostatitis according to sensitivity tests for a period of 2–3 weeks or in combination with antiphlogistic drugs in inflammatory epididymal diseases [50, 149, 425]. Nonsteroidal antiphlogistic therapy is recommended in inflammatory epididymal diseases in order to prevent local occlusions or the induction of local autoimmune phenomena. Furthermore, antiphlogistic therapy is indicated in patients with inflammatory testicular damage. The antiphlogistic drugs diclofenac, indomethacin, and aspirin are used for 3–6 weeks.

Immunmosuppressive treatment with corticosteroids at medium dosage is the therapy of choice in low-grade autoimmune orchitis, as determined by histological examination of tissue specimens [176]. In the treatment of antisperm antibodies, short-term administration of high doses of methylprednisolone is recommended (96 mg/day for 7 days, 3 weeks prior to the calculated date of ovulation) [367, 374]. However, other authors have questioned the effectiveness of steroids in the presence of antispermatozoal antibodies. During the past few years, IVF or ICSI has been recommended [72, 170, 287].

Kallikrein

Kallikrein is a kallidinogenase obtained from porcine pancreas and thus an enzyme from the group of kininogenases which lead to the release of kinins. The substance is approved for treatment of astheno-, oligo-, and oligoasthenozoospermia. Kallikrein is also contained in cryoprotectives, because it stimulates sperm motility in vitro. Its effects on spermatogenesis and motility remain to be clarified. Discussed are indirect effects on spermatogenesis, especially on Sertoli cells, and functional improvement of the accessory genital glands by increased blood supply. Direct effects on human sperm motility, which can be shown in vitro, are obviously irrelevant after oral administration, because kallikrein is not demonstrable in the seminal plasma under these conditions [275]. In a double-blind, placebo-controlled study of 90 subfertile men with sperm concentrations between 1 and 39×10^6/ml, Schill [344] observed increased total sperm count and motility after treatment with 3×200 kallikrein units (KU) daily for 7 weeks. In addition, the pregnancy rates differed significantly between the kallikrein group and the placebo group (38% versus 16%). Later double-blind, randomized, and placebo-controlled studies by other authors in more than 200 men did not confirm these observations [139, 207]. Therefore, kallikrein therapy is no longer accepted as being generally effective. In the treatment of oligozoospermia or asthenozoospermia, clear-cut criteria are lacking for selection of patients who might benefit from therapy. Therefore, kallikrein is not the drug of first choice, not least because of advances made in the assisted reproduction techniques.

Human Chorionic Gonadotropin (hCG)

hCG is a polypeptide with the action of luteinizing hormone (LH) which is released from the pituitary gland under physiological conditions. LH simulates testicular Leydig cells and thus the testosterone production. hCG is approved for ovulation induction in women, for treatment of undescended testis and retarded puberty in children, and for therapy of hypogonadotropic hypogonadism in adults. The usual dosage for hypogonadotropic hypogonadism is 1000–2500 IU hCG two to three times a week. During this therapy, serum testosterone concentrations return to normal and the testicular volume increases [214, 359]. In cases of hypogonadotropic hypogonadism and the wish for a child, hCG substitution is combined with the injection of human menopausal gonadotropin (hMG) and usually continued for several months (see below). A positive effect of hCG/hMG on the ejaculate quality in normogonadotropic men has not yet been demonstrated in controlled studies (see below; [216]). However, therapy with hCG was recommended for patients with sustained Leydig cell dysfunction after varicocelectomy [440]. hCG increases the testosterone concentration in cases of hypogonadotropic hypogonadism; in this indication, and combined with reduced ejaculate quality and the wish for a child, it can successfully be used together with hMG. In normogonadotropic men, hCG is not suitable for treatment of disturbed spermatogenesis, not even in combination with hMG.

Human Menopausal Gonadotropin (hMG)

hMG is obtained from the urine of menopausal women and possesses both FSH and LH activity. Highly purified FSH preparations and recombinant FSH (see below) have higher specific activities. Follicle-stimulating hormone (FSH), physiologically released from the pituitary gland, stimulates spermatogenesis via Sertoli cells, which produce androgen-binding protein (ABG) and inhibin. hMG is approved for women to support follicle growth and treatment of ovarian insufficiency. For men, approval is restricted to male sterility and induction of spermatogenesis in cases of hypogonadotropic or normogonadotropic hypogonadism. In cases of hypogonadotropic hypogonadism, hMG is applied in combination with hCG. The usual dosage is 75–150 IU hMG. In patients whose hypogonadotropic hypogonadism has remained untreated for a longer period or who have received testosterone substitution therapy, initial administration of hCG is recommended (see above) to stimulate the endogenous testicular testosterone production. hMG is then additionally given after 1–3 months. Spermatogenesis is restored in up to more than 90%, so that spermatozoa can be found in the ejaculate. Kliesch et al. [214] required average treatment periods of 6.7 months in men with hypogonadotropic hypogonadism subsequent to surgery or trauma. In men with idiopathic hypogonadotropic hypogonadism or Kallmann syndrome, the first spermatozoa reappeared after an average of 9 months. The therapy was sometimes continued for more than 2 years until pregnancy occurred. The combination with hCG also increased the testicular volume significantly. Comparing this treatment with pulsatile GnRH therapy, Schopohl [359] observed a more rapid restoration of spermatogenesis and a higher increase in testicular volume during GnRH therapy, while Kliesch et al. [214] and Buchter et al. [55] did not record significant differences. A controlled study in normogonadotropic men failed to achieve improved ejaculate quality during combined hCG and hMG therapy [216]. While hMG in combination with hCG reliably stimulates spermatogenesis in men with hypogonadotropic hypogonadism, its effectiveness in normogonadotropic men remains to be documented.

Pure and Recombinant FSH

Highly purified FSH and recombinant FSH have higher specific activities than hMG. The amino acid sequence of recombinant FSH is identical to that of natural FSH. Therefore, it possesses high purity and specific activity; there is no LH activity. It is approved for treatment of female infertility due to anovulation, as well as for controlled ovarian overstimulation prior to methods of assisted reproduction. Highly purified urinary FSH and recombinant FSH have also been approved for therapy of male hypogonadism. The mechanism of action is identical to that of hMG. The response rates concerning initiation of spermatogenesis with recombinant and highly purified FSH appear to be consistent with those of hMG [113, 253]. Acosta et al. [4] reported on the use of pure FSH in 24 men who had failed to fertilize in an IVF program (group 1) and 26 men with reduced ejaculate quality (group 2). The patients received 150 IU of pure FSH i.m. three times a week for at least 3 months. During this period, there were no significant changes in the ejaculate quality; however, the average fertilization rate in the FSH-treated group 1 increased from 2.2% to 54.4%, and in group 2 it was found to be 52.3%. These results implied effects of FSH therapy on sperm functions. In accordance with Acosta et al. [4], Glander and Kratzsch [138] did not observe effects on sperm quality after 10 weeks of therapy with pure FSH in 41 men with idiopathic infertility. On the other hand, a significant increase in sperm concentration and total motile sperm count was found in men who had shown lower FSH secretion after injection of GnRH. Like urinary FSH, recombinant FSH in combination with hCG seems to induce spermatogenesis in hypogonadotropic men [215]. Therefor, given the appropriate indications, pure and recombinant FSH can be used for the treatment of male hypogonadism.

Gonadotropin-Releasing Hormone (GnRH)

As a synthetic product GnRH is available as gonadorelin. Its structure is identical to that of native GnRH, which is secreted from the hypothalamus. It stimulates the release of LH and FSH from the pituitary gland. Under physiological conditions, pulsatile secretion of GnRH occurs every 60–120 min. The substance is approved as a solution for intranasal application in cases of unilateral or bilateral undescended testis, as an injection solution for diagnostic application in patients with hypothalamic, pituitary, or gonadal dysfunction, and for treatment of retarded puberty and tertiary hypogonadotropic hypogonadism in men with testicular dysfunction. Of highest andrological-therapeutic significance is currently the pulsatile subcutaneous administration by means of a portable infusion pump. It is indicated in cases of tertiary hypogonadotropic hypogonadism (e.g., Kallmann's syndrome or idiopathic hypogonadotropic hypogonadism) and retarded puberty. For these indications, the usual dosage is 5–20 μg gonadorelin per pulse every 120 min over several months. During this therapy, serum testosterone levels return to normal and an increase in testicular volume is achieved [214, 359]. Complete normalization of the ejaculate quality can be expected only rarely. In men with Kallmann's syndrome or idiopathic hypogonadotropic hypogonadism, the first spermatozoa have been redetected after an average of 9 months.

There is still controversy about the effectiveness of GnRH therapy compared with gonadotropins. Both treatment forms are efficacious; while Kliesch et al. [214] and Buchter et al. [55] did not find any differences, Schopohl et al. [359] observed higher testicular volumes and more rapid stimulation of spermatogenesis during GnRH therapy. GnRH is not effective in patients with disturbed spermatogenesis and a concomitant increase in FSH concentrations [26]. In addition, pulsatile GnRH administration does not improve semen parameters in patients with idiopathic normogonadotropic oligozoospermia [89]. Thus, pulsatile GnRH therapy is indicated in cases of tertiary hypogonadism, where it stimulates spermatogenesis, testicular volume and also the testosterone production. GnRH treatment is not indicated in patients with reduced ejaculate quality who have normal or elevated FSH levels.

Androgens

Androgens are used for substitution therapy of hypogonadism and its sequelae. Testosterone enanthate is an esterified form of endogenous testosterone, an anabolic steroid. Previously, the drug was used for release of a so-called rebound effect in oligozoospermic men; weekly injections resulted in azoospermia by suppression of gonadotropins. Thereafter, the injection therapy was interrupted until spermatogenesis was initiated. Today, this treatment must be considered obsolete.

Testosterone Undecanoate

Testosterone undecanoate is a testosterone that is esterified with undecanoic acid at position 17β. Testosterone undecanoate is approved for substitution therapy of hypogonadism, treatment of male climacteric symptoms, impaired spermatogenesis due to androgen deficiency, and osteoporosis associated with androgen deficiency. For substitution therapy, 80–160 mg testosterone undecanoate is administered daily. The effect on the ejaculate quality of patients with a normal hormone status is controversial. In a double-blind, randomized, placebo-controlled study of 60 men, Pusch [326] observed significantly increased sperm concentrations and a higher number of normally shaped spermatozoa after 100 days of therapy with 120 mg testosterone undecanoate daily. However, the pregnancy rates were not significantly different from those in the control group. Abdelmassih et al. [1] reported improved fertilization rates in an IVF program after the male partners had been treated with testosterone undecanoate. Later controlled studies, sometimes using higher concentrations (240 mg/day), failed to demonstrate positive therapeutic effects on sperm parameters and fertilizing capacity [78, 80, 81]. While testosterone undecanoate is suitable for substitution therapy of hypogonadism, for therapy of eugonadal infertile men, it is indicated only within the framework of clinical studies and for special indications (stimulation of epididymis or seminal vesicles).

Mesterolone

Mesterolone is the 1a-methyl compound of 5a-dihydrotestosterone which acts on androgen-dependent tissues as a testosterone metabolite. The substance is approved for treatment of relative or absolute androgen deficiency and its sequelae, such as renal anemia, vegetative psychiatric disorders, and decreased vitality in middle-aged and aged men. Inhibition of spermatogenesis is less pronounced during mesterolone therapy because of lower central inhibition of gonadotropins. Mesterolone has also been used for treatment of male fertility disorders. However, a significant effect on the pregnancy rates was not documented in controlled studies. In a double-blind, placebo-controlled trial, Gerris et al. [128] investigated the effects of mesterolone in 52 men with idiopathic oligozoospermia and/or teratozoospermia. The patients were given daily doses of 150 mg mesterolone for 12 months. While no improvement in sperm concentration was observed, the number of motile and morphologically normal spermatozoa increased in the group receiving mesterolone or placebo. The pregnancy rates were not significantly different. A more careful judgement resulted from a randomized, double-blind, and placebo-controlled study previously performed by the WHO [428]. A total of 157 men were treated with daily doses of 75 or 150 mg mesterolone for 6 months. No significant differences in ejaculate quality were seen, but there was a tendency towards higher pregnancy rates in the mesterolone-treated groups (control group 1: 11%; mesterolone 75 mg: 12%; mesterolone 150 mg: 19%). Thus, mesterolone is indicated in cases requiring targeted stimulation of dihydrotestosterone-dependent tissues (e.g., seminal vesicles). It is not suitable for sole stimulation in cases of hypogonadism. Given selected indications, it may also be used as a treatment attempt in male fertility disorders.

Midodrin

Midodrin is a long-acting a-sympathomimetic, approved for treatment of orthostatic hypotension, sensitivity to changes in the weather, and hypotension induced by psychotropic drugs. Since the autonomous innervation of the posterior urethra and bladder neck is regulated mainly via a-adrenergic receptors, midodrin has also been used for treatment of retrograde ejaculation. Smaller, partly controlled studies demonstrated the effectiveness of midodrin in retrograde ejaculation after oral (3×5 mg) or single i.v. administration (15–30 mg) prior to ejaculation [198, 220, 333]. Midodrin is effective in the treatment of partial and complete retrograde ejaculation. Since the drug is given mainly to patients with normal blood pressure, BP should be controlled after its administration.

Brompheniramine

Brompheniramine hydrogen maleate is an alkylamine antihistamine, approved for treatment of allergic reactions of the skin and mucous membranes. Because of its anticholinergic activity, the substance is also applied in patients with retrograde ejaculation. However, controlled studies are lacking. Information from the literature is restricted to case descriptions, some of them reporting pregnancies [348]. In andrological indications the recommended daily dosage is from 2×8 mg up to 3×8 mg brompheniramine hydrogen maleate daily for 1 week.

Imipramine

Imipramine is a tricyclic antidepressant, approved for treatment of depressive syndromes, long-term pain, enuresis, and pavor nocturnus. Because of its sympathomimetic active component the drug has also been used for therapy of retrograde ejaculation. However, controlled studies are lacking. Apart from case reports [134], the use of imipramine in larger patient groups has also been described in the literature. Plewa [322] investigated 117 patients with retrograde ejaculation of different genesis and achieved antegrade ejaculation in 58 men after therapy with this substance. In andrological indications, the daily dosage is up to 3×25 mg imipramine hydrochloride. Occasionally, antegrade ejaculation occurred within 1 day of therapy.

Medical Treatment of Hyperprolactinemia

Hyperprolactinemia may be caused by prolactin-producing pituitary tumors, drugs, tumors producing prolactin-releasing factors, renal insufficiency, hypothyroidism, or loss of the inhibitory effect of dopamine on pituitary prolactin production by pituitary or extrapituitary processes. It has to be distinguished from transitory prolactin level elevation, e.g., after a rich meal or by stress, which does not require treatment. Pathologically elevated serum prolactin levels may lead to erectile dysfunction and infertility. Most therapy knowledge has been gained with the dopamine agonist bromocriptine. In addition, hyperprolactinemia can also be treated with the dopaminergic serotonin receptor antagonist Metergolin, the longer-acting second-generation dopamine agonists Qinagolid and Cabergolin, or the dopamine agonist Lisurid.

Bromocriptine is an ergot derivative which acts as a dopamine agonist and stimulates hypothalamic dopaminergic receptors. Thereby it increases the release of prolactin-inhibiting factor, so that prolactin secretion from the anterior pituitary is reduced. The substance is approved for treatment of hyperprolactinema and its sequelae, idiopathic and postencephalitic Parkinson's disease, milk stasis, primary mastitis in the lactation period, inhibition of lactation after abortion, (prolactin-related) galactorrhea, amenorrhea, ovulation disorders,

sterility, premenstrual complaints, and acromegaly. For treatment of hyperprolactinemia, the initial dosage of bromocriptine is 1.25 mg daily. Because of its
hypotensive action the drug should preferably been taken in the evening. The
dosage is gradually increased by 1.25 mg up to 3×2.5 mg/day. The total daily
dosage should not exceed 30 mg. Bromocriptine appears to have had a positive
effect on the ejaculate quality of some hypogonadal patients with hyperprolactinemia [362, 363]. Bromocriptine has not been effective in oligozoospermic patients with normal serum prolactin levels [184]. Bromocriptine is an effective
drug for the reduction of pathologically elevated prolactin levels. While hyperprolactinemic patients may experience improvement of erectile dysfunction and
ejaculate quality, the therapeutic success rates have been inconsistent.

References

1. Abdelmassih R, Dhont M, Comhaire F (1992) Pilot study with 120 mg Andriol treat-
    ment for couples with a low fertilization rate during in-vitro fertilization. Hum Reprod
    7:267
2. Abdul-Aziz M, MacLusky NJ, Bhavnani BR, Casper RF (1995) Hyaluronidase activity in
    human semen: correlation with fertilization in vitro. Fertil Steril 64:1147
3. Aboulghar MA, Mansour RT, Serour GI, Sattar MA, Elattar I (1991) Cryopreservation
    of the occasionally improved semen samples for intrauterine insemination: a new
    approach in the treatment of idiopathic male infertility. Fertil Steril 56:1151
4. Acosta AA, Khalifa E, Oehninger S (1992) Pure human follicle stimulating hormone
    has a role in the treatment of severe male infertility by assisted reproduction: Norfolk's
    total experience. Hum Reprod 7:1067
5. Agarwal A, Ikemoto J, Loughlin KR (1994) Relationship of sperm parameters with lev-
    els of reactive oxygen species in semen specimens. J Urol 152:107
6. Aitken RJ (1990) Evaluation of human sperm function. Br Med Bull 46:654
7. Aitken RJ, Baker HWG (1995) Seminal leukocytes: passengers, terrorists or good Sa-
    maritans? Hum Reprod 10:1736
8. Aitken RJ, Brindle JP (1993) Analysis of the ability of three probes targeting the outer
    acrosomal membrane or acrosomal contents to detect the acrosome reaction in human
    spermatozoa. Hum Reprod 8:1663
9. Aitken RJ, Clarkson JS (1987) Cellular basis of defective sperm function and its asso-
    ciation with the genesis of reactive oxygen species by human spermatozoa. J Reprod
    Fertil 81:459
10. Aitken RJ, West KM (1990) Analysis of the relationship between reactive oxygen spe-
    cies production and leukocyte infiltration in fractions of human semen separated on
    Percoll gradients. Int J Androl 13:433
11. Aitken RJ, Thatcher S, Glaser AF, Clarkson JS, Wu FLW, Baird DT (1987) Relative abil-
    ity of modified versions of the hamster oocyte penetration test, incorporating hyperos-
    motic medium or the ionophore A 23187, to predict IVF outcome. Hum Reprod 2:227
12. Aitken RJ, Clarkson JS, Fishel S (1989) Generation of reactive oxygen species, lipid per-
    oxidation, and human sperm function. Biol Reprod 40:183
13. Aitken RJ, Clarkson JS, Hargreave TB, Irvine DS, Wu FCW (1989) Analysis of the rela-
    tionship between defective sperm function and the generation of reactive oxygen spe-
    cies in cases of oligozoospermia. J Androl 10:214
14. Akerlof E, Fredricsson B, Gustafson O, Lunell NO, Nylund L, Rosenborg L, Slotte H,
    Pousette A (1991) Sperm count and motility influence the results of human fertiliza-
    tion in vitro. Int J Androl 14:79
15. Akin JW (1993) The use of clomiphene citrate in the treatment of azoospermia second-
    ary to incomplete androgen resistance. Fertil Steril 59:223

16. Al-Shawaf T, Nolan A, Harper J, Serhal P, Craft I (1991) Pregnancy following gamete intra-fallopian transfer (GIFT) with cryopreserved semen from infertile men following therapy to lymphomas or testicular tumour: report of three cases. Hum Reprod 6:365

17. Anguiano A, Oates RD, Amos JA, Dean M, Gerrard B, Stewart C, Maher TA, White MB, Milunsky A (1992) Congenital bilateral absence of the vas deferens: a primarily genital form of cystic fibrosis. JAMA 267:1794

18. Aribarg A, Sukcharoen N (1995) Intrauterine insemination of washed spermatozoa for treatment with oligozoospermia. Int J Androl 18 [Suppl 1]:62

19. Arny M, Quagliarello J (1987) Semen quality before and after processing by a swim-up method: relationship to outcome of intrauterine insemination. Fertil Steril 48:643

20. Ashkenazi J, Bar-Hava I, Farhi J, Levy T, Feldberg D, Orvieto R, Ben-Rafael Z (1999) The role of purified follicle stimulating hormone therapy in the male partner before intracytoplasmic sperm injection. Fertil Steril 72:670

21. Aslam I, Fishel S, Green S, Campbell A, Garratt L, McDermott H, Dowell K, Thornton S (1998) Can we justify spermatid microinjection for severe male factor infertility? Hum Reprod Update 4:213

22. Auger J, Mesbah M, Huber C, Dadoune JP (1990) Aniline blue staining as a marker of sperm chromatin defects associated with different semen characteristics discriminates between proven fertile and suspected infertile men. Int J Androl 13:452

23. Avery S, Bolton VN, Mason BA (1990) An evaluation of the hypo-osmotic sperm swelling test as a predictor of fertilizing capacity in vitro. Int J Androl 13:93

24. Baker G, Brinsden P, Jouannet P, Loumaye E, Van Steirteghem A, Winston R (1993) Treatment of severe male infertility with pure follicle stimulating hormone (FSH) – the need for a properly controlled multicenter trial. Hum Reprod 8:500

25. Baker HWG, Kovacs GT (1985) Spontaneous improvement in semen quality: regression towards the mean. Int J Androl 8:421

26. Bals-Pratsch M, Knuth UA, Hönigl W, Klein HM, Bergmann M, Nieschlag E (1989) Pulsatile GnRH-therapy in oligozoospermic men does not improve seminal parameters despite decreased FSH levels. Clin Endocrinol 30:549

27. Barash A, Lurie S, Weissman A, Insler V (1995) Comparison of sperm parameters, in vitro fertilization results, and subsequent pregnency rates using sequential ejaculates, collected two hours apart, from oligoasthenozoospermic men. Fertil Steril 64:1008

28. Barkay J, Harpaz-Kerpel S, Ben-Ezra S, Gordon S, Zuckerman H (1984) The prostaglandin inhibitor effect of anti-inflammatory drugs in the therapy of male infertility. Fertil Steril 42:406

29. Barlow P, Delvigne A, Van Dromme J, Van Hoeck J, Vandenbosch K, Leroy F (1991) Predictive value of classical and automated sperm analysis for in-vitro fertilization. Hum Reprod 6:1119

30. Barratt CLR, Naeeni M, Clements S, Cooke ID (1995) Clinical value of sperm morphology for in-vivo fertility: comparison between World Health Organization criteria of 1987 and 1992. Hum Reprod 10:587

31. Bartoov B, Eltes F, Pansky M, Lederman H, Caspi E, Soffer Y (1993) Estimating fertility potential via semen analysis data. Hum Reprod 8:65

32. Bartoov B, Reichart M, Eltes F, Lederman H, Kedem P (1994) Relation of human sperm acrosin activity and fertilization in vitro. Andrologia 26:9

33. Beckerman H, Becker J, Lankhorst GJ (1993) The effectiveness of vibratory stimulation in anejaculatory men with spinal cord injury. Paraplegia 31:689

34. Behre HM, Nashan D, Nieschlag E (1989) Objective measurement of testicular volume by ultrasonography: evaluation of the technique and comparison with orchidometer estimates. Int J Androl 12:395

35. Behre HM, Kliesch S, Schädel F, Nieschlag E (1995) Clinical relevance of scrotal and transrectal ultrasonography in andrological patients. Int J Androl 18 [Suppl 2]:27

36. Behrendt H, Hilscher B, Passia D, Hofmann N, Hilscher W (1981) The occurrence of mast cells in the human testis. Acta Anat (Basel) 111:14

37. Belker AM, Sherins RJ, Bustillo M, Calvo L (1994) Pregnancy with microsurgical vas sperm aspiration from a patient with neurologic ejaculatory dysfunction. J Androl 15 [Suppl]:6 S

38. Belkien L, Bordt J, Freischem CW, Hano R, Knuth UA, Nieschlag E (1985) Prognostic value of the heterologous ovum penetration test for human in vitro fertilization. Int J Androl 8:275

39. Ben-Chetrit A, Senoz S, Greenblatt EM, Casper RF (1995) In vitro fertilization outcome in the presence of severe male factor infertility. Fertil Steril 63:1032

40. Benoff S, Cooper GW, Hurley I, Napolitano NB, Rosenfeld DL, Scholl GM, Hershlag A (1993) Human sperm fertilization potential in vitro is correlated with differential expression of a head-specific mannose ligand receptor. Fertil Steril 59:854

41. Bentivoglio G, Melica F, Cristoforoni F (1993) Folinic acid in the treatment of human male infertility. Fertil Steril 60:698

42. Berry WR, Gottesfeld RL, Alter HJ, Vierling JM (1987) Transmission of hepatitis B virus by artificial insemination. JAMA 257:1079

43. Biljan MM, Taylor CT, Manasse PR, Joughin EC, Kingsland CR, Lewis-Jones DI (1994) Evaluation of different sperm function tests as screening methods for male fertilization potential – the value of the sperm migration test. Fertil Steril 62:591

44. Bonduelle M, Legein J, Derde MP, Buysse A, Schietecatte J, Wisanto A, Devroee P, van Steirteghem A, Liebaers I (1995) Comparative follow-up study of 130 children born after intracytoplasmic sperm injection and 130 children born after in-vitro fertilization. Hum Reprod 10:3327

45. Bongso TA, Ng SC, Mok H, Lim MN, Teo HL, Wong PC, Ratnam SS (1989) Effect of sperm motility on human in vitro fertilization. Arch Androl 22:185

46. Bosman E, Fourie F Le R, van der Merwe JV (1990) Successful pregnancy despite retrograde ejaculation. A case report. S Afr Med J 77:368

47. Bostofte E, Serup J, Rebbe H (1982) Relation between sperm count and semen volume, and pregnancies obtained during a twenty-year follow-up period. Int J Androl 5:267

48. Bourne H, Watkins W, Speirs A, Baker HWG (1995) Pregnancies after intracytoplasmic injection of sperm collected by fine needle biopsy of the testis. Fertil Steril 64:433

49. Brandelli A, Miranda PV, Anón-Vazquez MG, Marín-Briggiler CI, Sanjurjo C, Gonzalez-Echeverría F, Blaquier JA, Tezón JG (1995) A new predictive test for in-vitro fertilization based on the induction of sperm acrosome reaction by N-acetylglucosamine-neoglycoprotein. Hum Reprod 10:1751

50. Branigan EF, Muller CH (1994) Efficacy of treatment and recurrence rate of leukocytospermia in infertile men with prostatitis. Fertil Steril 62:580

51. Brasch JG, Rawlins R, Tarchala S, Radwanska E (1994) The relationship between total motile sperm count and the success of intrauterine insemination. Fertil Steril 62:150

52. Brinsden PR, Avery SM, Marcus S, Macnamee MC (1997) Transrectal electroejaculation combined with in-vitro fertilization: effective treatment of anejaculatory infertility due to spinal cord injury. Hum Reprod 12:2687

53. Bruckert E (1991) Wie häufig ist ungewollte Kinderlosigkeit? Andrologia 23:245

54. Buch JP, Philips KA, Kolon TF (1994) Cryopreservation of microsurgically extracted ductal sperm: pentoxifylline enhancement of motility. Fertil Steril 62:418

55. Buchter D, Behre HM, Kliesch S, Nieschlag E (1998) Pulsatile GnRH or human chorionic gonadotropin/human menopausal gonadotropin as effective treatment for men with hypogonadotropic hypogonadism: a review of 42 cases. Eur J Endocrinol 139:298

56. Buckett WM, Luckas MJM, Aird IA, Farquharson RG, Kingsland CR, Lewis-Jones DI (1997) The hypo-osmotic swelling test in recurrent miscarriage. Fertil Steril 68:506

57. Burkman LJ, Coddington CC, Franken DR, Kruger TF, Rosenwaks W, Hodgen GD (1988) The hemozona assay (HZA): development of a diagnostic test for the binding of human spermatozoa to the human hemizona pellucida to predict fertilization potential. Fertil Steril 49:688

58. Calvo L, Vantman D, Banks SM, Tezon J, Koukoulis GN, Dennison L, Sherins RJ (1989) Follicular fluid-induced acrosome reaction distinguishes a subgroup of men with unexplained infertility not identified by semen analysis. Fertil Steril 52:1048

59. Calvo L, Dennison-Lagos L, Banks SM, Dorfmann A, Thorsell LP, Bustillo M, Schulman JD, Sherins RJ (1994) Acrosome reaction inducibility predicts fertilization success at in-vitro fertilization. Hum Reprod 9:1880

60. Chandley AC (1995) The genetic basis of male infertility. Reprod Med Rev 4:1

61. Check JH, Nowroozi K, Wu CH, Bollendorf A (1988) Correlation of semen analysis and hypoosmotic swelling test with subsequent pregnancies. Arch Androl 20:257

62. Check JH, Epstein R, Nowroozi K, Shanis BS, Wu CH, Bollendorf A (1989) The hypoosmotic swelling test as a useful adjunct to the semen analysis to predict fertility potential. Fertil Steril 52:159

63. Check JH, Bollendorf AM, Press MA, Breen EM (1990) Noninvasive techniques for improving fertility potential of retrograde ejaculates. Arch Androl 25:271

64. Chen D, Scobey MJ, Jeyendran RS (1995) Effects of urine on the functional quality of human spermatozoa. Fertil Steril 64:1216

65. Chitale AR, Rathaur RG (1995) Nuclear decondensation of sperm head and failure at in-vitro fertilization: an ultrastructural study. Hum Reprod 10:594

66. Chung PH, Yeko TR, Mayer JC, Sanford EJ, Maroulis GB (1995) Assisted fertility using electroejaculation in men with spinal cord injury – a review of literature. Fertil Steril 64:1

67. Chung PH, Palermo G, Schlegel PN, Veeck LL, Eid JF, Rosenwaks Z (1998) The use of intracytoplasmic sperm injection with electroejaculates from anejaculatory men. Hum Reprod 13:1854

68. Cintron RD, Wortham JW, Acosta A (1981) The association of semen factors with the recovery of Ureaplasma urealyticum. Fertil Steril 36:648

69. Cittadini E, Guastella G, Comparetto G, Gattuccio F, Chianchiano N (1988) IVF/ET and GIFT in andrology. Hum Reprod 3:101

70. Claassens OE, Menveld R, Franken DR, Pretorius E, Swart Y, Lombard CJ, Kruger TF (1992) The acridine orange test: determining the relationship between sperm morphology and fertilization in vitro. Hum Reprod 7:242

71. Clark RV, Sherins RJ (1989) Treatment of men with idiopathic oligozoospermic infertility using the aromatase inhibitor testolactone. Results of a double-blind, randomized, placebo-controlled trial with crossover. J Androl 10:240

72. Clarke GN, Bourne H, Baker HWG (1997) Intracytoplasmic sperm injection for treating infertility associated with sperm autoimmunity. Fertil Steril 68:112

73. Coddington CC, Oehninger SC, Olive DL, Franken DR, Kruger TF, Hodgen GD (1994) Hemizona index (HZI) demonstrates excellent predictability when evaluating sperm fertilizing capacity in in vitro fertilization patients. J Androl 15:250

74. Coetzee K, Kruger TF, Menkveld R, Swanson RJ, Lombard CJ, Acosta AA (1989) Usefulness of sperm penetration assay in fertility predictions. Arch Androl 23:207

75. Coetzee K, Kruger TF, Menkveld R, Lombard CJ, Swanson RJ (1989) Hypoosmotic swelling test in the prediction of male fertility. Arch Androl 23:131

76. Coetzee K, Kruger TF, Lombard CJ (1998) Predictive value of normal sperm morphology: a structured literature review. Hum Reprod Update 4:73

77. Cohen J, Edwards R, Fehilly C, Fishel S, Hewitt J, Purdy J, Rowland G, Steptoe P, Webster J (1985) In vitro fertilization: a treatment for male infertility. Fertil Steril 43:422

78. Comhaire F (1990) Treatment of idiopathic testicular failure with high-dose testosterone undecanoate: a double-blind pilot study. Fertil Steril 54:689

79. Comhaire FH, Verschraegen G, Vermeulen L (1980) Diagnosis of accessory gland infection and its possible role in male infertility. Int J Androl 3:32

80. Comhaire F, Milingos S, Liapi A, Gordts S, Campo R, Depypere H, Dhont M, Schoonjans F (1995) The effective cumulative pregnancy rate of different modes of treatment of male infertility. Andrologia 27:217

81. Comhaire F, Schoonjans F, Abdelmassih R, Gordts S, Campo R, Dhont M, Milingos S, Gerris J (1995) Does treatment with testosterone undecanoate improve the in-vitro fertilization capacity of spermatozoa in patients with idiopathic testicular failure? (results of a double blind study). Hum Reprod 10:2600

82. Cooper TG, Weidner W, Nieschlag E (1990) The influence of inflammation of the human male genital tract on secretion of the seminal markers α-glucosidase, glycerophosphocholine, carnitine, fructose and citric acid. Int J Androl 13:329

83. Cooper TG, Keck C, Oberdieck U, Nieschlag E (1993) Effects of multiple ejaculations after extended periods of sexual abstinence on total, motile and normal sperm numbers, as well as accessory gland secretions, from healthy normal and oligozoospermic men. Hum Reprod 8:1251

84. Cooper TG, Atkinson AD, Nieschlag E (1999) Experience with external quality control in spermatology. Hum Reprod 14:765

85. Costa M, Canale D, Filicori M, D'Iddio S, Lenzi A (1994) L-carnitine in idiopathic asthenozoospermia: a multicenter study. Italian Study Group on Carnitine and Male Infertility. Andrologia 26:155

86. Craft I, Tsirigotis M (1995) Simplified recovery, preparation and cryopreservation of testicular spermatozoa. Hum Reprod 10:1623

87. Crosignani PG, Collins J, Cooke ID, Diczfalusy E, Rubin B (1993) Unexplained infertility. Hum Reprod 8:977

88. Cross NL, Morales P, Overstreet JW, Hanson FW (1986) Two simple methods for detecting acrosome reacted sperm. Gamete Research 15:213

89. Crottaz B, Senn A, Reymond MJ, Rey F, Germond M, Gomez F (1992) Follicle-stimulating hormone bioactivity in idiopathic normogonadotropic oligoasthenozoospermia: double-blind trial with gonadotropin-releasing hormone. Fertil Steril 57:1034

90. Cummins JM, Pember SM, Jequier AM, Yovich JL, Hartmann PE (1991) A test of the human sperm acrosome reaction following ionophore challenge. J Androl 12:98

91. D'Agata RD, Vicari E, Moncada ML, Sidoti G, Calogero AE, Fornito MC, Minacapilli G, Mongioi A, Polosa P (1990) Generation of reactive oxygen species in subgroups of infertile men. Int J Androl 13:344

92. Dahlberg A, Ruutu M, Hovatta O (1995) Pregnancy results from a vibrator application, electroejaculation, and a vas aspiration programme in spinal-cord injured men. Hum Reprod 10:2305

93. De Jonge CJ, Mack SR, Zaneveld LJD (1989) Synchronous assay for human sperm capacitation and the acrosome reaction. J Androl 10:232

94. De Jonge CJ, Han HI, Mack SR, Zaneveld LJD (1991) Effect of phorbol diesters, synthetic diacylglycerols, and a protein kinase C inhibitor on the human sperm acrosome reaction. J Androl 12:62

95. De Jonge CJ, Han HL, Lawrie H, Mack SR, Zaneveld LJD (1991) Modulation of the human sperm acrosome reaction by effectors of the adenylate cyclase/cyclic AMP second messenger pathway. J Exp Zool 258:113

96. De Jonge CJ, Tarchala SM, Rawlins RG, Binor Z, Radwanska E (1993) Acrosin activity in human spermatozoa in relation to semen quality and in-vitro fertilization. Hum Reprod 8:253

97. Desai S, Cohen S, Khatamee M, Leiter E (1980) Ureaplasma urealyticum (T-mycoplasma) infection: does it have a role in male infertility? J Urol 124:469

98. Devroey P, Liu J, Nagy Z, Tournaye H, Silber SJ, van Steirteghem AC (1994) Normal fertilization of human oocytes after testicular sperm extraction and intracytoplasmic sperm injection. Fertil Steril 62:639

99. Devroey P, Liu J, Nagy Z, Goossens A, Tournaye H, Camus M, van Steirteghem A, Silber S (1995) Pregnancies after testicular sperm extraction and intracytoplasmic sperm injection in non-obstructive azoospermia. Hum Reprod 10:1457

100. Devroey P, Silber S, Nagy Z, Liu J, Tournaye H, Joris H, Verheyen G, van Steirteghem A (1995) Ongoing pregnancies and birth after intracytoplasmic sperm injection with frozen-thawed epididymal spermatozoa. Hum Reprod 10:903

101. Diamond MP, Rogers BJ, Vaughn WK, Wentz AC (1985) Effect of the number of inseminating sperm and the follicular stimulation protocol on in vitro fertilization of human oocytes in male factor and non-male factor couples. Fertil Steril 44:499

102. Dickey RP, Pyrzak R, Lu PY, Taylor SN, Rye PH (1999) Comparison of the sperm quality necessary for successful intrauterine insemination with World Health Organization threshold values for normal sperm. Fertil Steril 71:684

103. Donnelly ET, Lewis SEM, McNally JA, Thompson W (1998) In vitro fertilization and pregnancy rates: the influence of sperm motility and morphology on IVF outcome. Fertil Steril 70:305

104. Dony JMJ, Smals AGH, Rolland R, Fauser BCJM, Thomas CMG (1986) Effect of chronic aromatase inhibition by Δ^1-testolacton on pituitary-gonadal function in oligozoospermic men. Andrologia 18:69

105. Duleba AJ, Rowe TC, Ma P, Collins JA (1992) Prognostic factors in assessment and management of male infertility. Hum Reprod 7:1388

106. Duncan WW, Glew MJ, Wang XJ, Flaherty SP, Matthews CD (1993) Prediction of in vitro fertilization rates from semen variables. Fertil Steril 59:1233

107. Elliason R (1976) Clinical examination of infertile men. In: Hafez ESE (ed) Human semen and fertility regulation in men. Mosby, St. Louis, pp 321

108. El Mulla KF, Köhn FM, El Beheiry AH, Schill WB (1995) The effect of smoking and varicocele on human sperm acrosin activity and acrosome reaction. Hum Reprod 10:3190

109. Engel W, Murphy D, Schmid M (1996) Are there genetic risks associated with micro-assisted reproduction? Hum Reprod 11:2359

110. Enginsu ME, Pieters MHEC, Dumoulin JCM, Evers JLH, Geraedts JPM (1992) Male factor as determinant of in vitro fertilization outcome. Hum Reprod 7:1136

111. Enginsu ME, Dumoulin JCM, Pieters MHEC, Evers JLH, Geraedts JPM (1993) Predictive value of morphologically normal sperm concentration in the medium for in-vitro fertilization. Int J Androl 16:113

112. Englert Y, Delvigne A, Vekemans M, Lejeune B, Henlisz A, de-Maertelaer G, Leroy F (1989) Is fresh or frozen semen to be used in in vitro fertilization with donor sperm? Fertil Steril 51:661

113. European Metrodin HP Study Group (1998) Efficacy and safety of highly purified urinary follicle-stimulating hormone with human chorionic gonadotropin for treating men with isolated hypogonadotropic hypogonadism. Fertil Steril 70:256

114. Ezeh UIO, Moore HDM, Cooke ID (1998) A prospective study of multiple needle biopsies versus a single open biopsy for testicular sperm extraction in men with non-obstructive azoospermia. Hum Reprod 13:3075

115. Fénichel P, Donzeau M, Farahifar D, Basteris B, Ayraud N, Hsi BL (1991) Dynamics of human sperm acrosome reaction: relation with in vitro fertilization. Fertil Steril 55:994

116. Fisch B, Kaplan-Kracier R, Amit S, Zuckerman Z, Ovadia J, Tadir Y (1990) The relationship between sperm parameters and fertilizing capacity in vitro: a predictive role for swim-up migration. J In Vitro Fertil Embryo Transf 7:38

117. Ford WCL (1990) The role of oxygen free radicals in the pathology of human spermatozoa: Implications of IVF. In: Matson PL, Lieberman BA (eds) Clinical IVF Forum: current views in assisted reproduction. University Press, Manchester, pp 123–139

118. Francavilla F, Romano R, Santucci R, Poccia G (1990) Effect of sperm morphology and motile sperm count on outcome of intrauterine insemination in oligozoospermia and/or asthenozoospermia. Fertil Steril 53:892

119. Francavilla F, Romano R, Santucci R, Marrone V, Corrao G (1992) Failure of intrauterine insemination in male immunological infertility in cases in which all spermatozoa are antibody-coated. Fertil Steril 58:587

120. Francavilla S, Gabriele A, Romano R, Gianaroli L, Ferraretti AP, Francavilla F (1994) Sperm-zona pellucida binding of human sperm is correlated with the immunocytochemical presence of proacrosin and acrosin in the sperm heads but not with the proteolytic activity of acrosin. Fertil Steril 62:1226

121. Franken DR, Oehninger S, Burkman LJ, Coddington CC, Kruger TF, Rosenwaks L, Acosta AA, Hodgen GD (1989) The hemizona assay (HZA): a predictor of human sperm fertilizing potential in in vitro fertilization (IVF) treatment. J In Vitro Fertil Embryo Transf 6:44

122. Franken DR, Kruger TF, Oehninger S, Coddington CC, Lombard C, Smith K, Hodgen GD (1993) The ability of the hemizona assay to predict human fertilization in different and consecutive in-vitro fertilization cycles. Hum Reprod 8:1240

123. Franken DR, Acosta AA, Kruger TF, Lombard C, Oehninger S, Hodgen GD (1993) The hemizona assay: its role in identifying male factor infertility in assisted reproduction. Fertil Steril 59:1075

124. Fuse H, Takahara M, Ishii H, Sumiya H, Shimazaki J (1990) Measurement of testicular volume by ultrasonography. Int J Sonography 13:267

125. Gamzu R, Yogev L, Amit A, Lessing J, Homonnai ZT, Yavetz H (1994) The hemizona assay is of good prognostic value for the ability of sperm to fertilize oocytes in vitro. Fertil Steril 62:1056

126. Gavella M, Lipovac V, Marotti T (1991) Effect of pentoxifylline on superoxide anion production by human sperm. Int J Androl 14:320

127. Gerris JM, Delbeke LO, Punjabi U, Buytaert P (1987) The value of intrauterine insemination with washed husband's sperm in the treatment of infertility. Hum Reprod 2:315

128. Gerris J, Comhaire F, Hellemans P, Peeters K, Schoonjans F (1991) Placebo-controlled trial of high-dose Mesterolone treatment of idiopathic male infertility. Fertil Steril 55:603

129. Gerris J, van Royen E, Mangel-Schots K, Joostens M, de Vits A (1994) Pregnancy after intracytoplasmic sperm injection of metaphase II oocytes with spermatozoa from a man with complete retrograde ejaculation. Hum Reprod 9:1293

130. Geva E, Bartoov B, Zabludovsky N, Lessing JB, Lerna-Geva L, Amit A (1996) The effect of antioxidant treatment on human spermatozoa and fertilization rate in an in vitro fertilization program. Fertil Steril 66:430

131. Ghazzawi IM, Sarraf MG, Taher MR, Khalifa FA (1998) Comparison of the fertilizing capability of spermatozoa from ejaculates, epididymal aspirates and testicular biopsies using intracytoplasmic sperm injection. Hum Reprod 13:348

132. Ghazzawi IM, Al-Hasani S, Taher M, Souso S (1999) Reproductive capacity of round spermatids compared with mature spermatozoa in a population of azoospermic men. Hum Reprod 14:736

133. Giamarellou H, Tympanidis K, Bitos NA, Leonidas E, Daikos GK (1984) Infertility and chronic prostatitis. Andrologia 16:417

134. Gilja I, Parazajder J, Radej M, Cvitkovic P, Kovacic M (1994) Retrograde ejaculation and loss of emission: possibilities of conservative treatment. Eur Urol 25:226

135. Gil-Salom M, Mínguez Y, Rubio C, De los Santos MJ, Remohí J, Pellicer A (1995) Efficacy of intracytoplasmic sperm injection using testicular spermatozoa. Hum Reprod 10:3166

136. Gil-Salom M, Remohí J, Mínguez Y, Rubio C, Pellicer A (1995) Pregnancy in an azoospermic patient with markedly elevated serum follicle-stimulating hormone levels. Fertil Steril 64:1218

137. Girardi SK, Schlegel PN (1996) Microsurgical epididymal sperm aspiration: review of techniques, preoperative considerations, and results. J Androl 17:5

138. Glander HJ, Kratzsch J (1997) Effects of pure human follicle-stimulating hormone (pFSH) on sperm quality correlate with the hypophyseal response to gonadotrophin-releasing hormone (GnRH). Andrologia 29:23

139. Glezerman M, Lunenfeld E, Potashnik G, Huleihel M, Soffer Y, Segal S (1993) Efficacy of kallikrein in the treatment of oligozoospermia and asthenozoospermia: a double-blind trial. Fertil Steril 60:1052

140. Goldenberg M, Rabinovici J, Bider D, Lunenfeld B, Blankstein J, Weissenberg R (1992) Intra-uterine insemination with prepared sperm vs. unprepared first split ejaculates. A randomized study. Andrologia 24:135

141. Gottschalk-Sabag S, Weiss DB, Folb-Zarachow N, Zukerman Z (1995) Is one testicular specimen sufficient for quantitative evaluation of spermatogenesis? Fertil Steril 64:399

142. Gould JE, Overstreet JW, Yanagimachi H (1983) What functions of the sperm cell are measured by in vitro fertilization of zona-free hamster eggs? Fertil Steril 40:344

143. Greenberg SH, Lipshultz LI, Wein AJ (1978) Experience with 425 subfertile male patients. J Urol 119:507

144. Griveau JF, Dumont E, Renard P, Callegari JP, Le Lannou D (1995) Reactive oxygen species, lipid peroxidation and enzymatic defence systems in human spermatozoa. J Reprod Fertil 103:17

145. Grow DR, Oehninger S, Seltman HJ, Toner JP, Swanson RJ, Kruger TF, Muasher SJ (1994) Sperm morphology as diagnosed by strict criteria: probing the impact of teratozoospermia on fertilization rate and pregnancy outcome in a large in vitro fertilization population. Fertil Steril 62:559

146. Grunert JH, De Geyter C, Bordt J, Schneider HPG, Nieschlag E (1989) Does computerized image analysis of sperm movement enhance the predictive value of semen analysis for in-vitro fertilization results? Int J Androl 12:329

147. Guerin JF, Ben Ali H, Rollet J, Souchier C, Czyba JC (1986) α-Glucosidase as a specific epididymal marker. Its validity for the etiologic diagnosis of azoospermia. J Androl 7:156

148. Guerin JF, Ben Ali H, Cottinet D, Rollet J (1990) Seminal alpha-glucosidase activity as a marker of epididymal pathology in nonazoospermic men consulting for infertility. J Androl 11:240

149. Haidl G, Schill WB (1991) Guidelines for drug treatment of male infertility. Drugs 41:60

150. Haidl G, Schill WB (1994) Assessment of sperm chromatin condensation: an important test for prediction of IVF outcome. Arch Androl 32:263

151. Haidl G, Hartmann R, Hofmann N (1987) Morphological studies of spermatozoa in motility disorders. Andrologia 19:433

152. Haidl G, Becker A, Schill WB (1991) Poor development of outer dense fibres as a major cause of tail abnormalities in the spermatozoa of asthenoteratozoospermic men. Hum Reprod 6:1431

153. Haidl G, Rommel JD, Schill WB (1994) Sperm pooling as a possibility to increase the number of inseminating spermatozoa. Z Hautkrankheiten 69:95

154. Hakim LS, Lobel SM, Oates RD (1995) The achievement of pregnancies using assisted reproductive technologies for male factor infertility after retroperitoneal lymph node dissection for testicular carcinoma. Fertil Steril 64:1141

155. Hammadeh ME, Al-Hasani S, Stieber M, Rosenbaum P, Küpker D, Diedrich K, Schmidt W (1996) The effect of chromatin condensation (aniline blue staining) and morphology (strict criteria) of human spermatozoa on fertilization, cleavage and pregnancy rates in an intracytoplasmic sperm injection programme. Hum Reprod 11:2468

156. Hammadeh ME, Al-Hasani S, Doerr S, Stieber M, Rosenbaum P, Schmidt W, Diedrich K (1999) Comparison between chromatin condensation and morphology from testis biopsy extracted and ejaculated spermatozoa and their relationship to ICSI outcome. Hum Reprod 14:363

157. Harari O, Bourne H, Baker G, Gronow M, Johnston I (1995) High fertilization rate with intracytoplasmic sperm injection in mosaic Klinefelter's syndrome. Fertil Steril 63:182

158. Harari O, Bourne H, McDonald M, Richings N, Speirs AI, Johnston WIH, Baker HWG (1995) Intracytoplasmic sperm injection: a major advance in the management of severe male subfertility. Fertil Steril 64:360

159. Hargreave TB (1994) History and examination. In: Hargreave TB (ed) Male infertility. Springer, Berlin Heidelberg New York London, pp 17–36

160. Hargreave TB, Torrance M, Young H, Harris AB (1982) Isolation of Ureaplasma urealyticum from seminal plasma in relation to sperm antibody levels and sperm motility. Andrologia 14:223

161. Harrison KL, Callan VJ, Hennessey JF (1987) Stress and semen quality in an in vitro fertilization program. Fertil Steril 48:633

162. Hauser R, Temple-Smith PD, Southwick GJ, McFarlane J, de Kretser DM (1995) Pregnancies after microsurgical correction of partial epididymal and vasal obstruction. Hum Reprod 10:1152

163. Hauser R, Botchan A, Amit A, Ben Yosef D, Gamzu R, Paz G, Lessing JB, Yogev L, Yavetz H (1998) Multiple testicular sampling in non-obstructive azoospermia – is it necessary? Hum Reprod 13:3081

164. Henkel R, Müller C, Miska W, Gips H, Schill WB (1993) Determination of the acrosome reaction in human spermatozoa is predictive of fertilization in vitro. Hum Reprod 8:2128

165. Henkel R, Franken DR, Lombard CJ, Schill WB (1994) The selective capacity of glass wool filtration for normal chromatin condensed human spermatozoa: a possible therapeutic modality for male factor cases? J Assist Reprod Genet 11:395

166. Henkel R, Müller C, Miska W, Schill WB, Kleinstein J, Gips H (1995) Determination of the acrosin activity of human spermatozoa by means of a gelatinolytic technique. A simple, predictive method useful for IVF. J Androl 16:272

167. Hershlag A, Schiff SF, DeCherney AH (1991) Retrograde ejaculation. Hum Reprod 6:255

168. Hershlag A, Cooper GW, Benoff S (1995) Pregnancy following discontinuation of a calcium channel blocker in the male partner. Hum Reprod 10:599

169. Hinney B, Wilke G, Michelmann HW (1993) Prognostic value of an automated sperm analysis in IVF or insemination therapy. Andrologia 25:195

170. Hinting A, Vermeulen L, Comhaire F, Dhont M (1989) Pregnancy after in vitro fertilization and embryo transfer in severe immune male infertility. Andrologia 21:516

171. Hinting A, Comhaire F, Vermeulen L, Dhont M, Vermeulen A, Vandekerckhove D (1990) Possibilities and limitations of techniques of assisted reproduction for the treatment of male infertility. Hum Reprod 5:544

172. Hinting A, Comhaire F, Vermeulen L, Dhont M, Vermeulen A, Vandekerckhove D (1990) Value of sperm characteristics and the result of in-vitro fertilization for predicting the outcome of assisted reproduction. Int J Androl 13:59

173. Hirsh AV, Mills C, Bekir J, Dean N, Yovich JL, Tan SL (1994) Factors influencing the outcome of in-vitro fertilization with epididymal spermatozoa in irreversible obstructive azoospermia. Hum Reprod 9:1710

174. Ho PC, So WK, Chan YF, Yeung WSB (1992) Intrauterine insemination after ovarian stimulation as a treatment for subfertility because of subnormal semen: a prospective randomized controlled trial. Fertil Steril 58:995

175. Hofmann N, Hilscher B (1991) Use of aniline blue to assess chromatin condensation in morphologically normal spermatozoa in normal and infertile men. Hum Reprod 6:979

176. Hofmann N, Kuwert E (1979) Die chronische, nicht erregerbedingte Orchitis. Z Hautkrankheiten 54:173

177. Hofmann N, Hilscher B, Bierling C (1990) Quantitative studies on the correlation between disturbed chromatin condensation and sperm morphology. Fertilitat 6:208

178. Hofmann N, Hilscher B, Mörchen B, Schuppe HC, Bielfeld P (1995) Comparative studies on various modes of classification of morphology of sperm heads and results in in vitro fertilization – a preliminary report. Andrologia 27:19

179. Holden CA, Hyne RV, Sathananthan AH, Trounson AO (1990) Assessment of the human sperm acrosome reaction using Concanavalin A lectin. Mol Reprod Dev 25:247

180. Holland-Moritz H, Krause W (1990) Use of sperm cryopreservation by tumor patients. Hautarzt 41:204

181. Homonnai ZT, Yavetz H, Yogev L, Rotem R, Paz GF (1988) Clomiphene citrate treatment in oligozoospermia: comparison between two regimens of low-dose treatment. Fertil Steril 50:801

182. Horvarth PM, Bohrer M, Shelden RM, Kemmann E (1989) The relationship of sperm parameters to cycle fecundity in superovulated women undergoing intrauterine insemination. Fertil Steril 52:288

183. Hovatta O, von Schmitten K (1993) Sperm aspiration from vas deferens and in-vitro fertilization in cases of non-treatable anejaculation. Hum Reprod 8:1689

184. Hovatta O, Koskimies AI, Ranta T, Stenman UH, Seppala M (1979) Bromocriptine treatment of oligospermia: a double blind study. Clin Endocrinol (Oxf) 11:377

185. Hovatta O, Moilanen J, von Schmitten K, Reima I (1995) Testicular needle biopsy, open biopsy, epididymal aspiration and intracytoplasmic sperm injection in obstructive azoospermia. Hum Reprod 10:2595

186. Hulme VA, Stander FSH, Kruger TF, van der Merwe JP, Windt ML (1991) Retrograde ejaculation and pronuclear stage tubal transfer (PROST). Arch Androl 26:21

187. Hulting C, Rosenlund B, Törnbloom M, Sjöblom P, Garoff L, Nyman C, Hillensjö T (1995) Transrectal electroejaculation in combination with in-vitro fertilization: an effective treatment of anejaculatory infertility after testicular cancer. Hum Reprod 10:847

188. Huszar G, Vigue L, Morshedi M (1992) Sperm creatine phosphokinase M-isoform ratios and fertilizing potential of men: a blinded study of 84 couples treated with in vitro fertilization. Fertil Steril 57:882

189. Ibrahim ME, Moussa MAA, Pedersen H (1989) Efficacy of zona-free hamster egg sperm penetration assay as a predictor of in vitro fertilization. Arch Androl 23:267

190. Iwasaki A, Gagnon C (1992) Formation of reactive oxygen species in spermatozoa of infertile patients. Fertil Steril 31:531

191. Jequier AM, Ansell ID, Bullimore NJ (1985) Congenital absence of the vasa deferentia presenting with infertility. J Androl 6:15

192. Jeyendran RS, Van der Ven HH, Perez-Pelaez M, Crabo BG, Zaneveld LJD (1984) Development of an assay to assess the functional integrity of the human sperm membrane and its relationship to other semen characteristics. J Reprod Fertil 70:219

193. Jeyendran RS, Van der Ven HH, Kennedy WP, Heath E, Perez-Pelaez M, Sobrero AJ, Zaneveld LJD (1985) Acrosomeless sperm. A case of primary male infertility. Andrologia 17:31

194. Jezek D, Knuth UA, Schulze W (1998) Successful testicular sperm extraction (TESE) in spite of high serum follicle-stimulating hormone and azoospermia: correlation between testicular morphology, TESE results, semen analysis and serum hormone values in 103 infertile men. Hum Reprod 13:1230

195. Jimenez C, Grizard G, Pouly JP, Boucher D (1997) Birth after combination of cryopreservation of sperm recovered from urine and intracytoplasmic sperm injection in a case of complete retrograde ejaculation. Fertil Steril 68:542

196. Jochum M, Pabst W, Schill WB (1986) Granulocyte elastase as a sensitive diagnostic parameter of silent male genital tract inflammation. Andrologia 18:413

197. Johnson MD (1998) Genetic risks of intracytoplasmic sperm injection in the treatment of male infertility: recommendations for genetic counseling and screening. Fertil Steril 70:397

198. Jonas D, Linzbach P, Weber W (1979) The use of midodrin in the treatment of ejaculation disorders following retroperitoneal lymphadenectomy. Eur Urol 5:184

199. Jorgensen N, Auger J, Giwercman A, Irvine DS, Jensen TK, Jouannet P, Keiding N, Le Bon C, Macdonald E, Pekuri AM, Scheike T, Simonsen M, Suominen J, Skakkebek NE (1997) Semen analysis performed by different laboratory teams: an intervariation study. Int J Androl 20:201

200. Jow WW, Steckel J, Schlegel PN, Magid MS, Goldstein M (1993) Motile sperm in human testis biopsy specimens. J Androl 14:194

201. Kallajoki M, Suominen J (1984) An acrosomal antigen of human spermatozoa and spermatogenic cells characterized with a monoclonal antibody. Int J Androl 7:283

202. Kamischke A, Gromoll J, Simoni M, Behre HM, Nieschlag E (1999) Transmission of a Y chromosomal deletion involving the deleted in azoospermia (DAZ) and chromodomain (CDY1) genes from father to son through intracytoplasmic sperm injection. Hum Reprod 14:2320

203. Kanakas N, Mantzavinos T, Boufidou F, Koumentakou I, Creatsas G (1999) Ureaplasma urealyticum in semen: is there any effect on in vitro fertilization outcome? Fertil Steril 71:523

204. Kay VJ, Irvine DS (2000) Successful in-vitro fertilization pregnancy with spermatozoa from a patient with Kartagener's syndrome. Hum Reprod 15:135

205. Keating J, Grundy CE, Fivey PS, Elliott M, Robinson J (1997) Investigation of the association between the presence of cytoplasmic residues on the human sperm midpiece and defective sperm function. J Reprod Fertil 110:71

206. Keck C, Nieschlag E (1993) Cryopreservation of sperm as fertility reserve for oncologic patients. Internist (Berl) 34:775

207. Keck C, Behre HM, Jockenhövel F, Nieschlag E (1994) Ineffectiveness of kallikrein in treatment of idiopathic male infertility: a double-blind, randomized, placebo-controlled study. Hum Reprod 9:325

208. Kentenich H, Schmiady H, Radke E, Stief G, Blankau A (1992) The male IVF patient – psychosomatic considerations. Hum Reprod 7 [Suppl 1]:13

209. Kessopoulou E, Tomlinson MJ, Barratt CLR, Bolton AE, Cooke ID (1992) Origin of reactive oxygen species in human semen: spermatozoa or leucocytes? J Reprod Fertil 94:463

210. Kessopoulou E, Powers HJ, Sharma KK, Pearson MJ, Russel JM, Cooke ID, Barratt CLR (1995) A double-blind randomized placebo crossover controlled trial using the antioxidant vitamin E to treat reactive oxygen species associated male infertility. Fertil Steril 64:825

211. Kiefer D, Check JH, Katsoff D (1997) Evidence that oligoasthenozoospermia may be an etiologic factor for spontaneous abortion after in vitro fertilization-embryo transfer. Fertil Steril 68:545

212. Kim SJ, Han HD (1995) In vitro retrieval of epididymal sperm: a new approach to achievement of pregnancy for post-testicular azoospermia. Fertil Steril 63:656

213. Kirby RS, Kirby MG, Feneley MR, McNicholas T, McLean A, Well JA (1994) Screening for carcinoma of the prostate: a GP-based study. Br J Urol 74:64

214. Kliesch S, Behre HM, Nieschlag E (1994) High efficacy of gonadotropin or pulsatile gonadotropin-releasing hormone treatment in hypogonadotropic hypogonadal men. Eur J Endocrinol 131:347

215. Kliesch S, Behre HM, Nieschlag E (1995) Recombinant human follicle-stimulating hormone and human chorionic gonadotropin for induction of spermatogenesis in a hypogonadotropic male. Fertil Steril 63:1326

216. Knuth UA, Hönigl W, Bals-Pratsch M, Schleicher G, Nieschlag E (1987) Treatment of severe oligospermia with human chorionic gonadotropin/human menopausal gonadotropin: a placebo-controlled, double blind trial. J Clin Endocrinol Metab 65:1081

217. Knuth UA, Kühne J, Crosby J, Bals-Pratsch M, Kelly RW, Nieschlag E (1989) Indomethacin and oxaprozin lower seminal prostaglandin levels but do not influence sperm motion characteristics and serum hormones of young healthy men in a placebo-controlled double-blind trial. J Androl 10:108

218. Kobayashi T, Jinno M, Sugimura K, Nozawa S, Sugiyama T, Iida E (1991) Sperm morphological assessment based on strict criteria and in-vitro fertilization outcome. Hum Reprod 6:983

219. Köhn FM, Schill WB (1988) Kryospermabank München – Zwischenbilanz 1974–1986. Hautarzt 39:91

220. Köhn FM, Schill WB (1994) The alpha-sympathomimetic midodrin as a tool for diagnosis and treatment of sperm transport disturbances. Andrologia 26:283

221. Köhn FM, Schill WB, Schuppe HC, Jeyendran RS (1995) Hydrogen hexachloroplatinate reduces human sperm acrosome reaction. Int J Androl 18:321

222. Kotoulas IG, Cardamakis E, Michopoulos J, Mitropoulos D, Dounis A (1994) Tamoxifen treatment in male infertility. I. Effect on spermatozoa. Fertil Steril 61:911

223. Krause W (1993) Die Bedeutung des "Routine-Spermiogramms". Eine kritische Analyse. Hautarzt 44:269

224. Krause W, Brake A (1994) Utilization of cryopreserved semen in tumor patients. Urologia internationalis 52:65

225. Krausz C, Mills C, Rogers S, Tan SL, Aitken RJ (1994) Stimulation of oxidant generation by human sperm suspensions using phorbol esters and formyl peptides: relationships with motility and fertilization in vitro. Fertil Steril 62:599

226. Krausz C, Bonaccorsi L, Luconi M, Fuzzi B, Criscuoli L, Pellegrini S, Forti G, Baldi E (1995) Intracellular calcium increase and acrosome reaction in response to progesterone in human spermatozoa are correlated with in-vitro fertilization. Hum Reprod 10:120

227. Kret B, Milad M, Jeyendran RS (1995) New discriminatory level for glucosidase activity to diagnose epididymal obstruction or dysfunction. Arch Androl 35:29

228. Kruger TF, Menkveld R, Stander FSH, Lombard CJ, Van der Merwe JP, Van Zyl JA, Smith K (1986) Sperm morphologic features as a prognostic factor in in vitro fertilization. Fertil Steril 46:1118

229. Kruger TF, Acosta AA, Simmons KF, Swanson RJ, Matta JF, Oehninger S (1988) Predictive value of abnormal sperm morphology in in vitro fertilization. Fertil Steril 49:112

230. Kruger TF, Haque D, Acosta AA, Pleban P, Swanson RJ, Simmons KF, Matta JF, Morshedi M, Oehninger S (1988) Correlation between sperm morphology, acrosin, and fertilization in an IVF program. Arch Androl 20:237

231. Kynaston HG, Lewis-Jones DI, Lynch RV, Desmond AD (1988) Changes in seminal quality following oral zinc therapy. Andrologia 20:21

232. Lähteenmäki A, Veilahti J, Hovatta O (1995) Intra-uterine insemination versus cyclic, low-dose prednisolone in couples with male antisperm antibodies. Hum Reprod 10:142

233. Lalich RA, Marut EL, Prins GS, Scommegna A (1988) Life-table analysis of intrauterine insemination pregnancy rates. Am J Obstet Gynecol 158:980

234. Lanzendorf SE (1995) Experiences with intracytoplasmic sperm injection. Reprod Med Rev 4:75

235. Lee KO, Ng SC, Lee PS, Bongso AT, Taylor EA, Lin TK, Ratnam SS (1995) Effect of growth hormone therapy in men with severe idiopathic oligozoospermia. Eur J Endocrinol 132:159

236. Lehmann K, Simmler F, Schmucki O, Hauri D (1994) PSA in prostatic fluid. Urologe A 33:232

237. Leib Z, Bartoov B, Eltes F, Servadio C (1994) Reduced semen quality caused by chronic abacterial prostatitis: an enigma or reality? Fertil Steril 61:1109

238. Le Lannou D, Jezequel P, Blayau M, Dorval I, Lemoine P, Dabadie A, Roussey M, Le Marec B, Legall JY (1995) Obstructive azoospermia with agenesis of vas deferens or with bronchiectasia (Young's syndrome): a genetic approach. Hum Reprod 10:338

239. Lenzi A, Lombardo F, Gandini L, Culasso F, Dondero F (1992) Glutathione therapy for male infertility. Arch Androl 29:65

240. Lewis SEM, Moohan JM, Thompson W (1993) Effects of pentoxifylline on human sperm motility in normospermic individuals using computer-assisted analysis. Fertil Steril 59:418

241. Lewis SEM, Boyle PM, McKinney KA, Young IS, Thompson W (1995) Total antioxidant capacity of seminal plasma is different in fertile and infertile men. Fertil Steril 64:868

242. Liu DY, Baker HWG (1988) The proportion of human sperm with poor morphology but normal intact acrosomes detected with pisum sativum agglutinin correlates with fertilization in vitro. Fertil Steril 50:288

243. Liu DY, Baker HWG (1990) Relationships between human sperm acrosin, acrosomes, morphology and fertilization in vitro. Hum Reprod 5:298

244. Liu DY, Baker HWG (1992) Tests of human sperm function and fertilization in vitro. Fertil Steril 58:465

245. Liu DY, Baker HWG (1992) Sperm nuclear chromatin normality: relationship with sperm morphology, sperm-zona pellucida binding, and fertilization rates in vitro. Fertil Steril 58:1178

246. Liu DY, Baker HWG (1994) Disordered acrosome reaction of spermatozoa bound to the zona pellucida: a newly discovered sperm defect causing infertility with reduced sperm-zona pellucida penetration and reduced fertilization in vitro. Hum Reprod 9:1694

247. Liu DY, Baker HWG (1998) Calcium ionophore-induced acrosome reaction correlates with fertilization rates in vitro in patients with teratozoospermic semen. Hum Reprod 13:905

248. Liu DY, Clarke GN, Lopata A, Johnston WIH, Baker HWG (1989) A sperm-zona pellucida binding test and in vitro fertilization. Fertil Steril 52:281

249. Liu DY, Clarke GN, Lopata A, Johnston WIH, Baker HWG (1989) Human sperm-zona pellucida binding, sperm characteristics and in-vitro fertilization. Hum Reprod 4:696

250. Liu DY, Bourne H, Baker HWG (1997) High fertilization and pregnancy rates after intracytoplasmic sperm injection in patients with disordered zona pellucida-induced acrosome reaction. Fertil Steril 67:955

251. Liu DY, Bourne H, Baker HWG (1995) Fertilization and pregnancy with acrosome intact sperm by intracytoplasmic sperm injection in patients with disordered zona pellucida-induced acrosome reaction. Fertil Steril 64:116

252. Liu J, Nagy Z, Joris H, Tournaye H, Devroey P, Van Steirteghem A (1995) Successful fertilization and establishment of pregnancies after intracytoplasmic sperm injection in patients with globozoospermia. Hum Reprod 10:626

253. Liu PY, Turner L, Rushford D, McDonald J, Baker HWG, Conway AJ, Handelsman DJ (1999) Efficacy and safety of recombinant human follicle-stimulating hormone (Gonal-F) with urinary human chorionic gonadotrophin for induction of spermatogenesis and fertility in gonadotrophin-deficient men. Hum Reprod 14:1540

254. Lundin K, Sjögren A, Nilsson L, Hamberger L (1994) Fertilization and pregnancy after intracytoplasmic microinjection of acrosomeless spermatozoa. Fertil Steril 62:1266

255. Lunenfeld E, Shapiro BS, Sarov B, Sarov I, Insler V, De Cherney AH (1989) The association between chlamydial-specific IgG and IgA antibodies and pregnancy outcome in an in vitro fertilization program. J In Vitro Fertil Embryo Transf 6:222

256. Mac Leod J (1943) The role of oxygen in the metabolism and motility of human spermatozoa. Am J Physiol 138:512

257. Mac Leod J, Hotchkiss RS (1942) The distribution of spermatozoa and of certain chemical constituents in the human ejaculate. J Urol 48:225

258. Mahadevan MM, Trounson AO, Leeton JF (1983) Successful use of human semen cryobanking for in vitro fertilization. Fertil Steril 40:340

259. Mansour R (1998) Intracytoplasmic sperm injection: a state of the technique. Hum Reprod Update 4:43

260. Mansour RT, Aboulghar MA, Serour GI, Amin YM, Ramzi AM (1995) The effect of sperm parameters on the outcome of intracytoplasmic sperm injection. Fertil Steril 64:982

261. Margalioth EJ, Navot D, Laufer N, Lewin A, Rabinowitz R, Schenker JG (1986) Correlation between the zona-free hamster egg sperm penetration assay and human in vitro fertilization. Fertil Steril 45:665

262. Marmar JL, Katz S, Praiss DE, Debenedictis TJ (1975) Semen zinc levels in infertile and postvasectomy patients and patients with prostatitis. Fertil Steril 26:1057

263. Marshburn PB, McIntire D, Carr BR, Byrd W (1992) Spermatozoal characteristics from fresh and frozen donor semen and their correlation with fertility outcome after intrauterine insemination. Fertil Steril 58:179

264. Mashiach R, Fisch B, Eltes F, Tadir Y, Ovadia J, Bartoov B (1992) The relationship between sperm ultrastructural features and fertilizing capacity in vitro. Fertil Steril 57:1052

265. Matorras R, Corcostegui B, Perez C, Mandiola M, Mendoza R, Rodriguez-Escudero FJ (1995) Sperm morphology analysis (strict criteria) in male infertility is not a prognostic factor in intrauterine insemination with husband's sperm. Fertil Steril 63:608

266. Matthews GJ, Matthews ED, Goldstein M (1998) Induction of spermatogenesis and achievement of pregnancy after microsurgical varicocelectomy in men with azoospermia and severe oligoasthenozoospermia. Fertil Steril 70:71

267. McGovern P, Quagliarello J, Arny M (1989) Relationship of within-patient semen variability to outcome of intrauterine insemination. Fertil Steril 51:1019

268. Menchini-Fabris GF, Canale D, Izzo PL, Olivieri L, Bartelloni M (1984) Free L-carnitine in human semen: its variability in different andrologic pathologies. Fertil Steril 42:263

269. Meniru GI, Gorgy A, Batha S, Clarke RJ, Podsiadly BT, Craft IL (1998) Studies of percutaneous epididymal sperm aspiration (PESA) and intracytoplasmic sperm injection. Hum Reprod Update 4:57

270. Menkveld R, Rhemrev JPT, Franken DR, Vermeiden JPW, Kruger TF (1996) Acrosomal morphology as a novel criterion for male fertility diagnosis: relation with acrosin activity, morphology (strict criteria), and fertilization in vitro. Fertil Steril 65:637

271. Merino G, Carranza-Lira S (1995) Infection and male infertility: effect of different antibiotic regimens on semen quality. Arch Androl 35:209

272. Merino G, Carranza-Lira S, Murrieta S, Rodriguez L, Cuevas E, Moran C (1995) Bacterial infection and semen characteristics in infertile men. Arch Androl 35:43

273. Meschede D, de Geyter C, Nieschlag E, Horst J (1995) Genetic risk in micromanipulative assisted reproduction. Hum Reprod 10:2880

274. Mickle J, Milunsky A, Amos JA, Oates RD (1995) Congenital unilateral absence of the vas deferens: a heterogeneous disorder with two distinct subpopulations based upon aetiology and mutational status of the cystic fibrosis gene. Hum Reprod 10:1728

275. Miska W, Schill WB (1991) Resorptionsstudie mit Schweinepankreas-Kallikrein am Menschen. Arzneimittelforschung/Drug Res 41:1061

276. Mladenovic I, Micic S, Genbacev O, Papic N (1995) Hypoosmotic swelling test for quality control of sperm prepared for assisted reproduction. Arch Androl 34:163

277. Moghissi KS, Gruber JS, Evans S, Yanez J (1977) Homologous artificial insemination. a reappraisal. Am J Obstet Gynecol 129:909

278. Montagut JM, Lepretre S, Degoy J, Rousseau M (1991) Ureaplasma in semen and IVF. Hum Reprod 6:727

279. Moore DE, Ashley RL, Zarutskie PW, Coombs RW, Soules MR, Corey L (1989) Transmission of genital herpes by donor insemination. JAMA 261:3441

280. Moore HDM, Smith CA, Hartman TD, Bye AP (1987) Visualization and characterization of a the human acrosome reaction of human spermatozoa by immunolocalization with a monoclonal antibody. Gamete Res 17:245

281. Morgentaler A, Fung MY, Harris DH, Powers RD, Alper MM (1995) Sperm morphology and in vitro fertilization outcome: a direct comparison of World Health Organization and strict criteria methodologies. Fertil Steril 64:1177

282. Mortimer D (1991) Sperm preparation techniques and iatrogenic failures of in-vitro fertilization. Hum Reprod 6:173

283. Mortimer D, Curtis EF, Miller RG (1987) Specific labelling by peanut agglutinin of the outer acrosomal membrane of the human spermatozoon. J Reprod Fertil 81:127

284. Nagy B, Corradi G, Vajda Z, Gimes R, Csömör S (1989) The occurrence of Chlamydia trachomatis in the semen of men participating in an IVF programme. Hum Reprod 4:54

285. Nagy ZP, Liu J, Joris H, Verheyen G, Tournaye H, Camus M, Derde MP, Devroey P, Van Steirteghem AC (1995) The result of intracytoplasmic sperm injection is not related to any of the three basic sperm parameters. Hum Reprod 10:1123

286. Nagy Z, Liu J, Cecile J, Silber S, Devroey P, van Steirteghem A (1995) Using ejaculated, fresh, and frozen-thawed epididymal and testicular spermatozoa gives rise to comparable results after intracytoplasmic sperm injection. Fertil Steril 63:808

287. Nagy ZP, Verheyen G, Liu J, Joris H, Janssenswillen C, Wisanto A, Devroey P, Van Steirteghem AC (1995) Results of 55 intracytoplasmic sperm injection cycles in the treatment of male-immunological infertility. Hum Reprod 10:1775

288. Nagy ZP, Joris H, Verheyen G, Tournaye H, Devroey P, van Steirteghem AC (1998) Correlation between motility of testicular spermatozoa, testicular histology and the outcome of intracytoplasmic sperm injection. Hum Reprod 13:890

289. Nashan D, Behre HM, Grunert JH, Nieschlag E (1990) Diagnostic value of scrotal sonography in infertile men: report on 658 cases. Andrologia 22:387

290. Naz RK, Minhas BS (1995) Enhancement of sperm function for treatment of male infertility. J Androl 16:384
291. Nelson JR, Corson SL, Batzer FR, Gocial B, Huppert L, Go KJ, Maislin G (1993) Predicting success of gamete intrafallopian transfer. Fertil Steril 60:116
292. Neumann S, Jochum M (1984) Elastase-a^1-proteinase inhibitor complex. In: Bergmeyer HU, Bergmeyer J, Grassl M (eds) Methods of enzymatic analysis. Verlag Chemie, Weinheim, pp 184–195
293. Neumann PJ, Gharib SD, Weinstein MC (1994) The cost of a successful delivery with in vitro fertilization. N Engl J Med 331:239
294. Nikolettos N, Al-Hasani S, Baukloh V, Schöpper B, Demirel LC, Baban N, Sturm R, Rudolf K, Tomalak K, Tinneberg HR, Diedrich K (1999) The outcome of intracytoplasmic sperm injection in patients with retrograde ejaculation. Hum Reprod 14:2293
295. Oates RD, Amos JA (1994) The genetic basis of congenital bilateral absence of the vas deferens and cystic fibrosis. J Androl 15:1
296. Oehninger S, Acosta AA, Morshedi M, Veeck L, Swanson RJ, Simmons K, Rosenwaks Z (1988) Corrective measures and pregnancy outcome in in vitro fertilization in patients with severe sperm morphology abnormalities. Fertil Steril 50:283
297. Oehninger S, Coddington CC, Scott R, Franken DA, Burkman LJ, Acosta AA, Hodgen GD (1989) Hemizona assay: assessment of sperm dysfunction and prediction of in vitro fertilization outcome. Fertil Steril 51:665
298. Oehninger S, Franken D, Alexander N, Hodgen GD (1992) Hemizona assay and its impact on the identification and treatment of human sperm dysfunctions. Andrologia 24:307
299. Oehninger S, Veeck L, Lanzendorf S, Maloney M, Toner J, Muasher S (1995) Intracytoplasmic sperm injection: achievement of high pregnancy rates in couples with severe male factor infertility is dependent primarily upon female and not male factors. Fertil Steril 64:977
300. Oehninger S, Franken D, Kruger T (1997) Approaching the next millenium: how should we manage andrology diagnosis in the intracytoplasmic sperm injection era? Fertil Steril 67:434
301. Ohashi K, Saji F, Kato M, Okabe M, Mimura T, Tanizawa O (1992) Evaluation of acrosomal status using MH61-beads test and its clinical application. Fertil Steril 58:803
302. Ohashi K, Saji F, Wakimoto A, Tsutsui T, Nakazawa T, Okabe M, Mimura T, Tanizawa O (1994) Selection of acrosome-reacted sperm with MH61-immunobeads. J Androl 15:78
303. Ohl DA, Denil J, Bennett CJ, Randolph JF, Menge AC, McGabe M (1991) Electroejaculation following retroperitoneal lymphadenectomy. J Urol 145:980
304. Okabe M, Matzno S, Nagira M, Ying X, Kohama Y, Mimura T (1992) Collection of acrosome-reacted human sperm using monoclonal antibody-coated paramagnetic beads. Mol Reprod Dev 32:389
305. Ombelet W, Fourie FR, Vandeput H, Bosmans E, Cox A, Janssen M, Kruger T (1994) Teratozoospermia and in-vitro fertilization: a randomized prospective study. Hum Reprod 9:1479
306. Ombelet W, Menkveld R, Kruger TF, Steeno O (1995) Sperm morphology assessment: historical review in relation to fertility. Hum Reprod Update 1:543
307. Ombelet W, Vandeput H, Janssen M, Cox A, Vossen C, Pollet H, Steeno O, Bosmans E (1997) Treatment of male infertility due to sperm surface antibodies: IUI or IVF? Hum Reprod 12:1165
308. Ovesen P, Jorgensen JO, Kjaer T, Ho KK, Orskov H, Christiansen JS (1996) Impaired growth hormone secretion and increased growth hormone-binding protein levels in subfertile males. Fertil Steril 65:165
309. Ovesen P, Jorgensen JO, Ingerslev J, Ho KK, Orskov H, Christiansen JS (1996) Growth hormone treatment of subfertile males. Fertil Steril 66:292
310. Page DC, Silber S, Brown LG (1999) Men with infertility caused by AZFc deletion can produce sons by intracytoplasmic sperm injection, but are likely to transmit the deletion and infertility. Hum Reprod 14:1722

311. Palermo G, Joris H, Devroey P, Van Steirteghem AC (1992) Pregnancies after intracytoplasmic injection of a single spermatozoon into an oocyte. Lancet 340:17

312. Palermo G, Cohen J, Alikani M, Adler A, Rosenwaks Z (1995) Intracytoplasmic sperm injection: a novel treatment for all forms of male factor infertility. Fertil Steril 63:1231

313. Palermo GD, Schlegel PN, Hariprashad JJ, Ergün B, Mielnik A, Zaninovic N, Veeck LL, Rosenwaks Z (1999) Fertilization and pregnancy outcome with intracytoplasmic sperm injection for azoospermic men. Hum Reprod 14:741

314. Pampiglione JS, Tan SL, Campbell S (1993) The use of the stimulated acrosome reaction test as a test of fertilizing ability in human spermatozoa. Fertil Steril 59:1280

315. Parinaud J, Vieitez G, Moutaffian H, Richoilley G, Labal B (1995) Relevance of acrosome function in the evaluation of semen in vitro fertilizing ability. Fertil Steril 63:598

316. Patrizio P (1995) Intracytoplasmic sperm injection (ICSI): potential genetic concerns. Hum Reprod 10:2520

317. Patrizio P, Ord T, Silber SJ, Asch RH (1993) Cystic fibrosis mutations impair the fertilization rate of epididymal sperm from men with congenital absence of the vas deferens. Hum Reprod 8:1259

318. Patrizio P, Ord T, Silber SJ, Asch RH (1994) Correlation between epididymal length and fertilization rate in men with congenital absence of the vas deferens. Fertil Steril 61:265

319. Payne D, Flaherty SP, Jeffrey R, Warnes GM, Matthews CD (1994) Successful treatment of severe male factor infertility in 100 consecutive cycles using intracytoplasmic sperm injection. Hum Reprod 9:2051

320. Pellicer A, Ruiz M (1989) Fertilization in vitro of human oocytes by spermatozoa collected in different stressful situations. Hum Reprod 4:817

321. Plachot M, Mandelbaum J, Junca AM (1984) Acrosome reaction of human sperm used for in vitro fertilization. Fertil Steril 42:418

322. Plewa GF (1989) Die retrograde Ejakulation – Diagnose und Therapie. Dtsch Dermatologe 37:287

323. Pryor JP (1994) Erectile and ejaculatory problems in infertility. In: Hargreave TB (ed) Male infertility. Springer, Berlin Heidelberg New York London pp 319–336

324. Pryor JP, Hendry WF (1991) Ejaculatory duct obstruction in subfertile males: analysis of 87 patients. Fertil Steril 56:725

325. Purvis K, Christiansen E (1993) Infection in the male reproductive tract. Impact, diagnosis and treatment in relation to male infertility. Int J Androl 16:1

326. Pusch HH (1989) Oral treatment of oligozoospermia with testosterone-undecanoate: results of a double-blind-placebo-controlled trial. Andrologia 21:76

327. Rana N, Jeyendran RS, Holmgren WJ, Rotman C, Zaneveld LJD (1989) Glass wool-filtered spermatozoa and their oocyte penetrating capacity. J In Vitro Fertil Embryo Transf 6:280

328. Ranieri DM, Simonetti S, Vicino M, Cormio L, Selvaggi L (1995) Successful establishment of pregnancy by superovulation and intrauterine insemination with sperm recovered by a modified Hotchkiss procedure from a patient with retrograde ejaculation. Fertil Steril 64:1039

329. Rehan NE, Sobrero AJ, Fertig JW (1975) The semen of fertile men: statistical analysis of 1300 men. Fertil Steril 26:492

330. Reinhardt A, Haidl G, Schill WB (1995) Granulocyte elastase – significance for andrological diagnosis. Fertilitat 11:153

331. Riedel HH, Baukloh V, Mettler L (1984) Is the sperm bacteriology important for the results of in vitro fertilization? Andrologia 16:259

332. Riedel HH, Hübner F, Ensslen SC, Bieniek KW, Grillo M (1989) Minimal andrological requirements for in-vitro fertilization. Hum Reprod 4 [Suppl]:73

333. Riley AJ, Riley EJ (1982) Partial ejaculatory incompetence: the therapeutic effect of midodrine, an orally active selective alpha-adrenoceptor agonist. Eur Urol 8:155

334. Roberts KP (1998) Y-chromosome deletions and male infertility: state of the art and clinical implications. J Androl 19:255

335. Rodriguez-Rigau LJ, Ayala C, Grunert GM, Woodward RM, Lotze EC, Feste JR, Gibbons W, Smith KD, Steinberger E (1989) Relationship between the results of sperm analysis and GIFT. J Androl 10:139

336. Rolf C, Behre HM, Nieschlag E (1996) Tamoxifen bei männlicher Infertilität. Dtsch Med Wochenschr 121:33

337. Rolf C, Cooper TG, Yeung CH, Nieschlag E (1999) Antioxidant treatment of patients with asthenozoospermia or moderate oligoasthenozoospermia with high-dose vitamin C and vitamin E: a randomized, placebo-controlled, double-blind study. Hum Reprod 14:1028

338. Ron-EL R, Friedler S, Strassburger D, Komarovsky D, Schachter M, Raziel A (1999) Birth of a healthy neonate following the intracytoplasmic injection of testicular spermatozoa from a patient with Klinefelter's syndrome. Hum Reprod 14:368

339. Rossato M, Ferlin A, Garolla A, Pistorello M, Foresta C (1998) High fertilization rate in conventional in-vitro fertilization utilizing spermatozoa from an oligozoospermic subject presenting microdeletions of the Y chromosome long arm. Mol Hum Reprod 4:473

340. Saito K, Kinoshita Y, Yumura Y, Iwasaki A, Hosaka M (1998) Successful pregnancy with sperm retrieved from the bladder after the introduction of a low-electrolyte solution for retrograde ejaculation. Fertil Steril 69:1149

341. Saling PM, Storey BT (1979) Mouse gamete interactions during fertilization in vitro. Chlortetracycline as a fluorescent probe for the mouse sperm acrosome reaction. J Cell Biol 83:544

342. Salzbrunn A, Benson DM, Holstein AF, Schulze W (1996) A new concept for the extraction of testicular spermatozoa and their application in assisted fertilization (ICSI). Hum Reprod 11:752

343. Schill WB (1974) Quantitative determination of acrosin activity in human spermatozoa. Fertil Steril 25:25

344. Schill WB (1979) Treatment of idiopathic oligozoospermia by kallikrein: results of a double-blind study. Arch Androl 2:163

345. Schill WB (1981) Acrosin and seminal plasma proteinase inhibitors in the diagnostic workup of male infertility. In: Insler V, Bettendorf G (eds) Advances in diagnosis and treatment of infertility. Elsevier/North Holland, New York, pp 321–337

346. Schill WB (1984) Verwendung von Kryosperma für die In-vitro-Fertilisation (IVF). Hautarzt 35:313

347. Schill WB (1990) Determination of active, non-zymogen acrosin, proacrosin and total acrosin in different andrological patients. Arch Dermatol Res 282:335

348. Schill WB (1990) Pregnancy after brompheniramine treatment of a diabetic with incomplete emission failure. Arch Androl 25:101

349. Schill WB (1991) Some disturbances of acrosomal development and function in human spermatozoa. Hum Reprod 6:969

350. Schill WB (1993) Sperm function tests in the evaluation of male factor infertility. In: Moeloek FA, Affandi B, Trounson AO (eds) Advances in human reproduction. Parthenon, New York, pp 411–420

351. Schill WB (1995) Survey of medical therapy in andrology. Int J Androl [Suppl] 2:56

352. Schill WB, Dasilva M (1983) Results of spermiograms obtained close to conception. Fortschr Androl 8:27

353. Schill WB, Schneider J, Ring J (1986) The use of ketotifen, a mast cell blocker, for treatment of oligo- and asthenozoospermia. Andrologia 18:570

354. Schill WB, Korting HC, Schweikert HU (1987) Treatment of oligozoospermia by testolactone. Acta Endocrinol 114 [Suppl 283]:22

355. Schill WB, Haidl G (1993) Medical treatment of male infertility. In: Insler V, Lunenfeld B (eds) Infertility: male and female. Churchill Livingstone, Edinburgh, pp 575–622

356. Schill WB, Parsch EM, Miska W (1994) Inhibition of angiotensin-converting enzyme – a new concept of medical treatment of male infertility? Fertil Steril 61:1123

357. Schlegel PN (1999) Testicular sperm extraction: microdissection improves sperm yield with minimal tissue excision. Hum Reprod 14:131

358. Schlegel PN, Cohen J, Goldstein M, Alikani M, Adler A, Gilbert BR, Palermo GD, Rosenwaks Z (1995) Cystic fibrosis gene mutations do not affect sperm function during in vitro fertilization with micromanipulation for men with bilateral congenital absence of vas deferens. Fertil Steril 64:421

359. Schopohl J, Mehltretter G, von Zumbusch R, Eversmann T, von Werder K (1991) Comparison of gonadotropin-releasing hormone and gonadotropin therapy in male patients with idiopathic hypothalamic hypogonadism. Fertil Steril 56:1143

360. Schoysman R, Vanderzwalmen P, Nijs M, Segal L, Segal-Bertin G, Geerts L, van Roosendaal E, Schoysman-Deboeck A (1994) Pregnancy obtained with human testicular spermatozoa in an in vitro fertilization program. J Androl 15 [Suppl]:10 S

361. Schramm P, Simonis J (1991) Pentoxifyllin – 12 Jahre andrologische Therapie. Z Haut Geschlechtskrankh 66:868

362. Segal S, Polishuk WZ, Ben-David M (1976) Hyperprolactinemic male fertility. Fertil Steril 27:1425

363. Segal S, Yaffe H, Laufer N, Ben-David M Male (1979) Hyperprolactinemia: effects on fertility. Fertil Steril 32:556

364. Seidman DS, Madjar I, Levron J, Levran D, Mashiach S, Dor J (1999) Testicular sperm aspiration and intracytoplasmic sperm injection for persistent infection of the ejaculate. Fertil Steril 71:564

365. Senn A, Germond M, De Grandi P (1992) Immunofluorescence study of actin, acrosin, dynein, tubulin and hyaluronidase and their impact on in-vitro fertilization. Hum Reprod 7:841

366. Shangold GA, Cantor B, Schreiber JR (1990) Treatment of infertility due to retrograde ejaculation: a simple cost-effective method. Fertil Steril 54:175

367. Sharma KK, Barratt CLR, Pearson MJ, Cooke ID (1995) Oral steroid therapy for subfertile males with antisperm antibodies in the semen: prediction of the responders. Hum Reprod 10:103

368. Sharma R, Hogg J, Bromhan DR (1993) Is sperm acrosin a predictor of fertilization and embryo quality in the human? Fertil Steril 60:881

369. Sherins RJ, Thorsell LP, Dorfmann A, Dennison-Lagos L, Calvo LP, Krysa L, Coulam CB, Schulman JD (1995) Intracytoplasmic sperm injection facilitates fertilization even in the most severe forms of male infertility: pregnancy outcome correlates with maternal age and number of eggs available. Fertil Steril 64:369

370. Sherman JK (1987) Frozen semen: efficiency in artificial insemination and advantage in testing for aquired immune deficiency syndrome. Fertil Steril 47:19

371. Sheynkin YR, Ye Z, Menendez S, Liotta D, Veeck LL, Schlegel PN (1998) Controlled comparison of percutaneous and microsurgical sperm retrieval in men with obstructive azoospermia. Hum Reprod 13:3086

372. Shimonovitz S, Zacut D, Ben-Chetrit A, Ron M (1993) Growth hormone status in patients with maturation arrest of spermatogenesis. Hum Reprod 8:919

373. Shulman A, Feldman B, Madgar I, Levron J, Mashiach S, Dor J (1999) In-vitro fertilization treatment for severe male factor: the fertilization potential of immotile spermatozoa obtained by testicular extraction. Hum Reprod 14:749

374. Shulman JF, Shulman S (1982) Methylprednisolone treatment of immunologic infertility in the male. Fertil Steril 38:591

375. Shushan A, Eisenberg VH, Schenker JG (1995) Subfertility in the era of assisted reproduction: changes and consequences. Fertil Steril 64:459

376. Silbe SJ (1989) The relationship of abnormal semen parameters to male fertility. Hum Reprod 4:947

377. Silber SJ, Nagy ZP, Liu J, Godoy H, Devroey P, van Steirteghem AC (1994) Conventional in-vitro fertilization versus intracytoplasmic sperm injection for patients requiring microsurgical sperm aspiration. Hum Reprod 9:1705

378. Silber SJ, van Steirteghem AC, Liu J, Nagy Z, Tournaye H, Devroey P (1995) High fertilization and pregnancy rate after intracytoplasmic sperm injection with spermatozoa obtained from testicle biopsy. Hum Reprod 10:148

379. Silva PD, Meisch J, Schauberger CW (1989) Intrauterine insemination of cryopreserved donor semen. Fertil Steril 52:243

380. Simoni M, Kamischke A, Nieschlag E (1998) Current status of the molecular diagnosis of Y-chromosomal microdeletions in the workup of male infertility. Hum Reprod 13:1764

381. Soffer Y, Golan A, Herman A, Pansky M, Caspi E, Ron-El R (1992) Prediction of in vitro fertilization outcome by sperm penetration assay with TEST-yolk buffer preincubation. Fertil Steril 58:556

382. Sokol RZ, Madding CI, Handelsman DJ, Swerdloff RS (1986) The split ejaculate: assessment of fertility potential using two in vitro test systems. Andrologia 18:380

383. Spandorfer SD, Avrech OM, Colombero LT, Palermo GD, Rosenwaks Z (1998) Effect of parental age on fertilization and pregnancy characteristics in couples treated by intracytoplasmic sperm injection. Hum Reprod 13:334

384. Stalf T, Sanchez R, Köhn FM, Schalles U, Kleinstein J, Hinz V, Tielsch J, Khanaga O, Turley H, Gips H, Schill WB (1995) Pregnancy and birth after intracytoplasmic sperm injection with spermatozoa from a patient with tail stump syndrome. Hum Reprod 10:2112

385. Steinberger E, Smith KD (1973) Artificial insemination with fresh or frozen semen. JAMA 223:778

386. Stone SC, de la Maza LM, Peterson EM (1986) Recovery of microorganisms from the pelvic cavity after intracervical or intrauterine artificial insemination. Fertil Steril 46:61

387. Stone S, O'Mahony F, Khalaf Y, Taylor A, Braude P (2000) A normal livebirth after intracytoplasmic sperm injection for globozoospermia without assisted oocyte activation. Hum Reprod 15:139

388. Sukcharoen N, Keith J, Irvine DS, Aitken RJ (1995) Predicting the fertilizing potential of human sperm suspensions in vitro: importance of sperm morphology and leukocyte contamination. Fertil Steril 63:1293

389. Sukcharoen N, Keith J, Irvine DS, Aitken RJ (1995) Definition of the optimal criteria for identifying hyperactivated human spermatozoa at 25 Hz using in-vitro fertilization as a functional end-point. Hum Reprod 10:2928

390. Suleiman SA, Elamin Ali M, Zaki ZMS, El-Malik EMA, Nasr MA (1996) Lipid peroxidation and human sperm motility: protective role of vitmanin E. J Androl 17:530

391. Suominen JJO, Kilkku PP, Taina EJ, Puntala PV (1991) Successful treatment of infertility due to retrograde ejaculation by instillation of serum-containing medium into the bladder. A case report. Int J Androl 14:87

392. Takahashi K, Wetzels AMM, Goverde HJM, Bastiaans BA, Janssen HJG, Rolland R (1992) The kinetics of the acrosome reaction of human spermatozoa and its correlation with in vitro fertilization. Fertil Steril 57:889

393. Takihara H, Cosentino MJ, Cockett AT (1983) Effect of low-dose androgen and zinc sulfate on sperm motility and seminal zinc levels in infertile men. Urology 22:160

394. Takihara H, Cosentino MJ, Cockett AT (1987) Zinc sulfate therapy for infertile male with or without varicocelectomy. Urology 29:638

395. Talbot P, Chacon R (1980) A new procedure for rapidly scoring acrosome reactions of human sperm. Gamete Res 3:211

396. Tarlatzis BC, Bontis J, Kolibianakis EM, Sanopoulou T, Papadimas J, Lagos S, Mantalenakis S (1991) Evaluation of intrauterine insemination with washed spermatozoa from the husband in the treatment of infertility. Hum Reprod 6:1241

397. Tasdemir M, Tasdemir I, Kodama H, Tanaka T (1993) Pentoxifylline-enhanced acrosome reaction correlates with fertilization in vitro. Hum Reprod 8:2102

398. Tasdemir I, Tasdemir M, Tavukcuoglu S, Kahraman S, Biberoglu K (1997) Effect of abnormal sperm head morphology on the outcome of intracytoplasmic sperm injection in humans. Hum Reprod 12:1214

399. Terquem A, Dadoune JP (1983) Aniline blue staining of human spermatozoa chromatin: evaluation of nuclear maturation. In: André J (ed) The sperm cell. Martinus Nijhoff, The Hague, pp 249–252

400. Tesarik J, Mendoza C (1993) Sperm treatment with pentoxifylline improves the fertilizing ability in patients with acrosome reaction insufficiency. Fertil Steril 60:141

401. Toner JP, Mossad H, Grow DR, Morshedi M, Swanson RJ, Oehninger S (1995) Value of sperm morphology assessed by strict criteria for prediction of the outcome of artificial (intrauterine) insemination. Andrologia 27:143

402. Töpfer-Petersen E, Völcker C, Heissler E, Schill WB (1987) Absence of acrosome reaction in polyzoospermia. Andrologia 19:225

403. Torode HW, Wheeler PA, Saunders DM, McPetrie RA, Medcalf SC, Ackerman VP (1987) The role of chlamydial antibodies in an in vitro fertilization program. Fertil Steril 48:987

404. Tournaye H, Clasen K, Aytoz A, Nagy Z, Van Steirteghem A, Devroey P (1998) Fine-needle aspiration versus open biopsy for testicular sperm recovery: a controlled study in azoospermic patients with normal spermatogenesis. Hum Reprod 13:901

405. Tournaye H, Merdad T, Silber S, Joris H, Verheyen G, Devroey P, Van Steirteghem A (1999) No differences in outcome after intracytoplasmic sperm injection with fresh or with frozen-thawed epididymal spermatozoa.. Hum Reprod 14:90

406. Troup SA, Lieberman BA, Matson PL (1994) The acrosome reaction to ionophore challenge test: assay reproducibility, effect of sexual abstinence and results of fertile men. Hum Reprod 20:2079

407. Tsirigotis M, Craft I (1995) Sperm retrieval methods and ICSI for obstructive azoospermia. Hum Reprod 10:758

408. Tummon IS, Gore-Langton RE, Daniel SAJ, Deutsch A (1991) Total acrosin activity correlates with fertility potential after fertilization in vitro. Fertil Steril 56:933

409. Tummon IS, Gore-Langton RE, Daniel SAJ, Squires PM, Koval JJ, Alsalili MB, Martin JSB, Kaplan BR, Nisker JA, Yuzpe AA (1995) Randomized trial of partial zona dissection for male infertility. Fertil Steril 63:842

410. Tur-Kaspa I, Dudkiewicz A, Confino E, Gleicher N (1990) Pooled sequential ejaculates: a way to increase the total number of motile sperm from oligozoospermic men. Fertil Steril 54:906

411. Uchida A, Takahashi K, Kitao M (1992) Usefulness of the hypo-osmotic swelling test for evaluation of human sperm fertilization. Hum Reprod 7:1264

412. Van Der Ven HH, Jeyendran RS, Perez-Pelaez M, Al-Hasani S, Diedrich K, Krebs D (1987) Leucospermia and the fertilizing capacity of spermatozoa. Eur J Obstetr Gynecol Reprod Biol 4:49

413. Van Ranst H, Bocken G, Desmet B, Joris H, Vankeleccm AS, Liu J, Nagy ZP, Van Steirteghem AC (1994) Chromatin condensation assessment in spermatozoa used for intracytoplasmic sperm injection. Hum Reprod 9 [Suppl 4]:24

414. Vazquez-Levin M, Kaplan P, Sandler B, Garrisi GJ, Gordon J, Navot D (1990) The predictive value of zona-free hamster egg sperm penetration assay for failure of human in vitro fertilization and subsequent successful zona drilling. Fertil Steril 53:1055

415. Verheyen G, De Croo I, Tournaye H, Pletincx I, Devroey P, Van Steirteghem AC (1995) Comparison of four mechanical methods to retrieve spermatozoa from testicular tissue. Hum Reprod 10:2956

416. Verheyen G, Tournaye H, Staessen C, De Vos A, Vandervorst M, Van Steirteghem A (1999) Controlled comparison of conventional in-vitro fertilization and intracytoplasmic sperm injection in patients with asthenozoospermia. Hum Reprod 14:2313

417. Vernon M, Wilson E, Muse K, Estes S, Curry T (1988) Successful pregnancies from men with retrograde ejaculation with the use of washed sperm and gamete intrafallopian tube transfer (GIFT). Fertil Steril 50:822

418. Vitali G, Parente R, Melotti C (1995) Carnitine supplementation in human idiopathic asthenospermia: clinical results. Drugs Exp Clin Res 21:157

419. Vogt PH (1995) Genetic aspects of human infertility. Int J Androl 18 [Suppl 2]:3

420. Vogt PH, Edelmann A, Kirsch S, Henegariu O, Hirschmann P, Kiesewetter F, Köhn FM, Schill WB, Farah S, Ramos C, Hartmann M, Hartschuh W, Meschede D, Behre HM, Castel A, Nieschlag E, Weidner W, Grone HJ, Jung A, Engel W, Haidl G (1996) Human Y chromosome azoospermia factors (AZF) mapped to different subregions in Yq 11. Hum Mol Genet 5:933

421. Volpe A, Artini PG, Coukos G, Uccelli E, Marchini E, Genazzani AR (1992) Sperm retrieval for direct intraperitoneal insemination in a diabetic man with retrograde ejaculation: a case report. J Reprod Med Obstet Gynecol 37:219

422. Wang C, Lee GS, Leung A, Surrey ES, Chan SYW (1993) Human sperm hyperactivation and acrosome reaction and their relationships to human in vitro fertilization. Fertil Steril 59:1221

423. Weidner W, Krause W, Schiefer HG, Brunner H, Friedrich HJ (1985) Ureaplasmal infections of the male urogenital tract, in particular prostatitis, and semen quality. Urol Int 40:5

424. Weidner W, Jantos C, Schiefer HG, Haidl G, Friedrich HJ (1991) Semen parameters in men with and without proven chronic prostatitis. Arch Androl 26:173

425. Weidner W, Madsen PO, Schiefer HG (1994) Prostatitis. Etiopathology, diagnosis and therapy. Springer, Berlin Heidelberg New York

426. Weidner W, Schroeder-Printzen I, Weiske WH, Haidl G and the BMFT Study Group for Microsurgery, Giessen (1995) Microsurgical aspects of the treatment of azoospermia. Int J Androl 18 [Suppl 2]:63

427. Wheeler JJ, Walter JS, Culkin DJ, Canning JR (1988) Idiopathic anejaculation treated by vibratory stimulation. Fertil Steril 50:377

428. World Health Organization Task Force on the Diagnosis and Treatment of Infertility (1989) Mesterolone and idiopathic male infertility: a double-blind study. Int J Androl 12:254

429. World Health Organization (1991) Impact of the environment on reproductive health. Report and recommendations of a WHO international workshop. Dan Med Bull 38:425

430. World Health Organization (1992) A double-blind trial of clomiphene citrate for the treatment of idiopathic male infertility. Int J Androl 15:299

431. World Health Organization (1993) WHO manual for the standardized investigation and diagnosis for the infertile couple. Cambridge University Press, Cambridge

432. World Health Organization (1999) WHO laboratory manual for the examination of human semen and sperm-cervical mucus interaction, 4th edn. Cambridge University Press, Cambridge

433. Wolf DP, Boldt J, Byrd W, Bechtol K (1985) Acrosomal status evaluation in human ejaculated sperm with monoclonal antibodies. Biol Reprod 32:1157

434. Wolff H (1995) The biologic significance of white blood cells in semen. Fertil Steril 63:1143

435. Wolff H, Anderson DJ (1988) Evaluation of granulocyte elastase as a seminal plasma marker for leukocytospermia. Fertil Steril 50:129

436. Wolff H, Bezold G, Zebhauser M, Meurer M (1991) Impact of clinically silent inflammation on male genital tract organs as reflected by biochemical markers in semen. J Androl 12:331

437. Wong PC, Balmaceda JP, Blanco JD, Gibbs RS, Asch RH (1986) Sperm washing and swim-up technique using antibiotics removes microbes from human semen. Fertil Steril 45:97

438. Yamamoto M, Miyake K (1994) Successful use of interferon for male infertility. The Lancet 344:614

439. Yamamoto M, Takaba H, Hashimoto J, Miyake K, Mitsuya H (1986) Successful treatment of oligozoospermic and azoospermic men with α1-blocker and β-stimulator: new treatment for idiopathic male infertility. Fertil Steril 46:1162

440. Yamamoto M, Hibi H, Katsuno S, Miyake K (1995) Human chorionic gonadotropin adjuvant therapy for patients with Leydig cell dysfunction after varicocelectomy. Arch Androl 35:49

441. Yamamoto M, Hibi H, Miyake K (1995) New treatment of idiopathic severe oligozoospermia with mast cell blocker: results of a single-blind study. Fertil Steril 64:1221
442. Yamamoto M, Hibi H, Miyake K, Fukugaki H, Suganuma N, Tomoda Y (1995) Bulk sperm collection by epididymal micropuncture and stimulation of the spermatic nerve: a novel method for sperm retrieval for IVF for surgically irreparable vasal obstruction. Int J Androl 18:97
443. Yanagimachi R, Yanagimachi H, Rogers BJ (1976) The use of zona-free animal ova as a test-system for the assessment of the fertilization capacity of human spermatozoa. Biol Reprod 15:471
444. Yang YS, Chen SU, Ho HN, Chen HF, Lien YR, Lin HR, Huang SC, Lee TY (1994) Acrosin activity of human sperm did not correlate with IVF. Arch Androl 32:13
445. Yang YS, Chen SU, Ho HN, Chen HF, Chao KH, Lin HR, Huang SC, Lee TY (1995) Correlation between sperm morphology using strict criteria in original semen and swim-up inseminate and human in vitro fertilization. Arch Androl 34:105
446. Yavetz H, Yogev L, Hauser R, Lessing JB, Paz G, Homonnai ZT (1994) Retrograde ejaculation. Hum Reprod 9:381
447. Yemini M, Vanderzwalmen P, Mukaida T, Schoengold S, Birkenfeld A (1995) Intracytoplasmic sperm injection, fertilization, and embryo transfer after retrieval of spermatozoa by testicular biopsy from an azoospermic male with testicular tubular atrophy. Fertil Steril 63:1118
448. Yovich JM, Edirisinghe WR, Yovich JL (1994) Use of the acrosome reaction to ionophore challenge test in managing patients in an assisted reproduction program: a prospective, double blind, randomized controlled study. Fertil Steril 61:902
449. Yue Z, Meng FJ, Jorgensen N, Ziebe S, Nyboe Andersen A (1995) Sperm morphology using strict criteria after Percoll density separation: influence on cleavage and pregnancy rates after in-vitro fertilization. Hum Reprod 10:1781
450. Zaneveld LJR, De Jonge CJ, Anderson RA, Mack SR (1991) Human sperm capacitation and acrosome reaction. Hum Reprod 6:1265
451. Zaneveld LJD, Jeyendran RS (1992) Sperm function tests. In: Overstreet JW (ed) Male infertility. Saunders, Philadelphia, pp 353–371 (Infertility and reproductive medicine clinics of North America)
452. Zini A, DeLamirande E, Gagnon C (1993) Reactive oxygen species in semen of infertile patients: levels of superoxide dismutase- and catalase-like activities in seminal plasma and spermatozoa. Int J Androl 16:183

Mammalian Sex Preselection: Flow-cytometric Sorting of X and Y Spermatozoa Based on DNA Difference

L. A. Johnson, G. R. Welch

Introduction

The sex of one's offspring has occupied the imagination of mankind ever since the beginning of modern civilization. Theories abound as to how one can alter the sex of offspring. Early philosophers suggested that various body positions during intercourse could produce a child of one sex or the other. Still others suggested that parts of the male genital anatomy produced sperm specific to one particular sex. In mammals, X-chromosome-bearing sperm produce female offspring and Y-chromosome-bearing sperm produce male offspring, always in nearly equal numbers (50:50). Numerous investigations in animals have resulted in a significant body of literature on the skewing of this ratio. Claims for skewing of the sex ratio are commonplace, yet little if any verification has been offered to support them. Many of these protocols use one or more of the physical sperm measurements (size, shape, swimming speed, surface antigen, etc.) as the marker specific for X or Y sperm. A separation technique is then performed based on this "specific marker". None of the protocols based on these proposed markers of X or Y sperm has been shown to skew the sex ratio to any extent. The reader is guided to reviews which describe many of the "physical separation methods" in more detail than is possible here (Kiddy and Hafs 1971, Amann and Seidel 1982, Gledhill 1988, Johnson 1994, 1995).

Sex Preselection in Agriculturally Important Species

Controlling the sex of offspring through sperm separation is a valuable tool for the livestock producer. Males of high genetic merit can be more efficiently selected in order to propagate a large pool of offspring with improved genetic merit. Further, sex preselection offers the producer an important economic advantage, since better control of his or her product helps to maximize production efficiency. Since growth rate is sex-linked, preselecting the sex of cattle, swine, and sheep gives greater economic return to the producer, depending on the market. Controlling the sex of offspring in livestock has served as the impetus for developing a successful method of sex preselection. There are many instances where research on domestic animals for economic reasons has provided the foundation for the success of those biotechnologies in human application. Sex control is one of these areas, intracytoplasmic sperm injection is another. It also works in reverse, in that the first significant use of in vitro fertilization occurred in human beings, and the technique has now been applied in many animal species.

Sex Predetermination of Human Offspring

There is interest in the development of sex selection in human beings in conjunction with genetic testing for couples who risk transmitting a sex-linked disease to their offspring. There are approximately 6000 heritable defects in man. About 370 of these defects are known to be X-linked (McKusik 1992). Generally, the X-linked recessive disorders are expressed by the male child of carrier mothers who have inherited the X-chromosome with the defective gene. Common examples of X-linked recessives include hemophilia, Duchenne's muscular dystrophy, and X-linked hydrocephalus. Thus a female child would not express the X-linked recessive disorder in the majority of cases. In addition, there is the more controversial interest: that of preselecting the sex of offspring to maintain cultural traditions or for purposes of family balancing. It can be assumed that as long as civilization exists, the use of sex predetermination for these cosmetic reasons will engender controversy. However, we must also assume that if a method exists, people will desire to use it, irrespective of the social mores that may govern that aspect of family life and, to some extent, irrespective of the credibility of the method to do what it says it will do in terms of skewing the sex ratio. Evidence can be drawn from the use of the albumin-gradient semen sexing method (Ericsson et al. 1973) by those seeking some form of control over the sex of their offspring. Beernink et al. (1993) reported more than 500 births using this method in clinical circumstances, about 75% male. The method is based on swimming speed, the hypothesis being that Y sperm swim faster than X sperm. Scientific validation of the method is still not forthcoming, however. Actually, the most recent evidence using chromosome or DNA flow-sorting probe data suggests there is no reason to believe that there is any skewing of the sex ratio (Brandriff et al. 1986, Flaherty and Matthews 1996). The use of a more scientifically valid method, such as the DNA method reported in this paper, enhances the credibility of the use of sex predetermination in human beings but does not still the controversy associated with the use of sex preselection in man. A detailed description of the authors' method (Johnson et al. 1989) as adapted to high-speed cell-sorting instrumentation has recently been published (Johnson and Welch 1999).

DNA Difference as a Basis for Separating X and Y Sperm

Individual X- and Y-chromosome-bearing sperm carry DNA in constant amounts, characteristic of whether they are X or Y. The difference in X and Y sperm DNA is the only scientifically validated and measurable difference between X- and Y-chromosome-bearing sperm in mammals. Visual examination of the Y-chromosome illustrates its small size in comparison to the larger X-chromosome (Johnson and Clarke 1990). Autosomes, on the other hand, are also carried by both X- and Y-bearing sperm but are identical in DNA content. Thus the difference in X and Y sperm DNA is, for all practical purposes, the only difference between X and Y sperm. This fact attracted the attention of several investigators working with flow cytometry (Gledhill et al. 1976). They sought to measure the amount of DNA for purposes of monitoring mutational changes in human sperm. Their work showed, among other things, that there was an artifact associated with measuring DNA in sperm due to the differential fluorescence caused by sperm head shape. Advances in flow cytometry since those initial studies have made the analysis of cells in liquid suspension increasingly more sophisticated. Consistent with these advances have been those in the development and utilization of fluorochromes to identify various organelles within the cell. The primary challenge to be overcome in the DNA artifact was to orient the sperm head to the laser beam (Dean et al. 1978) so that the inherent variability associated with morphology (orientation artifact) and its influence on flow within a stream of fluid could be accounted for. Because of the small difference in DNA content (3–4%) between X and Y sperm, the differentiation of X and Y sperm in a sample of semen is difficult and requires that the coefficient of variation be reduced to about 1–1.5%.

Measurement of DNA in Sperm Heads for Analysis and Flow Sorting

Commercial flow cytometry/cell sorters provide the only alternative for measuring sperm DNA on a wider scale. The first commercial sorter to be adapted for sperm, using the beveled needle system to orient the sperm, was reported by Johnson and Pinkel (1986), who showed that commercial flow cytometry/cell sorter instrumentation (EPICS V; Coulter Corporation, Miami, Fla.) could be successfully modified, making it capable of overcoming the orientation artifact and routinely measuring the difference in X and Y sperm DNA. The modified system led to the use of that instrumentation for routine sperm DNA analysis (Johnson et al. 1987a,b, Welch and Johnson 1999). More importantly, from a method development standpoint, it led to the sorting of sperm heads that maintained their ability to fertilize eggs (Johnson and Clarke 1988, Johnson 1995). The shape and the compact chromatin structure within the nucleus require specialized staining procedures. The differentiating of small DNA variations for purposes of separation requires ideal conditions in terms of stain type and processing. The Hoechst 33 342 stain was found to provide excellent permeability and specific binding to DNA (Johnson 1984), bringing improved uniformity of staining and cleaner separation of the bimodal X and Y peak (Fig. 1). Not only was it superior in staining uniformity; it also penetrated the sperm membrane very readily and faster than any other stain. A multitude of stains have been tested in succeeding years for this specific application, but none have come close to displacing Hoechst 33 342 as the stain of choice for this application. This discovery was followed by improved stain

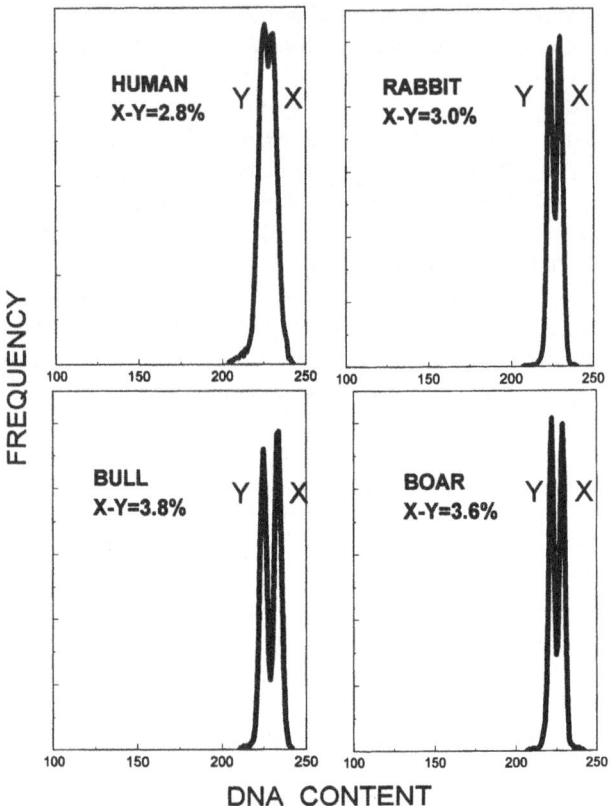

Fig. 1. Histograms representing frequency distributions of X and Y sperm for several species. Sperm from each species carry a different amount of DNA according to their X and Y chromosome content, and thus the differential DNA content between X and Y is also different. The depth of the split between the bimodal peaks is an indication of the ease at which the particular species X and Y sperm can be sorted into separate populations. In this grouping, human sperm have the smallest difference and are the most difficult to sort into separate populations at high purity. (Modified from Johnson 1995)

and preparation protocols (Johnson et al. 1987a) that resulted in fertilization using intracytoplasmic sperm injection (ICSI) of sorted sperm nuclei (Johnson and Clarke 1988). This work demonstrated that sperm treated with Hoechst 33342 stain and put through the sorting process could form pronuclei in hamster eggs, thus showing that the DNA of the sperm could withstand the effects of the staining and sorting process.

Successful Development of a Method to Sort Viable X and Y Sperm

Success with sperm nuclei, and the finding that staining intact sperm could be accomplished relatively rapidly without compromising viability, led to the development of a method to flow-sort intact, viable X and Y sperm that were functionally sound, so as to carry out normal fertilization and to produce normal offspring. A key part of this process was the finding that sperm with their tails intact (Johnson et al. 1989) could indeed be sorted into separate populations with 80–90% purity of X and Y sperm. This finding overturned the previously held view that only sperm heads could be oriented well enough to sort (Pinkel et al. 1982, Johnson and Pinkel 1986, Johnson and Clarke 1988).

The rabbit was chosen as the first experimental animal in which to demonstrate the skewing of the sex ratio (Johnson et al. 1989). This initial study involved the staining of the living sperm DNA with Hoechst 33342, flow-sorting of the stained X and Y sperm based on the fact that they differ in DNA content by about 3.0% (specific for the rabbit), and the subsequent insemination of the sorted sperm into the tip of the uterus via surgical means. Litters resulting from insemination of X-bearing sperm were 94% female. Correspondingly, the litters resulting from insemination of Y bearing sperm were 81% male. The validity of this DNA sexing method was further demonstrated with the production of litters of pigs that showed a skewing of the sex ratio (Johnson 1991). Swine X and Y sperm differ in DNA content by about 3.6%, which should have made the skewing of the sex ratio of the resulting litters easier to achieve than was the case in the rabbit. This was not the case, however, in that females averaged 74% while males averaged 68%. We found that swine sperm do not orient themselves to the laser beam as well as rabbit sperm, for example, and consequently in this initial study it was more difficult to achieve a high purity of X or Y sperm in the respective sorts used for surgical insemination. Since then, however, we have improved the sorting of the swine sperm, so that 95% skewing of the sex ratio can easily be achieved using our standard protocols (Johnson et al. 1999).

Since these initial demonstration studies, the usefulness of the DNA sexing method, termed the Beltsville Sperm Sexing Technology for producing offspring, particularly in combination with in vitro fertilization (IVF), has also been demonstrated in cattle. The initial study with cattle (Cran et al. 1993) produced six calves, all of the predicted sex. The second study, a field trial designed to produce male calves from sorted Y sperm, produced 41 calves from 106 embryo transfers. Of the 41 calves, 37 were male, equivalent to a 90% skewing of the sex ratio (Cran et al. 1995). We have also sought to adapt the DNA sexing method to swine using IVF. The methodology of IVF is not as well developed for swine as it is for cattle. However, we have demonstrated in an initial study (Rath et al. 1997) that one can effectively produce females from IVF embryos produced from X sperm sorted for high purity (>90%). Ten pigs (all female) were born from two sows in whom embryos had been produced from X-sorted sperm and transferred surgically. Unassisted fertilization with viable and intact X or Y sperm, flow-cytometrically sorted on the basis of DNA content difference, was the final confirmation of the validity of the DNA-based method for sex preselection. The DNA sexing method for intracervical insemination shows promise for application in numerous livestock situations if the numbers of sperm required for fertilization can be reduced. A total of 2×10^5 sperm has proven effective with cattle when used with deep uterine insemination (Seidel et al. 1997). Extensive field trials have now been conducted using sexed sperm in cattle (Seidel et al. 1999) and demonstrate the widespread efficacy of the technology in combination with artificial insemination.

Flow-cytometric Sorting of Human Sperm

Although the sperm sexing method described above was developed for livestock sperm, it has wide application to other mammalian species (Fig. 2). Any mammal carrying about 2.5% or greater amounts of DNA in the X sperm than in the Y sperm has the inherent potential for sorting into nearly pure X and Y sperm populations. In 1993 we reported (Johnson et al. 1993) the results of studies in which we were able to demonstrate the feasibility of using this tech-

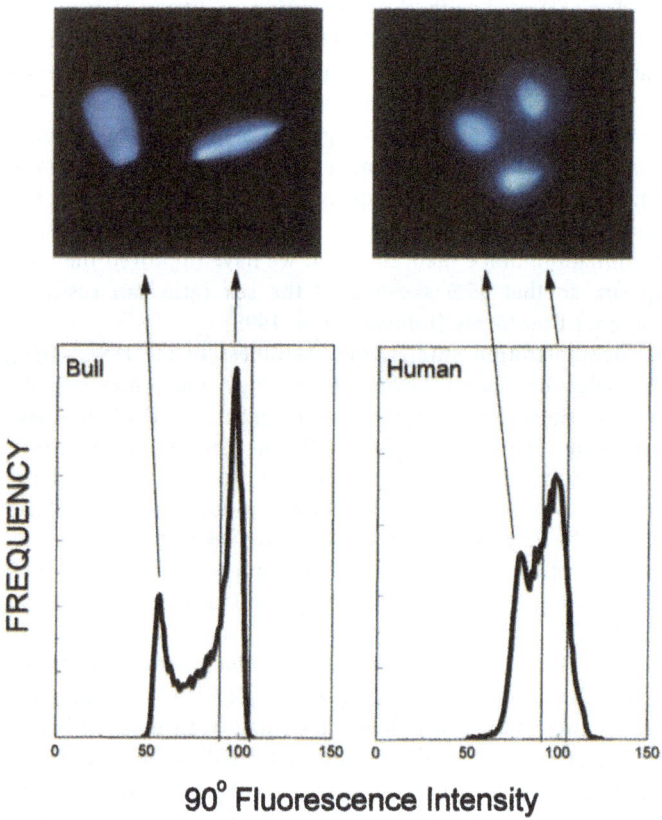

Fig. 2. Histograms from the bull and the human being demonstrate the population of sperm that orient properly. Sperm falling within the *lined gates* are properly oriented and correspond to the edge of the sperm, as shown in the respective pictures. *Left*, bull sperm heads; *right*, human sperm heads. Note that each demonstrates the brighter fluorescence from the edge of the sperm head

nology for human sperm, particularly for those couples who were at risk for transmitting a sex-linked genetic disease. The Genetics and IVF Institute in Fairfax, Va., collaborated on this project. By adapting the sorting technology to a somewhat higher level of detection, we were able to repeatedly sort the X and Y human sperm into separate populations. Human sperm is somewhat more difficult to sort to high purity because the X sperm carries only about 2.8% more DNA than the Y sperm. Our studies showed that we could repeatedly separate X sperm to 82% purity and Y sperm to 76% purity (Johnson et al. 1993). In these studies we were interested more in proving that it could be done than in achieving the highest purity. Fine tuning of the protocols may lead to still higher purities of X or Y human sperm (Fugger et al. 1998).

Fluorescence In Situ Hybridization (FISH) to Validate Human X and Y Sperm

In livestock semen sexing work we have always used "sort reanalysis" (Welch and Johnson 1999) of the sperm populations for DNA to determine the proportions of final sorted X or Y sperm. In man, however, the X and Y DNA difference is so small (2.8%) that it is difficult to consistently reanalyze the sorted sperm with unquestioned accuracy. We thus decided to test the sorting system using FISH technology in combination with microsatellite DNA probes (Johnson et al. 1993, Leif et al. 1971). In this study we used both X and Y probes to eliminate the possibility of counting false positives. The FISH technology has proved to be an effective method for assessing the proportions of X and Y sperm (Vidal et al. 1998). It also compares favorably with sort reanalysis (Kawarasaki et al. 1998, Welch and Johnson 1999) and PCR of single sperm (Welch et al. 1995). Validation of a sorted X or Y sperm population before using it to produce embryos by IVF for transfer or by insemination intracervically, intratubally, or into the uterus is essential to knowing the outcome. Using these monitoring techniques one can avoid the expense and consequences of the undesired sex.

Following the initial demonstration that human sperm could be separated into X and Y populations based on DNA difference (Johnson et al. 1993) and flow-cytometric cell sorting, clinical trials were initiated using this technology (now called MicroSort when used in human beings). The success of this application was reported by Fugger et al. (1998), when initial clinical trial results were published showing the skewing of the offspring sex ratio from 50% female to 92% female when sperm sorted for the X chromosome were used for impregnation. This landmark work has produced more than 50 births of healthy normal children (Fugger 1999). The sorting technology applied to human beings is termed MicroSort, and it is being used in continued clinical trials to produce offspring in families seeking to avoid X-linked disease and for families seeking to balance the sex of their children.

Flow-cytometric Sorting of Sperm Based on DNA:
Beltsville Sperm Sexing Technology

Effective sperm sorting is dependent on a combination of factors. Among them are uniformity of staining, orientation of the sperm head to the laser beam, and maintenance of conditions to ensure the viability of the sperm. Mammalian sperm come in all shapes and sizes; generally, all stain quite readily with a DNA-specific fluorochrome. Our development work for the Beltsville DNA sexing method began in 1982. The purpose for doing the research was to enhance the efficiency of producing livestock that are used for human consumption and to provide the consumer with a higher quality product. Therefore, the development work was done with domestic animal sperm, most of which have a flat, paddle-shaped head. The paddle-shaped head is ovoid, about 3–4 µm wide, 8–10 µm long, and 0.3–0.4 µm thick. Once the method had been proven, we chose to apply the technology to human sperm. Human sperm have a more angular head shape and appear not to have the definitive edge seen in the sperm of many domestic animals, especially the livestock species (bovine, porcine, ovine, equine, lagomorph). Once we had established that the human sperm also exhibited differential fluorescence between the flat, though angular, head (Fig. 2) and a less defined edge, we were able to optimize and fine-tune the flow-sorting system to also measure human X and Y sperm DNA. Differential fluorescence is due to preferential emission of light in the plane of the sperm head (from the edge), which is caused by a difference in refractive index between the sperm head and the surrounding medium (Fig. 3). The orientation, as mentioned earlier, is critical to resolving the small differences in DNA found between X and Y sperm in most mammalian species.

The instrumentation modifications for the DNA sexing method are shown in Fig. 3. This illustration is of a flow cytometer/cell sorter modified specifically for sperm DNA analysis and flow sorting (Johnson and Pinkel 1986). The modification consists of installing a beveled needle in place of the standard cylindrical needle, and then replacing the more typical light-scatter detector (positioned in the forward or 0° position in relation to the laser beam) with another fluorescence detector (Johnson and Pinkel 1986), similar to the fluorescence detector found at the 90° position in relation to the laser beam. We have recently found a more effective means of orienting sperm. Rens et al. (1998) showed the effectiveness of using an orienting nozzle in place of the beveled needle. This increases the percentage of sperm that are oriented by a factor of 2–3. We have also adapted this improved nozzle to the high-speed sorting system (Johnson et al. 1999). The modification of the flow cytometer/cell sorter is essential for attaining separate populations of X- and Y-chromosome-bearing sperm based on DNA content difference, and for reanalyzing sorted sperm to determine the proportions of X or Y sperm in a given sorted sample (Johnson et al. 1987b, 1989).

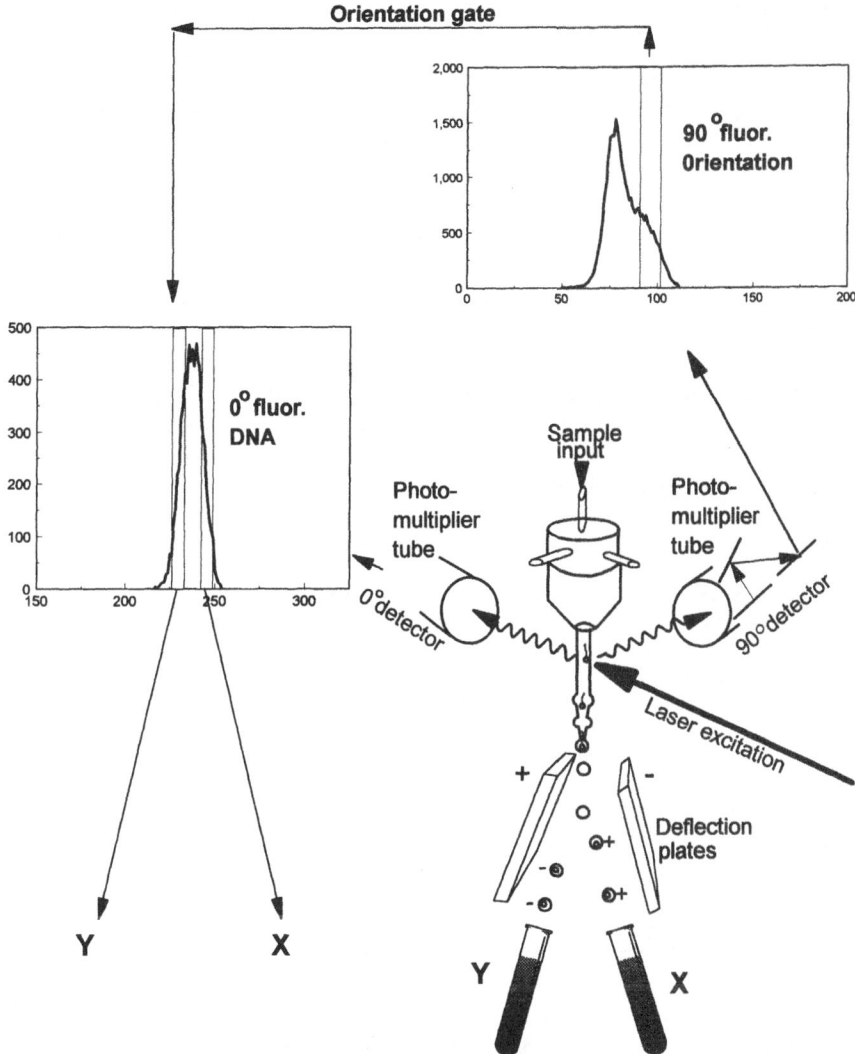

Fig. 3. The flow cytometry/cell sorting system that has been modified specifically for the analysis of sperm DNA as well as for the sorting of sperm into X and Y populations. The system includes a sample injection needle that is beveled at the exit orifice so that fluid will exit the needle in a flat stream, rather than in the cylindrical stream common to most flow systems. The system also contains the additional fluorescence detector in the forward or 0° position. The presence of both of these modifications allows the sperm to be selected on the basis of its orientation to the laser beam. Properly oriented sperm show their edge to the 90° detector and the flat face to the 0° detector. Those sperm falling within the orientation gate are then seen by the 0° detector. Sperm are sorted (within a droplet) to respective tubes for insemination. Sperm sorted for FISH determination are sorted onto slides. (Modified from Johnson 1995)

High-speed Sorting for Improved Production of Sexed Sperm

Separation of X and Y sperm by flow-cytometric sorting is accomplished on a sperm-by-sperm basis. This leads to inherent limits as to the rate of production of X and Y populations. Under the constraints of flow-cytometric sorting, sorting rates have recently been increased by the introduction of commercially available, high-speed cell sorters. Soon after their introduction in 1996, we modified a high-speed cell sorter, MoFlo (Cytomation Inc., Ft. Collins, Colo.), for sperm sorting based on our earlier reports (Johnson and Pinkel 1986). With the standard-speed sorters typical production rates were in the area of 350 000 sperm/h; with the high-speed system we are producing 6 million each of X and Y sperm/h under routine sorting conditions (Johnson et al. 1999, Johnson and Welch 1999). This system is also equipped with the improved orienting nozzle or tip (Rens et al. 1998; Fig. 4). Sort purities continue to be 90% or higher for each sex. We have used the system on many species, and it works effectively for all sperm including human (L.A. Johnson and G.R. Welch, unpublished data).

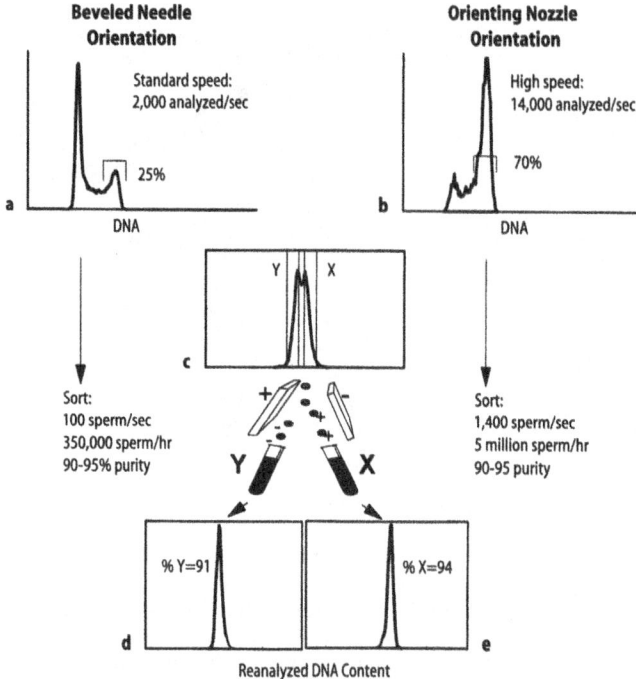

Fig. 4a–e. Two advances in sperm-sorting technology produce a 10- to 15-fold increase in sorting efficiency. (a) Standard-speed cell sorter analyzes about 2000 sperm/s, of which about 20–30% are properly oriented for DNA analysis (c). (b) High-speed sorting analyzes about 20 000 sperm/s, of which 60–70% are properly oriented for DNA analysis. In both cases X and Y sperm of about 90% purity (d, e) are collected, but at rates of 6–10 million/h for the orienting nozzle under high-speed conditions vs 350 000/h

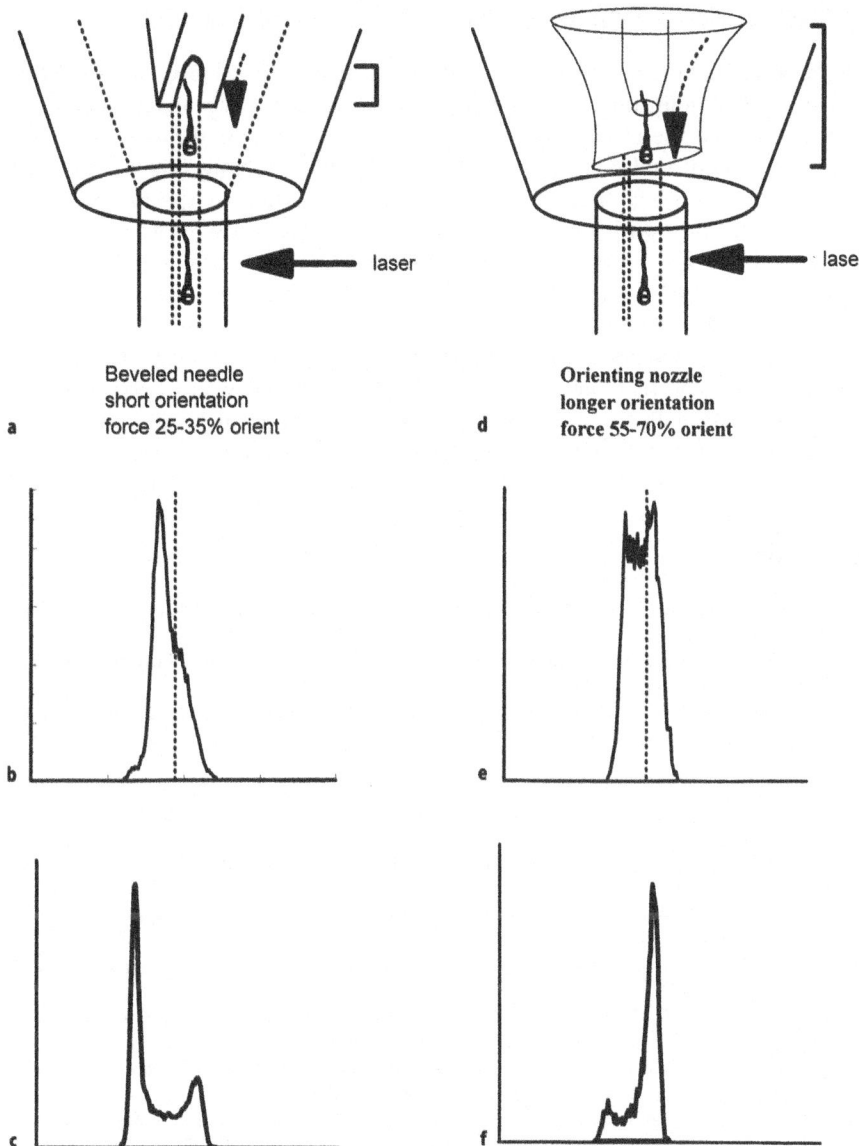

Fig. 5 a–f. Fluid forces are used to properly orient the sperm head to the laser beam to enable the resolution of X and Y sperm. Two methods of applying a fluid-orienting force have been used. The first (**a**) involved injecting the sperm into the flow stream through a beveled needle, which created a ribbon-shaped sample core stream. The beveled needle provided enough force at the point of laser interrogation to orient only 25–35% of the sperm, depending on the species (**b** human, **c** bull). The more recently developed orienting nozzle (**d**) creates a force which acts on the sperm lower in its assembly, closer to the point of laser interrogation, thus orienting 50–70% of the sperm, again depending on the species (**e** human, **f** bull)

Protocol for Flow-cytometric Sorting of X and Y Human Sperm

The protocol for human semen is based on procedures developed earlier (Johnson et al. 1989, Johnson 1991, Johnson et al. 1993). Numerous adaptations must be made for the use of high-speed sorting, since sperm pass through the sorter much faster than under conditions of standard speed sorting (Fig. 5). Detailed protocols for livestock sperm that can be applied to human sperm have been presented recently with respect to high-speed sorting (Johnson and Welch 1999), and specific protocols for human sperm sorting using standard-speed sorting (MicroSort) under clinical conditions have also been published (Fugger et al. 1998; Fugger 1999).

The methods described in this paper require a significant degree of understanding and expertise due to the sophisticated technology involved. However, once familiarity with the protocol is achieved, separation of X and Y mammalian sperm by flow-cytometric sorting can be done on a routine basis.

References

Amann RP, Seidel GE (eds) (1982) Prospects for sexing mammalian sperm. Colorado University Press, Boulder

Beernink FJ, Dmowski WP, Ericsson RJ (1993) Sex preselection through albumin separation of sperm. Fertil Steril 59:382–386

Brandriff BF, Gordon LA, Haendel S, Singer S, Moore DH, Gledhill BL (1986) Sex chromosome ratios determined by karyotypic analysis in albumin-isolated human sperm. Fertil Steril 46:678–685

Cran DG, Johnson LA, Miller NGA, Cochrane D, Polge C (1993) Production of bovine calves following separation of X- and Y-chromosome bearing sperm and in vitro fertilisation. Vet Rec 132:40–41

Cran DG, Johnson LA, Polge C (1995) Sex preselection in cattle: a field trial. Vet Rec 136:495–496

Dean PN, Pinkel D, Mendelsohn ML (1978) Hydrodynamic orientation of sperm heads for flow cytometry. Biophys J 23:7–13

Ericsson RJ, Langevin CN, Nishino M (1973) Isolation of fractions rich in human Y sperm. Nature 246:421–424

Flaherty S, Mathews J, Mathews CD (1996) Application of modern molecular techniques to evaluate sperm sex selection methods. Mol Hum Reprod 2:937–942

Fugger EF (1999) Clinical experience with flow cytometric separation of X-and Y-chromosome bearing sperm in humans. Theriogenology 52:1435–1440

Fugger EF, Black SH, Keyvanfar K, Schulman JD (1998) Births of normal daughters after MicroSort sperm separation and intrauterine insemination, in vitro fertilization, or intracytoplasmic sperm injection. Hum Reprod 13:2367–2370

Gledhill BL (1988) Gender preselection: historical, technical, and ethical perspectives. Semin Reprod Endocrinol 6:385–395

Gledhill BL, Lake S, Steinmetz LL, Gray JW, Crawford JR, Dean PN, Van Dilla MA (1976) Flow microfluorometric analysis of sperm DNA content: effect of cell shape on the fluorescence distribution. J Cell Physiol 87:367–376

Johnson LA (1984) Relative DNA content of X and Y chromosome-bearing chinchilla and porcine spermatozoa stained with Hoechst 33342. Proc 10th Int. Conf Analyt Cytol A-11. Soc for Analyt Cytol, Breckenridge, Colo

Johnson LA (1991) Sex preselection in swine: altered sex ratios in offspring following surgical insemination of flow sorted X- and Y-bearing sperm. Reprod Domest Anim 26:309–314

Johnson LA (1994) Isolation of X- and Y-bearing sperm for sex preselection. In: Charlton HH (ed) Oxford Reviews of Reproductive Biology 16:303–326, Oxford University Press, Oxford, UK

Johnson LA (1995) Sex preselection by flow cytometric separation of X and Y-chromosome-bearing sperm based on DNA difference: a review. Reprod Fertil Dev 7:1–11

Johnson LA, Clarke RN (1988) Flow sorting of X- and Y-chromosome-bearing mammalian sperm: activation and pronuclear development of sorted bull, boar and ram sperm microinjected into hamster oocytes. Gamete Res 21:335–343

Johnson LA, Clarke RN (1990) Sperm DNA and sex chromosome differences between two geographical populations of the creeping vole, Microtus oregoni. Mol Reprod Dev 27:159–162

Johnson LA, Pinkel D (1986) Modification of a laser-based flow cytometer for high-resolution DNA analysis of mammalian spermatozoa. Cytometry 7:268–273

Johnson LA, Welch GR (1999) Sex preselection: high-speed flow cytometric sorting of X and Y sperm for maximum efficiency. Theriogenology 52:1323–1341

Johnson LA, Flook JP, Look MV (1987a) Flow cytometry of X- and Y-chromosome-bearing sperm for DNA using an improved preparation method and staining with Hoechst 33 342. Gamete Res 17:203–212

Johnson LA, Flook JP, Look MV, Pinkel D (1987b) Flow sorting of X- and Y-chromosome-bearing spermatozoa into two populations. Gamete Res 16:1–9

Johnson LA, Flook JP, Hawk HW (1989) Sex preselection in rabbits: live births from X and Y sperm separated by DNA and cell sorting. Biol Reprod 41:199–203

Johnson LA, Welch GR, Keyvanfar K, Dorfmann A, Fugger EF, Schulman JD (1993) Gender preselection in humans? Flow cytometric separation of X and Y spermatozoa for the prevention of X-linked diseases. Hum Reprod 8:1733–1739

Johnson LA, Welch GR, Rens W (1999) The Beltsville sperm sexing technology: high-speed sperm sorting gives improved sperm output for in vitro fertilization and AI. J Anim Sci 77:213–220

Kawarasaki T, Welch GR, Long CR, Yoshida M, Johnson LA (1998) Verification of flow cytometrically-sorted X- and Y-bearing porcine spermatozoa and reanalysis of spermatozoa for DNA content using the fluorescence in situ hybridization (FISH) technique. Theriogenology 50:625–635

Kiddy CA, Hafs HD (eds) (1971) Sex ratio at birth – prospects for control. J Anim Sci Symp-Suppl Am Soc Anim Sci, Champaign, Ill

Leif RC, Easter HM, Warters RL, Thomas RA, Dunlap LA (1971) I. A quantitative technique for the preparation of glutaraldehyde-fixed cells for the light and scanning electron microscope. J Histochem Cytochem 19:203–215

McKusick VA (1992) Mendelian inheritance in man. Johns Hopkins University Press, Baltimore, Md.

Pinkel D, Gledhill BL, Van Dilla MA, Stephenson D, Watchmaker G (1982) High-resolution DNA measurements of mammalian sperm. Cytometry 3:1–9

Rath D, Johnson LA, Dobrinsky JR, Welch GR, Niemann H (1997) Production of piglets preselected for sex following in vitro fertilization with X- and Y-chromosome-bearing spermatozoa sorted by flow cytometry. Theriogenology 47:795–800

Rens W, Welch GR, Johnson LA (1998) A novel nozzle for more efficient sperm orientation to improve sorting efficiency of X- and Y-chromosome-bearing sperm. Cytometry 33:476–481

Seidel GE Jr, Allen CH, Johnson LA, Holland MD, Brink Z, Welch GR, Graham JE, Cattell MB (1997) Uterine horn insemination of heifers with very low numbers of nonfrozen and sexed spermatozoa. Theriogenology 48:1255–1265

Seidel GE Jr, Schenk JL, Herickhoff LA, Doyle SP, Brink Z, Green RD, Cran DG (1999) Insemination of heifers with sexed sperm. Theriogenology 52:1407–1420

Vidal F, Fugger EF, Blanco J (1998) Efficiency of MicroSort flow cytometry for producing sperm populations enriched in X- or Y-chromosome haplotypes: a blind trial assessed by double and triple colour fluorescence in-situ-hybridization. Hum Reprod 13:308–312

Welch GR, Johnson LA (1999) Sex preselection: laboratory validation of the sperm sex ratio of flow sorted X and Y sperm by sort reanalysis for DNA. Theriogenology 52:1343–1352

Welch GR, Waldbieser GC, Wall RJ, Johnson LA (1995) Flow cytometric sperm sorting and PCR to confirm separation of X- and Y-chromosome-bearing bovine sperm. Anim Biotechnol 6:131–139

Assessment of Oocyte and Early Embryo Morphology with Regard to Embryonic Development and the Outcome of Assisted Reproduction

A. Herrler, H. M. Beier

Evaluation of Oocytes and the Cumulus-Oocyte Complex

Ovarian hormone stimulation is accompanied in most assisted reproduction therapies by the monitoring of follicular growth using ultrasonographic investigations. In addition, the amount of estrogen and luteinizing hormone in peripheral blood plasma is assessed to determine the optimal time for ovulation induction. The therapeutic goal is to achieve an appropriate number of mature oocytes, for example, for in vitro fertilization or intracytoplasmic sperm injection (ICSI), because these seem to guarantee superior-quality embryos. However, well-monitored ovarian stimulation does not necessarily always guarantee mature oocytes. Since no reliable biochemical tests are available to assess follicular fluid components in the punctured fluid material, direct microscopic assessment of the morphology of the oocytes remains the most practical and promising method of evaluation. This assessment leads to a scoring of the oocyte and the resulting embryos, which bears a relation to the subsequent pregnancies. The use of a widely accepted score and photo/video documentation would be an accurate base for a comparison between different laboratories. The cumulus-oocyte complex, which has to be seen as a functional unit, contains the cumulus cells, the densely packed corona radiata cells, and the oocyte itself with the zona pellucida (Fig. 1).

The Cumulus Oophorus

The cumulus cells are the follicular epithelial cells released from the follicle by the process of ovulation together with the oocyte. The innermost layer of cells directly surrounding the oocyte are referred to as "corona radiata". These are densely packed epithelial cells. The surrounding cumulus shows a typical appearance in relation to the maturity of the oocyte and has to be assessed separately, as its function differs from that of the corona radiata.

Characteristic of immature oocytes is a dense cumulus, sometimes appearing very dark under the microscope, hiding the oocyte. The most favorable appearance of a "mature" cumulus-oocyte complex shows all signs of "dissociation": the follicular cells (synonym: granulosa cells) are expanded as single cells in a wide network of matrix filaments. The more pronounced this dissociation is,

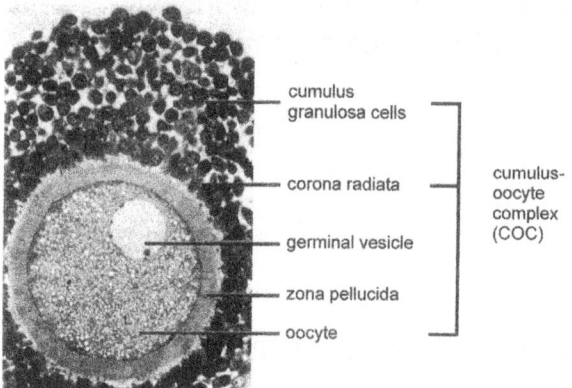

Fig. 1. Structure of a cumulus-oocyte complex. Semi-thin section, light microscopy

the more mature is the oocyte for fertilization. Because the granulosa cells lose contact they become apoptotic, as sometimes visible under light microscopy (Fig. 2e). These cells become dense and dark, located as clumps within a mass of extracellular matrix.

The corona radiata has to be assessed separately. These cells are closely associated with the oocyte and the zona pellucida during the entire period of development. They influence directly the cytoplasmic and nuclear maturation of the oocyte (see also Küpker and Diedrich, this volume). During development one can distinguish either a tightly packed corona radiata or a process of slight loosening of the corona cells, although they remain apposed to the oocyte. In old or overmature oocytes, some corona cells are still present at the zona pellucida while most of them have been pinched off. In these oocytes further maturation is impossible.

The Oocyte

When the cumulus is beginning its dissociation, the oocyte can be seen under the microscope. Three distinct morphological structures can be assessed: the nucleus, the ooplasm, and the zona pellucida. In addition, particular attention should be paid to the polar body, as it develops in parallel to the meiosis. During meiosis the oocyte is arrested in prophase I (until peak gonadotropin release), and later at metaphase II (until fertilization). As can be demonstrated very clearly, the oocyte therefore displays the following morphological parameters:

- No polar body and a germinal vesicle (prophase I, first block)
- No polar body and no nucleus (metaphase I)
- Extrusion of the first polar body (metaphase II, second block).

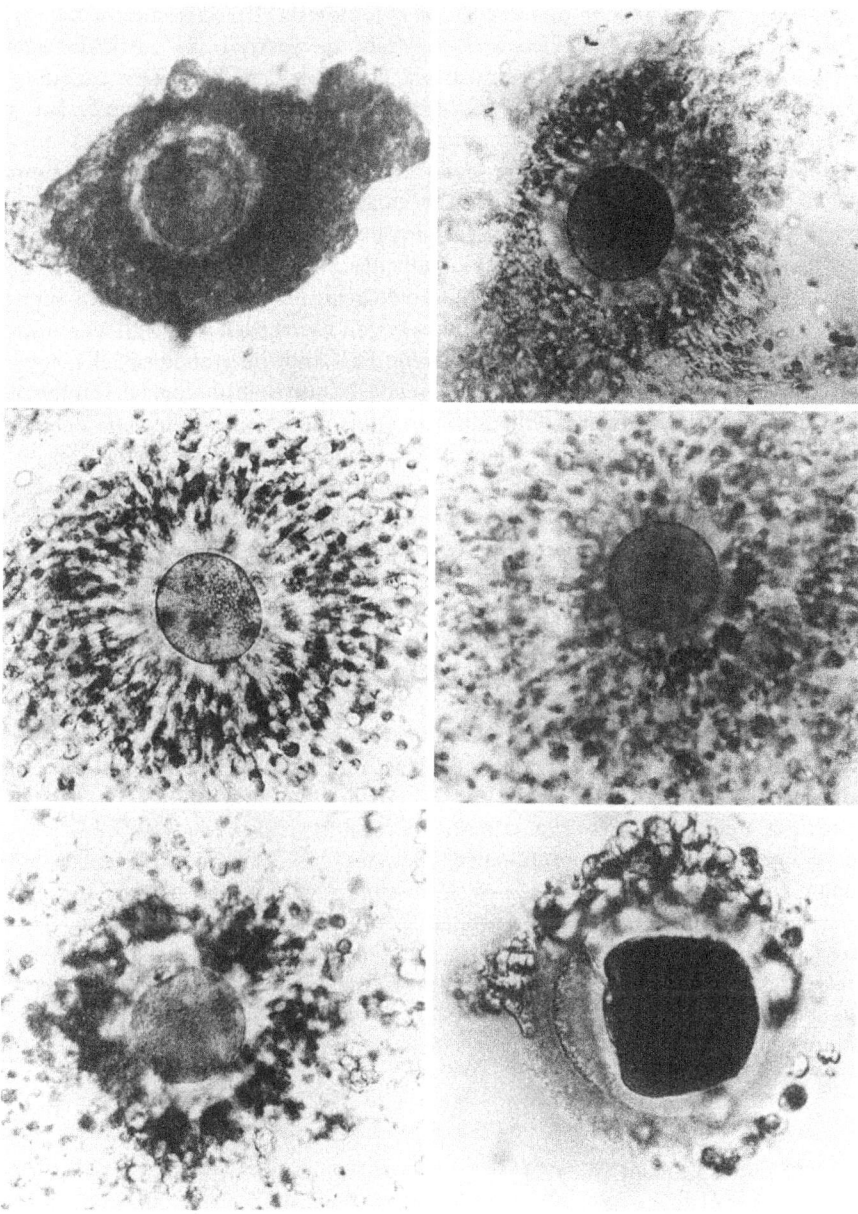

Fig. 2a–f. Grading of oocytes: **a** Grade 1, immature, prophase; **b** grade 2, nearly mature, metaphase I; **c** grade 3, mature, metaphase II; **d** grade 3, preovulatory, metaphase II; **e** grade 4, postmature; **f** grade 5, nonviable. (With kind permission from Veeck 1986)

Assessment should next be directed to the cytoplasmic characteristics of the oocyte, which easily can be visualized by light microscopy; in particular one should focus on the color and granulation. The color depends on the transmission of light, but it usually appears light yellow to gray and normally has a homogeneous appearance. The presence of dark granules of various sizes may be interpreted as denaturation or signs of coagulation of proteins at various stages. Coarse granulation is found in overmature or pathologically altered oocytes. The overall shape and size of an oocyte is assessed simultaneously with the shape and appearance of the zona pellucida. The evenly round oocyte body measures 100–150 μm in diameter, the zona pellucida usually varies in thickness from 10 to 30 μm. The zona pellucida is an extracellular matrix surrounding the oocyte and is formed by the oocyte itself and the granulosa cells, composed of three proteins (ZP1, ZP2, ZP3). The typical morphological feature of the human zona is a "fuzzy" outer surface. The significance of the zona pellucida's thickness is controversial. Chan (1987) reported a positive correlation between the zona thickness and the in vitro fertilization rate, while Bertrand et al. (1995) observed a clear negative correlation. Concerning this, the kind of hormone treatment seems to be of interest. The importance of the zona pellucida during fertilization will be discussed later on. Furthermore, it has to be noted that a very thick zona pellucida might inhibit embryo hatching later on in embryo development (for review see De Vos and Van Steirteghem 2000). Additionally, zona hardening during in vitro maturation would hinder sperm penetration.

The parameters listed in Table 1 have been accepted for assessing the maturity of a human oocyte. Hill et al. (1989) have proposed a grading system which has been established in several IVF laboratories. Because of their nonviable condition, neither oocytes from cumulus-oocyte complexes of grade 5 nor fractured oocytes should be inseminated. Oocytes are sometimes observed that cannot be categorized to grades 1–4. A possible reason is that nuclear and cellular maturity are not necessarily concurrent events (Eppig et al. 1994). Particularly in FSH-stimulated cycles, oocytes can be observed which include a germinal vesicle and no polar body and are surrounded by a highly expanded cumulus and corona radiata. Development is always poor if the discrepancy between oocyte and cumulus morphology is very extreme, although maturation may progress up to metaphase II.

In Vitro Maturation of Oocytes

The germinal vesicle breakdown, i.e., the final oocyte maturation, normally occurs in response to the peak in luteinizing hormone. If there are immature oocytes, insemination should be delayed until extrusion of the first polar body is visible. In particular, grade-2 oocytes can be cultured in vitro for up to 15 h to allow them to complete the nuclear and cytoplasmic maturation. Maturation of grade-1 oocytes occurs within about 24 h (20–28 h). Insemination is recommended 2–6 h after the first polar body is extruded. If the nuclear assessment

Table 1. Oocyte grading (Hill et al. 1989)

Grade	Characteristics
Grade 1 (immature oocyte, prophase I; Fig. 2a)	Dense and compact-appearing cumulus cells, tightly packed all around the oocyte Shows a centrally located germinal vesicle on light microscopy No polar body present
Grade 2 (nearly mature, metaphase I; Fig 2b)	Oocyte exhibits an expanded cumulus mass, but corona radiata is closely apposed to the zona pellucida No polar body, no germinal vesicle Ooplasm is lightly colored, sometimes slightly granular Diameter of extended, dissociated cumulus complex is 400–600 μm (equivalent 3–5 oocyte diameters)
Grade 3 (mature/preovulatory, metaphase II; Fig. 2c, d)	Very expanded cumulus, looking "fluffy" in a thin web of fibrils of matrix mass Corona radiata is still associated to the zona, sometimes appearing loosely aggregated Extruded polar body (often hardy to visualize), no nucleus Clear ooplasm, homogeneously granulated
Grade 4 (postmature; Fig. 2e)	Cumulus is clumped, sometimes absent Corona may be extremely expanded, partly missing or clumped; darkened and irregular cells Polar body is still intact or fragmented Ooplasm may be slightly darkened, mainly granulated Oocyte is still round and even
Grade 5 (atretic, nonviable; Fig. 2f)	Atresia occurs in all oocytes from early immature to postmature stages Cumulus cell mass is missing Corona radiata is present, clumped and irregular Polar body and nucleus are degenerated, if present Ooplasm is dark and vacuolated Uneven surface and very irregular shape of the oocyte; a perivitelline space is obvious Clearly visible, dark (brush-like) zona pellucida

is not clear because of a tightly packed cumulus, insemination about 29 h after the oocyte pick-up generally results in a favorable outcome. If insemination is performed too early, the oocytes are cytoplasmically immature, which means that the cortical granules are not yet located close enough to the oocyte cell membrane. Extrusion of the cortical granules results in the block to polyspermy (see below). If this extrusion does not take place, more than one sperm penetrates, resulting in a polyspermic oocyte.

The possibility of maturing immature oocytes in vitro has been discussed for a long time, especially for those couples in whom a factor is the reason for infertility, or for patients at risk for developing a hyperstimulation syndrome or polycystic ovaries. In this cases follicles which are mainly immature can be punctured without hormone treatment throughout a normal cycle. The disadvantage has been the low pregnancy rates resulting from in vitro matured oocytes (Salha et al. 1998). Mikkelsen (1999) recently reported a pregnancy rate of 11% following oocyte collection from non-hormone-treated women and in vitro maturation. Although these pregnancy rates are still low this is a very promising method for special cases without hormone treatment.

Fertilization Cascade

Fertilization occurs stepwise (Beier 1992). The first step is the binding of the sperm to the zona pellucida initiated by ZP3 (mouse, Saling 1989), resulting in the acrosome reaction (Larson and Miller 1997). Consecutively, the sperm bind also to ZP2 (Bleil and Wassarman 1986). The importance of the zona pellucida, i.e., ZP3 for fertilization in vivo, was shown by Rankin et al. (1996). In female mice lacking the ZP3 gene an in vivo fertilization was never observed. The reorganization of the zona pellucida by transformation of ZP3 (-/-) mice with hZP3 did restore the fertilization competence (Rankin et al. 1998). Similar to this observation in mice is the report of a patient with repeatedly unsuccessful IVF cycles; it was realized later on that all oocytes were zona-free. ICSI finally resulted in normal embryo development, making it very possible that the missing zona was the reason for the unsuccessful in vitro fertilization (P. M. Wassarman, personal communication). Zona-free oocytes are generally discarded, but Ding et al. (1999) recently reported that such oocytes can be fertilized by ICSI and develop up to the blastocyst stage.

Hypermotility of the sperm leads to a penetration of the zona pellucida (Bedford 1998), followed by the fusion with the oocyte cell membrane. This causes a depolarization of the oocyte membrane (Edwards 1980) and an increase of Ca^{++} concentration, followed by the extrusion of cortical granules into the perivitelline space (Hyttel et al. 1988). The depolarization initially prevents fusion of further sperm, while the long-term block to polyspermy is caused by transformation of ZP3 to ZP3f by cortical granule material (Wassarman 1987). This block is insufficient in immature and overmature oocytes, leading to polyspermic fertilization. Penetration by a sperm allows the proteolytic enzymes of the acrosome to overcome the metaphase II block. Subsequently, the second polar body is extruded and the male and female pronuclei form, with the male pronucleus often larger than the female. The paternal pronucleus moves towards the fixed maternal one, and both align before the germinal vesicle breakdown. Furthermore, a clockwise rotation of the cortical cytoplasm can frequently be observed before the second polar body is extruded. Long cytoplasmic waves seem to be important, as they are correlated to embryo quality (for review see Edwards and Beard 1997). This knowledge led Scott and Smith

(1998) to assess prezygotes and transfer pronuclear embryos 24–26 h post insemination. They scored alignment of the pronuclei 16–17 h after insemination, as well as the shape of the cytoplasm (ideal: heterogeneous, a clear halo around the edges, a dark ring in the middle, occasionally a clear area around the pronuclei). At the time of embryo transfer, germinal vesicle breakdown had occurred, with a loss of the halo effect. When two to six embryos were transferred with a score of >15 each (out of 25 possible) an implantation rate of 28% was reported. Scoring of prezygotes and transfer 24 h following insemination circumvents negative in vitro effects with reasonable transfer results.

Assessment of Fertilization

Light-microscopic evaluation of a successful fertilization should be performed 16–18 h after insemination. The following should be seen:
- Two polar bodies
- Two pronuclei with several nucleoli
- Pronuclei aligned
- Fine granulated cytoplasm, with a dark ring and a halo in the outer part
- Spherical oocyte with a narrow perivitelline space
- Several sperm detectable within the zona pellucida and the perivitelline space.

For clear evaluation, the oocyte sometimes must be freed from remaining cumulus and corona cells by gentle "up- and -down pipetting". The time for the assessment procedure should be kept as short as possible. Light, especially the UV wavelengths, generates free radicals (Wang and Nixon 1978) and causes DNA damage (Peak et al. 1991). Furthermore, changes in pH and temperature are harmful to early embryo development (Fischer et al. 1988, Schuhmacher and Fisher 1988).

However, the assessment of oocytes during fertilization is very important, as prezygotes with three or more pronuclei (Fig. 3c) are able to develop to morphologically normal appearing cleavage stages (Balakier and Casper 1991). Plachot and Crozet (1992) reported that 6.5% of fertilized oocytes show three pronuclei. The surplus pronucleus may be derived from an additional spermatozoon (delayed polyspermy block) or from a nonextruded second polar body. Two maternally derived pronuclei have been reported, particularly following ICSI (Palermo et al. 1993, Flaherty et al. 1995), because of damage to the spindle apparatus. Male and female pronuclei can be distinguished by their size. In 82% of trinucleate prezygotes at least one cleavage can be observed, and 25% may even reach the blastocyst stage (Plachot et al. 1989). Balakier and Casper (1991) often observed triploid and tetraploid cleavage stages with a normal morphology. While those four-cell to eight-cell embryos seem normal, most blastocysts show developmental abnormalities (Plachot and Mandelbaum 1990), which explains the increased incidence of spontaneous abortions following transfer of such embryos. Possible reasons for tripronucleated prezygotes include immature or overmature oocytes (van der Ven et al. 1985), high sperm concentration (Wolf et al. 1984), defects of the zona pellucida (Englert et al.

Fig. 3a–c. Oocytes 16–18 h after insemination. a Unfertilized oocyte, one polar body, no pronucleus; b Fertilized oocyte, two pronuclei, two polar bodies; c polyspermy, three pronuclei. (With kind permission from Veeck 1986)

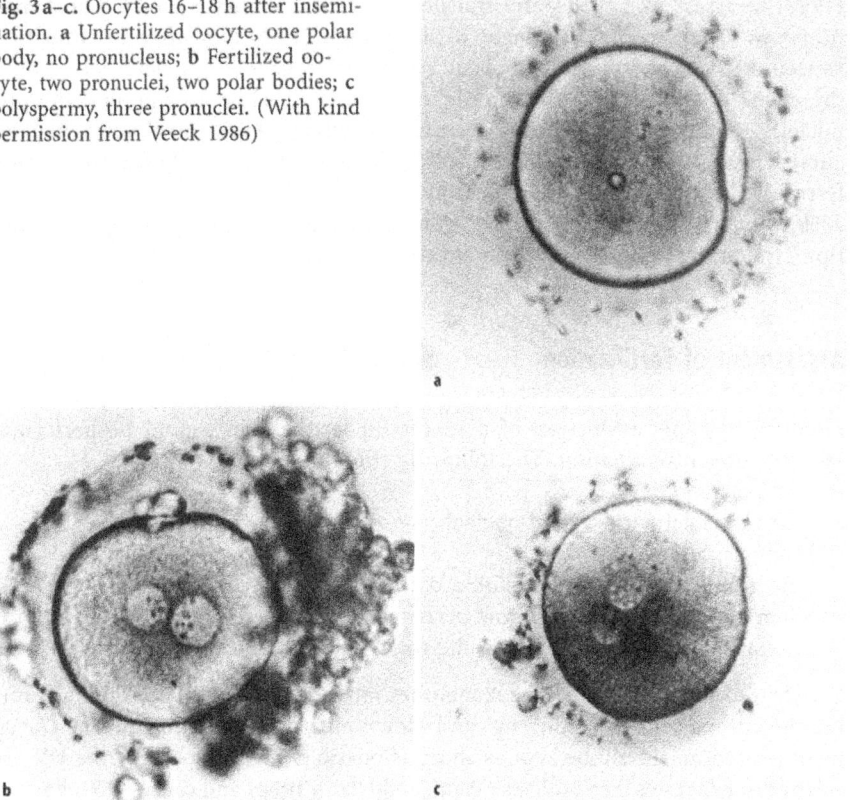

1986), and the failure of cortical granule extrusion (Sathananthan et al. 1985). Deciding whether to transfer an embryo originating from a tripronucleated prezygote is difficult; one fears causing an abnormal pregnancy. Furthermore, the abortion of a polyploid embryo would also lead to the loss of a co-transferred normal embryo. On the other hand, embryos originating from trinucleate prezygotes show a diploid karyotype in 32%, a triploid in 24%, and a mosaic in 29% of cases (Plachot et al. 1989).

Another abnormal fertilization phenomenon is the appearance of only a single pronucleus (Fig. 3a). Penetration by a spermatozoon may have occurred despite this feature. Plachot et al. (1987, Plachot and Crozet 1992) have shown that 80% of virtually "unfertilized" oocytes have sperm chromosomes. The male pronucleus was not visible in these prezygotes because of premature sperm chromosome condensation (PCC), which seems to be induced by an ooplasmic factor (Flaherty et al. 1995). The incidence of PCC is 34% in immature oocytes. It is higher following FSH than after hMG treatment (30% vs. 11%). It also has been reported that oocytes which failed fertilization cleaved up to the blastocyst stage (Plachot and Crozet 1992). Of these oocytes, 77% proceeded to the two- or four-cell stage. Within 7 days 30% had reached the expanded blastocyst stage. Of the two-cell to eight-cell embryos, 16.9% showed a haploid set of chromosomes (30% diploid due to nonextrusion of the second polar body, 18% mosaic).

Veeck (1986) described cases in which cleavage stages were obtained directly from the follicle and oocytes which underwent division without fertilization. Although it is possible to induce such divisions by stressing factors such as acidic solutions and high vacuum pressure, a cytosolic sperm factor is normally responsible for activating oocyte division (Swann et al. 1994, Dozortsev et al. 1995). In ICSI it has been shown that spermatozoa can be rejected again by the oocyte after more than 20 min (Flaherty et al. 1995). This explains one aspect of haploid embryos, as Dozortsev et al. (1995) demonstrated that 4% of sham-injected (ICSI) oocytes are able to cleave at least once. A cleavage of haploid nonfertilized oocytes is therefore possible. These 'embryos' will never result in an ongoing pregnancy.

In addition to the number of pronuclei, their alignment should be considered 16 h post insemination (Fig. 3 b), as well as the feature of the cytoplasm for the assessment of fertilization, as has been reported by Scott and Smith (1998).

Evaluation of the Early Embryo

The cleavage stages are often retransferred 48–72 h after insemination. Shortly before transfer they are normally assessed for the following features:
- Number of blastomeres
- Morphology of blastomeres
- Cytoplasm of blastomeres
- Attachment of blastomeres
- Size and content of the perivitelline space
- Fragmentation of blastomeres
- Zona pellucida.

They are also graded (Table 2) to evaluate the success of in vitro fertilization and culture. Two-cell stages are observed 22–44 h after insemination (usually around 24 h). Four-cell stages are expected at 46 h post insemination (36–50 h). Eight-cell stages are seen after 48 h. Blastomeres may undergo asynchronous cleavage, and embryos with consecutive numbers of blastomeres are therefore observed. As blastomeres divide without any preceding cytoplasmic production, ongoing cleavage results in smaller blastomeres. Therefore, different sizes of blastomeres are also observed regularly within one embryo (Roux et al. 1995).

According to Hill et al. (1989), four embryonic grades can be distinguished (see Table 2, Fig. 4). Such assessment provides the possibility of judging the embryos immediately prior to transfer. Videotaping and photographing the embryo allows retrospective analyses of several parameters with higher accuracy.

Table 2. Embryo grading (Hill et al. 1989)

Grade	Characteristics
Grade A (high-quality embryo; Fig. 4a)	Blastomeres evenly sized, nearly spherical
	Cytoplasm uniform, slightly granulated
	Four blastomeres (48 h after insemination), eight blastomeres (72 h after insemination)
	Blastomeres symmetrically located within the zona pellucida
	No fragmentation
	Zona pellucida looks pale; some corona cells may remain; some spermatozoa are visible within the zona
Grade B (good embryo; Fig. 4b)	Blastomeres slightly uneven or irregularly shaped
	Cytoplasm with uneven granules
	Reduced blastomere adherence
	Up to 10% fragmented blastomeres
Grade C (sufficient embryo; Fig. 4c)	Blastomeres of uneven size and appearance
	Reduced blastomere adherence
	Cytoplasm shows large dark granules and vacuoles
	Blastomere membrane appears 'patchy'
	Blastomeres are located nonsymmetrically within the zona, enlarged perivitelline space
	Up to 50% fragmented blastomeres
Grade D (bad embryo; Fig. 4d)	At least one blastomere should be visible
	Blastomeres are very uneven
	Cytoplasm shows large dark granules and vacuoles
	Blastomere membrane looks 'patchy', reduced blastomere adherence
	Extensive fragmentation

Blastocyst Culture

The benefits and pitfalls of the culture of embryos up to the blastocyst stage (Fig. 5) have been the subject of controversy recently (Tsirigotis 1998, Gardner and Schoolcraft 1998, Desai 1998, Behr 1999, Edwards and Beard 1999, Sakkas 1999). There are several advantages in favor culture to the blastocyst stage, but the disadvantages should also be discussed. One major goal has been to distinguish between viable embryos and those that develop initially but die later, which often show genetic defects (Edwards and Hollands 1988, Menezo and Ben-Khalifa 1995). These embryos also might be the reason for several implantation failures, leading to false expectations for the patients. To distinguish such embryos, blastocyst culture systems have been considered favorable (Bolton et al. 1991, Tarin and Handyside 1993, Gardner and Lane 1997). Embryos with proven viability consequently led to excellent implantation rates (50.5%; Gardner et al. 1998). Furthermore, comparison of day-3 and day-5 transfers showed

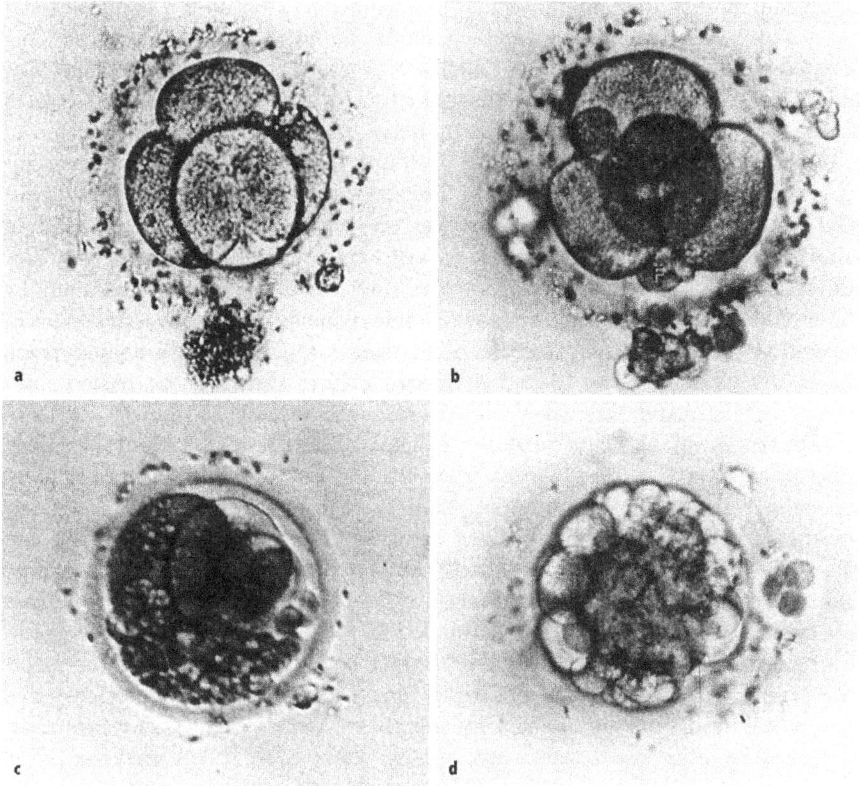

Fig. 4a–d. Grading of embryos 48 h after insemination. **a** Grade A; **b** grade B, some fragmentation; **c** grade C, 50% fragmentation; **d** grade D, total fragmentation. (With kind permission from Veeck 1986)

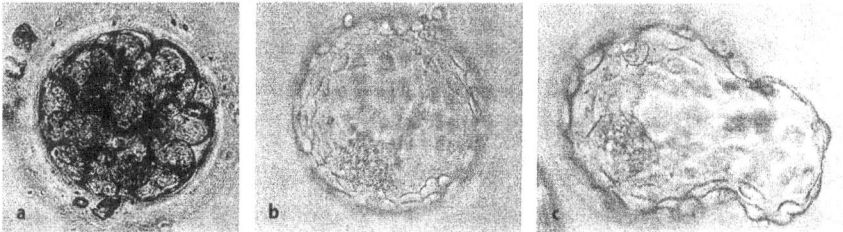

Fig. 5a–c. Embryos cultured for 5 days (**a** morula) or 6 days (**b** blastocyst, **c** hatching blastocyst)

significant higher implantation rates following day-5 blastocyst transfer (fetal heart 30.1% vs. 50.5%, respectively). It should be noted that in these cases only selected patients with at least ten follicles > 12 mm diameter were included. Another very important benefit is the reduction of multiple pregnancies, which occurs mainly in good responders. In these cases the number of transferred embryos can be reduced to two, and even only one, given a good embryo culture system (ECS) for blastocysts in the near future (Gardner and Schoolcraft 1998). Additional culture conditions are very important. For development of embryos up to the blastocyst stage, in vitro culture conditions have been improved. Each little fault during in vitro culture would increase exponentially by the end of culture, affecting the embryo and reducing pregnancy rates. A well-controlled (for example by culture of F1-mouse zygotes; > 85% should reach the blastocyst stage by 96 h) and developed culture system is the basic condition for a successful blastocyst culture. Recently, several laboratories have reported successful blastocyst culture systems (Gardner and Lane 1997, 1998, Jones et al. 1998, Behr et al. 1999). The common rationale is the use of sequential culture media for the different requirements of early/oviductal and later/ uterine embryos. In general, oviductal embryos utilize mainly pyruvate and lactate, while glucose seems to be toxic; however, glucose is the major energy source for uterine embryos. Furthermore, the medium for early embryos does not contain essential amino acids. This led to the development of the G1 medium (early embryos up to the eight-cell stage) and G2 medium (from the eight-cell to the blastocyst stage) by Gardner and Lane (1997). They reported that 75% of cultured embryos reached the blastocyst stage by day 5 after insemination, leading to an implantation rate of 50%. Jones et al. (1998) used the IVF50 and G2, while Behr et al. (1999) have used P1 and a more complex, glucose-containing blastocyst medium. Two media for the prolonged embryo culture are now commercially available: G2.2 (Scandinavian IVF Science AB, Sweden) and M_3 (Medicult a/s, Denmark).

One further advantage of the blastocyst culture is that more than two cells can be obtained for a preimplantation genetic diagnosis by trophectoderm biopsy (see also Liebaers et al., this volume). Preimplantation genetic diagnosis using trophectoderm biopsies might therefore be more accurate and efficient, because of the much higher number of cells/RNA available. Furthermore, the trophectoderm is a nonembryonic tissue, which might make this technology attractive for certain religious groups.

On the other hand, there may be several pitfalls. One point has been discussed before, i.e., the culture conditions. Faults will accumulate over time and reduce pregnancy rates. Also factors such as air and water (Cohen et al. 1998), UV light, temperature, and pH have to be considered (Fischer et al. 1988, Schumacher et al. 1988). Furthermore, the birth of large offspring from sheep and cows has been reported frequently after extended in vitro embryo culture (Walker et al. 1992, Behboodi et al. 1995, Farin and Farin 1995, Thompson et al. 1995, Holm et al. 1996). A much quicker development of embryos in in vitro culture than in vivo has already been observed (Walker et al. 1992). Serum is discussed as one cause of this syndrome (Thompson et al. 1995, Thompson

Table 3. Criteria for blastocyst culture

Factor	Criteria
Patient	At least 10 follicles >12 mm
Culture	Sequential culture media
	Change at the 8-cell stage
	Regular check of culture system (F1-mice zygote culture)
Embryo	Blastocyst formation by day 5 post insemination
	Distinct inner cell mass

1997). Another factor is the IGF-I, which is known to enhance embryo development (Harvey and Kaye 1992) by reducing apoptosis (Herrler et al. 1998), leading to even larger embryos than in in vivo controls (Grundker and Kirchner 1996). Furthermore, bFGF has been proposed as favoring the development of the embryonic disc, which might lead to larger fetuses and offspring (Hrabe de Angelis et al. 1995). Both factors are detectable within serum and albumin products, sometimes in high amounts. Therefore, serum- and albumin-free media have been developed by replacing them with polyvinyl alcohol or polyvinylpyrrolidone (Bavister 1995). Recently, Gardner and Lane (1998) recommended the use of synthetic hyaluronate (0.5 mg/ml), which might avoid the problems described above.

A further disadvantage might be the "loss" of embryos during prolonged in vitro culture. Scholtes and Zeilmacker (1998) reported that in 40% of patients no blastocysts were available for transfer, in contrast to Gardner et al. (1998) with only 5%. The reason might be the selection of patients with at least ten follicles, as well as the culture conditions. Therefore, in cases where there are only two embryos and those with repeated failure of development to the blastocyst stage, an early transfer to the uterus, which is also not the physiological place for an eight-cell embryo to be, has to be considered. It is still controversial whether the premature transfer of an embryo to the uterus or its culture in vitro in medium that is only adapted to nature is superior. There is no doubt that the culture of embryos offers several very interesting advantages, if certain criteria regarding the selection of patients, embryos, and culture are followed (Table 3).

Finally, each stage of transfer used in the clinic – whether pronuclear embryos, as proposed by Scott and Smith (1998), eight-cell embryos using the cumulative embryo score (Steer et al. 1992), or the blastocyst – has its own benefits.

Prediction of Assisted Reproduction Outcome

The factors affecting the outcome of pregnancy include oocyte maturity, success of fertilization, and quality of embryos. According to Hill et al. (1989), grade-2 and -3 oocytes are more likely to develop into grade-A embryos. The transfer of grade-A embryos resulted in the highest pregnancy rates (38%). Steer et al. (1992) presented a simple cumulative embryo score (CES) to determine which and how many embryos should be transferred. They multiplied the number of blastomeres by the morphological grade of an embryo, finally summing the score of all transferred embryos. The highest pregnancy rate with the lowest rate of multiple pregnancy was observed with a CES of 35–42. Increasing the CES, i.e., the transfer of more 'good' embryos, also increased the incidence of multiple pregnancies.

Reducing the number of transferred embryos from three to two in order to reduce multiple pregnancies might also increase the incidence of pregnancy failure, but if only "high-quality embryos" are transferred, this incidence would be kept to a minimum. Therefore, transferring two "good" embryos is the best method (Puissant et al. 1987 Kodama et al. 1995). In addition to morphological criteria, the assessment of embryos includes the cleavage rate per time. Giorgetti et al. (1995) have clearly demonstrated that four-cell embryos (48 h after insemination) resulted in significant higher pregnancy rates than embryos with fewer or even more blastomeres (15.6% vs. 7.4%, respectively). Both slowly and rapidly cleaving embryos resulted in fewer pregnancies than those that reached the four-cell stage within 40 h after insemination (Cummins et al. 1986, Claman et al. 1987).

Regarding morphological criteria, irregular blastomeres and fragments play the most important role in predicting further development (Grillo et al. 1991, Morgan et al. 1995, Giorgetti et al. 1995). Either an abnormal cleavage of blastomeres (Roux et al. 1995) or fragmentation should lead to an inferior grading of the embryo. The cell fragments often observed in embryos are signs of degenerated blastomeres, the result of programmed cell death (PCD; Jurisicova et al. 1996, Warner et al. 1998). The chromatin of these cells becomes segregated during apoptosis, the nucleus is fragmented, and at least the cell disintegrates into several membrane-wrapped bodies, sometimes with nuclear components (Kerr et al. 1994). Since blastomeres are not able to phagocytose apoptotic bodies, the fragments remain visible for a long time. In early embryos apoptotic bodies persist and may become necrotic. Further research is required to determine whether this can damage the remaining cells or if they should be removed microsurgically.

Chemical criteria have also been investigated in the search for a correlation to pregnancy outcome. Pyruvate uptake has been shown to be correlated with the developmental competence of human embryos (Leese et al. 1986), although the authors were unable to verify this in individual embryos (Conaghan et al. 1993). Oxygen consumption has been shown not to be a good parameter (Magnusson et al. 1986). It has been suggested that platelet-activating factor is produced in higher amounts by embryos which subsequently result in ongoing pregnancies (O'Neil et al. 1987, Nakatsuka et al. 1992). Clark et al. (1989) described an embryo-associated suppressor factor. None of these parameters has shown itself to be of practical means for assessment of in vitro fertilization in the laboratory. The morphology of embryos thus remains the most useful, practical, and reliable indicator of their quality.

References

Balakier H, Caspar RF (1991) A morphologic study of unfertilized oocytes and abnormal embryos in human in vitro fertilization. J In Vitro Fertil Embryo Transf 8:73–79

Bavister BD (1995) Culture of preimplantation embryos: facts and artefacts Hum Reprod Update 1:91–148

Bedford JM (1998) Mammalian fertilization misread? Sperm penetration of the eutherian zona pellucida is unlikely to be a lytic event. Biol Reprod 59:1275–1287

Behboodi E, Anderson GB, Bondurant RH, Cargil SL, Kreuscher BR, Medrano JF, Murray JD (1995) Birth of large calves that developed from in-vitro-derived bovine embryos. Theriogenology 44:227–232

Behr B (1999) Blastocyst culture and transfer. Hum Reprod 14:5–6

Behr B, Pool TB, Milki AA, Moore D, Gebhardt J, Dasig D (1999) Preliminary clinical experience with human blastocyst development in vitro without co-culture. Hum Reprod 14:454–457

Beier HM (1992) Die molekulare Biologie der Befruchtungskaskade und der beginnenden Embryonalentwicklung. Ann Anat 174:491–508

Bertrand E, Van Den Bergh M, Englert Y (1995) Does zona pellucida thickness influence the fertilization rate? Hum Reprod 10:1189–1193

Bleil JD, Wassarman PM (1986) Autoradiographic visualization of the mouse egg's sperm receptor bound to sperm. J Cell Biol 102:1363–1371

Bolton VN, Wren ME, Parsons JH (1991) Pregnancies after in vitro fertilization and transfer of human blastocysts. Fertil Steril 55:830–832

Chan PJ (1987) Developmental potential of human oocytes according to zona pellucida thickness. J In Vitro Fertil Embryo Transf 4:237–241

Claman P, Armant DR, Seibel MM, Wang TA, Oskowitz SP, Taymor ML (1987) The impact of embryo quality and quantity on implantation and the establishment of viable pregnancies. J In Vitro Fertil Embryo Transf 4:218–222

Clark DA, Lee S, Fishell S (1989) Immunosuppressive activity in human in-vitro fertilization (IVF) culture supernatants and prediction of outcome of embryo transfer: a multicenter trial. J In Vitro Fertil Embryo Transf 6:51–58

Cohen J, Gilligan A, Willadsen S (1998) Culture and quality control of embryos. Hum Reprod 13 [Suppl 3]:137–144

Conaghan J, Hardy K, Handyside AH, Winston RML, Leese HJ (1993) Selection criteria for human embryo transfer – a comparison of pyruvate uptake and morphology. J Assist Reprod Genet 10:21–30

Cummins JM, Breen TM, Harrison KL, Shaw JM, Wilson LM, Hennessey JF (1986) A formula for scoring human embryo growth rates in in vitro fertilization: its value in predicting pregnancy and in comparison with visual estimates of embryo quality. J In Vitro Fertil Embryo Transf 3:284–295

Desai NN (1998) The road of blastocyst transfer. Hum Reprod 13:3292–3295

De Vos A, Van Steirteghem A (2000) Tona hardening, zona drilling and assisted hatching – new achievements in assisted reproduction. Cells Tissue Organs 166:220–227

Ding J, Rana N, Dmowski WP (1999) Intracytoplasmic sperm injection into zona-free human oocytes results in normal fertilization and blastocyst development. Hum Reprod 14:476–478

Dozortsev D, Rybouchkin A, De Sutter P, Qian C, Dhont M (1995) Human oocyte activation following intracytoplasmic injection: the role of sperm cell. Hum Reprod 10:403–407

Edwards RG (1980) Conception in the human female. Academic, London

Edwards RG, Hollands P (1988) New advances in human embryology: implications of the preimplantation diagnosis of genetic disease. Hum Reprod 3:549–556

Edwards RG, Beard HK (1997) Oocyte polarity and cell determination in early mammalian embryos. Mol Hum Reprod 3:863–905

Edwards RG, Beard HK (1999) Is the success of human IVF more a matter of genetics and evolution than growing blastocysts? Hum Reprod 14:1–4

Englert Y, Puissant F, Camus M, Degueldre M, Leroy F (1986) Factors leading to tripronucleate eggs during human in-vitro fertilization. Hum Reprod 1:117–119

Eppig JJ, Schultz RM, O'Brien M, Chesnel F (1994) Relationship between the developmental programs controlling nuclear and cytoplasmic maturation of mouse oocytes. Develop Biol 164:1–9

Farin PW, Farin CE (1995) Transfer of bovine embryos produced in vivo or in vitro: survival and fetal development. Biol Reprod 52:676–682

Fischer B, Schumacher A, Hegele-Hartung C, Beier HM (1988) Potential risk of light and room temperature exposure to preimplantation embryos. Fertil Steril 50:938–944

Flaherty SP, Payne D, Swann NJ, Matthews CD (1995) Aetiology of failed and abnormal fertilization after intracytoplasmic sperm injection. Hum Reprod 10:2623–2629

Gardner DK, Lane M (1997) Culture and selection of viable blastocysts: a feasible proposition for human IVF? Hum Reprod Update 3:367–382

Gardner DK, Lane M (1998) Culture of viable human blastocysts in defined sequential serum-free media. Hum Reprod 13 [Suppl 3]:148–159

Gardner DK, Schoolcraft WB (1998) No longer neglected: the human blastocyst. Hum Reprod 13:3289–3292

Gardner DK, Schoolcraft WB, Wagley L, Schlenker T, Stevens J, Hesla J (1998) A prospective randomized trial of blastocyst culture and transfer in in-vitro fertilization. Hum Reprod 13:3434–3440

Giorgetti C, Terriou P, Auquier P, Hans E, Spach J-L, Salzmann J, Roulier R (1995) Embryo score to predict implantation after in-vitro fertilization: based on 957 single embryo transfers. Hum Reprod 10:2427–2431

Grillo JM, Gamerre M, Lacroix O, Noizet A, Vitry G (1991) Influence of the morphological aspect of embryos obtained by in vitro fertilization on their implantation rate. J In Vitro Fertil Embryo Transf 8:317–321

Grundker C, Kirchner C (1996) Influence of uterine growth factors on blastocyst expansion and trophoblast knob formation in the rabbit. Early Pregnancy 2:264–270

Harvey MB, Kaye PL (1992) Insulin-like growth factor-1 stimulates growth of mouse preimplantation embryos in vitro. Mol Reprod Dev 31:195–199

Herrler A, Krusche CA, Beier HM (1998) Insulin and insulin-like growth factor-I promote rabbit blastocyst development and prevent apoptosis. Biol Reprod 59:1302–1310

Hill GA, Freeman M, Bastias MC, Rogers BJ, Herbert CM III, Osteen KG, Wentz AC (1989) The influence of oocyte maturity and embryo quality on pregnancy rate in a program for in vitro fertilization-embryo transfer. Fertil Steril 52:801–806

Holm P, Walker SK, Seamark RF (1996) Embryo viability, duration of gestation and birth weight in sheep after transfer of in vitro matured and in vitro fertilized zygotes cultured in vitro or in vivo. J Reprod Fertil 107:175–181

Hrabe de Angelis M, Grundker C, Herrmann BG, Kispert A, Kirchner C (1995) Promotion of gastrulation by maternal growth factor in cultured rabbit blastocysts. Cell Tissue Res 282:147–154

Hyttel P, Greve T, Callesen H (1988) Ultrastructure of in-vivo fertilization in superovulated cattle. J Reprod Fertil 82:1–13

Jones GM, Trounson AO, Gardner DK, Kausche A, Lolatgis N, Wood C (1998) Evolution of a culture protocol for successful blastocyst development and pregnancy. Hum Reprod 13:169–177

Jurisicova A, Varmuza S, Casper RF (1996) Programmed cell death and human embryo fragmentation. Mol Hum Reprod 2:93–98

Kerr JFR, Winterford CM, Harmon BV (1994) Morphological criteria for identifying apoptosis. In: Celis JE (ed) Cell biology: a laboratory handbook. Academic, New York, pp 319–329

Kodama H, Fukuda J, Karube H, Matsui T, Shimizu Y, Tasdemir M, Tasdemir I, Tanaka T (1995) Prospective evaluation of simple morphological criteria for embryo selection in double embryo transfer cycles. Hum Reprod 10:2999–3003

Larson JL, Miller DJ (1997) Sperm from a variety of mammalian species express beta 1,4-galactosyltransferase on their surface. Biol Reprod 57:442–453

Leese HJ, Hooper MAK, Edwards RG, Ashwood-Smith MJ (1986) Uptake of pyruvate by early human embryos determined by a non-invasive technique. Hum Reprod 1:181–182

Magnusson C, Hillensjö T, Hamberger L, Nilsson L (1986) Oxygen consumption by human oocytes and blastocysts grown in vitro. Hum Reprod 1:183–184

Menezo YJ, Ben Khalifa M (1995) Cytogenetic and cryobiology of human cocultured embryos: a 3-year experience. J Assist Reprod Genet 12:35–40

Mikkelsen AL (1999) IVM research bears fruit. FertiNet 2:http://ferti.net, special interest

Morgan K, Wiemer K, Steuerwald N, Hoffman D, Maxson W, Godke R (1995) Use of video-cinematography to assess morphological qualities of conventionally cultured and cocultured embryos. Hum Reprod 10:2371–2376

Nakatsuka M, Yoshida N, Kudo T (1992) Platelet activating factor in culture media as an indicator of human embryonic development after in-vitro fertilization. Hum Reprod 7:1435–1439

O'Neill C, Gidley-Baird AA, Pike IL, Saunders DM (1987) A bio-assay for embryo-derived platelet activating factor as a means of assessing quality and pregnancy potential of human embryos. Fertil Steril 47:969–975

Palermo G, Joris H, Derde M-P, Camus M, Devroey P, Van Steirteghem AC (1993) Sperm characteristics and outcome of human assisted fertilization by subzonal insemination and intracytoplasmic sperm injection. Fertil Steril 59:826–835

Peak JG, Pilas B, Dudek EJ, Peak MJ (1991) DNA breaks caused by monochromatic 365 nm ultraviolet-A radiation or hydrogen peroxide and their repair in human epithelioid and xeroderma pigmentosum cells. Photochem Photobiol 54:197–203

Plachot M, Mandelbaum J (1990) Oocyte maturation, fertilization and embryonic growth in vitro. Br Med Bull 46:675–694

Plachot M, Crozet N (1992) Fertilization abnormalities in human in vitro fertilization. Hum Reprod 7 [Suppl]:89–94

Plachot M, de Grouchy J, Junca AM, Mandelbaum J, Turleau C, Couillin P, Cohen J, Salat-Baroux J (1987) From oocyte to embryo: a model, deduced from in vitro fertilization, for natural selection against chromosome abnormalities. Ann Genet 30:22–32

Plachot M, Mandelbaum J, Junca A-M, de Grouchy J, Salat-Baroux J, Cohen J (1989) Cytogenetic analysis and developmental capacity of normal and abnormal embryos after IVF. Hum Reprod 4 [Suppl]:99–103

Puissant F, Van Rysselberge M, Barlow P, Deweze J, Leroy F (1987) Embryo scoring as a prognostic tool in IVF treatment. Hum Reprod 2:705–708

Rankin T, Familari M, Lee E, Ginsberg A, Dwyer N, Blanchette-Mackie J, Drago J, Westphal H, Dean J (1996) Mice homozygous for an insertional mutation in the Zp3 gene lack a zona pellucida and are infertile. Development 122:2903–2910

Rankin TL, Tong ZB, Castle PE, Lee E, Gore-Langton R, Nelson LM, Dean J (1998) Human Zp3 restores fertility in Zp3 null mice without affecting order-specific sperm binding. Development 125:2415–2424

Roux C, Borodkine R, Joanne C, Bresson JL, Agnani G (1995) Morphological classification of human in-vitro fertilization embryos based on the regularity of the asynchronous division process. Hum Reprod Update 1:488–496

Sakkas D (1999) The use of blastocyst culture to avoid inheritance of an abnormal paternal genome after ICSI. Hum Reprod 14:4–5

Salha O, Abusheika N, Sharma V (1998) Dynamics of human follicular growth and in-vitro oocyte maturation. Hum Reprod Update 4:816–832

Saling MP (1989) Mammalian sperm interaction with extracellular matrices of the egg. In: Milligan SR (ed) Oxford reviews of reproductive biology 11. Oxford University Press, Oxford, pp 339–388

Sathananthan AH, Ng SC, Chia CM, Lay HY, Edirisinghe WR, Raiman SS (1985) The origin and distribution of cortical granules in human oocytes with reference to Golgi nucleolar and microfilament activity. Ann NY Acad Sci 442:251–264

Scholtes MCW, Zeilmaker GH (1998) Blastocyst transfer in day-5 embryo transfer depends primarily on the number of oocytes retrieved and not on age. Fertil Steril 69:78–83

Schumacher A, Fischer B (1988) Influence of visible light and room temperature on cell proliferation in preimplantation rabbit embryos. J Reprod Fertil 84:197–204

Scott LA, Smith S (1998) The successful use of pronuclear embryo transfers the day following oocyte retrieval. Hum Reprod 13:1003–1013

Steer CV, Mills CL, Tan SL, Campbell S, Edwards RG (1992) The cumulative embryo score: a predictive embryo scoring technique to select the optimal number of embryos to transfer in an in-vitro fertilization and embryo transfer programme. Hum Reprod 7:117–119

Swann K, Homa S, Carroll J (1994) An inside job: the results of injecting whole sperm into eggs support one view of signal transduction at fertilization. Hum Reprod 9:978–980

Tarin JJ, Handyside AH (1993) Embryo biopsy strategies for preimplantation diagnosis. Fertil Steril 59:943–952

Thompson JG (1997) Comparison between in vivo-derived and in vitro-produced pre-elongation embryos from domestic ruminants. Reprod Fertil Dev 9:341–354

Thompson JG, Gardner DK, Pugh PA, McMillan WH, Tervit HR (1995) Lamb birth weight is affected by culture system utilized during in vitro pre-elongation development of ovine embryos. Biol Reprod 53:1385–1391

Tsirigotis M (1998) Blastocyst stage transfer: pitfalls and benefits. Too soon to abandon current practice. Hum Reprod 13:3285–3289

Van der Ven NH, Al-Hasani S, Dietrich K, Hamerich U, Lehmann F, Krebs D (1985) Polyspermy in in vitro fertilization of human oocytes: frequency and possible causes. Ann NY Acad Sci 442:88–95

Veeck L (ed) (1986) Atlas of the human oocyte and early conceptus. Williams & Wilkins, Baltimore, pp 1–331

Walker SK, Heard TM, Seamark RF (1992) In-vitro culture of sheep embryos without coculture: successes and perspectives. Theriogenology 37:111–126

Wang RJ, Nixon BR (1978) Identification of hydrogen peroxide as a photoproduct toxic to human cells in tissue-culture medium irradiated with "daylight" fluorescent light. In Vitro 14:715–722

Warner CM, Cao W, Exley GE, McElhinny AS, Alikani M, Cohen J, Scott RT, Brenner CA (1998) Genetic regulation of egg and embryo survival. Hum Reprod 13 [Suppl 3]:178–190

Wassarman PM (1987) Early events in mammalian fertilization. Annu Rev Cell Biol 3:109–142

Wolf DP, Byrd W, Dandkar P, Quigley MM (1984) Sperm concentration and the fertilization of human eggs in vitro. Biol Reprod 31:837–848

Predicting Embryo Development

L. Scott

Introduction

The ability to sustain mammalian gametes outside the body, to perform in vitro fertilization and embryo culture and subsequently to transfer the developing embryo back to the uterus with establishment of a viable pregnancy has been a reality for many decades. With the landmark success of Steptoe and Edwards in 1978, it became feasible to apply this technique to human beings. To date, the birth of tens of thousands of babies worldwide through the in vitro production (IVP) of embryos has revolutionized the whole field of infertility treatment. Society has come to accept the treatment as standard practice. Over the past 20 years the field has expanded, and today the types of treatment include techniques for almost every form of infertility. However, there is one major factor that still imposes limits on the techniques available for treatment: the oocyte. The quality of the oocyte and its ability to grow into a viable embryo, capable of implanting, is paramount to IVP success, as outlined in detail for many species and orders by Edwards and Beard (Edwards and Beard 1997). As ovarian stimulation protocols improved with the development of more efficacious drugs, it became possible to harvest more and more mature oocytes. This gave practitioners the ability to grow embryos further out in development and allowed the laboratory "choice" regarding which embryos were transferred. This resulted in increased success in pregnancy rates. However, no matter how good the laboratory has become, what techniques are available for delivering the sperm to the egg, what culture media are available, or what transfer catheters and techniques are used, it is still not possible to take a poor-quality oocyte and make it into a high-quality one in the laboratory. Thus, the rate-limiting step in the IVP of human embryos is the oocyte.

The Oocyte

The oocytes that are recruited for development in a natural or exogenously stimulated cycle began their development in the fetus after the deposition of the primordial germ cells into the developing ovary (Tsafriri 1988). During fetal development the primordial cells begin to divide; they become oogonia and some enter into meiosis, thus forming the first oocytes (Eppig et al. 1996). By birth, all of the oogonia have entered meiosis, which is arrested at the dictyate stage. At the same time as the oogonia are entering meiosis a layer of somatic cells surround them, forming the primordial follicle (Anderson and Hirshfield 1992). Most of these follicles will degenerate over the lifetime of the female or are recruited into development for ovulation. Development is triggered by an unknown signal and is accompanied by proliferation of the surrounding somatic cells and an increase in size and protein content of the oocyte (Eppig et al. 1996, Lintern-Moore and Moore 1979, Schultz and Wassarman 1977). The resulting structure is the preantral follicle, an oocyte surrounded by three layers of granulosa cells. These oocytes are not mature enough to resume meiosis (Sorenson and Wassarman 1976). During this growth phase the oocyte increases in size about 300-fold and the zona pellucida is laid down. The granulosa cells proliferate and an antrum, or fluid-filled sac, forms in the follicle in which the oocyte, surrounded by two layers of granulosa cells, is suspended. The granulosa cells closest to the oocyte form gap junctions with it and are known as the corona radiata. The mature ovary contains pools of these fully grown oocytes arrested in prophase of the first meiotic division.

It is only these follicles that respond to stimulation with the resumption of meiosis in the oocyte. It is postulated that cAMP, delivered to the oocyte via the granulosa cells, holds the oocyte in an arrested state of meiosis (Eppig 1990). To resume meiosis the oocyte needs to first undergo further growth. During this growth the germinal vesicle also increases in size, altering the nuclear-to-cytoplasmic ratio. Ribosomal RNA synthesis is initiated, as evidenced by the increase in size of the nucleoli (Baker and Franchi 1967). Nucleoli form within the nucleus at areas known as the "nucleolus-organizing regions". The nucleolus-organizing regions are located on the chromosomes where the genes coding for ribosomal RNA are located and are the sites where pre-rRNA is synthesized. The number and location of nucleolus-organizing regions are species specific but the nucleoli differ according to the cell type, cellular activity, and the stage of development in any one species (Goessens 1984). Nucleoli are comprised of chromatin and ribosomal nuclear protein portions. The nucleoli in oocytes in antral follicles are well defined and actively synthesize rRNA, a process that is essential for attaining full meiotic competence (Motlik et al. 1984 a, b).

As the oocyte grows the metabolism changes; mitochondria change from being elongated with transverse cisternae to oval with columnar cisternae containing vacuoles (Baker and Franchi 1967, Balakier 1978). Further, the Golgi structures change in shape, and small membrane-bound vesicles involved in fertilization, known as the cortical granules, move to a subcortical region (Balakier and Czolowska 1977). The number of ribosomes increases dramatically (Biggers 1971).

The granulosa cells adjacent to the oocyte secrete hyaluronic acid in cumulus expansion or mucification, and the cells in the follicle wall begin to change. These processes are stimulated by FSH and LH. The gap junctions formed between the oocyte, the corona radiata, and the cells in the follicle wall are essential for the final phases of oocyte maturation (Eppig 1990). Oocyte maturation, with the resumption of meiosis, occurs when the flow of the meiosis-arresting factor cAMP (Eppig 1990) to the oocyte is decreased or stopped. At this point meiosis begins, with germinal vesicle breakdown and nuclear progression from the dictyate stage of the first meiotic prophase to metaphase II of the second meiotic division (first meiotic reduction), with expulsion of the first polar body.

It is thought that the granulosa cells produce a substance that overcomes the meiosis-arresting action of cAMP (Eppig 1990) and that this stimulated by either FSH or epidermal growth factor or both. The gap junctions decrease in number but do not entirely disappear.

As the follicles grow to the preantral and antral stages the blood supply increases. This is vital for the normal development of the oocyte since the blood brings in oxygen for oxidative phosphorylation, which the oocyte and growing follicle deep in the ovary utilize for their metabolic needs. Oocytes derived from follicles that have abnormal or poor capillary development are nonviable (Gregory et al. 1994, Hartshorne 1989). Furthermore, decreased blood flow leading to hypoxia results in decreased fertilization rates, increased spindle defects, and chromosomal abnormalities (Van Blerkom et al. 1997). Hypoxia in the follicle has also been related to disorganized cytoplasm, lower cytosolic pH, and lower ATP content in mature metaphase II oocytes (Van Blerkom and Henry 1992, Van Blerkom et al. 1995). Oocytes that have a lower ATP content (<0.2 pmol) fail to develop normally and do not establish successful pregnancies, even if they do implant (Van Blerkom et al. 1995).

The events of nuclear and cytoplasmic maturation in the oocyte and the growth and differentiation of the follicle somatic cells all play crucial and linked roles in the formation of a mature functional oocyte. If all the events of somatic cell follicle development have not occurred systematically, aspects of the final stages of maturation and oocyte feeding will not occur correctly. If the events of nuclear maturation, including the resumption of the first meiotic division and progression to metaphase II, are disrupted or not coordinated with cytoplasmic development the oocyte will be abnormal. Cytoplasmic maturation is crucial and includes all the events that prepare the oocyte for successful fertilization, including zona pellucida acquisition, cortical granule formation and the ability to release them and calcium, mitochondrial changes, protein synthesis involved in growth, and cytoskeletal changes. Each of these events can proceed independently with the production of seemingly normal follicles containing an oocyte that can be fertilized but will be abnormal (Anderson and Hirshfield 1992, Eppig et al. 1994, 1996). Thus, the production of a mature oocyte capable of being fertilized with potential for further development is a complex and coordinated series of events involving numerous cellular processes and structures and occurring over an extended time period in the ovary. The complex and coordinated development of the oocyte within the follicle ends with ovulation, when the oocyte surrounded by the cumulus cells enters the oviduct and awaits fertilization.

Fertilization and the Zygote

When the sperm enters the oocyte (by normal fertilization or ICSI) a series of complex events ensues. Initially the cortical granules are released and calcium is mobilized. As the sperm head begins to decondense, the centriole, or microtubule-organizing center forms. In human beings the centriole is sperm derived (Sathananthan et al. 1991; Schatten 1984). The microtubules arising from the centriole are responsible for bringing the newly formed male pronucleus and the female pronuclei together. If this does not occur normally development cannot continue (Sathananthan et al. 1991, Schatten 1984). As the oocyte matures and is ovulated rRNA synthesis decreases and the nucleoli become small and scattered (Crozet et al. 1986). When the oocyte is fertilized and the pronuclei form, rRNA synthesis resumes with the re-formation and growth of the nucleoli. There is also evidence that they begin to coalesce as more synthesis occurs. Nucleoli also grow in the male pronucleus (King et al. 1988, Tesarik and Kopecny 1989a,b, 1990). Ovulated oocytes and the early embryo rely exclusively on maternal RNA that was synthesized prior to ovulation. However, as the nucleoli begin to form in the male and female pronuclei, new rRNA can be synthesized, as evidenced by the appearance of the nucleoli. As the embryonic gene becomes active the rRNA being synthesized by the new unique embryo can take over, which occurs in the human being at about the four-cell stage (Braude et al. 1988). The timely and sequential initiation of events leading to rRNA synthesis in the zygote is therefore essential for subsequent development.

Nucleoli have a tendency to fuse (Goessens 1984, Tesarik and Kopecny 1989a), which is related to the cell cycle. There are more nucleoli present at the beginning of the G1 phase, and during the cell cycle they fuse, until by the S phase there should be only one or two per nucleus. During a mitotic cycle, daughter cells display synchrony in their nuclei content, daughter cells being indicative of aberrant chromosomal function. Asynchrony and inequality between the male and female pronucleus in the human zygote are evidence of either chromosomal abnormalities or an asynchrony between the nuclear events of meiosis. Either situation would lead to a breakdown of normal development with lack of embryonic implantation.

Early Embryo Culture, Extended Culture, and Blastocyst Development

Once the oocyte is fertilized in vitro it can be transferred to the uterus as a pronuclear one-cell embryo or cultured for 2, 3, or 5 days and transferred as cleaving stages or blastocysts. In vivo a human embryo reaches the uterus as a compacting morula only approximately 3 days after fertilization (72 or 96 h after ovulation). Placing an earlier-stage embryo into the uterine environment is unphysiologic, yet it is clearly successful in the human being, pregnancies having been attained after pronuclear one-cell-stage transfers (Ahuja et al. 1985, Scott and Smith 1998) and at the four- to eight-cell stages (Dawson et al. 1995, Edwards et al. 1980, Scholtes and Zeilmaker 1996, Tan et al. 1992). The practice of transferring day-

5 blastocysts is a recent development in the field of human IVP (Gardner and Lane 1997, Gardner et al. 1998), brought about by the development of specific culture media designed to meet the dynamic metabolic needs of embryos in vitro (Barnett and Bavister 1996, Bavister 1995, Gardner and Lane 1993, Gardner and Sakkas 1993, Leese 1991, Leese 1995, Leese et al. 1993).

In all aspects of human IVP, embryos are chosen for transfer based on their appearance, their morphology. Cleaving-stage embryos are graded according to cell number and the evenness of the blastomeres in the embryo. Human cleavage stage embryos routinely "bleb" and sometimes fragment. The degree of blebbing and fragmentation is also accounted for in the scoring systems. Initially embryos were routinely transferred on day 2, 48 h after insemination at the four-cell stage. With the development of more efficacious drugs, allowing better ovulation induction and therefore more oocytes, and a better understanding of the human embryo's needs in vitro it became more common to transfer embryos on day 3, at the eight-cell stage. This led to an increase in pregnancy rates, which was due to the ability to select those embryos that were more advanced and morphologically of better quality (Dawson et al. 1995). However, there was a dramatic increase in the incidence of higher-order multiple pregnancies. In countries where the process of IVP is at considerable cost to the patient, the idea of mandating a limit on the numbers of embryos replaced was not feasible. With the introduction of extended culture and day-5 transfers it was feasible to add a further level of embryo selection to the process, since only 30–40% of all zygotes actually reach the blastocyst stage. Using day-5 transfers it has been possible to almost double the implantation rate using far fewer embryos (Scholtes and Zeilmaker 1996, Gardner et al. 1998).

Of great concern to all in the practice of IVP when using day-5 blastocyst transfers is the fact that in some instances there is no blastocyst for transfer. The question remains as to whether embryos that do not grow in vitro in the media currently available would be able to implant if transferred at an earlier stage. Another aspect of IVP that has not improved, even with the introduction of day-5 transfers and increased implantation per embryo, is the overall efficacy of human IVP when one considers how many oocytes are needed to attain one baby. The efficiency in good programs remains at approximately 10%, which is very low (Scott and Smith 1998, Edwards and Beard 1999). Clearly, the oocyte holds the key to this low success. Screening oocytes and the early events of development may contribute to increasing the overall efficacy of human IVP.

Embryo Scoring

The Zygote

It has become evident that the earliest event of human embryo development can be used to assess developmental potential and implantation (Scott and Smith 1998, Tesarik and Greco 1999). Two separate pronuclear morphology scoring systems have been described in which the number, size, and distribution of nucleoli in the male and female pronuclei of human zygotes has been correlated with ability to implant and establish a successful pregnancy. The data have been retrospective in nature but recently, with the ability to grow embryos to the blastocyst stage, it has become possible to also correlate the zygote morphology with later development in vitro, resulting in improved embryo selection for transfer.

Zygote scoring involves looking very critically at the progress of the pronuclei, their size, shape, and the nucleolar structures within them, as shown in Figs. 1–4. Initially, the alignment of the pronuclei at 16–18 h post insemination needs to be recorded. Ideally they should be aligned or appearing to touch. Since the centrioles and microtubules bring the nuclei together, failure in this event is indicative of failure of one or several fertilization events (Schatten 1984, Sathananthan et al. 1991). These embryos do not progress well and rarely form blastocysts in vitro (Fig. 4b).

The actual size of the pronuclei is also of utmost importance. Human embryos have been shown to have an aneuploidy rate of anywhere from 20% to 40% (Plachot et al. 1987, Munne et al. 1997), although the reported aneuploidy rate may be high due to mosaicism (Munne and Cohen 1998). However, the incidence of chromosomal abnormalities in embryos deriving from zygotes in which there is a marked size difference in the pronuclei (Fig. 4a) is on the order of 87% (Munne and Cohen 1998, Sadowy et al. 1998). Thus, any zygotes

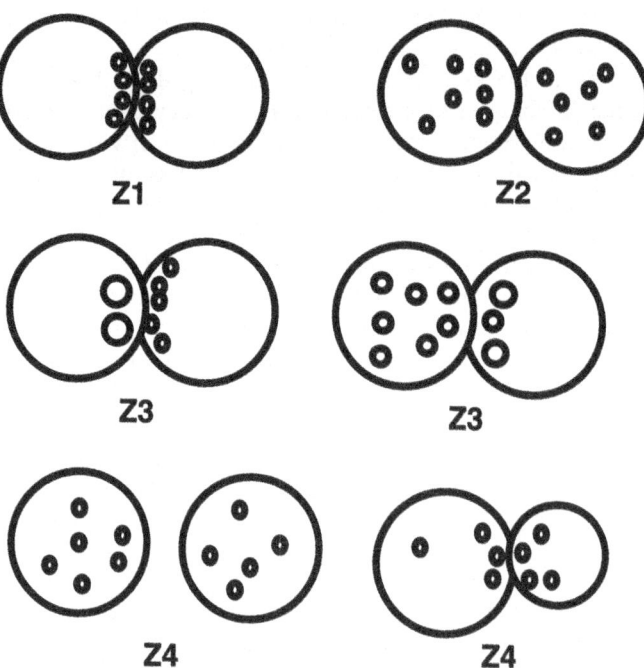

Fig. 1. Zygote scoring system

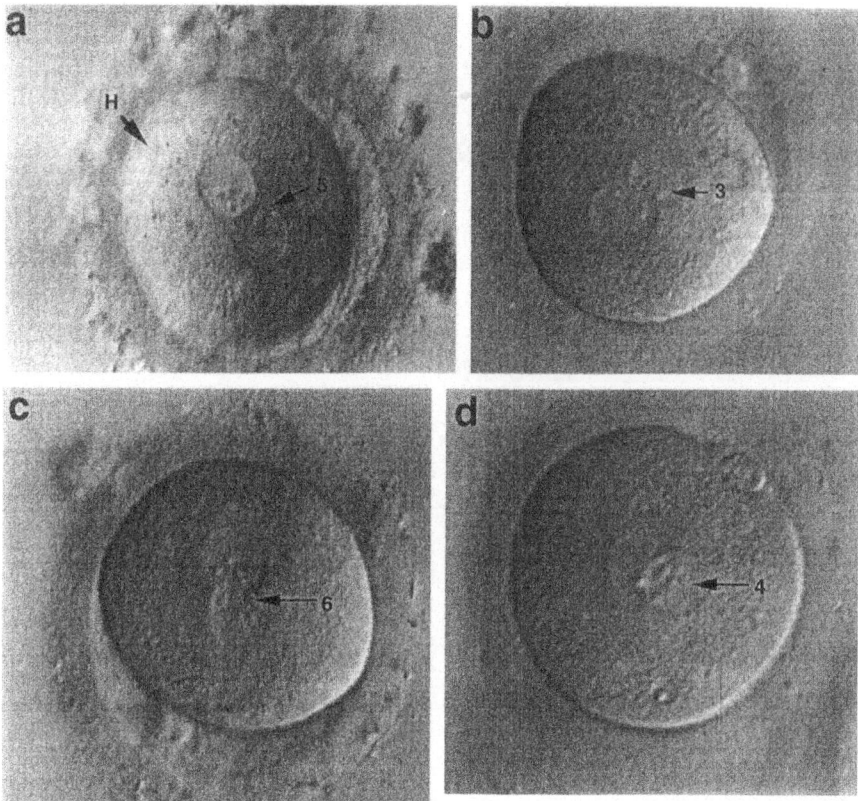

Fig. 2a-d. Zygotes optimal for development and implantation: **a,b** with alignment at pronuclear junction – designated Z1; **c,d** with nucleoli still scattered – Z2. *Numbers and arrows* indicate number of nucleoli, *H* "halo" effect

that have nonaligned pronuclei or pronuclei that are of distinctly different sizes are probably abnormal in some way and should not be considered for transfer. A grading scheme has been developed (Scott, unpublished data) in which these zygotes are designated Z-4 (Fig. 1).

As described above, the nucleoli begin to grow in the newly formed nuclei and are indicative of early rRNA activity. The state of these nucleoli forms the central aspect of zygote scoring. A scoring system accounting for the number, size, and distribution within the nucleoli can be used to grade them, as depicted in Fig. 1 (Scott, unpublished data).

The number of nucleoli should ideally be between 3 and 7 per nucleus (see Fig. 2a-d). The presence of fewer nucleoli at 16-18 h after insemination has not been associated with pregnancies (Figs. 3, 4c,d) Zygotes with many small pinpoint nucleoli are probably delayed in nuclear events and the formation of the nucleolar organizing centers (Fig. 3f). These zygotes are slow in development and routinely result in suboptimal embryos and only 10–15% blastocyst forma-

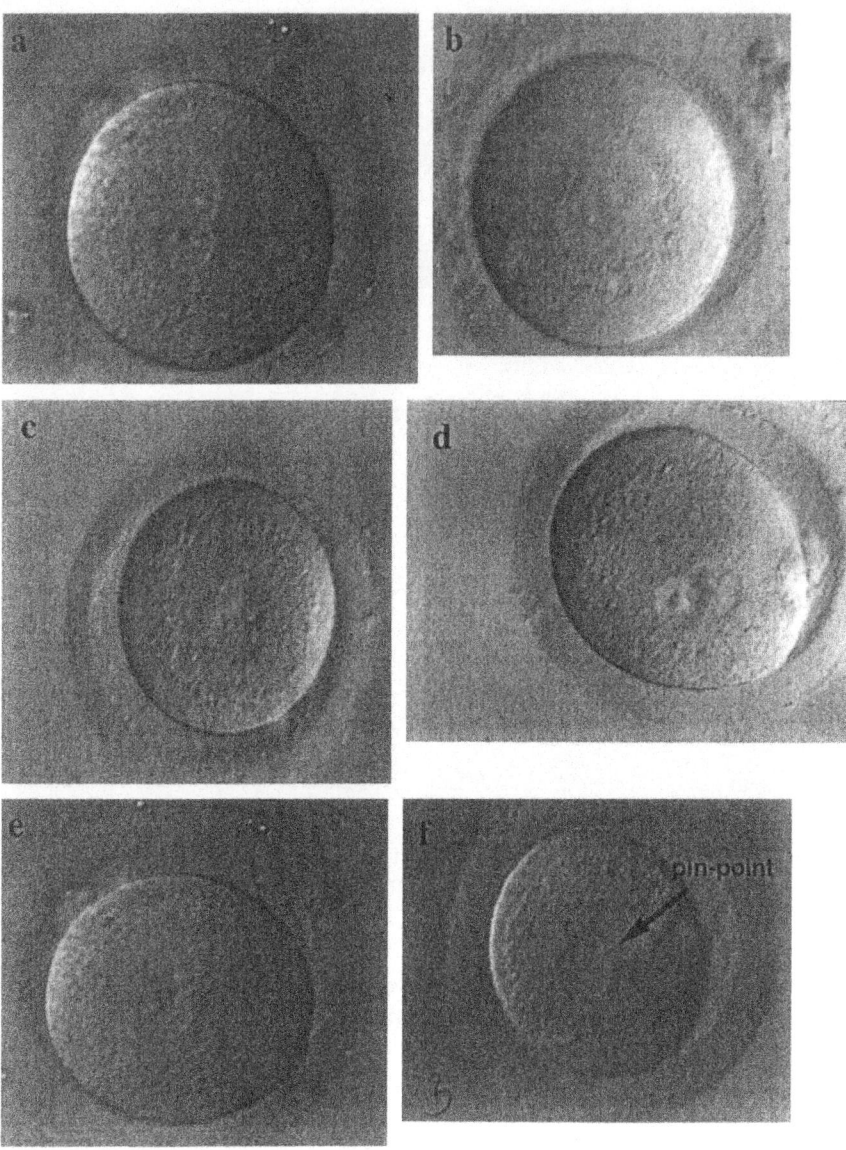

Fig. 3 a–f. Zygotes less suited for transfer, scored Z3, have fewer nucleoli and in some cases many small *pin-point* nucleoli

tion (unpublished data). Some women routinely present with all zygotes in this form and, even after repeated attempts at IVP with day-3 or day-5 embryo transfers, fail to achieve a pregnancy. Zygotes of this form are designated Z3.

The alignment of the nucleoli at the pronuclear junction is important for the metabolic status of the embryo and for the ability of the nuclei to fuse and form

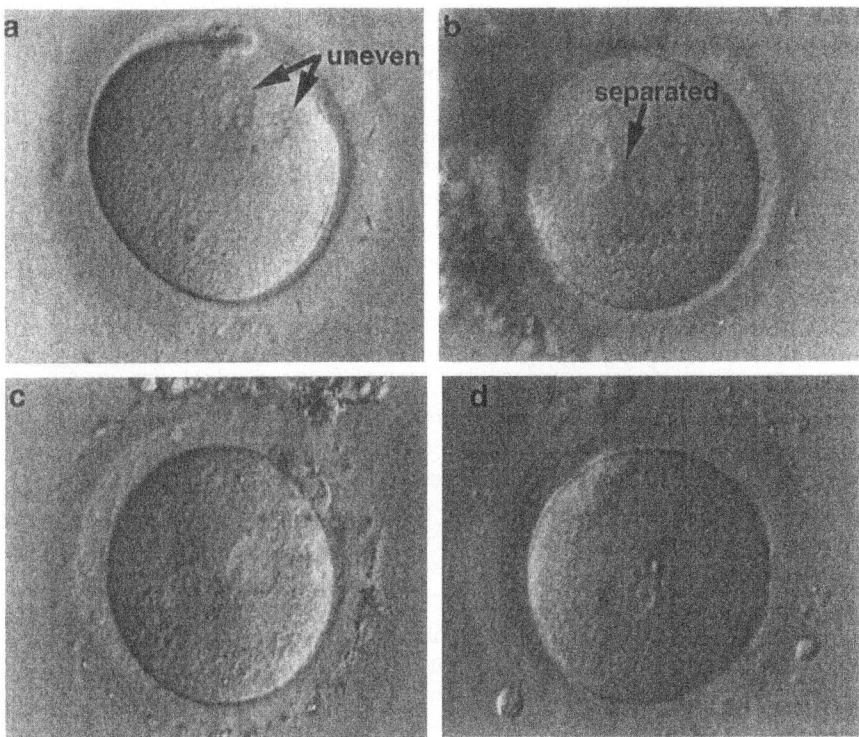

Fig. 4a–d. Zygotes unsuited for transfer have fewer nucleoli and show a marked size difference in the pronuclei

the unique embryonic genome (Van Blerkom 1990, Van Blerkom and Henry 1992, Van Blerkom and Runner 1984). The pH gradient between the two sets of nucleoli is lower than elsewhere and is an important factor in this fusion event. Failure to align or the inequality of nuclei could drastically alter this gradient which could lead to abnormal development when the male and female genomes combine.

Zygotes with inequality in the nucleoli also have reduced developmental potential (Fig. 3). Those with unequal numbers or unequal sizes of nucleoli probably display asynchrony between male and female pronuclei. Since the nucleoli progress from small centers to coalesce and align at the pronuclear junction, any inequality between them will lead to aberrant development. In the scoring system these would also be designated Z3.

Zygotes with equal numbers of nucleoli that are of even size, between 3 and about 7 per pronucleus, have been shown to give optimal development and implantation (Scott, unpublished data). Those in which there is alignment at the pronuclear junction are designated Z1 (Fig. 2 a, b), and those whose nucleoli are still scattered are designated Z2 (Fig. 2 c, d).

The appearance of the cytoplasm can also be used to assess the zygotes. The presence of a "halo" effect (Scott and Smith 1998) is generally associated with zygotes that lead to high-quality embryos on day 3 and day 5 (Fig. 2a). It is not necessarily associated with any particular Z-score but is consistently linked to cohorts of zygotes that developed to good-quality blastocysts. This clearing of the cytoplasm, or cytoplasmic streaming (Payne et al. 1997), is most likely associated with mitochondrial movement within the zygote. Both mouse (Muggleton-Harris and Brown 1988) and hamster (Barnett et al. 1996) one-cell fertilized embryos display differential mitochondrial distribution that is cell-cycle related. In the mouse the mitochondria migrate to the periphery of the cell, whereas in the hamster they migrate and aggregate in the center of the cell, around the pronuclei. A pattern equivalent to that in the hamster can be seen in human zygotes (Payne et al. 1997, Scott and Smith 1998) and is associated with increased developmental potential. If it were indeed the mitochondria that are migrating, it would seem reasonable that they are aggregating at the site of most intense activity, the pronuclei, for maximum metabolic use. Zygotes in which this movement is not so pronounced or does not occur could be metabolically compromised, which will ultimately lead to poor development.

The Cleaving Embryo

Cleaving-embryo morphology traditionally relies on cell number, evenness of cleavage, and the degree of fragmentation (Pruissant et al. 1987, Steer et al. 1992). Fragmentation has been associated with mosaicism but not so much with aneuploidy (Munne and Cohen 1998, Plachot et al. 1987). The rate of development of human embryos is slower in vitro than in vivo. However, rapid entry into the first cleavage division has been shown to be associated with increased rates of implantation with day-3 transfers (Shoukir et al. 1997). When zygote scoring was applied, the subsequent rapid entry of Z1 or Z2 zygotes to the first cleavage division was always associated with increased blastocyst formation and increased implantation rates. However, the rapid entry of zygotes with one or two large nucleoli was associated with high day-3 morphology but very low blastocyst development.

Since so many human embryos are chromosomally abnormal, checking the ploidy at the cleaving stages is also important. At the two- to eight-cell stage the nuclei in the blastomeres can easily be seen. Embryos containing one or two blastomeres with two or more nucleoli are most likely to be mosaics at best and totally aneuploid at worst and should not be used for embryo transfer (Munne and Cohen 1998). There appears to be no association between Z score and blastomere ploidy.

The cell-cell contact between the blastomeres in an eight-cell embryo is almost more important than the state of fragmentation. Embryos with the blastomeres beginning to flatten and form tight junctions result in higher implantation rates than those that are perfectly rounded with little cell-cell contact. If these embryos have been cultured in a glucose-free system up to this point, a short exposure to a glucose- and amino acid-containing medium results in greatly increased implantation rates (Scott, unpublished data). Embryos at earlier stages or those that do not display the cell flattening do not appear to benefit from this treatment. This phenomenon is probably related to the metabolic switch the embryo is undergoing at this stage of development. Until it reaches the eight-cell stage the human embryo relies almost exclusively on oxidative phosphorylation for all its metabolic needs. Glycolysis is initiated at this stage, allowing for the use of glucose. The embryo also begins to compact and grow with the production of new proteins (Barnett and Bavister 1996, Bavister 1995, Leese 1990, Leese 1991, Leese 1995, Leese et al. 1993, Scott and Smith 1998, Scott and Whittingham 1996). It could be that by being briefly exposed to a combination of glucose and amino acids they are able to switch into "high gear", giving them an advantage over the other embryos.

Blastocysts

Only certain blastocysts have the potential to implant. A high-grade blastocyst must have reached this stage by the morning of the fifth day of culture. There should be >40 cells in the blastocyst, a well-defined inner cell mass, and a continuous, even trophectoderm (Fig. 5a, b). The blastocyst should be free of degenerate cells in the blastocoele, be free of spidery projections traversing the blastocoele (Fig. 5c), and have no large cells which are clearly arrested from earlier cleavage stages (Fig. 5d). The trophectoderm should be continuous, with a sufficient number of evenly sized cells such that no one cell needs to stretch to form contact with the next cell. All blastocysts should have arisen from embryos that cleaved on an appropriate time course from the one-cell to the blastocyst stage.

Zygote, Embryo, and Blastocyst Morphology and Implantation

When human zygotes are scored using the zygote scoring system, Z1–Z4, there is a fairly even spread of zygotes between Z1, Z2, and Z3 types, with no differences seen for age or infertility presentation (Fig. 6). Fewer than 10% of all zygotes are of the Z4 type, with nonaligned nuclei or grossly unevenly sized nuclei. Often these embryos can develop normally (see Fig. 6), but since they are so abnormal they should not be considered for transfer. The correlation between Z score and day-3 morphology is not significant, although there is a trend for the Z1 and Z2 zygotes to produce more eight-cell embryos that are not fragmenting as much. Since the equality of nucleoli between male and female pronuclei should be important for synchronous development in the embryo (see above), this observation seems logical.

When embryos are placed in extended culture a significant difference is observed in the extent of blastocyst development between Z1, Z2, and Z3 zygotes (Fig. 7). Greater than 60% of all Z1 zygotes develop into good-grade blastocysts compared with 36% of Z2 zygotes and 28% of Z3 zygotes. Again, if the role of the nucleoli in embryonic development is considered, this is a predictable out-

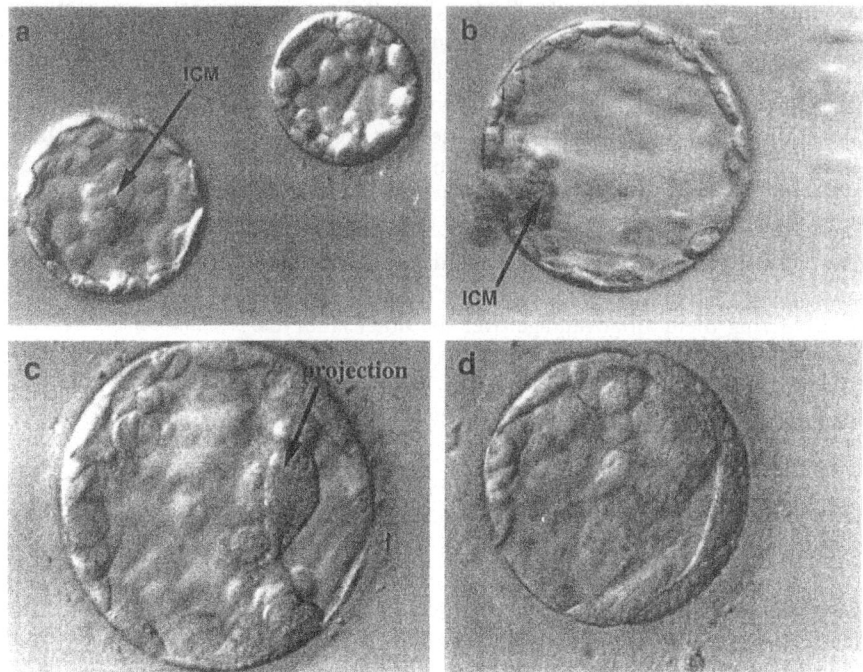

Fig. 5 a–d. High- (**a,b**) and low-grade (**c,d**) blastocysts. *ICM* inner cell mass

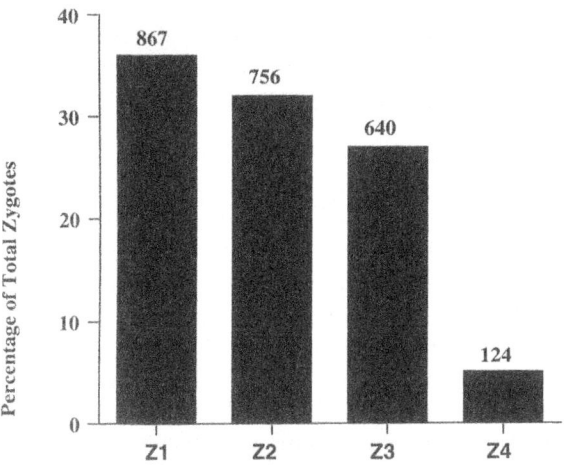

Fig. 6. Distribution of Z types for 2387 scored zygotes

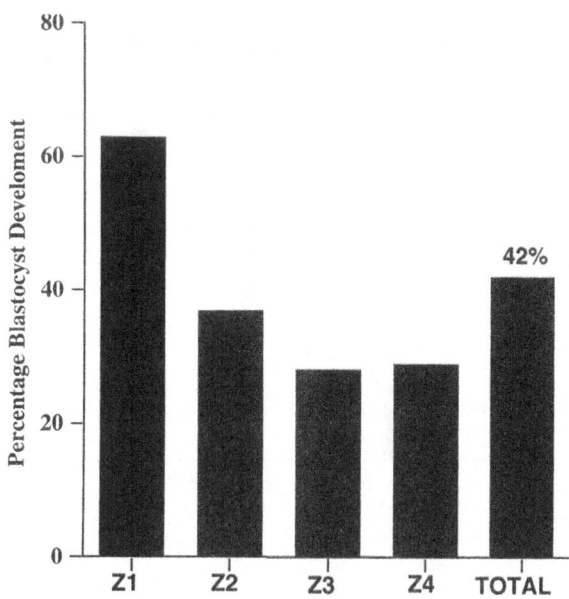

Fig. 7. Blastocyst development from each Z score

come. Embryos in which there is asynchrony between the nuclei are more likely to have chromosomal and cellular aberrations which will compromise their development. If the alignment of nucleoli at the nuclei junction is important for metabolism, failure to progress to this stage will result in a metabolically compromised embryo, lacking the ability to grow to the blastocyst stage (Van Blerkom 1990, Van Blerkom and Henry 1992, Van Blerkom and Runner 1984). Further, if there is abnormal syngamy due to lack of nucleoli alignment the embryos will be chromosomally abnormal.

This shows that there is a clear correlation between the zygote morphology and ability to grow to the blastocyst stage. The implantation rates quoted for blastocyst transfers are far greater than those reported for day-2 and day-3 transfers (Gardner et al. 1998, Scholtes and Zeilmaker 1996). It is clear that most of the good-grade blastocysts arise from Z1 zygotes. Thus, it stands to reason that there should be a correlation between zygote score and implantation on any day of transfer. When this is analyzed for both day-3 and day-5 transfers the difference in pregnancy and implantation are highly significant between zygote-scored and nonscored cycles (Fig. 8). If embryos are selected on day 3 based initially on zygote score and secondarily on day-3 morphology, the implantation rate can be doubled, from 19% to 31%, as can the pregnancy rate, from 33% to 57%. The mean number of embryos required to achieve this is also significantly less for scored cycles compared with nonscored cycles (2.8 vs. 3.3, $p < 0.01$; Scott unpublished data). The data from day-5 blastocyst transfers are not as dramatic. Overall, there is an increase in both implantation and pregnancy compared with day-3 transfers, as has been previously reported. The dif-

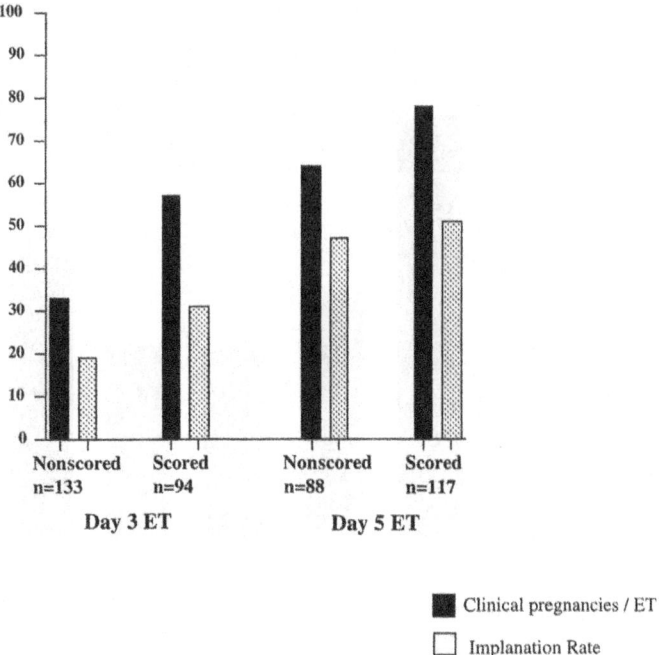

Fig. 8. Implantation and pregnancy data resulting from the transfer of embryos derived from Z-scored or nonscored zygotes

ference between scored and nonscored cycles is not significant. This is not surprising, since the majority of good-grade blastocysts arise from Z1 embryos. It therefore follows that scored and nonscored cycles will not be too different.

An interesting observation is that the implantation rate of blastocysts arising from Z1 zygotes is >60%, compared with <40% for Z2 blastocysts. To date there have been no recorded ongoing pregnancies achieved from the transfer of only Z3 blastocysts. Thus, even if the Z3 embryos are able to grow to the blastocyst stage they are abnormal in some way that is not morphologically apparent and cannot continue growing.

Another very important observation is the development of embryos in vitro related to their Z score. Cleaving embryos resulting from zygotes that have numerous very small, scattered nucleoli do not develop well in the extended culture media currently available and do not form blastocysts. To date, the author has recorded two pregnancies in 2 years from such embryos, although both ended in early miscarriage. It may be expedient, when zygotes present with this morphology, to transfer them as early as possible, in an attempt to stress them as little as possible in the artificial systems we have available.

Zygotes that have only two or three very large nucleoli do not grow well to the blastocyst stage. However, as long as there is an equal number of nucleoli per nucleus they form very high grade day-3 embryos. Further, the implantation rate of these embryos, when transferred on day 3 after exposure to extended culture media for a few hours, is >60%. If they are beginning to flatten and compact it is best to transfer only two embryos, since the implantation rate is so high. The explanation for this phenomenon may be metabolic. It could be that these embryos are advancing very rapidly with very rapid coalescence of the nucleoli. They may burn out too soon metabolically or just be unable to grow in the systems that are currently available for in vitro culture. Thus scoring them and transferring them on day 3 could realize their potential better than using day-5 transfer.

Conclusion

Human reproduction is very inefficient. Using very careful and defined scoring at every stage of development increases the chances of a woman's getting pregnant and reduces the need for large cohorts of embryos. Zygote scoring, blastomere screening for multinucleation, and selective day-3 or day-5 transfers maximize the potential of every embryo and reduce the incidence of high-order multiple pregnancies. However, until we are able to alter the quality of the oocyte we will always have a highly inefficient system. Not all fertilized embryos have the same potential. Embryos with little or no potential can be selected out and not used for either embryo transfer or cryopreservation. Figure 9 illustrates the scoring and fallout at each step, starting with an unfertilized oocyte. What is obvious is that no matter how good we become at selecting embryos and get-

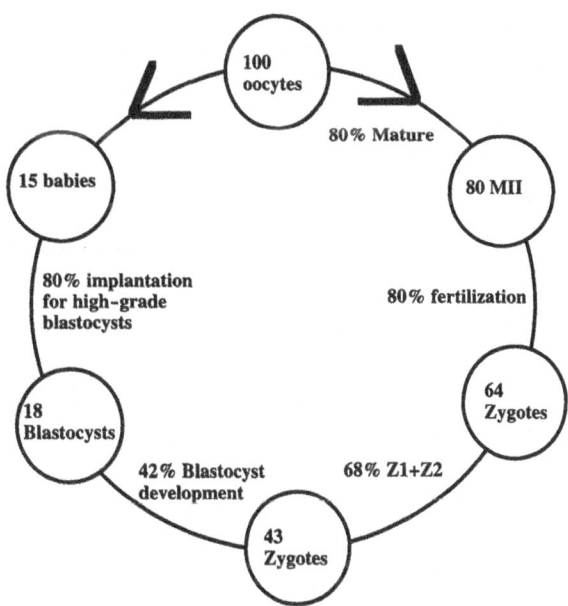

Fig. 9. Human reproductive inefficiency. *MII* metaphase II

ting women pregnant, large cohorts of oocytes are needed to attain this goal. Better methods of stimulation are required, as is a deeper understanding of what controls the complicated events of oocyte growth and maturation.

References

Ahuja KK, Smith W, Tucker M, Craft I (1985) Successful pregnancies from the transfer of pronuclear embryos in an outpatient in vitro fertilization program. Fertil Steril 44:181–184

Anderson LD, Hirshfield AN (1992) An overview of follicular development in the ovary: From embryo to the fertilized ovum in vitro. Md Med J 41:614–620

Baker T, Franchi L (1967) The structure of the chromosomes in human primordial oocytes. Chromosoma 22:358–377

Balakier H (1978) Induction of maturation in small oocytes from sexually immature mice by fusion with mitotic cells. Exp Cell Res 112:137–141

Balakier H, Czolowska R (1977) Cytoplasmic control of nuclear maturation in mouse oocytes. Exp Cell Res 110:466–469

Barnett DK, Bavister BD (1996) What is the relationship between the metabolism of preimplantation embryos and their developmental competence. Mol Reprod Dev 43:105–133

Barnett DK, Kimura J, Bavister BD (1996) Translocation of active mitochondria during hamster preimplantation embryo development studied by confocal laser scanning microscopy. Dev Dyn 205:64–72

Bavister BD (1995) Culture of preimplantation embryos: facts and artifacts. Hum Reprod Update 1:91–148

Biggers JD (1971) New observations on the nutrition of the mammalian oocyte and the preimplantation embryo. University of Chicago Press, Chicago, pp 319–325

Braude P, Bolton V, Moore S (1988) Human gene expression first occurs between the four and eight-cell stages of preimplantation development. Nature 332:459–461

Crozet N, Kanka J, Motlik J, Fulka J (1986) Nucleolar fine structure and RNA synthesis in bovine oocytes from antral follicles. Gamete Res 14:65–73

Dawson KJ, Conaghan J, Ostera GR, Winston RML, Hardy K (1995) Delaying transfer to the third day post-insemination, to select non-arrested embryos, increases development to the fetal heart stage. Hum Reprod 10:177–182

Edwards RG, Beard HK (1997) Oocyte polarity and cell determination in early mammalian embryos. Mol Hum Reprod 3:863–905

Edwards RG, Beard HK (1999) Blastocyst stage transfer: pitfalls and benefits. Hum Reprod 14:1–6

Edwards RG, Steptoe PC, Purdy JM (1980) Establishing full term human pregnancies using cleaving embryos grown in vitro. Br J Obstet Gynaecol 87:737–757

Eppig JJ (1990) The induction of oocyte maturation. In: Serono symposia, vol 66. Springer, New York, pp 77–86

Eppig JJ, Schultz RM, O'Brien M, Chesnal F, Smith A (1994) Relationship between the developmental programs controlling nuclear and cytoplasmic maturation of mouse oocytes. Dev Biol 164:1–9

Eppig JJ, O'Brien M, Wigglesworth K (1996) Mammalian oocyte growth and development in vitro. Mol Reprod Dev 44:260–273

Gardner DK, Lane M (1993) Amino acids and ammonium regulate mouse embryo development in culture. Biol Reprod 48:377–385

Gardner DK, Lane M (1997) Culture and selection of viable blastocysts: a feasible proposition for human IVF? Hum Reprod Update 3:367–382

Gardner DK, Sakkas D (1993) Mouse embryo cleavage, metabolism and viability: role of medium composition. Hum Reprod 8:288–295

Gardner DK, Vella P, Lane M (1998) Culture and transfer of blastocysts increases implantation rates and reduces the need for multiple embryo transfers. Fertil Steril 69:84–88

Goessens G (1984) Nucleolar structure. Int Rev Cytol 87:107–158

Gregory L, Booth A, Wells C, Walker S (1994) A study of the cumulus-corona cell complex in in vitro fertilization and embryo transfer; a prognostic indicator of the failure of implantation. Hum Reprod 9:1308–1317

Hartshorne G (1989) Steroid production by the cumulus: relationship to fertilization in vitro. Hum Reprod 7:742–745

King WA, Nair I, Chartrain KJ, Betteridge KJ, Guay P (1988) Nucleolus organizer regions and nucleoli in preattachment bovine embryos. J Reprod Fertil 82:87–95

Leese HJ (1990) The environment of the preimplantation embryo. In: Edwards RG (ed) Establishing a successful human pregnancy. Serono Symposium, vol 66, pp 143–154

Leese HJ (1991) Metabolism of the preimplantation mammalian embryo. In: Mulligan SR (ed) Oxford reviews of reproductive biology, vol 13. Oxford University Press, Oxford, pp 35–72

Leese HJ (1995) Metabolic control during preimplantation mammalian development. Hum Reprod Update 1:63–72

Leese HJ, Conaghan J, Martin KL, Hardy K (1993) Early human embryo metabolism. Bioessays 15:259–264

Lintern-Moore A, Moore GP (1979) The initiation of follicle and oocyte growth in the mouse ovary. Biol Reprod 20:773–778

Motlik J, Crozet N, Fulka J (1984a) Meiotic competence in vitro of pig oocytes isolated from early antral follicles. J Reprod Fertil 72:323–328

Motlik J, Kopecny V, Pivko J (1984b) RNA synthesis in pig follicular oocytes. Autoradiographic and cytochemical study. Biol Cell 50:229–236

Muggleton-Harris AL, Brown JJG (1988) Cytoplasmic factors influence mitochondrial reorganization and resumption of cleavage during culture of early mouse embryos. Hum Reprod 3:1020–1028

Munne S, Cohen J (1998) Chromosome abnormalities in human embryos. Hum Reprod Update 4:842–855

Munne S, Magli C, Adler A (1997) Treatment-related chromosome abnormalities in human embryos. Hum Reprod 12:780–784

Payne D, Flaherty SP, Barry MF, Mathews CD (1997) Preliminary observations on polar body extrusion and pronuclear formation in human oocytes using time-lapse video cinematography. Hum Reprod 12:532–541

Plachot M, Junca AM, Mandelbaum J, Grouchy JD, Salat-Baroux J, Cohen J (1987) Chromosome investigations in early life. II. Human preimplantation embryos. Hum Reprod 2:29–35

Pruissant F, Van Rysselberg M, Barlow P, Deweze J, Levoy F (1987) Embryo scoring as a prognostic tool in IVF treatment. Hum Reprod 2:705–708

Sadowy S, Tomkin G, Munne S (1998) Impaired development of zygotes with uneven pronuclear size. Zygote 63:137–141

Sathananthan AH, Kola I, Trounson A, Ng SC, Bongso A (1991) Centrioles in the beginning of human development. Proc Natl Acad Sci USA 88:4806–4810

Schatten G (1984) The centrosome and its mode of inheritance: the reduction of the centrosome during gametogenesis and its restoration during fertilization. Dev Biol 165:299–335

Scholtes MC, Zeilmaker GH (1996) A prospective, randomized study of embryo transfer results after 3 or 5 days of embryo culture in in vitro fertilization. 65:1245–1248

Schultz RM, Wassarman PM (1977) Biochemical studies of mammalian oogenesis: protein synthesis during oocyte growth and meiotic maturation in the mouse. J Cell Sci 24:167–194

Scott LA, Smith S (1998) The successful use of pronuclear embryo transfers the day after oocyte retrieval. Hum Reprod 13:1003–1013

Scott LA, Whittingham DG (1996) The influence of genetic background and media components on the development of mouse embryos in vitro. Mol Reprod Dev 43:336–346

Shoukir Y, Campana A, Farley T, Sakkas D (1997) Early cleavage of in-vitro fertilized human embryos to the 2-cell stage: a novel indicator of embryo quality and viability. Hum Reprod 12:1531–1536

Sorenson RA, Wassarman PM (1976) Relationship between growth and meiotic maturation of the mouse oocyte. Dev Biol 50:531–536

Steer CV, Mills CL, Tan SL, Campbell S, Edwards RG (1992) The cumulative embryo score: a predictive embryo scoring technique to select the optimal number of embryos to transfer in an in-vitro fertilization and embryo transfer programme. Hum Reprod 7:117–119

Tan SL, Royston P, Campbell S (1992) Cumulative conception and live birth rates after in-vitro fertilization. Lancet 339:1390–1394

Tesarik J, Greco E (1999) The probability of abnormal preimplantation development can be predicted by a single static observation on pronuclear stage morphology. Hum Reprod 14:1318–1323

Tesarik J, Kopecny V (1989a) Development of human male pronucleus: Ultrastructure and timing. Gamete Research 24:135–149

Tesarik J, Kopecny V (1989b) Developmental control of the human male pronucleus by ooplasmic factors. Hum Reprod 4:962–968

Tesarik J, Kopecny V (1990) Assembly of the nuclear precursor bodies in human male pronuclei is correlated with an early RNA synthetic activity. Exp Cell Res 191:153–156

Tsafriri A (1988) Local nonsteroidal regulators of ovarian function. In: Knobil E, Neil JD (eds) The physiology of reproduction, vol 1. Raven, New York, pp 527–565

Van Blerkom J (1990) Occurrence and developmental consequences of aberrant cellular organization in meiotically mature human oocytes after exogenous ovarian hyperstimulation. J Electron Microsc Tech 16:324–346

Van Blerkom J, Henry G (1992) Oocyte dysmorphism and aneuploidy in meiotically mature human oocytes after ovulation stimulation. Hum Reprod 7:379–390

Van Blerkom J, Runner MN (1984) Mitochondrial reorganisation during resumption of arrested meiosis in the mouse oocyte. Am J Anat 171:335–355

Van Blerkom J, Davis PW, Lee J (1995) ATP content of human oocytes and developmental potential and outcome after in vitro fertilization and embryo transfer. Hum Reprod 10:415–424

Van Blerkom J, Antczak M, Schrader R (1997) The developmental potential of the human oocyte is related to the dissolved oxygen content of follicular fluid: association with vascular endothelial growth factor levels and perifollicular blood flow characteristic. Hum Reprod 12:1047–1055

Cryoconservation: Sperms and Oocytes

G. Verheyen, J. Van der Elst, A. Van Steirteghem

General Introduction

From the moment of fertilization onwards, life processes run by the rhythm of a biological clock. The technology of cryopreservation gives us the possibility of interfering with the clockwork by stopping biological time. Cryopreservation of a cell therefore involves the cooling of a cell and storage at a temperature where all metabolic processes are arrested. In practice, frozen cells are stored at -196°C in liquid nitrogen. The ultimate challenge associated with cryopreservation would be the realization of whole-body freezing. As beautiful and romantic as this may be depicted in motion pictures such as "Forever Young", the reality is that the cryopreservation of single cells and small pieces of tissue is where we stand today. The freezing of single cells is considered cryobiologically the simplest, since only the physicochemical characteristics of one specific type of cell have to be taken into account in predictions of the response to freezing. Paradoxically, sperm cells and oocytes are single cells but seem rather sensitive to cryopreservation stress. This may be related to their highly specialized structure, and to their function of reconstituting an entire organism from the fusion of two single cells. In the following chapter we give an overview of the current status of oocyte and sperm freezing.

Cryoconservation of Oocytes

Historical Background

The pioneers of oocyte cryoconservation set out their goals almost 50 years ago. It is therefore surprising that by the year 1999, near the turn of the twenty-first century, there was still no successful method for the efficient cryoconservation of the human oocyte. In this chapter we shall try to explore reasons for this and, if possible, to provide an idea of what the prospects for the near future are.

In 1949, a paper by Polge et al. appeared in *Nature*, describing the first successful cryopreservation of fowl spermatozoa with glycerol. It is worth mentioning that this discovery was made in a rather pragmatic and serendipitous way, since the experiments leading to this discovery were designed primarily to investigate the aiding effect of sugars on vitrification. The cryoconservation of the female gamete, however, was to require more than pragmatism and good fortune.

In 1957, Lin, Sherman, and Willet demonstrated that the mouse oocyte can survive cooling to $-5\,°C$ in a medium containing 5% glycerol. In 1958, Sherman and Lin reported the birth of live young following in vitro fertilization of mouse oocytes that had been "frozen" at $-10\,°C$ in a medium containing 5% glycerol. However, no oocytes survived exposure at a temperature of $-20\,°C$. The question with regard to these experiments is whether the oocytes were really frozen at $-10\,°C$ or whether they were reduced to a supercooled state. Protocols that involved a lower storage temperature of $-79\,°C$ were applied by Smith and Parkes in 1951 and by Parkes in 1958 for the cryopreservation of ovarian sections rather than for the ovulated oocyte. They found that although all graafian follicles had degenerated after thawing, a few primordial follicles had survived. In 1960, Parrott was able to obtain live young from transplanted ovarian wedges that had been frozen with glycerol to $-79\,°C$.

A breakthrough in oocyte freezing did not occur, however, and this line of research was rather abandoned. It was another breakthrough that was to renew interest in cryoconservation of the female gamete. In 1978 the world was startled by the birth of the first test-tube baby, Louise Brown. This revolution in medicine and biology was possible only through the pioneering work of Robert G. Edwards and the late Patrick Steptoe (Steptoe and Edwards 1978, Edwards et al. 1980), who combined biology and gynecology in an extremely symbiotic way. An important consequence of the establishment of the technique of in vitro fertilization was that the human ovum was made accessible during an extracorporeal bypass between the ovary and the uterus. This possibility gave a vast new impulse to the interest in human oocyte cryoconservation.

It was not the human oocyte, however, but the human embryo that was first to be successfully cryopreserved. Indeed, within an approximately 20-year period (1960–1980) cryobiology had been raised from the level of pragmatism to science by pioneers of mathematical cryobiology such as Peter Mazur (Mazur 1970, 1984) and Stanley Leibo (Leibo 1977, 1980, Leibo et al. 1978). These authors had set up mathematical models for the freezing of biological systems based on the physicochemical characteristics of cells, such as membrane permeability and surface-to-volume ratio. In 1972, David Whittingham and co-workers applied mathematically based cryopreservation protocols to mouse embryos, so leading to the first report of the birth of live young after storage of mouse embryos at $-196\,°C$ in liquid nitrogen (Whittingham et al. 1972). The protocols that had been shown to work well with mouse embryos were largely copied for the human embryo, and it was in 1983 that the first paper on a pregnancy from a cryopreserved human embryo was published by Trounson and Mohr (1983). Unfortunately, a live birth did not ensue and it was the Dutch group of Zeilmaker and colleagues (1984) who reported the first recorded live birth after cryopreservation of human embryos on Boxing Day, 1983.

It was again David Whittingham (1977) who reported on the first successful cryoconservation of the mouse oocyte at $-196\,°C$ in liquid nitrogen followed by the birth of live young. Based on these protocols, and encouraged by the successful start of human embryo cryopreservation, several teams started to investigate the cryoconservation of the human oocyte. It was Chen who reported the first birth ensuing from a pregnancy obtained from a frozen oocyte in 1986. A limited number of live births were announced in the following years (van Uem et al. 1987, Chen 1988, 1989, Kolodziej et al. 1991). Despite the early successes, oocyte cryopreservation did not find widespread clinical application. The reasons for this were that the efficiency of oocyte cryopreservation was low due to low survival rates and that alarming reports questioning the genetic safety appeared in the literature. It was found that the degree of polyploidy increased significantly after cryopreservation of the mouse oocyte (Glenister et al. 1987) and of human oocytes (Al-Hasani et al. 1987). Oocyte cryopreservation was stopped in almost all clinical settings, while a few research teams continued to investigate the effects of cryopreservation on the oocyte. A comprehensive review of problems encountered with oocyte cryopreservation is given by Bernard and Fuller (1996). Recently, oocyte cryopreservation has been moved back to the clinic following reports by Gook et al. (1993, 1995) that proposed a workable protocol for cryopreservation of human oocytes. Using the proposed protocols, some successful pregnancies following oocyte cryopreservation have been obtained recently (Porcu et al. 1997, 1998, Borini et al. 1998, Polak de Fried et al. 1998). Questions remain, however, as to whether oocyte cryopreservation can safely and efficiently be offered to a couple, rather than managing a fresh replacement cycle with cryopreservation of supernumerary embryos.

The problems encountered in the freezing of mature oocytes stimulated research on the cryopreservation of immature oocytes in the germinal vesicle stage. In this stage the chromosomes are in the prophase of the first meiotic division and are protected within a nuclear membrane, rather than being exposed in a condensed state on an assembled spindle. It was estimated, therefore, that cryopreservation of the oocyte in the germinal vesicle stage would be less problematic in terms of spindle damage and genetic risk. It has been shown that the freezing of immature mouse and bovine oocytes can be followed by in vitro maturation, in vitro fertilization, embryo development, and even the production of live offspring (Schroeder et al. 1990, Van der Elst et al. 1992a, 1993b, Candy et al. 1994, Martino et al. 1996). The cryopreservation of human immature oocytes has been shown to be more problematic in terms of survival and maturation to the MII stage (Mandelbaum et al. 1988, Toth et al. 1994; Son et al. 1996). A limited number of pregnancies have been achieved from in vitro matured human oocytes derived from fresh ovarian biopsies, collected during IVF treatment cycles or from unstimulated ovaries (Trounson et al. 1994; Cha and Chian 1998, Russell 1998). One human pregnancy has been established so far from cryopreserved immature human germinal vesicle-stage oocytes (Tucker et al. 1998). With time, improvements in in vitro maturation culture techniques may make it possible for frozen immature human oocytes to be used in clinical practice.

The Need for Oocyte Cryopreservation

Autoconservation of Oocytes

In the routine of assisted procreation, oocyte cryopreservation can be of importance in the case of cycles where transfer of embryos to the uterus is counterindicated due to an increased risk for severe ovarian hyperstimulation syndrome, or where no sperm can be produced at the moment of pick-up.

At present, the greatest interest in oocyte cryopreservation comes from the field of oncological medicine. With the progress in screening and improved treatments for several types of cancers, an increased survival prognosis and eventually total cure have become possibilities. However, cancer treatment by radiotherapy, often in combination with chemotherapy, puts a serious burden on the function of reproductive organs. It is often the case that systemic cancer treatment leads to ovary burnout, so that the frequently young patient loses any hope of ever becoming pregnant, at least with her genetically own child. Chemotherapy for breast cancer may induce amenorrhea in up to 62% of patients (Collichio and Pandya 1994). As long-term survival rates for young women with cancer tend to improve, more attention is being focused on prevention of detrimental effects of radio- or chemotherapy on the patient's germinal cells (Ash 1980, Apperley and Reddy 1995).

Oocyte cryopreservation prior to anticancer treatment is therefore the only resort for young patients without a partner. In analogy to cryopreservation of human sperm, freezing of mature oocytes was considered an elegant option for preservation of fertility. Although interest in mature oocyte cryopreservation recently seemed to be renewed, clinical practice has proven it to be rather disappointing, resulting in only a handful of successful pregnancies (Chen 1986, 1988, 1989, Kolodziej et al. 1991; Porcu et al. 1997, 1998, Borini et al. 1998, Polak de Fried et al. 1998). Furthermore, the medical and psychological burden of ovarian stimulation and the delay it causes in starting cancer treatment prevents this attitude from being widely applied. Cryopreservation of embryos is an existing technique, although impossible to apply in children and women without a partner. Furthermore, in case of the patient's death, the existing "orphan embryo" can cause a moral debate. A remaining option is to cryopreserve cortical ovarian tissue prior to cancer treatment and to perform transplantation once therapy is finished. The cryopreservation and banking of ovarian cortical tissue containing primordial follicles announces itself as a promising new technique for the preservation of ovarian function in young female cancer patients.

Donor Oocyte Cryopreservation

Oocyte cryopreservation would also be a great tool in cases of oocyte donation. In the current situation oocyte donation is often cumbersome, not only as a result of the psychological aspects involved, but also because of the strict endocrinological requirements for synchronization of the ovarian cycles of the donor and the acceptor. The preservation of the oocyte until the appropriate moment of fertilization and embryo transfer would circumvent elegantly this now-mandatory synchronization system.

Oocyte Cryopreservation for Legal, Ethical, or Religious Indications

It is of interest to note that clinical oocyte cryopreservation was investigated intensively by German teams. This is not an accidental matter but is linked to the fact that in Germany, as in many other countries, the cryopreservation of embryos is prohibited by law (Embryonen-Schütz Gewalt) or is strongly disapproved of by religious and ethical guidelines. For countries or groups with objections to embryo freezing, the cryopreservation of oocytes is the only way out. Thus it is clear that the challenge to and necessity for establishing oocyte cryopreservation are still very prevalent.

Cryobiological Factors Influencing Cryoefficiency

Cell Survival

Cryopreservation of a cell involves the cooling of this cell to a subzero temperature at which all metabolic processes are arrested, followed by the return from this frozen condition to a physiologically active state. In other words, cryopreservation comes down to stopping biological time. In practice, cells are stored in liquid nitrogen at $-196\,°C$. The real challenge associated with cryopreservation is not to survive storage at $-196\,°C$ but to avoid intracellular ice formation in the transition across a temperature zone between $-15\,°C$ and $-60\,°C$, where intracellular ice formation is possible (Mazur 1984). Cells have to pass this zone twice, once during cooling and once during thawing. As will become clear from the following, it is absolutely necessary to control the cooling and thawing rate in this zone. Another prerequisite for cell survival is the presence of cryoprotective agents in the freezing medium. Evidence is accumulating for the occurrence of cryoprotective agents as part of a natural defense system. The discovery of the cryoprotectant glycoprotein in the circulation fluid of arctic fish is a living example of this (Rubinsky et al. 1991).

The Addition of Cryoprotectants

As stated above, glycerol was discovered to act as a cryoprotective agent in 1949. Since then several other chemical substances have been found to have a cryoprotective action (Ashwood-Smith 1967, 1986, Ashwood-Smith and Friedmann 1979, Boutron and Kaufmann 1979, Mazur 1970, 1984, McGann 1978). The most commonly used cryoprotectants besides glycerol are dimethylsulfoxide (DMSO) and 1,2-propanediol (PROH).

Cryoprotectants are highly miscible with water and have a low molecular weight, so that they can readily permeate the cell. Cryoprotectants are commonly used in concentrations of 1–2 M and can exert a prefreezing dehydrating effect due to the hypertonicity they bring to the freezing medium. Often, non-permeating cryoprotectants such as sucrose are used to promote prefreeze dehydration. Furthermore, cryoprotectants cause a freezing-point depression so that the temperature at which the cellular contents will freeze is lowered. In addition, cryoprotectants exhibit a high glass-forming tendency upon freezing. Also, at any time during cooling, cryoprotectants reduce the absolute concentration of salts that remain in the unfrozen solution. Thus, we can say that cryoprotectants confer protection by reducing the risks of intracellular ice formation and of solution effects. However, the use of cryoprotectants must be considered a knife that cuts two ways: as well as affording cryoprotection, cryoprotectants can also become toxic when exposure conditions are inappropriate.

Control of Cooling and Thawing Rate

Consider a cell that is suspended in an isotonic medium. When the temperature drops below 0 °C, the medium and the cell will initially remain unfrozen but supercooled, i.e., in a liquid state below the freezing point. Since the cell contains no efficient ice nucleators, ice will form first in the extracellular medium. Due to this extracellular ice formation, the extracellular concentration of solutes will increase. The cell will respond osmotically, and water will start to leave the cell to restore the chemical water potential. In other words, the cell will start to dehydrate, and this is the cell's first step in the prevention of intracellular ice formation.

All further physical events can be described in terms of the cooling rate. If the cycle of dehydration can be repeated often enough, i.e., if the cooling rate is slow enough, the cell will have lost all freezable water by the time the cell freezing point is reached. If cooling is done rapidly or ultrarapidly, water cannot leave the cell fast enough to restore the osmotic equilibrium and the equilibrium will be restored by a sudden and fast intracellular freezing, so that intra- and extracellular solute concentrations will match again. It therefore seems imperative to cool a cell slowly. If this is done, the question then is how to thaw this cell. What happens if a slowly frozen cell that is almost fully dehydrated is thawed rapidly? The extracellular water will melt massively and due to the large solute gradient with the hypertonic cell, water will rush into the cell and cause lysis of the cell through osmotic burst. If thawing is done slowly, the rehydration of the cell can take place gradually. Slow cooling therefore requires slow thawing. Cooling and thawing may not be too slow, however, since then the cellular components are exposed for a long time to high concentrations of salts, which may be harmful in terms of lipid and protein destabilization. This type of injury is referred to as solution effects.

If cooling is done very rapidly or slowly but to a high subzero temperature such as –30 °C, small ice crystals will be present when the cell is plunged into liquid nitrogen. It is imperative then to thaw rapidly so that the typical ice crystal aggregation tendency is overcome by quick melting of the ice crystals.

In conclusion, the challenge is to find a cooling rate that is slow enough to prevent intracellular ice formation and fast enough to prevent solution effects according to the two-factor hypothesis proposed by Mazur (1984). Every cell type will have an optimal cooling rate dictated by conditions of cell permeability and surface-to-volume ratio. For the oocyte, which is a large cell, the optimal cooling rate is below 1 °C/min. In practice, cooling and thawing are done with computer-controlled biological freezers. To make sure that the cycle of dehydration is started, the necessary triggering of extracellular ice formation is induced manually by touching the solution with a cooled tool. This is called "seeding".

Equilibrium and Nonequilibrium Freezing

Equilibrium freezing refers to the above-described procedures. It means that during the cooling and thawing phases the aim is to maintain chemical equilibrium between intra- and extracellular water potential. The cryoprotectants are used in 1–2 M concentrations and prefreeze exposure times are on the order of 10–20 min. Cryodamage is done either through intracellular ice formation or through solution effects.

Nonequilibrium freezing is a total departure from classic freezing theories. It is characterized by high concentrations of permeating cryoprotectants in combination with nonpermeating cryoprotectants, by short prefreeze exposure times of less than 5 min, and by immediate high cooling rates (Mazur 1990). Plunging into liquid nitrogen is done directly after the short exposure time. A distinction can be made between ultrarapid freezing and vitrification, which are both types of nonequilibrium freezing. In ultrarapid freezing, one permeating cryoprotectant in combination with a nonpermeating agent such as sucrose is often used. In vitrification, a mixture of different cryoprotective agents in combination with a nonpermeating agent is used. The concept of vitrification (literally: glass formation) was introduced as early as the late 1930s and 1940s (Ashwood-Smith 1986) and was rediscovered by Rall and Fahy in 1985. Vitrification is a process of solidification whereby an aqueous, viscous solution does not crystallize upon cooling but immediately forms a glass.

Equilibrium Freezing of Oocytes

In the first successful experiment on mouse oocyte cryopreservation, reported by Whittingham (1977), a slow-cooling equilibrium-freezing method was used with 1.5 M DMSO as the cryoprotectant. Oocytes were equilibrated in 1.5 M DMSO at 0 °C and cooled slowly at a rate of less than 1 °C/min to −80 °C; this was followed by storage in liquid nitrogen and slow thawing at a rate of 8°/min. A survival rate of approximately 70% was obtained and in vitro fertilizability was lower than for unfrozen control oocytes, but live young were obtained after transfer of embryos at the two-cell or blastocyst stage to pseudopregnant foster mice. In a randomized study on mouse oocyte cryopreservation with DMSO, Trounson and Kirby (1989) compared protocols with prefreeze equilibration at 0 °C or at room temperature and with slow and rapid thawing phases. They concluded that the best results were obtained with the addition of DMSO at 0 °C and slow cooling–slow thawing, which is the condition closest to the original protocol used by Whittingham (1977). This very protocol, however, was shown to induce increased polyploidy in pronuclear-stage mouse oocytes, where the chromosome complement of the male and female pronuclei have not yet fused (Glenister et al. 1987).

The use of PROH as a cryoprotectant for mouse and other animal oocytes has been far less successful. Comparative studies by Siebzehrübl (1989), Siebzehrübl et al. (1989), Todorow et al. (1989a,b) and Van der Elst (1992) pointed out that the protocols with PROH were less successful in particular in terms of mouse oocyte survival. Furthermore, it was demonstrated that PROH can cause parthenogenetic activation of the mouse oocyte (Shaw and Trounson 1989, Van der Elst et al. 1992b).

In the first successful attempt at human oocyte cryopreservation by Chen (1986) a modification of the technique by Whittingham (1977) was used. The prefreeze equilibration was done similarly in 1.5 M DMSO at 0 °C followed by slow cooling, but at –32 °C the oocytes were plunged into liquid nitrogen, followed by rapid thawing. Two other experiments with cryopreservation of the human oocyte also used DMSO as a cryoprotectant (Al-Hasani et al. 1987, van Uem et al. 1987). One human pregnancy was reported from a thawed oocyte where PROH was used as the cryoprotectant (Kolodziej et al. 1991). A new wave of research reports by Gook et al. (1993, 1995) in the 1990s proposed a workable protocol for cryopreservation of human oocytes. The freezing of human oocytes with PROH was advocated, linked to the use of intracytoplasmic sperm injection (ICSI) (Gook et al. 1995, Kazem et al. 1995), making it possible to obtain high levels of fertilization and embryo cleavage rates. The risk of chromosomal abnormalities did not seem to be increased (Gook et al. 1994, Bos Mikich and Whittingham 1995, Bos-Mikich et al. 1995). Using the proposed protocols, a few pregnancies following oocyte cryopreservation have recently been obtained (Tucker et al. 1996, Porcu et al. 1997, 1998, Borini et al. 1998, Polak de Fried et al. 1998).

Nonequilibrium Freezing of Oocytes

Ultrarapid Freezing. Ultrarapid freezing was introduced to the field of modern reproductive biology by Trounson et al. (1987) for mouse embryos. The technique was revolutionary, easy to perform, and much cheaper in terms of equipment than the slow-freezing techniques which require a programmable biological freezer.

In the case of mouse oocytes, the effect of ultrarapid freezing with both DMSO and PROH on oocyte ultrastructure was evaluated by Sathananthan

(1988). Survival rates of 34% and 33% and blastocyst formation rates of 15% and 7% were reported for DMSO and PROH, respectively. Surrey and Quinn (1990) reported a high survival rate of 61% and an oocyte-to-blastocyst transition rate of 59% for ultrarapid freezing of mouse oocytes with 3.5 M DMSO. Van der Elst et al. (1993a) used the protocol described by Surrey and Quinn (1990) and were also able to obtain high survival rates, but they reported increased polyploidy in pronuclear embryos and decreased cell numbers in blastocysts.

Results on ultrarapid freezing of the human oocyte have been very scarce until now. Trounson (1986) reported survival rates of around 50% upon thawing, but after culture the oocytes degenerated. Feichtinger (1987) reported a 12% survival rate, while Al-Hasani et al. (1987) found only one of 25 oocytes surviving. Pensis et al. (1989) engineered a protocol for optimal survival of human oocytes after ultrarapid freezing, but fertilization was not attempted.

Vitrification. Nakagata (1989) reported a very high survival rate of 88% and a two-cell formation rate of 78% using a modification of the original vitrification solution of Rall and Fahy (1985). Kono et al. (1991) published comparable results. Very different data were reported by Kola et al. (1988), who stated that vitrification of mouse oocytes resulted in increased aneuploidy and malformed fetuses. Wood et al. (1991) reported very high survival rates for mouse and hamster oocytes but decreased rates of implantation and development. Shaw et al. (1991) proposed an optimization of mouse oocyte vitrification by reducing the osmotically induced damage.

Vitrification of the human oocyte was investigated by Trounson (1986), Feichtinger (1987), and Hunter et al. (1995). Good survival rates have been reported, but embryonic development seems limited.

In conclusion, different cryobiological systems have been tried out on the oocyte, be it slow equilibrium freezing or rapid nonequilibrium freezing. Results in terms of survival and fertilization rates tend to be quite variable. Numerous studies on animal oocyte cryopreservation have been conducted with varying success, and there are some excellent reviews (Parks and Ruffing 1992, Rall 1992, Van Blerkom 1991, Vincent and Johnson 1992). Some general conclusions can be drawn, however: generally, fertilization rates seem lower and disturbances to the genetic integrity of the resulting embryos have been found. In the next section we will explore studies that have tried to find a reason for the problems observed in the cryopreservation of animal and human oocytes.

Oocyte Structures Affected by Cryopreservation

Whatever type of cryopreservation was used for the oocyte, be it equilibrium or nonequilibrium freezing, the freezing efficiency and genetic safety were under review. The oocyte is a highly unique structure containing the information for the body plan of the organism. Several research teams have been investigating which type of structure(s) in the oocyte are sensitive to the stresses imposed by cryopreservation. Several targets have been studied: microtubules, the zona pellucida, the fertilization machinery (parthenogenetic activation), and the chromosomes.

Microtubules

Microtubules are structures essential to intracellular architecture. Since microtubules are highly dynamic structures, they can rapidly assemble and disassemble in response to external stimuli. The oocyte contains a highly structured microtubular system in the form of the meiotic spindle, which carries the chromosomes at the metaphase plate. The microtubules of the spindle are in a steady-state equilibrium with the pool of free tubulin in the cytoplasm.

Cryopreservation involves cooling and exposure to cryoprotectants. Microtubules are sensitive to cooling (depolymerization) and to chemical agents that interfere greatly with the water hydrogen bonds which, in particular, are also involved in building microtubules. Since microtubules are essential to the architecture of the oocyte as well as to normal fertilization and development (Maro et al. 1984), it is important to consider that damage to the microtubules during freezing may have an effect on further development.

Magistrini and Szöllösi (1980) demonstrated in an ultrastructural study that the cooling of oocytes causes depolymerization of the spindle microtubules and that rewarming allowed repolymerization and reformation of spindle structures. This depolymerizing effect was confirmed and detailed further on whole oocyte mounts both by immunofluorescence by the Cambridge group (Pickering and Johnson 1987) and by immunogold cytochemistry by the Brussels group (Van der Elst et al. 1988). After recuperation from cooling, most of the depolymerization was restored but in some oocytes there was chromosome dispersal. Oocytes can thus recover from cooling, but the longer the exposure, the lower the chance of full restoration. The human oocyte seems more sensitive to cooling, and the degree of reversibility is less than in the mouse oocyte (Pickering et al. 1990). Bernard et al. (1992) demonstrated that human oocytes cooled to 0 °C and returned to culture conditions were capable of subsequent development.

The effects on microtubules by exposing oocytes to cryoprotectants were studied by different groups. The Cambridge group (Johnson and Pickering 1987) and the Brussels group (Van der Elst et al. 1988) showed that for the combination of cooling and exposure to DMSO the depolymerizing effect of cooling can be counteracted to a certain extent (for mouse oocytes), given that the exposure time is not too long. The best results in terms of spindle repolymerization and chromosomal scattering were obtained for exposure of mouse oocytes to DMSO at 4 °C (Johnson and Pickering 1987, Vincent and Johnson 1992).

A totally different picture was described by Van der Elst et al. (1988) for exposure of mouse oocytes to PROH. Although initially a protective effect from PROH on spindle depolymerization by temperature lowering was found, a big difference between the effect of DMSO and that of PROH became evident as regards the dilution of the cryoprotectant from the oocytes. Where for DMSO a restoration of spindle morphology was seen in the majority of oocytes, PROH caused the disappearance of the spindle after dilution and recovery. A parthenogenetic activation of the mouse oocyte by PROH was hypothesized and confirmed on the basis of these results (Shaw and Trounson 1989, Van der Elst et al. 1992b). For the human oocyte this oocyte activating effect of PROH was not found (Joly et al. 1992, Gook et al. 1993, Bernard et al. 1985).

The effect of ultrarapid freezing on the spindle was investigated by Aigner et al. (1992). It was shown that ultrarapid freezing with DMSO preserves spindle morphology even better than slow freezing. Spindle analysis of in vitro matured mouse oocytes that were cryopreserved in the germinal vesicle stage demonstrated only a few abnormalities incompatible with further development (Van der Elst et al. 1992a, Frydman et al. 1997).

In conclusion, cooling and cryoprotectants have an influence on the organization of the microtubular system of the oocyte, but restoration of the normal condition can be obtained. With this knowledge it seems possible to design optimal conditions of exposure (George and Johnson 1993).

Zona pellucida

The zona pellucida is a very characteristic integument of the oocyte and is of primordial importance in the sperm's interaction with the oocyte (Wassarman, 1990) and in the prevention of polyspermy by means of the zona reaction. The zona reaction leads, after the penetration of one sperm in the oocyte, to release of the content of the oocyte's submembranous cortical granules in order to alter the glycoproteins of the zona coat, so causing zona hardening.

It has been demonstrated that both cooling (Johnson et al. 1988) and exposure to DMSO (Johnson 1989) can cause premature zona hardening and reduced fertilization in mouse (Johnson 1989, Vincent et al. 1990) and human oocytes (Pickering et al. 1991). Again, the best conditions with the least effect on the zona involved exposure to DMSO at 4 °C for the mouse oocyte (Johnson 1989, George and Johnson 1993) as well as for the human oocyte (Bernard et al. 1992, Hunter et al. 1991). The use of fetal bovine serum in the freezing medium also seems to be beneficial in preventing premature zona reaction (Carroll et al. 1993, Vincent and Johnson 1992).

Chromosomes

Since the cytoskeletal integrity of the oocyte can be altered by cryopreservation, and since the chromosomes in particular are carried by the spindle consisting of microtubules, the induction of genetic abnormalities by cryopreservation is a major concern. It was demonstrated by Glenister et al. (1987) that slow freezing of mouse oocytes with DMSO induced increased polyploidy in the first-cleavage embryos. A more recent report by Bouquet et al. (1992) has confirmed this finding. The increased polyploidy seemed to be triploidy of the digynic type caused by retention of the second polar body (Carroll et al. 1989, Bouquet et al. 1992). For ultrarapid freezing of mouse oocytes it was demonstrated by Van der Elst et al. (1993a) that, as for slow freezing, increased polyploidy occurred in the first-cleavage embryos. The most important finding from these studies, however, is that there was no increase in the frequency of aneuploidy. Only Kola et al. (1988) reported a threefold increase in the degree of aneuploidy after vitrification of the mouse oocyte. Bos Mikich et al. (1995) reported that the frequency of aneuploidy in vitrified mouse oocytes was not increased, provided that the time of exposure to the cryoprotectant was carefully controlled.

For the human oocyte the data are scarce. The birth of healthy children, however few, indicates that normal fertilization and normal human development without chromosomal abnormalities are possible after freezing of the human oocyte. Recently, Van Blerkom and Davies (1994) reported that there was no increase in the frequency of aneuploidy in cryopreserved mature human oocytes. Moreover, Gook et al. (1994) reported that after cryopreservation of the human oocyte with PROH there were no abnormal karyotypes in pronuclear embryos.

Parthenogenetic Activation

Since the cytoskeleton is involved in the steps of fertilization, it was useful to consider the effect of cryopreservation on the possible precocious activation of the fertilization machinery. It was indeed shown by Shaw and Trounson (1989) and by Van der Elst et al. (1992) that PROH can cause activation of the mouse oocyte but that the degree of activation can be controlled by lowering the temperature and time of exposure for concentrations of up to 1.5 M. For DMSO no parthenogenetic activating activity has been demonstrated (Shaw and Trounson 1989).

For the human oocyte, no increased frequency of activation has been demonstrated after freezing with DMSO (Hunter et al. 1991), after vitrification (Hunter et al. 1992, 1995, Pensis et al. 1989), or after freezing with PROH (Gook et al. 1994).

Freezing of Ovarian Tissue

The latest development in oocyte cryopreservation is the freezing of human ovarian cortical tissue. The ovarian cortex houses a vast supply of primordial follicles. In the 1950s and 1960s, cryopreservation of ovarian sections with the birth of live young was reported (Parrott 1960). The renewed interest in cryopreservation of ovarian tissue results from the search by oncologists for a way to preserve the fertility of young cancer patients before they have to undergo sterilizing anticancer treatment.

The ovarian cortex in young women contains hundreds of thousands of primordial follicles which, because of their small size, are suitable for cryopreser-

vation. Cryopreservation of ovarian cortical tissue followed by orthotopic transplantation has already led to embryo development and/or pregnancies in mice
(Parrott 1960, Cox et al. 1996, Gunasena et al. 1997), sheep (Gosden et al.
1994a) and rats (Aubard et al. 1998). Follicular development was observed in
ovine and feline (Gosden et al. 1994b) and cryopreserved marmoset tissue
(Candy et al. 1995) after xenografting in SCID mice. Cryopreservation of human ovarian cortical tissue has demonstrated that morphologically normal follicles are present in the thawed tissue (Hovatta et al. 1996). Xenografting of frozen-thawed human ovarian cortical tissue under the kidney capsule of immuno-
deficient SCID mice has shown that follicle survival after transplantation can be
obtained (Newton et al. 1996). Oktay et al. (1998) showed that gonadotropic
stimulation of human xenografts in hypogonadal mice can lead to the growth
of follicles to the antral stage. Even more recently, it was shown by Van den
Broecke et al. (1999) that cryopreserved human ovarian xenografts remain susceptible to gonadotropic stimulation after grafting under the kidney capsule of
recipient SCID mice. Extensive reviews on ovarian tissue transplantation have
been published by Nugent et al. (1997) and Newton (1998), in which strategies
for the use of frozen-banked tissue for assisted reproduction are explored thoroughly.

Practical Aspects

To give an idea of the practice of oocyte cryopreservation we shall now detail
three protocols, one for slow and one for ultrarapid freezing of mouse oocytes
with DMSO, and one for slow freezing of ovarian cortical tissue with DMSO.

Slow Freezing of Mature Oocytes with DMSO

Media

- Oocyte collection medium: HEPES-buffered Earle's medium (Hogan et al.
  1986) supplemented with 0.5% bovine serum albumin (BSA) fraction V
- Freezing medium: HEPES-buffered Earle's medium supplemented with 0.5%
  crystalline BSA and 1.5 M DMSO
- Thawing medium: HEPES-buffered Earle's medium supplemented with crystalline 0.5% BSA.

Prefreeze Cryoprotectant Equilibration

- Equilibrate oocyte cumuli in groups of three to five for 10 min in 2.5 ml collection medium precooled at 0 °C.
- Transfer the cumuli in a minimal volume of medium to 2.5 ml freezing medium precooled at 0 °C and equilibrate for 15 min.

- Load straws (Industrie de Médecine Vétérinaire, I.M.V., France) as follows in the meantime: 100 μl freezing medium near the cotton plug end, a 100-μl air bubble, 100 μl freezing medium in the middle section to contain the oocytes, a 100-μl air bubble, and 100 μl freezing medium at the end to be plugged. Keep the straws cooled on crushed ice.

Cooling and Storage

- Transfer the cumuli in a minimal volume of medium to the middle section of a cooled straw with the aid of a finely-drawn pipette. Straws are plugged with polyvinyl powder (I.M.V., l'Aigle, France). Bring the straws, still on crushed ice, to the programmable freezer pre-set at 0 °C.
- Cooling at –2 °C/min to –6 °C.
- Seed manually by touching the end of the middle section with a liquid nitrogen-cooled forceps and observe whitening of the medium.
- Hold for 1 min at –6 °C.
- Cool at –0.3 °C/min to –80 °C.
- Transfer the straws to liquid nitrogen.

Thawing

- Remove straws from liquid nitrogen, transport them in a small container with liquid nitrogen, and transfer them quickly to the programmable freezer pre-set at –80 °C.
- Hold at –80 °C for 15 min.
- Warm at 10 °C/min to –20 °C.
- Hold at –20 °C for 15 min.
- Warm at 10 °C/min to 0 °C.
- Remove the straws from the freezer while keeping them on crushed ice.
- Allow the straws to equilibrate to ambient temperature on the bench of a laminar flow (22 °C).

Cryoprotectant Removal

- Expel the thawed content of a straw in 2.5 ml thawing medium.
- Equilibrate for 15 min at ambient temperature.
- Rinse twice in collection medium.
- Transfer cumuli to droplets of 100 μl culture medium Earle's medium (Hogan et al. 1986) with 0.5% BSA at 37 °C for 1 h of post-thaw recuperation before insemination.

Ultrarapid Freezing of Mature Oocytes with DMSO

Media

- Oocyte collection medium: HEPES-buffered Earle's medium supplemented with 0.5% BSA
- Prefreeze media:
  - HEPES-buffered Earle's medium supplemented with 20% bovine calf serum (BCS) and 0.25 M sucrose
  - HEPES-buffered Earle's medium supplemented with 20% BCS and 0.50 M sucrose
- Freezing medium: HEPES-buffered Earle's medium supplemented with 20% BCS, 0.50 M sucrose and 3.5 M DMSO
- Thawing media:
  - HEPES-buffered Earle's medium supplemented with 20% BCS and 0.25 M sucrose
  - HEPES-buffered Earle's medium supplemented with 20% BCS and 0.50 M sucrose.

Cooling and Storage

- Remove cumulus with 0.1% (w/v) hyaluronidase and rinse cumulus-free oocytes three times in 2.5 ml collection medium.
- Predehydrate oocytes in serial concentrations of sucrose: 0.25 M and 0.50 M in HEPES-buffered Earle's medium with 20% BCS for 5 min each at ambient temperature.
- Add the oocytes to droplets (250 µl) of freezing medium.
- Load the straws as described above and transfer the oocytes to the middle section. Leave the straws horizontally on the bench at ambient temperature.
- After a total of 2.5 min of contact between the oocytes and the freezing medium, straws are plunged immediately into liquid nitrogen.

Thawing

- Agitate straws in a water bath at 37 °C for 5–6 s.

Cryoprotectant Removal

- Expel the thawed content of a straw into a 35-mm Petri dish containing 2.5 ml thawing medium with 0.5 M sucrose and equilibrate for 5 min.
- Transfer the oocytes to 2.5 ml thawing medium with 0.25 M sucrose for 5 min.
- Remove sucrose by rinsing twice in 2.5 ml HEPES-buffered Earle's medium +0.5% BSA for 5 min.

- Transfer the surviving oocytes to 100-μl droplets of Earle's medium +0.5% BSA at 37 °C for 1 h of recuperation before insemination.

Slow Freezing of Ovarian Cortical Tissue with DMSO

Media

- Transfer tissue cubes to Leibovitz L-15 medium supplemented with 10% (v/v) fetal bovine serum (FBS) and 1.5 M DMSO.

Cooling and Storage

- Incubate the tissue cubes for 30 min in the freezing medium at 0 °C in cryogenic vials that are gently shaken.
- Transfer vials into a programmable biological freezer at the end of the incubation time.
- Cooling at –2 °C/min to –9 °C
- Manual seeding at –9 °C
- Cooling at –0.3 °C/min to –40 °C
- Cooling to –140 °C at –10 °C/min, followed by transfer to liquid nitrogen (–196 °C).

Thawing

- Swirl the vials containing the tissue cubes in water at room temperature for about 1 min.

Cryoprotectant Removal

- Expel the content of the vials in Leibovitz L-15 medium with 10% FBS.
- Rinse two to three times in Leibovitz L-15 medium with 10% FBS.

Future Prospects

From the numerous research reports listed in this chapter it must become clear that the search for clinical application of oocyte cryopreservation is still going on. We can only applaud the fact that the investigation of possible damage to the oocyte is being given this much attention in current reproductive research projects. A few teams have taken up the clinical practice of mature oocyte cryopreservation again but the general attitude is one of caution, since in particular the efficiency of the procedure is still questionable. As for the cryopreservation of immature oocytes, this is even more under question since only one success-ful pregnancy has been reported to date.

The newest evolution in the field of cryopreservation of oocytes is the freez-ing of ovarian cortical tissue to restore fertility in young cancer patients. Although first results look promising, we must be careful to stay realistic about the possibilities of this technique to actually restore natural fertility.

A major task for the future will be the establishment of proven, safe cryopre-servation protocols designed specifically for human oocytes or ovarian tissue. Furthermore, techniques to prevent transmission of infectious organisms dur-ing cryostorage should be given great attention. Finally, the long-term follow-up of children originating from cryopreserved gametes or tissues has to be well or-ganized in order to monitor the long-term effect of freezing on the offspring. Keeping in mind the enormous impact assisted reproduction has had in the field of human procreation during the final decades of the last century of the second millennium, we now must enter the third millennium with a spirit of both endeavor and caution.

Cryoconservation of Sperm

Historical Background

More than two centuries ago, in 1776, Spallanzani was the first to report the maintenance of motility of human spermatozoa after exposure to low tempera-tures. In 1866, Mantagazza suggested sperm banks for frozen human sperm. In 1949, Polge and colleagues discovered the effectiveness of glycerol as a cryopro-tective agent for fowl spermatozoa. In the following period, more attention was paid to sperm cryopreservation of farm animals. Freezing of human spermato-zoa was reported shortly afterwards by Sherman and Bunge (1953), who ob-served that human spermatozoa, after freezing on dry ice followed by thawing, were able to fertilize the egg and to produce normal embryonic development and offspring. The first birth obtained after freezing human spermatozoa with glycerol in liquid nitrogen vapor was described by the same group (Perloff et al. 1964).

The development of human sperm cryobanks in the 1970s gave rise to a growing need for standardization. Especially in the United States, commercial and university sperm banks were established to ensure later fertility prior to vasectomy. The first association of human sperm banks was set up in France (CECOS: Centre d' Etude et de Conservation du Sperme) in 1973, followed by the creation of the American Association of Tissue Banks (AATB) in 1976, which also covered cryopreservation of gametes. The growing use of cryopre-served human semen led to the First International Meeting on Human Semen Cryopreservation, held in Paris in 1978.

The Need for Sperm Cryopreservation

Frozen human sperm can be divided into two main categories, i.e., semen for autoconservation and donor semen. There are various reasons for autoconservation in both short-term and long-term storage of sperm.

Autoconservation

Long-term (more than 5 years) cryopreservation of sperm is designed to ensure later fertility in men who are to undergo (a) radio- or chemotherapy which might lead to sterility or (b) surgical sterilization by vasectomy. Prior to the introduction of ICSI, only semen samples of reasonable quality could be stored and successfully used for assisted reproduction. However, the concept of "one oocyte – one vital spermatozoon" for ICSI considerably changed the criteria for freezability of human semen samples. A low sperm yield is no longer a major obstacle to offering cryopreservation to the patients (Botchan et al. 1997). In theory, all sperm suspensions, whatever the origin or quality, may be frozen and used for assisted fertilization once motile (vital) spermatozoa have been observed.

Short-term (1–5 years) storage of sperm can be useful in cases of (a) stress with regard to collection of semen on demand on the day of intrauterine insemination (IUI), IVF, or ICSI; (b) absence of the husband during the wife's treatment; and (c) large intraindividual variations in semen quality. Since 1993, *surgically obtained spermatozoa*, too, have been used for assisted fertilization (Schoysman et al. 1993, Tournaye et al. 1994, Devroey et al. 1994). Epididymal or testicular spermatozoa obtained after diagnostic surgery or after sperm retrieval for use in a therapeutic ICSI may be frozen in order to avoid repeated surgery in following ICSI cycles (Nagy et al. 1995). Ejaculates obtained *after electroejaculation* from spinal-cord injured men may also be frozen for later use in an ICSI treatment cycle.

Donor Sperm Conservation

Freezing and storage of donor sperm allows repeated testing of the donors for acquired immune deficiency syndrome (AIDS), hepatitis B, and other sexually transmitted diseases and in this way avoids the risk of infecting the recipient. A quarantine period of at least 6 months is respected, according to the Guidelines of the American Society for Reproductive Medicine (1998). Another important advantage of using frozen sperm is the ready availability of different donor genotypes and phenotypes, so as to match as closely as possible the infertile male partner.

Cryobiological Factors Influencing Cryoefficiency

Compared with human oocytes and compared with sperm of other mammalian species, human spermatozoa are more resistant to cold shocks and osmotic stress. This is due partly to their small dimensions and partly to the low surface-to-volume ratio of the sperm head. Nevertheless, the spermatozoon is a highly differentiated and specialized cell type, with many functions to be maintained after freezing and thawing. Various factors affect the success of cryopreservation of human spermatozoa. 'Motility' is generally preferred as the primary parameter for evaluating freeze-thawing efficiency, although it is not the only parameter to be correlated with post-thaw functionality in general and, more specifically, with the fertilizing ability of frozen spermatozoa. Percentage recovery of motility (PR) is defined as the final post-thaw percentage motility × 100/initial fresh percentage motility.

The Cryoprotectant and Cryomedia

When human spermatozoa are frozen without addition of a cryoprotectant, their survival rate is less than 15% (Lucena and Obando 1986). Important functions of the cryoprotectant are to depress the freezing point, to reduce the electrolyte concentration and maintain the pH. The commonly used cryoprotectant for human sperm is glycerol, first described by Polge and colleagues in 1949, and found to be used ideally in a final concentration of 5% to 10%, giving minimal toxicity and maximal cryoprotection (Sherman 1973).

DMSO is not recommended for the cryopreservation of human semen because of its higher toxicity before freezing and after thawing in terms of motility (Sherman 1964) as compared with glycerol (Serafini and Marrs 1986, Serafini et al. 1986), while PROH has no application in sperm cryopreservation.

A higher cryosurvival can be obtained by adding various components, called extenders, to the cryoprotective agent glycerol. The precise mechanism by which these compounds protect the spermatozoa during the freezing and thawing process is not fully understood. Some of their functions are (a) to optimize osmotic pressure and pH, (b) to provide an energy source, (c) to prevent bacterial contamination, and (d) to stabilize the cell membrane.

Several complex cryobuffers are described and compared in the literature. One of the common components is egg yolk, which protects the sperm membrane against freezing damage by increasing its fluidity. The most widely used media are:
- Glycerol–egg yolk–citrate medium (GEYC), buffered by citrate and glycine (Behrman and Ackerman 1969)
- TES–Tris–egg yolk buffer with (TESTCY) or without citrate (TYB), buffered by the zwitterionic buffers TES and Tris (Jeyendran et al. 1984)
- Human sperm preservation medium (HSPM), buffered by N-2 hydroxyethyl piperazine N-2 ethane sulfonic acid (HEPES) (Mahadevan and Trounson 1983.)

A comparative study of eight buffer systems with glycerol (6–16%) and without glycerol for sperm freezing revealed the highest post-thaw recovery of motility

(>80%) from the use of the TESTCY buffer with glycerol, while eliminating glycerol reduced the recovery rate to only 20% (Prins and Weidel 1986).

The Freezing Method

The standard liquid-nitrogen-vapor technique was introduced by Sherman in 1954 and is still widely employed around the world. Straws are horizontally placed about 15 cm above the liquid nitrogen surface for 50 min and afterwards plunged into liquid nitrogen (-196 °C). Modifications of the static fast vapor freezing method were introduced later. According to the size of the straws, one- or two-step cooling is preferred. Two-hundred and fifty microliter straws are placed 25 cm above the liquid level for 25 min, while 500-µl straws are preferably placed at 35 cm for 15 min and at 15 cm for another 15 min (Mortimer 1994).

Controlled-rate freezing of sperm gained popularity with increased equipment availability in the 1980s. The optimal sperm cooling rate (cooling = decrease in temperature from room temperature to +5 °C) was found to be -0.5 ° to -1 °C/min and the optimal freezing rate (freezing = decrease in temperature from +5 °C to -30 °C) -10 °C/min (Mahadevan and Trounson 1984a). Although programmed freezing is essential for embryo cryopreservation, there is still controversy in the literature about its beneficial effect on human spermatozoa. While some investigators found computer-controlled freezing to preserve sperm motility and vitality better than vapor freezing (Serafini and Marrs 1986, McLaughlin et al. 1990), especially when lower-quality sperm is involved (Ragni et al. 1990), others were unable to prove its advantage (Thachill and Jewett 1981, Wolf and Patton 1989, Verheyen et al. 1993) and therefore advocated vapor freezing, taking into account differences in cost, time of execution, and practical implications.

The Thawing Procedure

Sperm thawing at room temperature or at 37 °C preserves motility, vitality (Taylor et al. 1982, Mahadevan and Trounson 1984a), and fertilizing ability (Cohen et al. 1981) better than slower thawing in ice baths or faster thawing in warm-water baths. According to others, the optimal thawing or warming rate is dependent on the cooling rate, slow cooling requiring slow thawing and vice-versa (Verheyen et al. 1993, Gao et al. 1992, Henry et al. 1993).

Prefreeze Addition and Post-thaw Washing Procedures

While the addition of glycerol is indispensable for cryosurvival of spermatozoa, sperm cells are subjected to hyperosmotic stress when exposed to the cryoprotectant, due to its high osmolarity. To minimize osmotic injury and prevent severe dehydration, the cryoprotectant solution should be added dropwise or by multistep addition (McLaughlin et al. 1990, Gao et al. 1992). Spermatozoa show a very high permeability to glycerol that is temperature dependent. An osmotic equilibrium is obtained within a few minutes at room temperature or at 37 °C, while equilibration is delayed at lower temperatures. Gao and colleagues described an increased spermolysis when glycerol was added at 0 °C or 8 °C (Gao et al. 1993). On the other hand, prolonged exposure of spermatozoa to glycerol can cause chemical toxicity to the sperm cells, which is more pronounced at higher temperatures. To find the optimal balance between minimizing hyperosmotic injury and reducing the potential chemical toxicity of glycerol, further investigation is needed (Gao et al. 1992).

The chemical toxicity of glycerol requires its removal after thawing, before the sperm can be used with safety in an IUI, IVF, or ICSI program. Spermatozoa have to be returned to isotonic conditions by dilution with isotonic media. To prevent severe hypo-osmotic stress, dilution should again be carried out dropwise or by multistep addition. Only little information on the detrimental effects of post-thawing dilution on sperm quality is available (Verheyen et al. 1993, Gao et al. 1993, Graczykowski and Siegel 1991). In a previous study, we found a 50% loss in progressive motility from freezing and thawing, which was in turn reduced by another 50% by dilution and washing of the sperm (Verheyen et al. 1993). A comparable decrease was observed for light-microscopic morphology parameters, where additional impairment was manifested especially by increased bending and curling of the tail (Verheyen et al. 1993, Gao et al. 1993).

Sperm Functions Affected by Cryopreservation

Freezing and thawing of human spermatozoa is undoubtedly associated with a decrease in sperm quality. The most intensively studied adverse effects are impairment of sperm motility, viability, and morphology. Influences on ultrastructural morphology, fertilizing capacity, chromosomal abnormalities, and pregnancy rate have also been described. Ejaculates, obtained after masturbation or after electroejaculation, are most commonly frozen in the presence of seminal plasma. Surgically obtained epididymal sperm is suspended into culture medium before addition of the cryoprotectant medium. In both conditions, however, the mature spermatozoon is the highly predominant cell type. The situation is different for surgically retrieved testicular tissue, which is composed of a very heterogeneous cell population. Freezing of testicular sperm, as a novel application, is therefore discussed in a separate chapter. The studies on the different parameters discussed in this chapter are all carried out with ejaculated sperm.

Sperm Motility

Although motility is not completely related to fertilizing capacity, it is generally accepted to be a sensitive parameter by which to evaluate freeze-thawing success (Cross and Hanks 1991).

A wide individual variability in percentage recovery of sperm motility (PR) after freezing and thawing is reported, ranging from 10% to 95% (Serres et al. 1980). In most papers, a mean PR of 40–60% immediately after thawing has been observed when an appropriate cryoprotective medium was used. As previously described, this percentage is further decreased after preparation of the sperm for IUI, IVF, or ICSI (Verheyen et al. 1993). According to Serres et al. (1980), two thirds of the post-thaw decrease in motility is due to cryoaggression and one third to hyperosmotic stress induced by glycerol addition. As reported by the same group, an inverse relationship exists between the initial concentration of spermatozoa in the fresh ejaculate and the PR, as well as between the initial percentage motility or normal morphology and the PR (David and Czyglik 1977).

Sperm Morphology

Cryopreservation of sperm significantly reduces the percentage of spermatozoa with normal morphology. Light-microscopic analysis has clearly shown an increase in bent and coiled tails (Verheyen et al. 1993, Gao et al. 1993; Mahadevan and Trounson 1984b). As early as 1971, Pedersen and Lebech described severe impairment of sperm in terms of ultrastructural morphology. Several investigators have confirmed this damage at the level of the membranes and acrosomes after freezing (Mahadevan and Trounson 1984b, Cross and Hanks 1991, Henry et al. 1993). Mahadevan and Trounson (1984) reported post-thaw recoveries of spermatozoa with intact membranes and with intact acrosomes of only 27.7% and 40.8%, respectively, while the average motility recovery for the same group of donors was 69.2%. These results indicate that morphological damage is even more pronounced than the impairment of motility. However, spermatozoa which showed mechanically intact acrosomes after thawing maintained their acrosomal function (McLaughlin et al. 1993).

Sperm Chromosomal Constitution and Chromatin Structure

Cytogenetic analysis after fusion of hamster oocytes with human sperm did not reveal any difference in type or frequency of chromosomal abnormalities between fresh and frozen sperm (Chernos and Martin 1989). However, overcondensation of sperm chromatin after freezing and thawing has been raised as a hypothesis by other investigators (Hamamah et al. 1993).

Sperm Fertilizing Capacity and Pregnancy Rate

The literature does not provide well-controlled studies comparing the fertilizing ability of fresh and frozen-thawed spermatozoa. Reliable results can be obtained only when alternating oocytes of one patient collected in an IVF cycle are inseminated either with fresh or with frozen-thawed sperm from the same donor or the husband. The use of fresh donor sperm is unjustified, however, because of the risk of transmitting severe diseases (HIV, hepatitis B, and other sexually transmitted diseases).

The few properly controlled studies on the fertilizing ability of ejaculated fresh, as compared with frozen-thawed, spermatozoa have been carried out in vitro by means of the zona-free hamster oocyte penetration test (HOPT). While one group described an individual variability in the post-thaw maintenance of fertilizing capacity, with a mean fertilization rate decreasing from 75% with fresh to 51% with frozen sperm (Cohen et al. 1981), others found no difference for normozoospermic samples but a decreased fertilizing ability for oligozoospermic samples after freezing and thawing (Yoshida et al. 1990). In vivo studies carried out in the 1980s, when fresh donor insemination was still carried out, compared the fertilizing ability of sperm from different donors, either fresh or frozen, in different recipients and separate cycles, and therefore lack any clear and reliable control. Others even compared the efficiency of fresh husband with frozen donor sperm in different cycles and patients. In any case, the conclusions are contradictory, in that some groups found no differences between fresh and frozen sperm as regards fertilization rate (Mahadevan and Trounson 1983, Cohen et al. 1985), while others observed impaired fertilizing capacity with frozen-thawed sperm (Englert et al. 1989, Morroll et al. 1990, Yavetz et al. 1991).

It is remarkable, however, that the same investigators unanimously found similar pregnancy rates after replacement of embryos derived from insemination with either fresh or frozen sperm. This has led to the hypothesis that freezing and thawing acts more aggressively on a subpopulation of weaker, probably infertile spermatozoa (Englert et al. 1989), and to the conclusion that frozen sperm can be used without compromising pregnancy chances.

Freezing of Testicular Sperm

Although testicular spermatozoa have been used successfully for ICSI since 1993 (Schoysman et al. 1993), a few years passed before the use of frozen-thawed testicular sperm for ICSI was introduced (Romero et al. 1996). Several factors indeed hampered the use of cryopreserved testicular sperm. First, testicular biopsies usually contain low numbers of motile spermatozoa, especially in cases of testicular failure (nonobstructive azoospermia), in which even the fresh tissue may be explored for hours in order to gather the appropriate number of 'motile' (live) spermatozoa. Second, the tissue is composed of a very heterogeneous cell population. Besides mature spermatozoa, all different stages of spermatogenic cells, Sertoli cells, red and white blood cells, and interstitial cells are present. Because of the unique environment, the question arose whether to freeze the tissue as an intact biopsy or as a heterogeneous cell suspension.

Freezing of the Intact Testicular Biopsy or the Suspension

The low amount of testicular tissue available for research and the limited numbers and quality of spermatozoa present hardly permit reliable comparisons of freezing protocols, cryoprotectants, freezing environments, and preparation methods before and after freezing. The freezing conditions for testicular spermatozoa are therefore based completely on the experience with ejaculated spermatozoa, without considering the physicochemical characteristics of the different cell types present in testicular tissue. One of the questions arising was whether the tissue needs some preparation in order to improve the efficiency of cryopreservation. A controlled comparative study on testicular biopsies derived from 14 patients with obstructive azoospermia revealed that freezing of testicular sperm in suspension after mincing (Verheyen et al. 1995) preserves their quality (motility and vitality) better than freezing of the intact biopsies (Crabbé et al. 1999). Suspensions may be frozen in straws, with glycerol as cryoprotectant and use of the conventional vapor freezing program as used for ejaculates.

Quality of Frozen-Thawed Testicular Sperm

Because of the low tissue availability and its limited quality, the number of reported controlled studies comparing the prefreeze and post-thaw quality of testicular spermatozoa is very limited. Verheyen et al. (1997) found that motility decreased from 21% before freezing to 6% after thawing, and vitality from 68% before freezing to 22% after thawing. These observations were based on 29 biopsies derived from patients with obstructive azoospermia.

Nogueira et al. (1999) compared the ultrastructural morphology of fresh and frozen-thawed testicular biopsies. They observed morphological damage by freezing and thawing which was comparable to that of ejaculated spermatozoa: rupture of the plasma membranes and inner or outer acrosomal membranes, loss of the acrosomal content, but intactness of the nuclear membranes and chromatin.

Fertilizing Capacity of Frozen-Thawed Testicular Sperm

Despite the lack of experimental data, several reports are available on the use of frozen-thawed testicular sperm for therapeutic ICSI (Romero et al. 1996, Gil-Salom et al. 1996, Oates et al. 1997, Friedler et al. 1997, De Croo et al. 1998). Satisfying results have been obtained in terms of fertilization rates (44–68%) and pregnancy rates (16–33%), especially in cases of obstruction which mostly show normal spermatogenesis. The efficiency of frozen-thawed testicular sperm for ICSI derived from nonobstructive cases, however, depends largely on the severity of testicular failure and on the quality criteria and limits for testicular sperm freezing, defined in a different way by each individual ART center.

In general, the use of frozen-thawed testicular sperm for ICSI may be efficient as long as motile sperm is found after thawing. For cases with severe testicular failure, preference should be given to fresh testicular sperm for ICSI in order to maximize the chances for the couple (own experience, unpublished results). However, this approach is associated with a high risk (Tournaye et al., 1997) of being faced with testicular sperm retrieval failure on the day of oocyte retrieval. An alternative approach is to routinely freeze the diagnostic testicular biopsies and to only allow a couple for ICSI treatment based on the quality of fresh and/or frozen-thawed biopsies (Salzbrunn et al. 1996, Ben-Yosef et al. 1999). This approach, however, may result in an increased rate of patients who will be refused entry to the ICSI program.

Practical Aspects

Composition of Cryoprotective Media

Formulations for 100 ml of commonly used cryoprotective media to be added to the sperm in a 1:1 dilution are summarized here, as described by Mortimer (1994):

Glycerol-Egg Yolk-Citrate Buffer (GEC).
- 20 ml egg yolk (Bacto Egg-Yolk Enrichment, Difco Labs., Cat.No. 3347–72)
- 15 ml glycerol
- 1.3 g glucose
- 1.15 g sodium citrate
- 65 ml milli-Q water

Heat-inactivate at 56 °C for 30 min. Add after cooling to room temperature:
- 1 g glycine
- 100 000 IU penicillin
- 0.1 g streptomycin
- Adjust the pH to 7.2.

TES-Tris-Egg Yolk Buffer (TYB).
- 3.46 g TES
- 0.822 g Tris
- 0.16 g dextrose
- 20 ml heat-inactivated fresh egg yolk
- 15 ml glycerol
- 65 ml milli-Q water
- 100 000 IU penicillin
- 0.1 g streptomycin.

Centrifuge at 1000 µg for 10 min and discard the pellet; adjust the pH to 7.35–7.45 with Tris and the osmolarity to 290–320 mOsm.

Human Sperm Preservation Medium (HSPM).
- 0.58 g NaCl
- 0.04 g KCl

- 2.721 mM CaCl$_2 \cdot$2H$_2$O
- 0.492 mM MgCl$_2 \cdot$6H$_2$O
- 12.856 mM Na-lactate
- 0.321 mM NaH$_2$PO$_4 \cdot$2H$_2$O
- 0.26 g NaHCO$_3$
- 0.477 g HEPES-free acid
- 1.718 g sucrose
- 1 g glycine
- 0.1 g glucose
- 15 ml glycerol
- 0.49 g human serum albumin
- 0.005 g kanamycin sulfate or other antibiotics
- Make up to 100 ml with milli-Q water.

After preparation, the medium is divided into aliquots of 5 ml in sterile tubes and stored frozen at –20 °C until needed. Thawing is carried out at room temperature or at 37 °C.

TESTCY medium can also be purchased commercially from Irvine Scientific (Santa Ana, Calif., USA; cat. no. 9971). Other media without egg yolk are available from Medi-Cult (Copenhagen, Denmark) and from FertiPro (Beernem, Belgium).

Addition of the Cryoprotectant Medium and Loading of Straws

Semen is produced in a sterile container by masturbation. After liquefaction, the volume of the ejaculate is measured with a disposable pipette or a syringe. Basic semen analysis is carried out and the results are recorded. Semen is diluted 1:1 (v/v) with the cryoprotectant medium, which is added dropwise (over 10 min) to minimize hyperosmotic stress, while the container is shaken continuously. The mixture is placed in a thermostatic water bath at 37 °C for 10 min for equilibration.

Straws are most widely used to store human sperm. For many years, plastic, nonsterile straws designed for veterinary use have been employed to freeze also human semen. However, these straws proved to have a low mechanical resistance at low temperatures. It has been shown that damage to the straw may cause leakage and thus diffusion and allow exchange of viruses through the liquid nitrogen. For this reason, I.M.V. (Instruments de Médecine Vétérinaire, 61300 l' Aigle, France) developed a separate production unit for high-security straws and devices to store human tissue and cells in a safe way. Cryo Bio System (I.M.V. Division, 61300 l' Aigle, France) provides sterile straws which are mechanically resistant to high pressure, composed of physiochemical inert material that may be heat-sealed safely. The company also provides the material to fill, heat-seal, and label the straws. At our center, we are currently introducing the use of this type of straw for both sperm and embryo cryostorage.

Cooling and Freezing of Sperm

Sperm can be cooled and frozen either by the static vapor method or by the computer-controlled method. Vapor freezing is most widely applied for reasons of low cost, and for practical considerations, and because it is as convenient and effective as programmed freezing.

Vapor Freezing. The straws are placed horizontally as a single layer in a copper-mesh tray, which is placed in an aluminum-mesh basket at a level of 35 cm (14 in) above the liquid-nitrogen surface, and left for 15 min. The basket is then moved down to a level of 15 cm (6 in) above the liquid surface and left for another 15 min. Finally, the straws are immersed in liquid nitrogen (-196 °C). For storage, straws of one ejaculate are collected in a visotube (IMV, cat. nos. PA005 and PA006), which is marked with the name of the donor and the date of semen production, or with the identification data (name, file number, date) of the patient. More details concerning this procedure and the organization of the sperm bank are described by Mortimer (1994).

Computer-controlled Freezing. The procedure of preparing the semen sample for freezing is the same as the preparation for vapor freezing. Several biological freezers are available, and different programs for sperm freezing are described in the literature. A currently applied program is composed of the following steps:
1. -1 °C/min from room temperature to +5 °C
2. -10 °C/min from +5 °C to -80 °C
3. -25 °C/min from -80 °C to -130 °C
4. Hold for 1 h at -130 °C; during this period, straws are removed from the freezer and immediately immersed in liquid nitrogen.

The storage of the straws in visotubes is the same as for vapor freezing.

Thawing of Sperm

According to the freezing procedure, straws are thawed either at 37 °C for 10 min (vapor freezing) or at room temperature for 10 min (programmed freezing). After analysis, the sperm is either immediately introduced intracervically (ICX), or immediately prepared for intrauterine insemination (IUI) or in vitro insemination (IVF) or injection (ICSI).

Testicular Tissue Preparation Before Freezing

While some labs freeze whole biopsies (Salzbrunn et al. 1996), most freeze the morseled tissue (Gil-Salom et al. 1996, Friedler et al. 1997, Crabbé et al. 1999).

In order to obtain the tissue suspension before freezing and in order to be able to assess the quality of the tissue, the biopsy is shredded with two sterile microscopic glass slides. Fine pincers are used for further mincing (Verheyen et al. 1995), in order to prevent obstruction of the straw during aspiration. Multiple biopsies are pooled two or three to a tube, depending on the size of the biopsies. The suspensions are centrifuged at 500 μg for 5 min. Following aspiration of the supernatant, the pellets are resuspended in 0.5–1 ml medium. A 5-ll droplet (aspirated in between the remaining tissue fractions) is used to evaluate concentration and motility of spermatozoa and late spermatids in the Neubauer chamber. If the concentration is $>0.5 \times 10^6$/ml, the suspension may be further diluted in order to obtain more straws (for more cycles) for the patient.

If no sperm is found after mechanical mincing of the biopsies, enzymatic digestion of the remaining tissue fractions may be carried out using collagenase type IV (1000 IU/ml) (Crabbé et al. 1997, 1998). This procedure allows concentration of the free cell suspension into a limited volume of medium and makes it possible to find sperm in 25% of the cases where mechanical treatment was insufficient to find the few sperm present (Crabbé et al. 1998). Some centers that freeze biopsies use enzymatic digestion with collagenase IA to treat the thawed specimens (Salzbrunn et al. 1996, Fischer et al. 1996).

Future Prospects

Although a great many investigations have been carried out in order to understand the basic fundamentals of sperm freezing and the processes causing sperm damage, cryoefficiency is still limited. Further research and an understanding of the osmotic tolerance of human spermatozoa and the potential chemical toxicity of glycerol to the cells in terms of time, temperature, and glycerol concentration may lead to improved cryoefficiency of human spermatozoa (Gao et al. 1992).

Ejaculated as well as epididymal and testicular spermatozoa are currently frozen as a routine for reasons of convenience or to ensure later fertility. With the development of ICSI (one oocyte – one sperm), the storage of sperm from whatever source and of whatever quality has become worthwhile, which is of particular importance for young cancer patients in order to preserve their fertility chances. A challenge for the future is the development of an efficient cryostorage protocol for spermatogonial stem cells of prepubertal cancer patients who need to undergo intensive cancer therapy. Cryopreservation of spermatogonia followed by their transplantation at later age might reconstitute spermatogenesis and fertility. Experimental work on isolation, cryopreservation, and transplantation of spermatogonia is currently being carried out in mice (Brinster and Avarbock 1994, Avarbock et al. 1996), but there is still a long way to go before its application in the human will be possible.

In the field of gamete and embryo cryobanking, safety is currently a major responsibility and concern for the near future. All precautions should be taken to identify individual straws carefully and correctly, to ensure optimal cryoprotocols and cryostorage conditions, and to avoid exchange of viruses through liquid nitrogen. Important suggestions are the use of safe straws, separate storage of potential infectious material (each patient should be screened for infectious diseases), and storage in the vapor phase of liquid nitrogen instead of in the liquid phase itself, the latter being currently applied for human tissue storage.

References

Aigner S, Van der Elst J, Siebzehnrübl E, Eichenlaub-Ritter U, Todorow S, Wildt L, Van Steirteghem AC (1992) The influence of slow and ultra-rapid freezing on the organization of the meiotic spindle of the mouse oocyte. Hum Reprod 7:857–864

Al-Hasani S, Diedrich K, van der Ven H, Reinecke A, Hartje M, Krebs D (1987) Cryopreservation of human oocytes. Hum Reprod 2:695–700

American Society for Reproductive Medicine (1998) Guidelines for therapeutic donor insemination: sperm. Fertil Steril 70 [Suppl 3]:1S-13S

Apperley JF, Reddy N (1995) Mechanism and management of treatment-related gonadal failure in recipients of high dose chemotherapy. Blood Rev 9:93–116

Ash P (1980) The influence of radiation on fertility in man. Br J Radiol 53:271–278

Ashwood-Smith MJ (1967) Radioprotective and cryoprotective properties of dimethylsulphoxide in cellular systems. Ann NY Acad Sci 141:45–46

Ashwood-Smith MJ (1986) The cryopreservation of human embryos. Hum Reprod 1:319–332

Ashwood-Smith MJ, Friedmann GB (1979) Lethal and chromosomal effects of freezing, thawing, storage time and X-radiation on mammalian cells preserved at -196 °C in dimethyl sulfoxide. Cryobiology 16:132–140

Aubard Y, Newton H, Scheffer G et al (1998) Conservation of the follicular population in irradiated rats by the cryopreservation and orthotopic autografting of ovarian tissue. Eur J Obstet Gynecol. Reprod Biol 79:83–87

Avarbock MR, Brinster CJ, Brinster RL (1996) Reconstitution of spermatogenesis from frozen spermatogonial stem cells. Nature Med 2:693–696

Behrman SJ, Ackerman DR (1969) Freeze preservation of human sperm. Am J Obstet Gynecol 103:654

Ben-Yosef D, Yogev L, Hauser R, Yavetz H, Azem F, Yovel I, Lessing JB, Amit A (1999) Testicular sperm retrieval and cryopreservation prior to initiating ovarian stimulation as the first line approach in patients with non-obstructive azoospermia. Hum Reprod 14:1794–1801

Bernard A, Fuller BJ (1996) Cryopreservation of human oocytes: a review of current problems and perspectives. Hum Reprod Update 2:193–207

Bernard A, Imoedemhe DA, Shaw RW, Fuller BJ (1985) Effects of cryoprotectants on human oocytes. Lancet 1:632–633

Bernard A, Hunter JE, Fuller BJ, Imoedemhe D, Curtis P, Jackson A (1992) Fertilisation and embryonic development of human oocytes after cooling. Hum Reprod 7:1447–1450

Borini A, Bafaro MG, Bonu MA, Di Stratis V, Sereni E, Sciajno R, Serrao L (1998) Pregnancies after oocyte freezing and thawing. Preliminary data. Hum Reprod 13 (Abstract book 1):124–125

Bos-Mikich A, Whittingham DG (1995) Analysis of the chromosome complement of frozen-thawed mouse oocytes after parthenogenetic activation. Mol Reprod Dev 42:254–260

Bos-Mikich A, Wood MJ, Candy CJ, Whittingham DG (1995) Cytogenetical analysis and developmental potential of vitrified mouse oocytes. Biol Reprod 53:780–785

Botchan A, Huaser R, Yogev L, Gamzu R, Paz G, Lessing JB, Yavetz H (1997) Testicular cancer and spermatogenesis. Hum Reprod 12:755–758

Bouquet M, Selva J, Auroux L (1992) The incidence of chromosomal abnormalities in frozen-thawed mouse oocytes after in vitro fertilization. Hum Reprod 7:76–80

Boutron P, Kaufmann A (1979) Stability of the amorphous state in the system water-1,2-propanediol. Cryobiology 16:557–568

Brinster RL, Avarbock MR (1994) Germline transmission of donor haplotype following spermatogonial transplantation. Proc Natl Acad Sci USA 91:11303–11307

Candy CJ, Wood MJ, Whittingham DG, Merriman JA, Choudhury N (1994) Cryopreservation of immature mouse oocytes. Hum Reprod 9:1738–1742

Candy CJ, Wood MJ, Whittingham DG (1995) Follicular development in cryopreserved marmoset ovarian tissue after transplantation. Hum Reprod 10:2334–2338

Carroll J, Warnes GM, Matthews CD (1989) Increase in digyny explains polyploidy after invitro fertilization of frozen-thawed mouse oocytes. J Reprod Fert 85:489–494

Carroll J, Wood MJ, Whittingham DG (1993) Normal fertilisation and development of frozen-thawed mouse oocytes: protective action of certain macromolecules. Biol Reprod 48:606–612

Cha KY, Chian RC (1998) Maturation in vitro of immature human oocytes for clinical use. Hum Reprod Up 4:103–120

Chen C (1986) Pregnancy after human oocyte cryopreservation. Lancet 1:884–886

Chen C (1988) Pregnancies after human oocyte cryopreservation. Ann NY Acad Sci 541:541–549

Chen C (1989) Oocyte freezing. In: Wood C, Trounson A (eds) Clinical in vitro fertilization. Springer, Berlin Heidelberg New York London, pp 113–126

Chernos JE, Martin RH (1989) A cytogenetic investigation of the effects of cryopreservation on human sperm. Am J Hum Genet 45:766–777

Cohen J, Felten P, Zeilmaker GH (1981) In vitro fertilizing capacity of fresh and cryopreserved human spermatozoa: a comparative study of freezing and thawing procedures. Fertil Steril 36:356–362

Cohen J, Edwards RG, Fehilly CB, Fishel SB, Hewitt J, Rowland GF, Steptoe PC, Walters, DE, Webster J (1985) In vitro fertilization using cryopreserved donor semen in cases where both partners are infertile. Fertil Steril 43:570–574

Collichio F, Pandya K (1994) Amenorrhea following chemotherapy for breast cancer: effect on disease-free survival. Oncology 8:45–52

Cox SL, Shaw J, Jenkin G (1996) Transplantation of cryopreserved fetal ovarian tissue to adult recipients in mice. J Reprod Fertil 107:315–322

Crabbé E, Verheyen G, Tournaye H, Van Steirteghem A (1997) The use of enymatic procedures to recover testicular germ cells. Hum Reprod 12:1682–1687

Crabbé E, Verheyen G, Tournaye H, Van de Velde H, Goossens A, Van Steirteghem A (1998) Enzymatic digestion of testicular tissue may rescue the intracytoplasmic sperm injection cycle in some patients with non-obstructive azoospermia. Hum Reprod 13:2791–2796

Crabbé E, Verheyen G, Tournaye H, Van Steirteghem A (1999) Freezing testicular tissue as a minced suspension preserves sperm quality better than whole-biopsy freezing when glycerol is used as cryoprotectant. Int J Androl 22:43–48

Cross NL, Hanks SE (1991) Effects of cryopreservation on human sperm acrosomes. Hum Reprod 6:1279–1283

David G, Czyglik F (1977) Tolérance à la congélation du sperme humain en fonction de la qualité initiale du sperme. J Gynecol Obstet Biol Reprod 6:601–610

De Croo I, Van der Elst J, Everaert K et al (1998) Fertilization, pregnancy and embryo implantation rates after ICSI with fresh and frozen-thawed testicular spermatozoa. Hum Reprod 13:1893–1897

Devroey P, Liu J, Nagy Z, Tournaye H, Silber, Van Steirteghem AC (1994) Normal fertilization of human oocytes after testicular sperm extraction and intracytoplasmic sperm injection. Fertil Steril 62:639–641

Edwards RG, Steptoe P, Purdy JM (1980) Establishing full-term pregnancies with cleaving embryos grown in vitro. Br J Obstet Gynaec 887:757–768

Englert Y, Delvigne A, Vekemans M, Lejeune B, Henlisz A, de Maertelaer G, Leroy F (1989) Is fresh or frozen sperm to be used in in vitro fertilization with donor sperm? Fertil Steril 51:661–664

Feichtinger W, Benkö I, Kemeter P Freezing human oocytes using rapid methods. (1987) In: Feichtinger W, Kemeter P (eds) Future aspects of human in vitro fertilization. Springer, Berlin Heidelberg New York, pp 101–110

Fischer R, Baukloh V, Naether OGJ, Schulze W, Salzbrunn A, Benson DM (1996) Pregnancy after intracytoplasmic sperm injection of spermatozoa extracted from frozen-thawed testicular biopsy. Hum Reprod 11:2197–2199

Friedler S, Raziel A, Soffer Y, Strassburger D, Komarovsky D, Ron-El R (1997) Intracytoplasmic sperm injection of fresh and cryopreserved testicular spermatozoa in patients with nonobstructive azoospermia – a comparative study. Fertil Steril 68:892–897

Frydman N, Selva J, Bergère M, Auroux M, Maro B (1997) Cryopreserved immature mouse oocytes: a chromosomal and spindle study. J Assist Reprod Genet 14:617–623

Gao DY, Mazur P, Kleinhans FW, Watson PF, Noiles EE, Critser JK (1992) Glycerol permeability of human spermatozoa and its activation energy. Cryobiology 29:657–667

Gao DY, Ashworth E, Watson PF, Kleinhans FW, Mazur P, Critser JK (1993) Hyperosmotic tolerance of human spermatozoa: separate effects of glycerol, sodium chloride, and sucrose on spermolysis. Biol Reprod 49:112–123

George MA, Johnson MH (1993) Cytoskeletal organisation and zona sensitivity to digestion by chymotrypsin of frozen-thawed mouse oocytes. Hum Reprod 8:612–620

Gil-Salom M, Romero J, Minguez Y, Rubio C, De Los Santos MJ, Remohi J, Pellicer A (1996) Pregnancies after intracytoplasmic sperm injection with cryopreserved testicular spermatozoa. Hum Reprod 11:1309–1313

Glenister PH, Wood MJ, Kirby C, Whittingham DG (1987) Incidence of chromosome anomalies in first-cleavage mouse embryos obtained from frozen-thawed oocytes fertilized in vitro. Gamete Res 16:205–216

Gook DA, Osborn SM, Johnston WIH (1993) Cryopreservation of mouse and human oocytes using 1,2-propanediol and the configuration of the meiotic spindle. Hum Reprod 8:1101–1109

Gook DA, Osborn SM, Bourne H, Johnston WIH (1994) Fertilisation of human oocytes following cryopreservation: normal karyotypes and absence of stray chromosomes. Hum Reprod 9:684–691

Gook DA, Schiewe MC, Osborn SM, Asch R, Jansen RPS, Johnston WIH (1995) Intracytoplasmic sperm injection and embryo development of human oocytes cryopreserved using 1,2-propanediol. Hum Reprod 10:2637–2641

Gosden RG, Baird DT, Wade JC et al (1994a) Restoration of fertility to oophorectomized sheep by ovarian autografts stored at −196 °C. Hum Reprod 9:597–603

Gosden RG, Boulton MI, Grant K, Webb R (1994b) Follicular development of ovarian xenografts in SCID mice. J Reprod Fertil 101:619–623

Graczykowski JW, Siegel MS (1991) Motile sperm recovery from fresh and frozen-thawed ejaculates using a swim-up procedure. Fertil Steril 55:841–843

Gunasena KT, Villines PM, Critser ES, Critser JK (1997) Live births after autologous transplant of cryopreserved mouse ovaries. Hum Reprod 12:101–106

Hamamah S, Royere D, Nicolle JC, Paquignon M, Lansac J (1993) Effects of freezing-thawing on the spermatozoon nucleus: a comparative chromatin cytophotometric study in the porcine and human species. Reprod Nutr Dev 30:59–64

Henry MA, Noiles EE, Gao D, Mazur P, Critser JK (1993) Cryopreservation of human spermatozoa. IV. The effects of cooling rate and warming rate on the maintenance of motility, plasma membrane integrity, and mitochondrial function. Fertil Steril 60:911–918

Hogan B, Costantini F, Lacy E (1986) Manipulating the mouse embryo: a laboratory manual. Cold Spring Harbor Laboratory Press, Cold Spring Harbor, pp 245–268

Hovatta O, Silye R, Krausz T, Abir R, Margara R, Trew G, Lass A, Winston RM (1996) Cryopreservation of human ovarian tissue using dimethylsulphoxide and propanediol-sucrose as cryoprotectants. Hum Reprod 11:1268–1272

Hunter JE, Bernard A, Fuller B, Amso N, Shaw RS (1991) Fertilization and development of the human oocyte following exposure to cryoprotectants, low temperatures and cryopreservation: a comparison of two techniques. Hum Reprod 6:1460–1465

Hunter JE, Bernard AG, Fuller BJ (1992) Vitrification of the unfertilised human oocyte. Cryobiology 29:756

Hunter JE, Fuller BJ, Bernard A, Jackson A, Shaw RW (1995) Vitrification of human oocytes following minimal exposure to cryoprotectants: initial studies on fertilisation and embryonic development. Hum Reprod 10:1184–1188

Jeyendran RS, Van der Ven HH, Kennedy W, Perez-Pelaez M, Zaneveld LJD (1984) Comparison of glycerol and a zwitterion buffer system as cryoprotective media for human spermatozoa. J Androl 5:1

Johnson MH (1989) The effect on fertilization of exposure of mouse oocytes to dimethylsulphoxide: an optimal protocol. J In vitro Fertil Embryo Transf 6:168–175

Johnson MH, Pickering SJ (1987) The effect of dimethylsulphoxide on the microtubular system of the mouse oocyte. Development 100:313–324

Johnson MH, Pickering SJ, George MA (1988) The influence of cooling on the properties of the zona pellucida of the mouse oocyte. Hum Reprod 3:383–387

Joly C, Bchini O, Boulekbache H, Testart J, Maro B (1992) Effects of 1,2-propanediol on the cytoskeletal organization of the mouse oocyte. Hum Reprod 7:374–378

Kazem R, Thompson LA, Srikantharajah A, Laing MA, Hamilton MPR, Templeton A (1995) Cryopreservation of human oocytes and fertilisation by two techniques: in-vitro fertilisation and intracytoplasmic sperm injection. Hum Reprod 10:2650–2654

Kola I, Kirby C, Shaw J, Davey A, Trounson A (1988) Vitrification of mouse oocytes results in aneuploid zygotes and malformed fetuses. Teratology 38:467–474

Kolodziej FB, Katzorke T, Propping D (1991) Cryopreservation of human oocytes and pronuclei embryos – first results. Reproduction in Domestic Animals, Zuchthygiene, 24. Jahrestagung über Physiologie und Pathologie der Fortpflanzung, 16. Veterinar-Humanmedizinische Gemeinschaftstagung, Leipzig

Kono T, Kwon OY, Nakahara T (1991) Development of vitrified mouse oocytes after in vitro fertilization. Cryobiology 28:50–54

Leibo SP (1977) Fundamental cryobiology of mouse ova and embryos. In: Eliott K, Whelan J (eds) The freezing of mammalian embryos. Ciba Foundation Symposium no 52. Elsevier, Amsterdam, pp 69–92

Leibo SP (1980) Water permeability and its activation energy of fertilized and unfertilized mouse ova. J Membr Biol 53:179–188

Leibo SP, McGrath JJ, Cravalho EG (1978) Microscopic observation of intracellular ice formation in unfertilized mouse ova as a function of cooling rate. Cryobiology 15:257–271

Lin TP, Sherman JK, Willett EL (1957) Survival of unfertilized mouse eggs in media containing glycerol and glycine. J Exp Zool 134:275–292

Lucena E, Obando H (1986) Comparative analysis of different glycerol levels when used as cryoprotective agents on human spermatozoa. In: Paulson JD (ed) Andrology: male fertility and sterility. Academic, New York, p 553

Magistrini M, Szöllösi D (1980) Effects of cold and of isopropyl-N-phenylcarbamate on the second meiotic spindle of mouse oocytes. Eur J Cell Biol 22:699–707

Mahadevan M, Trounson AD (1983) Effect of cryoprotective media and dilution methods on the preservation of human spermatozoa. Andrologia 15:355–366

Mahadevan M, Trounson AD (1984a) Effect of cooling, freezing and thawing rates and storage conditions on preservation of human spermatozoa. Andrologia 16:52–60

Mahadevan MM, Trounson AO (1984b) Relationship of fine structure of sperm head to fertility of frozen human semen. Fertil Steril 41:287–293

Mahadevan MM, Trounson AO, Leeton JF (1983) Successful use of semen cryobanking for in vitro fertilization. Fertil Steril 40:340–343

Mandelbaum J, Junca AM, Plachot M, Alnot MO, Salat-Baroux J, Alvarez S, Tibi C, Cohen J, Debache C, Tesquier L (1988) Cryopreservation of human embryos and oocytes. Hum Reprod 3:117–119

Mantagazza P (1866) Sullo sperma umano. Rendic Reale Inst Lomb 3:183

Maro B, Johnson MH, Pickering S, Flach G (1984) Changes in actin distribution during fertilisation of the mouse egg. J Embryol Exp Morph 81:1–237

Martino A, Songsasen N, Leibo SP (1996) Development into blastocysts of bovine oocytes cryopreserved by ultra-rapid cooling. Biol Reprod 54:1059–1069

Mazur P (1970) Cryobiology: the freezing of biological systems. Science 168:939–949

Mazur P (1984) Freezing of living cells: mechanisms and implications. Am J Physiol 247:C125-C142

Mazur P (1990) Equilibrium, quasi-equilibrium, and nonequilibrium freezing of mammalian embryos. Cell Biophysics 17:53-92

McGann LE (1978) Differing actions of penetrating and nonpenetrating cryoprotective agents. Cryobiology 15:382-390

McLaughlin EA, Ford WCL, Hull MGR (1990) A comparison of the freezing of human semen in the uncirculated vapour above liquid nitrogen and in a semi-programmable freezer. Hum Reprod 5:724-728

McLaughlin EA, Ford WC, Hull MG (1993) Effects of cryopreservation on the human sperm acrosome and its response to A23187. J Reprod Fertil 99:71-76

Morroll DR, Matson PL, Troup SA, Izzard H, Prior JR, Burslem RW, Lieberman BA (1990) The cryopreservation of donor semen by a simplified method: use in an IVF and GIFT programme. Int J Androl 13:352-360

Mortimer D (1994) Semen cryopreservation. In: Mortimer D (ed) Practical laboratory andrology. Oxford University Press, Oxford, pp 301-323

Nagy Z, Liu J, Joris H, Verheyen G, Tournaye H, Camus M, Derde M-P, Devroey P, Van Steirteghem A (1995) The result of intracytoplasmic sperm injection is not related to any of the three basic sperm parameters. Hum Reprod 10:1123-1129

Nakagata N (1989) High survival rate of unfertilized mouse oocytes after vitrification. J Reprod Fertil 87:479-483

Newton H (1998) The cryopreservation of ovarian tissue as a strategy for preserving the fertility of cancer patients. Hum Reprod Up 4:237-247

Newton H, Aubard Y, Rutherford A Sharma V, Gosden R (1996) Low temperature storage and grafting of human ovarian tissue. Hum Reprod 11:1487-1491

Nogueira D, Bourgain C, Verheyen G, Van Steirteghem A (1999) Light and electron microscopic analysis of human testicular spermatozoa and spermatids from frozen and thawed testicular biopsies. Hum Reprod 14:2041-2048

Nugent D, Meirow D, Brook PF, Aubard Y, Gosden R (1997) Transplantation in reproductive medicine: previous experience, present knowledge and future prospects. Hum Reprod Update 3:267-280

Oates RD, Mulhall J, Burgess C, Cunningham D, Carson R (1997) Fertilization and pregnancy using intentionally cryopreserved testicular tissue as the sperm source for intracytoplasmic sperm injection in 10 men with non-obstructive azoospermia. Hum Reprod 12:734-739

Oktay K, Newton H, Mullan J, Gosden R (1998) Development of human primordial follicles in SCID/hpg mice stimulated with follicle stimulating hormone. Hum Reprod 13:1133-1138

Parkes AS (1958) Factors affecting the viability of frozen ovarian tissue. J Endocrinol 17:337-346

Parks JE, Ruffing NA (1992) Factors affecting low temperature survival of mammalian oocytes. Theriogenology 37:59-73

Parrott DMV (1960) The fertility of mice with orthotopic ovarian grafts derived from frozen tissue. J Reprod Fertil 1:230-241

Pedersen H, Lebech PE (1971) Ultrastructural changes in the human spermatozoon after freezing for artificial insemination. Fertil Steril 22:125-133

Pensis M, Loumaye E, Psalti I (1989) Screening of conditions for rapid freezing of human oocytes: preliminary study toward their cryopreservation. Fertil Steril 52:787-794

Perloff WH, Steinberger E, Sherman JK (1964) Conception with human spermatozoa frozen by nitrogen vapour technique. Fertil Steril 15:501

Pickering SJ, Johnson MH (1987) The influence of cooling on the organization of the meiotic spindle of the mouse oocyte. Hum Reprod 2:207-216

Pickering SJ, Braude PR, Johnson MJ, Cant A, Currie J (1990) Transient cooling to room temperature can cause irreversible disruption of the meiotic spindle in the human oocyte. Fertil Steril 54:102-108

Pickering SJ, Braude PR, Johnson MH (1991) Cryopreservation of human oocytes: inappropriate exposure to DMSO reduces fertilization rates. Hum Reprod 6:142–143

Polak de Fried E, Notrica J, Rubinstein M, Marazzi A, Gomez Gonzalez M (1998) Pregnancy after human donor oocyte cryopreservation and thawing in association with intracytoplasmic sperm injection in a patient with ovarian failure. Fertil Steril 69:555–557

Polge C, Smith AU, Parkes AS (1949) Revival of spermatozoa after vitrification and dehydration at low temperatures. Nature 164:666

Porcu E, Fabbri R, Seracchioli R, Ciotti PM, Magrini O, Flamigni C (1997) Birth of a healthy female after intracytoplasmic sperm injection of cryopreserved human oocytes. Fertil Steril 68:724–726

Porcu E, Fabbri R, Seracchioli R, Ciotti PM, Petracchi S, Savelli L, Ghi T, Flamigni C (1998) Birth of six healthy children after intracytoplasmic sperm injection of cryopreserved human oocytes. Hum Reprod 13:124

Prins GS, Weidel L (1986) A comparative study of buffer systems as cryoprotectants for human spermatozoa. Fertil Steril 46:147–149

Ragni GR, Caccamo AM, Dalla Serra A, Guercilena S (1990) Computerized slow-staged freezing of semen from men with testicular tumors or Hodgkin's disease preserves sperm better than standard vapour freezing. Fertil Steril 53:1072–1075

Rall WF (1992) Cryopreservation of oocytes and embryos: methods and applications. Anim Reprod Sci 28:237–245

Rall WF, Fahy GM (1985) Ice-free cryopreservation of mouse embryos at −196 °C by vitrification. Nature 313:573–575

Romero J, Remohi J, Minguez Y, Rubio C, Pellicer A, Gil-Salom M (1996) Fertilization after intracytoplasmic sperm injection with cryopreserved testicular spermatozoa. Fertil Steril 65:877–879

Rubinsky B, Arav A, Devries AL (1991) Cryopreservation of oocytes using directional cooling and antifreeze glycoproteins. Cryo Letts 12:93–106

Russell JB (1998) Immature oocyte retrieval combined with in-vitro maturation. Hum Reprod 13 [Suppl 3]:63–75

Salzbrunn A, Benson DM, Holstein AF, Schulze W (1996) A new concept for the extraction of testicular spermatozoa as a tool for assisted fertilization (ICSI). Hum Reprod 11:752–755

Sathananthan AH, Ng SC, Trounson AO, Bongso A, Ratnam SS, Ho J, Mok H, Lee MN (1988) The effects of ultra-rapid freezing on meiotic and mitotic spindles of mouse oocytes and embryos. Gamete Res 21:385–401

Schoysman R, Vanderzwalmen P, Nijs M, Segal-Bertin G, Geerts L et al (1993) Pregnancy after fertilisation with human testicular spermatozoa. Lancet 342:1237

Schroeder AC, Champlin AK, Mobraaten LE, Eppig JJ (1990) Developmental capacity of mouse oocytes cryopreserved before and after maturation in vitro. J Reprod Fertil 89:43–50

Serafini P, Marrs RP (1986) Computerized staged-freezing technique improves sperm survival and preserves penetration of zona-free hamster ova. Fertil Steril 45:854–858

Serafini P, Hauser D, Moyer D, Marrs RP (1986) Cryopreservation of human spermatozoa: correlations of ultrastructural sperm head configuration with sperm motility and ability to penetrate zona-free hamster ova. Fertil Steril 46:691–695

Serres C, Jouannet P, Czyglik F, David G (1980) Effects of freezing on spermatozoa motility. In: David G, Price WS (eds) Human artificial insemination and semen preservation. Plenum, NewYork, pp 147–161

Shaw JM, Trounson AO (1989) Parthenogenetic activation of unfertilized mouse oocytes by exposure to 1,2-propanediol is influenced by temperature, oocyte age and cumulus removal. Gamete Res 24:269–279

Shaw PW, Fuller BJ Bernard A, Shaw RW (1991) Vitrification of the mouse oocyte: improved rates of survival, fertilization, and development to blastocysts. Mol Reprod Dev 29:373–378

Sherman JK (1954) Freezing and freeze-drying of human spermatozoa. Fertil Steril 5:357

Sherman JK (1964) Dimethyl sulfoxide as a protective agent during freezing and thawing of human spermatozoa. Proc Soc Exp Biol Med 117:261

Sherman JK (1973) Synopsis of the use of frozen semen since 1964: state of the art of human semen banking. Fertil Steril 24:397–412

Sherman JK, Bunge RG (1953) Observations on preservation of human spermatozoa at low temperatures. Proc Soc Exp Biol Med 82:686

Sherman JK, Lin TP (1958) Effect of glycerol and low temperature on survival of unfertilized mouse eggs. Nature 4611:785–786

Siebzehnrübl ER (1989) Cryopreservation of gametes and cleavage stage embryos. Hum Reprod 4:105–110

Siebzehnrübl ER, Todorow S, van Uem J, Koch R, Wildt L, Lang N (1989) Cryopreservation of human and rabbit oocytes and one-cell embryos: a comparison of DMSO and propanediol. Hum Reprod 4:312–317

Smith AU, Parkes AS (1951) Preservation of ovarian tissue at low temperatures. Lancet:570

Son WY, Park SE, Lee KA, Lee WS, Ko JJ, Yoon TK, Cha KY (1996) Effects of 1,2-propanediol and freezing-thawing on the in vitro developmental capacity of human immature oocytes. Fertil Steril 66:995–999

Spallanzani L (1776) Opuscoli di fisca. Animale e vegetabile opusculo. II. Osservazioni, e sperienze intorno ai vermicelli spermatici dell'uomo e degli animali. Modena

Steptoe PC, Edwards RG (1978) Birth after the reimplantation of a human embryo. Lancet 2:336

Surrey EC, Quinn PJ (1990) Successful ultra-rapid freezing of unfertilized oocytes. J In Vitro Fertil Embryo Transf 7:262–266

Taylor PJ, Wilson J, Laycock R, Weger J (1982) A comparison of freezing and thawing methods for the cryopreservation of human semen. Fertil Steril 37:100–103

Thachill JV, Jewett MAS (1981) Preservation techniques for human semen. Fertil Steril 35:546–548

Todorow SJ, Siebzehnrübl ER, Koch R, Wildt L, Lang N (1989a) Comparative results on survival of human and animal eggs using different cryoprotectants and freeze-thawing regimens. I. Mouse and hamster. Hum Reprod 4:805–811

Todorow SJ, Siebzehnrübl ER, Spitzer M, Koch R, Wildt L, Lang N (1989b) Comparative results on survival of human and animal eggs using different cryoprotectants and freeze-thawing regimens. II. Human. Hum Reprod 4:812–816

Toth TL, Baka SG, Veeck LL, Jones, HW jr, Muasher S, Lanzendorf SE (1994) Fertilisation and in vitro development of cryopreserved human prophase I oocytes. Fertil Steril 61:891–894

Tournaye H, Devroey P, Liu J, Nagy Z, Lissens W, Van Steirteghem A (1994) Microsurgical epididymal sperm aspiration and intracytoplasmic sperm injection: a new effective approach to infertility as a result of congenital absence of the vas deferens. Fertil Steril 61:1045–1051

Tournaye H, Verheyen G, Nagy P, Ubaldi F, Goossens A, Silber S, Van Steirteghem AC, Devroey P (1997) Are there any predictive factors for successful testicular sperm recovery in azoospermic patients? Hum Reprod 12:80–86

Trounson A (1986) Preservation of human eggs and embryos. Fertil Steril 46:1–12

Trounson A, Kirby C (1989) Problems in the cryopreservation of unfertilized eggs by slow cooling in dimethyl sulfoxide. Fertil Steril 52:778–786

Trounson A, Mohr L (1983) Human pregnancy following cryopreservation, thawing and transfer of an eight-cell embryo. Nature 305:707–709

Trounson A, Peura A, Kirby C (1987) Ultra-rapid freezing: a new low-cost and effective method of embryo cryopreservation. Fertil Steril 48:843–850

Trounson A, Wood C, Kausche A (1994) In vitro maturation, fertilization and developmental competence of oocytes recovered from untreated polycystic ovarian patients. Fertil Steril 62:353–362

Tucker M, Wright G, Morton P et al (1996) Preliminary experience with human oocyte cryopreservation using 1,2-propanediol and sucrose. Hum Reprod 11:1513–1515

Tucker MJ, Wright G, Morton PC, Massey JB (1998) Birth after cryopreservation of immature oocytes with subsequent in vitro maturation. Fertil Steril 70:578–579

Van Blerkom J (1991) Cryopreservation of the mammalian oocyte. In: Pedersen RA, McLaren A, First NL (eds) Animal applications of research in mammalian development. Cold Spring Harbor Laboratory Press, Cold Spring Harbor, pp 83–119

Van Blerkom J, Davies PW (1994) Cytogenetic, cellular, and developmental consequences of cryopreservation of immature and mature mouse and human oocytes. Microsc Res Tech 27:165–193

Van den Broecke R, Van der Elst J, Dumortier F, Liu J, Schelfhout V, Kaufman J, Serreyn R, Dhont M (1999) Follicular growth in cryopreserved human ovarian xenografts in ovariectomized CID mice stimulated with follicle-stimulating hormone. Hum Reprod 14 (Abstract Book 1):29

Van der Elst J (1992) Cryopreservation of the mouse oocyte. Doctoral dissertation, Dutch-speaking Brussels Free University

Van der Elst J, Van den Abbeel E, Jacobs R, Wisse E, Van Steirteghem A (1988) Effect of 1,2-propanediol and dimethylsulphoxide on the meiotic spindle of the mouse oocyte. Hum Reprod 3:960–967

Van der Elst J, Nerinckx S, Van Steirteghem AC (1992a) In vitro maturation of mouse germinal vesicle-stage oocytes following cooling, exposure to cryoprotectants and ultra-rapid freezing: limited effect on the morphology of the second meiotic spindle. Hum Reprod 7:1440–1446

Van der Elst J, Van den Abbeel E, Nerinckx S, Van Steirteghem AC (1992b) Parthenogenetic activation pattern and microtubular organisation of the mouse oocyte after exposure to 1,2-propanediol. Cryobiology 29:549–562

Van der Elst J, Nerinckx S, Van Steirteghem AC (1993a) Association of ultra-rapid freezing of mouse oocytes with increased polyploidy at the pronucleate stage, reduced cell numbers in blastocysts and impaired fetal development. J Reprod Fertil 99:25–32

Van der Elst J, Nerinckx S, Van Steirteghem AC (1993b) Slow and ultra-rapid freezing of fully-grown germinal vesicle-stage mouse oocytes: optimal survival rate outweighed by defective blastocyst formation. J Assist Reprod Genet 10:202–212

van Uem JF, Siebzehnrübl ER, Schuh B, Koch R, Trotnow S, Lang N (1987) Birth after cryopreservation of unfertilized oocytes (letter). Lancet 1:752–753

Verheyen G, Pletincx I, Van Steirteghem A (1993) Effect of freezing method, thawing temperature and post-thaw dilution/washing on motility (CASA) and morphology characteristics of high-quality human sperm. Hum Reprod 8:1678–1684

Verheyen G, De Croo I, Tournaye H, Pletincx I, Devroey P, Van Steirteghem AC (1995) Comparison of four mechanical methods to retrieve spermatozoa from testicular tissue. Hum Reprod 10:2956–2959

Verheyen G, Nagy Z, Joris H, De Croo I, Tournaye H, Van Steirteghem AC (1997) Quality of frozen-thawed testicular sperm and its preclinical use for intracytoplasmic sperm injection into in-vitro matured germinal-vesicle stage oocytes. Fertil Steril 67:74–80

Vincent C, Johnson MH (1992) Cooling, cryoprotectants and the cytoskeleton of the mammalian oocyte. Oxf Rev Reprod Biol 14:73–100

Vincent C, Pickering SJ, Johnson MH (1990) The hardening effects of dimethylsulphoxide on the mouse zona pellucida requires the presence of an oocyte and is associated with a reduction in the number of cortical granules present. J Reprod Fertil 89:253–259

Wassarman PM (1990) Profile of a mammalian sperm receptor. Development 108:1–17

Whittingham DG (1977) Fertilization in vitro and development to term of unfertilized mouse oocytes previously stored at −196 °C. J Reprod Fertil 49:89–94

Whittingham DG, Leibo SP, Mazur P (1972) Survival of mouse embryos frozen to −196 °C and −269 °C. Science 178:414

Wolf DP, Patton PE (1989) Sperm cryopreservation: state of art. J In Vitro Fertil Embryo Transf 6:325–327

Wood MJ, Carroll JC, Whittingham DG, Barros C, Candy C (1991) Vitrification of mouse and hamster oocytes. Cryobiology 28:515–516

Yavetz H, Lessing JB, Niv Y, Amit A, Barak Y, Yovel I, David MP, Peyser MR, Yogev L, Homonnai Z, Paz G (1991) The efficiency of cryopreserved semen versus fresh semen for in vitro fertilization/embryo transfer. J In Vitro Fertil Embryo Transf 8:145–148

Yoshida H, Hoshiai H, Fukaya T, Ohi T, Kakuta C, Tozawa H, Mandai Y, Murakami T, Mansfield C, Yajima A (1990) Fertilizability of fresh and frozen human spermatozoa. ARTA 1:164–172

Zeilmaker GH, Alberda AT, van Gent I, Rijkmans CMPM, Drogendijk AC (1984) Two pregnancies following transfer of intact frozen-thawed embryos. Fertil Steril 42:293–296

Microinjection

A. Van Steirteghem, P. Devroey, I. Liebaers

Introduction

Since the birth of Louise Brown in July 1978 in vitro fertilization (IVF) has been successful in the treatment of long-standing infertility due to tubal disease and idiopathic and male-factor infertility. It is a well documented that the results of IVF in male infertility are not as good as those in patients with normal semen parameters. In andrological infertility the fertilization rate of the inseminated oocytes is much lower than in patients with tubal infertility and normal semen parameters (Tournaye et al. 1992). Absence of fertilization occurs in about one-third of the cycles. It has been the experience of all centers for reproductive medicine, including our own, that a certain number of patients with andrological infertility cannot be helped by standard IVF treatment. Furthermore, a sizeable number of couples cannot be accepted for IVF if the number of progressively motile spermatozoa with normal morphology available for insemination is below a certain threshold number such as 500000. The latter group includes, of course, the patients with obstructive and nonobstructive azoospermia.

In the past decade assisted fertilization procedures have been developed to circumvent the barriers that prevent sperm access to the ooplasma, namely the zona pellucida and the ooplasmic membrane. Successful fertilization, embryo development, pregnancies and births have been reported after partial zona dissection (PZD) and subzonal insemination (SUZI; Cohen et al. 1992; Fishel et al. 1992; Ng et al. 1991).

In 1992 the first pregnancies and births obtained by a novel procedure of assisted fertilization, i.e., intracytoplasmic sperm injection (ICSI) were reported by our group (Palermo et al. 1992). In rabbits and cattle, embryos obtained by ICSI have been transferred to recipient mothers and live offspring have resulted (Iritani et al. 1991). Very recently ICSI was also successful in the mouse when a piezo-driven micropipette was used instead of a mechanically driven conventional pipette (Kimura and Yanagimachi 1995). The results of the first 600 cycles of assisted fertilization by SUZI and ICSI at the Brussels Free University Center, as well as a controlled comparison on 144 oocytes in 11 cycles, indicated that the normal fertilization rate after ICSI is substantially higher than after SUZI, while the further in vitro development to transferable or freezable embryos is quite similar for the two procedures. The higher fertilization rate and similar cleavage rate resulted in more embryos for replacement after ICSI and high implantation rates have been obtained (Palermo et al. 1993; Van Steirteghem et al. 1993a; Van Steirteghem et al. 1993b; Van Steirteghem et al. 1993c). These results were further confirmed in the review of 1275 ICSI treatment cycles carried out from October 1991 until December (Tournaye et al. 1995).

This chapter summarizes the intracytoplasmic sperm injection procedure. Full details of the ICSI protocol were recently published on CD-ROM (Van Steirteghem et al. 1995). We also review the outcome of 2853 planned ICSI treatment cycles in 1953 infertile couples. These ICSI cycles were carried out between January 1991 and December 1994. ICSI was carried out in 2820 cycles since in 33 planned cycles there were no oocytes or no spermatozoa available for the assisted fertilization procedure. Three types of spermatozoa were used for the ICSI: (a) ejaculated spermatozoa (91% of the cycles), (b) epididymal spermatozoa (5% of the cycles), and (c) testicular spermatozoa (4% of the cycles).

Patient Selection and Management

ICSI can be carried in couples who have undergone at least one but more frequently more cycles of standard IVF procedure; after juxtaposition of the cumulus-oocyte complexes with 200 000 or more progressively motile spermatozoa per milliliter, fertilization did not occur or occurred in a limited number of the inseminated oocytes. ICSI can also be carried out in couples with semen parameters too impaired to be accepted for standard IVF because after semen preparation fewer than, e.g., 500 000 progressively motile spermatozoa with normal morphology were present in the total ejaculate.

ICSI can also be carried out with fresh and frozen-thawed epididymal or testicular spermatozoa in couples with obstructive azoospermia due to congenital bilateral absence of the vas deferens or failed vasovasostomy and vasoepididymostomy (Silber et al. 1994; Tournaye et al. 1994; Devroey et al. 1994, 1995a; Silber et al. 1995). ICSI can also be carried out in some couples with nonobstructive azoospermia due, e.g., to Sertoli cell only syndrome or maturation arrest (Devroey et al. 1995b).

The couples were fully informed about the novelty of the ICSI procedure and about its many unknown aspects. After extensive counseling they agreed and signed a consent form to have prenatal diagnosis and to participate in a prospective follow-up study of the children born after ICSI (Bonduelle et al. 1994, 1995a,b, 1996; Liebaers et al. 1995a; Wisanto et al. 1995).

Oocytes and Spermatozoa for Intracytoplasmic Sperm Injection

Ovarian stimulation was carried out by a combination of gonadotropin-releasing hormone agonist and human menopausal gonadotropins. The ovulation was induced with human chorionic gonadotropins when at least three follicles measured 18 mm or more in diameter and when serum oestradiol concentration were at least 1000 ng/l. The luteal phase was supplemented with intravaginally administered micronized progesterone (Smitz et al. 1988; Smitz et al. 1992; Smitz et al. 1993).

Oocyte retrieval was carried out by vaginal ultrasound-guided follicular puncture 36 h after HCG. In all 36425 cumulus-oocyte complexes were retrieved in these 2820 cycles, i.e., a mean of 12.9 complexes per cycle. Inspection of these complexes under the inverted microscope revealed that in almost all cases the cumulus and corona cells were well dispersed. These complexes were transferred into 5-ml Falcon tubes with one ml of preequilibrated Earle's medium and transported in a thermobox at 37 °C to the microinjection laboratory, which is located at a distance of about 500 m.

The cells of the cumulus and corona cells were removed by a combination of an enzymatic and mechanical procedure: (a) incubation for about 1 min in HEPES-buffered Earle's medium with about 60 IU hyaluronidase/ml and (b) thereafter aspiration of the cumulus-corona-oocyte complexes in and out of hand-drawn glass pipettes with two different diameters, first with an opening of 250–300 μm and then with an opening of 200 μm. Afterwards the oocytes were rinsed several times in droplets of HEPES-buffered Earle's and B_2 medium and then carefully observed under the inverted microscope at ×200 magnification. This included an assessment of the zona pellucida and the oocyte as well as noting the presence or absence of a germinal vesicle or the first polar body. Of the 36425 complexes, 34572 (95%) contained an intact oocyte with an intact zona pellucida and clear cytoplasm. Analysis of the nuclear status revealed 81% of the cumulus-oocytes complexes contained metaphase II oocytes which had extruded the first polar body, 10% germinal-vesicle-stage oocytes and 4% metaphase I oocytes which had undergone breakdown of the germinal vesicle but had not yet extruded the first polar body. The oocytes were then incubated in 25-μl microdrops of B_2 medium covered by mineral oil at 37 °C in an atmosphere of 5% O_2, 5% CO_2, and 90% N_2. ICSI was carried out on all metaphase II oocytes.

Before the start of the treatment cycle semen analysis and a semen selection procedure were carried out to verify whether enough spermatozoa were present to carry out ICSI. Semen analysis included the assessment of conventional semen characteristics by the procedures recommended by the World Health Organization (1992) except for sperm morphology, which was assessed by strict Tygerberg criteria after Shorr staining (Kruger et al. 1986). Semen values were considered normal if (a) sperm concentration was at least 20×106/ml, (2) progressive sperm motility was at least 40%, and (c) normal sperm morphology was at least 14%. The distribution of the semen characteristics of freshly ejaculated semen used for ICSI in 2524 cycles revealed that (a) normal semen parameters were present in 7% of the cycles, (b) a single sperm defect was present in 15% of the cycles, (c) a double sperm defect was present in 29% of the cycles, and (d) oligo-astheno-teratozoospermia was present in 49% of the cycles.

The preparation of the ejaculated sperm for ICSI involved the following steps: (a) removal of the seminal fluid by washing with medium, by centrifugation at 1800 g for 5 min and removal of the supernatant, (b) a passage through two or three layers of a discontinuous Percoll gradient, and (c) a final centrifugation step just prior to microinjection (Liu et al. 1994; Van Steirteghem et al. 1995).

Epididymal sperm was usually recovered by microsurgery from the most proximal part of the caput of the epididymis. During the microsurgical epididymal sperm aspiration several sperm fractions were collected into separate tubes. Sperm fractions with similar concentration and motility were pooled and then treated in the same way as ejaculated semen. Whenever possible, a part of the freshly recovered sperm was frozen for later use to avoid surgery in subsequent cycles (Silber et al. 1994; Tournaye et al. 1994; Devroey et al. 1995a). After thawing epididymal sperm was put on a discontinuous Percoll gradient and thereafter treated as ejaculated semen (Van Steirteghem et al. 1995).

Testicular spermatozoa were isolated from a testicular biopsy specimen. The testicular biopsy tissue was transferred into a petri dish with HEPES-buffered Earle's medium and shredded into small pieces with sterile microscope slides on the heated stage of a stereomicroscope. The presence of spermatozoa was assessed on the inverted microscope. The pieces of the biopsy tissue were removed and the medium was centrifuged at 300 g for 5 min. The pellet was then resuspended for the intracytoplasmic sperm injection procedure (Devroey et al. 1994; Nagy et al. 1995a; Silber et al. 1995; Van Steirteghem et al. 1995).

Intracytoplasmic Sperm Injection Procedure

The details of microtool preparation and microinjection procedure have been described in detail (Van Steirteghem et al. 1993a,b, 1995). Holding and injection pipettes were made from washed borosilicate glass capillary tubes which were first pulled on a horizontal microelectrode puller and then with the help of a microgrinder and microforge a sharp opening was made at the end of the injection pipette. The injection pipette had a 5–6 µm inner and 7–8 µm outer diameter while the holding pipette had a 10–20 µm inner and 60–80 µm outer diameter respectively. Both needles were bent to an angle of about 40°.

The injection dish contained 8 droplets of 5 µl HEPES-buffered Earle's medium surrounding a central droplet of medium with 10% polyvinyl-pyrrolidone and 1 µl of the resuspended sperm droplet. The intracytoplasmic sperm injection procedure was carried out on the heated stage of an inverted microscope at ×400 magnification using the Hoffman Modulation Contrast system. The holding and injection pipettes were fixed into a tool holder and were connected to a micrometer-type microinjector. The movement of the pipettes was coordinated by two coarse positioning manipulators and with two three-dimensional hydraulic remote-control micromanipulators.

A single, living, immobilized spermatozoon was aspirated tail first into the injection pipette. The oocyte was fixed on the holding pipette in a way that the polar body was situated at 6 o'clock while the injection pipette was pushed through the zona pellucida at the 3 o'clock position and into the cytoplasm, where the sperm was delivered together with the smallest possible amount of medium (Nagy et al. 1995b).

After injection the oocytes were washed and stored in 25 µl microdrops of B_2 medium in a petri dish and stored at 37 °C in an incubator containing 5% CO_2, 5% O_2, and 90% N_2.

Fertilization and Embryo Development After Intracytoplasmic Sperm Injection

Oocytes were inspected 16–18 h after microinjection for intactness and fertilization (Nagy et al. 1994). The number and aspect of polar bodies and pronuclei were recorded. Oocytes were considered to be normally fertilized when two individualized or fragmented polar bodies were present together with two clearly visible pronuclei. In these 2820 cycles ICSI was carried out on 29 415 metaphase II oocytes, i.e., a mean of 10.4 oocytes per cycle. The number of intact oocytes after ICSI was 26 228, i.e., 89.2% of the injected oocytes. The mean number of successfully injected oocytes was 9.3 per treatment cycle. The number of normally fertilized oocytes was 18 364, i.e., 70% of the successfully injected oocytes, 62.4% of the injected metaphase II oocytes and 50.4% of the retrieved cumulus-oocyte complexes. The number of abnormally fertilized oocytes was 991 one-pronuclear oocytes (3.8% of the intact oocytes) and 1194 three-pronuclear oocytes (4.6% of the intact oocytes). One-pronuclear oocytes were reassessed for their pronuclear status a few hours after the initial observation. In contrast to our standard IVF program, no change in pronuclear status was observed at the time of the second microscopic observation (Staessen et al. 1993a). If these abnormally fertilized oocytes cleave they are not transferred. This parthenogenetic activation may be due to mechanical or chemical factors. It may come as a surprise to observe three-pronuclear oocytes after the injection of only one spermatozoon into the ooplasm. We carefully observed the polar bodies at the time of fertilization, and it is obvious that the three pronuclei were mostly due to nonextrusion of the second polar body at the time of fertilization.

Damage, normal fertilization rates, and embryo development after ICSI were analyzed for the three types of sperm used to carry out ICSI (Table 1). The proportion of intact oocytes was 89% or 90%, and the normal fertilization rate varied from 58% to 71% of the intact oocytes. The percentage of normally fertilized oocytes was significantly higher with ejaculated semen (71%) than with fresh or frozen-thawed epididymal sperm (58%) or testicular sperm (60%; Table 1).

The exceptional circumstances in which none of the injected oocytes were normally fertilized occurred when (a) only one metaphase II oocyte was available for ICSI, (b) only totally immotile spermatozoa were available for the injection, (c) gross abnormalities were present in the oocytes, (d) round-headed spermatozoa were injected, and (e) when all oocytes were damaged by the injection procedure. The majority of these patients achieved fertilization in a subsequent cycle (Liu et al. 1995).

The embryo cleavage of the two-pronuclear oocytes was evaluated after a further 24 h of in vitro culture. The cleaving embryos were scored according to the equality of size of the blastomeres and the number of anucleate fragments.

Table 1. Damage, fertilization, and embryo development after ICSI with ejaculated, epididymal, and testicular spermatozoa

	Ejaculated	Epididymal	Testicular
Cycles	2572	128	120
Oocytes injected	26343	1628	1444
% intact after ICSI	89	90	89
% of intact oocytes with 2PN	1[a]	58[a]	60[a]
2-PN embryos	16758	844	767
Percent transferable embryos	74[b]	67[b]	71[b]
Percent embryos transferred or frozen	65	63	68

[a] $p = 0.0001$ by χ^2 contingency table, [b] $p=0.0001$ by χ^2 contingency table

These embryos were classified into three categories according to the percentage of anucleate fragments: (a) excellent type A embryos (without anucleate fragments), (b) good-quality type B embryos (between 1% and 20% of the volume filled with anucleate fragments), and (c) fair-quality type C embryos (between 21% and 50% anucleate fragments). Cleaved embryos with less than half of their volume filled with anucleate fragments were eligible for transfer. If supernumerary embryos with less than 20% anucleate fragments were available, they were cryopreserved on day 2 or 3 after oocyte retrieval using the slow-freezing protocol with dimethylsulfoxide (Van Steirteghem et al. 1994; Van der Elst et al. 1995).

The total number of embryos of sufficient quality to be transferred, i.e., those with less than 50% anucleate fragments was 13479, i.e., 73.4% of the two-pronuclear oocytes, 51.4% of the successfully injected oocytes, 45.8% of the injected metaphase II oocytes and 37.0% of the retrieved cumulus-oocyte complexes.

The percentages of two-pronuclear oocytes which developed to transferable embryos and which were actually transferred or frozen when ICSI was carried out with ejaculated, epididymal, and testicular spermatozoa are summarized in Table 1. The percentage of transferable embryos was higher after ICSI with ejaculated semen (74%) than after ICSI with epididymal (67%) or testicular spermatozoa (71%). The percentage of embryos which were acutally transferred or frozen were similar for the three types of spermatozoa used in the ICSI procedure. There was no difference in the percentage of excellent quality type A embryos (7–9%), good-quality type B embryos (46–53%) and fair-quality type C embryos (13–14%) when ICSI was carried out with ejaculated, epididymal, or testicular spermatozoa.

The total number of embryos, which were actually transferred or frozen (less than 20% anucleate fragments) was 11983, i.e., 65.3% of the two-pronuclear oocytes, 45.7% of the successfully injected oocytes, 40.7% of the injected metaphase II oocytes and 32.9% of the retrieved cumulus-oocyte complexes.

Outcome of Embryo Transfers, Obstetrical Outcome, Prenatal Diagnosis, and Children Follow-Up

An embryo replacement was possible in 2608 of the 2820 treatment cycles (92.6%). This is a high transfer rate for couples with previous fertilization failure in standard IVF, with ejaculated sperm too poor to be included in IVF or with obstructive or nonobstructive azoospermia. As indicated in Table 2 the percentage of transfers was similar in the four groups of ejaculated semen parameters; the transfer rate varied from 92% to 94% of the cycles. The distribution of transfers with one, two, three, or more than three embryos was also similar in the four groups of semen parameters. Except for some patients older than 40, the number of embryos replaced was limited to a maximum of two or three embryos (Staessen et al. 1993b).

The number of patients with positive serum HCG was 964, i.e., a 36.9% pregnancy rate per transfer and 34.2% per started cycle. As indicated in Table 3, the pregnancy rate per transfer was similar for ICSI with ejaculated (37%), epididymal (43%), and testicular sperm (40%). The pregnancy rate was especially high when an elective transfer of two or three embryos could be carried out.

Because of the novelty and the many unknown aspects of ICSI, the couples were asked after extensive counseling to adhere to the follow-up conditions, which include genetic counseling, agreement to prenatal testing and participation in a prospective clinical follow-up study of the children (Bonduelle et al. 1994, 1995a,b, 1996; Liebaers et al. 1995a; Wisanto et al. 1995).

As of September 1995, 585 prenatal diagnoses have been carried out in pregnancies after ICSI. Of these 585 samples obtained through either chorionic villus sampling or amniocentesis, six (1%) chromosomal anomalies were observed. Five were sex-chromosomal aberrations; two were 47, XXY, one was 47, XXX, one was 47, XYY, and one was a mosaic 46, XX/47, XXX; the remaining one was a trisomy 21. These data show that there might indeed be a slightly increased risk of sex chromosomal anomalies in children conceived after ICSI as compared with the incidence of the general population or at prenatal diagnosis carried out because of maternal age. The six abnormal karyotypes were observed in children from women between 25 and 32 years old except the 46, XX/47, XXX and the 47, XY+21 which occurred in women 44 and 41 years old. Two pregnancies were ter-

Table 2. ICSI and number of embryos transferred in relation to the ejaculated sperm parameters: sperm parameters

	Cycles	Transfers		1		2		3		>3	
	n	n	%	n	%	n	%	n	%	n	%
Normal	175	162	93	18	11	45	28	87	54	12	7
1 anomaly	377	350	93	22	6	115	33	192	55	21	6
2 anomalies	731	685	94	52	8	236	35	360	53	37	5
3 anomalies	1241	1139	92	105	9	405	36	575	51	54	5

Table 3. Sperm origin and outcome of embryo transfer after ICSI

	Ejaculated		Epididymal		Testicular	
	n	%	*n*	%	*n*	%
Cycles	2572	–	128	–	120	–
Transfers	2382	93	117	91	108	90
Pregnancies/transfers						
1 embryo	21/204	10	1/7	14	2/14	14
2 embryos	78/321	24	3/15	20	4/13	32
2 embryos (elective)	218/488	45	3/14	21	3/12	25
3 embryos	253/694	36	17/37	46	10/21	48
3 embryos (elective)	254/544	47	17/24	71	11/20	55
>3 embryos	47/131	36	9/20	45	13/28	46
	871/2382	37	50/117	43	43/108	40
Pregnancies/cycle	–	34	–	39	–	36

minated: the 47, XX+21 and one of the 47, XXY's. The pregnancy with the mosaic karyotype ended at 38 weeks' gestation with an intrauterine death for no apparent reason; necropsy failed to reveal any abnormality.

As of September 1995, in 877 children born after ICSI, 23 (2.6%) of major malformations leading to functional impairment or necessitating surgery have been observed. This malformation rate is similar to the numbers observed in population surveys or in children born after assisted procreation procedures other than ICSI (Liebaers et al. 1995b).

Although there is no indication of an increase in major congenital malformations after replacement of embryos obtained after ICSI, it is important to continue this careful prospective follow-up study of the children in different centers practicing ICSI. This is one of the goals of the Task Force on ICSI established by the European Society of Human Reproduction and Embryology (Bonduelle et al. 1995b).

Acknowledgements. The authors are indebted to their many colleagues of the Center for Reproductive Medicine and the Center for Medical Genetics. Special thanks go to (a) Geertrui Bocken, An Vankelecom, Heidi Van Ranst, Bart Desmet, and Nadine Franceus of the microinjection team, (b) research nurses Marleen Magnus, Andrea Buysse, and Pascale Dekoninck for collecting the data on pregnancy and pediatric follow-up, (c) Viviane De Wolf for typesetting the manuscript, and (d) Michael Whitburn of the Language Education Center for correcting the manuscript. This work is supported by grants from the Belgian Fund for Medical Research and from Organon International.

References

Bonduelle M, Desmyttere S, Buysse A, Van Assche E, Schiettecatte J, Devroey P, Van Steirteghem A, Liebaers I (1994) Prospective follow-up study of 55 children born after subzonal insemination and intracytoplasmic sperm injection. Hum Reprod 9:1765-1769

Bonduelle M, Legein J, Derde MP, Buysse A, Schiettecatte J, Wisanto A, Devroey P, Van Steirteghem A, Liebaers I (1995a) Comparative follow-up study of 130 children born after ICSI and 130 children born after IVF. Hum Reprod in press

Bonduelle M, Hamberger L, Joris H, Tarlatzis BC, Van Steirteghem AC (1995b) Assisted reproduction by intracytoplasmic sperm injection: an ESHRE survey of clinical experiences until 31 December 1993. Hum Reprod Update 1, no 3, CD-ROM

Bonduelle M, Legein J, Buysse A, Van Assche E, Wisanto A, Devroey P, Van Steirteghem A, Liebaers I (1996) Prospective follow-up study of 423 children born after intracytoplasmic sperm injection. Hum Reprod, in press

Cohen J, Alikani M, Adler A, Berkely A, Davis O, Ferrara TA, Graf M, Grifo J, Liu HC, Malter HE, Reing AM, Suzman M, Talansky BE, Trowbridge J, Rosenwaks Z (1992) Microsurgical fertilization procedures: the absence of stringent criteria for patient selection. J Assist Reprod Genet 9:197-206

Devroey P, Liu J, Nagy Z, Tournaye H, Silber SJ, Van Steirteghem AC (1994) Normal fertilization of human oocytes after testicular sperm extraction and intracytoplasmic sperm injection. Fertil Steril 62:639-641

Devroey P, Silber SJ, Nagy Z, Liu J, Tournaye H, Joris H, Verheyen G, Van Steirteghem AC (1995a) Ongoing pregnancies and birth after intracytoplasmic sperm injection with frozen-thawed epididymal spermatozoa. Hum Reprod 10:903-906

Devroey P, Liu J, Nagy Z, Goossens A, Tournaye H, Camus M, Van Steirteghem A (1995b) Pregnancies after testicular sperm extraction and intracytoplasmic sperm injection in non-obstructive azoospermia. Hum Reprod 10:1457-1460

Fishel S, Timson J, Lisi F, Rinaldi L (1992) Evaluation of 225 patients undergoing subzonal insemination for the procurement of fertilization in vitro. Fertil Steril 57:840-849

Iritani A (1991) Micromanipulation of gametes for in vitro assisted fertilization. Mol Reprod Develop 28:199-207

Kimura Y, Yanagimachi R (1995) Intracytoplasmic sperm injection in the mouse. Biol Reprod 52:709-720

Kruger TF, Menkveld R, Stander FSH, Lombard CJ, Van der Merwe JP, van Zyl JA, Smith K (1986) Sperm morphologic features as a prognostic factor in in vitro fertilization. Fertil Steril 46:1118-1123

Liebaers I, Bonduelle M, Legein J, Wilikens A, Van Assche E, Buysse A, Wisanto A, Devroey P, Van Steirteghem AC (1995a) Follow-up of children born after intracytoplasmic sperm injection. In: Hedon B, Bringer J, Mares P (eds) Fertility and sterility. A current overview. Proceedings of the 15th World Congress on Fertility and Sterility, Montpellier, France, 17-22 September 1995. Parthenon, London, pp 409-412

Liebaers I, Bonduelle M, Van Assche E, Devroey P, Van Steirteghem A (1995b) Sex chromosome abnormalities after intracytoplasmic sperm injection. Lancet 346:1095

Liu J, Nagy Z, Joris H, Tournaye H, Devroey P, Van Steirteghem AC (1994) Intracytoplasmic sperm injection does not require special treatment of the spermatozoa. Hum Reprod 9:1127-1130

Liu J, Nagy Z, Joris H, Tournaye H, Smitz J, Camus M, Devroey P, Van Steirteghem A (1995) Analysis of 76 total fertilization failure cycles out of 2732 intracytoplasmic sperm injection cycles. Hum Reprod 10:2630-2636

Nagy ZP, Liu J, Joris H, Devroey P, Van Steirteghem A (1994) Time-course of oocyte activation, pronucleus formation and cleavage in human oocytes fertilized by intracytoplasmic sperm injection. Hum Reprod 9:1743-1748

Nagy Z, Liu J, Janssenswillen C, Silber S, Devroey P, Van Steirteghem AC (1995a) Using ejaculated, fresh and frozen-thawed epididymal and testicular spermatozoa gives rise to comparable results after intracytoplasmic sperm injection. Fertil Steril 63:808-815

Nagy ZP, Liu J, Joris H, Bocken G, Desmet B, Van Ranst H, Vankelecom A, Devroey P, Van Steirteghem AC (1995b) The influence of the site of sperm deposition and mode of oolemma breakage at intracytoplasmic sperm injection on fertilization and embryo development rates. Hum Reprod 10:3171-3177

Ng SC, Bongso A, Ratnam SS (1991) Microinjection of human oocytes: a technique for severe oligoasthenoteratozoospermia. Fertil Steril 56:1117-1123

Palermo G, Joris H, Devroey P, Van Steirteghem AC (1992) Pregnancies after intracytoplasmic injection of single spermatozoon into an oocyte. Lancet 340:17-18

Palermo G, Joris H, Derde MP, Camus M, Devroey P, Van Steirteghem AC (1993) Sperm characteristics and outcome of human assisted fertilization by subzonal insemination and intracytoplasmic sperm injection. Fertil Steril 59:826-835

Silber SJ, Nagy ZP, Liu J, Godoy H, Devroey P, Van Steirteghem AC (1994) Conventional in-vitro fertilization versus intracytoplasmic sperm injection for patients requiring microsurgical sperm aspiration. Hum Reprod 9:1705-1709

Silber SJ, Van Steirteghem AC, Liu J, Nagy Z, Tournaye H, Devroey P (1995) High fertilization and pregnancy rate after intracytoplasmic sperm injection with spermatozoa obtained from testicle biopsy. Hum Reprod 10:148-152

Smitz J, Devroey P, Camus M, Deschacht J, Khan I, Staessen C, Van Waesberghe L, Wisanto A, Van Steirteghem AC (1988) The luteal phase and early pregnancy after combined GnRH-agonist/HMG treatment for superovulation in IVF or GIFT. Hum Reprod 3:585-590

Smitz J, Devroey P, Faguer B, Bourgain C, Camus M, Van Steirteghem AC (1992) A prospective randomized comparison of intramuscular or intravaginal progesterone as a luteal phase and early pregnancy supplement. Hum Reprod 7:168-175

Smitz J, Bourgain C, Van Waesberghe L, Camus M, Devroey P, Van Steirteghem AC (1993) A prospective randomized study on oestradiol valerate supplementation in addition to intravaginal micronized progesterone in buserelin and HMG induced superovulation. Hum Reprod 8:40-45

Staessen C, Janssenswillen C, Devroey P, Van Steirteghem AC (1993a) Cytogenetic and morphological observations of single pronucleated human oocytes after in-vitro fertilization. Hum Reprod 8:221-223

Staessen C, Janssenswillen C, Van den Abbeel E, Devroey P, Van Steirteghem AC (1993b) Avoidance of triplet pregnancies by elective transfer of two good quality embryos. Hum Reprod 8:1650-1653

Tournaye H, Devroey P, Camus M, Staessen C, Bollen N, Smitz J, Van Steirteghem AC (1992) Comparison of in-vitro fertilization in male and tubal infertility: a 3 year survey. Hum Reprod 7:218-222

Tournaye H, Devroey P, Liu J, Nagy Z, Lissens W, Van Steirteghem AC (1994) Microsurgical epididymal sperm aspiration and intracytoplasmic sperm injection: a new effective approoach to infertility as a result of congenital bilateral absence of the vas deferens. Fertil Steril 61:1045-1051

Tournaye H, Liu J, Nagy Z, Joris H, Wisanto A, Bonduelle M, Van der Elst J, Staessen C, Smitz J, Silber S, Devroey P, Liebaers I, Van Steirteghem A (1995) Intracytoplasmic sperm injection (ICSI): the Brussels experience. Reprod Fertil Dev 7:269-279

Van der Elst J, Camus M, Van den Abbeel E, Maes R, Devroey P, Van Steirteghem AC (1995) Prospective randomized study on the cryopreservation of human embryos with dimethylsulfoxide or 1,2-propanediol protocols. Fertil Steril 63:92-100

Van Steirteghem AC, Liu J, Joris H, Nagy Z, Janssenswillen C, Tournaye H, Derde M-P, Van Assche E, Devroey P (1993a) Higher success rate by intracytoplasmic sperm injection than by subzonal insemination. Report of a second series of 300 consecutive treatment cycles. Hum Reprod 8:1055-1060

Van Steirteghem AC, Nagy Z, Joris H, Liu J, Staessen C, Smitz J, Wisanto A, Devroey P (1993b) High fertilization and implantation rates after intracytoplasmic sperm injection. Hum Reprod 8:1061-1066

Van Steirteghem AC, Liu J, Nagy Z, Joris H, Tournaye H, Liebaers I, Devroey P (1993c) Use of assisted fertilization. Hum Reprod 8:1784-1785

Van Steirteghem AC, Van der Elst J, Van den Abbeel E, Joris H, Camus M, Devroey P (1994) Cryopreservation of supernumerary multicellular human embryos obtained after intracytoplasmic sperm injection. Fertil Steril 62:775–780

Van Steirteghem AC, Joris H, Liu J, Nagy Z, Bocken G, Vankelecom A, Desmet B, Van Ranst H, Franceus N (1995) Protocol for intracytoplasmic sperm injection. Hum Reprod Update 1:no 3: CD-ROM

Wisanto A, Magnus M, Bonduelle M, Liu J, Camus M, Tournaye H, Liebaers I, Van Steirteghem AC, Devroey P (1995) Obstetric outcome of 424 pregnancies after intracytoplasmic sperm injection (ICSI). Hum Reprod 10:2713–2718

World Health Organization (1992) WHO laboratory manual for the examination of human semen and sperm cervical mucus interaction. Cambridge University Press, Cambridge

-

In Vitro Fertilization

T. Rabe, K. Diedrich, I. Eberhardt, S. Al-Hasani

Introduction

The short report by Steptoe and Edwards that appeared in the *Lancet* in 1978, entitled "Birth after the reimplantation of a human embryo", marked the culmination of a long development in the field of reproductive medicine and the beginning of in vitro fertilization (IVF) as a routine method of infertility treatment (Table 1). IVF means the fertilization of an oocyte with sperm outside the body. IVF treatment involves the collection of mature oocytes, their fertilization and cultivation as embryos, and their subsequent transfer into the uterus (Fig. 1).

Some recommendations made in this chapter are based on the following: Acosta et al. (1990), Beier and Lindner (1983), Bettendorf and Breckwoldt (1989), Wood and Trounson (1989), Edwards and Livingstone (1990), Edwards and Brody (1995), Fishel (1986), Fischl (1995), Hinrichsen (1990), Jones et al. (1986), Ludwig and Tauber (1978), Krebs and Al-Hasani (1984), Rabe and Runnebaum (1994), Schill and Bollmann (1986), Veeck (1987, 1991), WHO Technical Report Series (1992), and the WHO Laborhandbuch zur Beurteilung des menschlichen Ejakulates und der Spermien-Zervikalschleim-Interaktion (1993).

Follicular Aspiration

For in vitro fertilization follicles were initially aspirated by the laparoscopic route, normally under general anesthesia. Since several aspirations are often necessary to achieve pregnancy, puncturing methods have been developed which reduce the strain on the patient. The first ultrasound-guided follicular aspirations were performed in the early 1980s. Transvesical, transurethral, and transvaginal methods initially involved placing the transducer on the lower abdomen and visualizing the organs of the small pelvis through the full bladder, serving as a sound window. These techniques required considerable experience on the part of the physician performing the aspiration. The medical profession was reluctant to apply them routinely, and they are now considered obsolete.

The introduction of vaginal transducers made it possible to perform transvaginal follicular aspiration under ultrasound guidance, which increased the acceptance of ultrasound-guided follicular aspiration considerably. Even under adverse conditions (e.g., obesity), the ovaries can normally be visualized easily.

Table 1. Historical development of new techniques in reproductive medicine

Year	Technique	Author
1878	IVF of rabbit and guinea pig oocytes	Schenk (1878)
1890	First heterologous transfer of mammalian embryos	Heape (1980)
1909	Human pregnancy with donar semen	Hard (1909)
1944	IVF of a human oocyte	Rock and Menkin (1944)
1970	Laparoscopic oocyte harvest	Steptoe and Edwards (1970)
1973	Transient B-hCG rise after transfer of IVF embryos	de Kretzer et al. (1973)
1976	Extrauterine pregnancy after IVF	Steptoe and Edwards (1976)
1978	Birth after reimplantation of a human embryo	Steptoe and Edwards (1978)
1980	IVF-ET: term pregnancy after unexplained infertility	Lopata et al. (1980)
1981	IVF-ET pregnancy after stimulation with clomiphene citrate	Trounson et al. (1981)
	Laparoscopic oocyte collection under ultrasound control	Lenz et al. (1981)
1982	Birth after gamete transfer (oocyte/sperm) into the uterus	Craft et al. (1982)
1983	IVF-ET treatment in patient with endometriosis	Mahadevan et al. (1983)
1984	Intrauterine insemination with prepared sperm	Kerin et al. (1984)
	Pregnancy in a woman with premature ovarian insufficiency after transfer of an IVF donar embryo	Lutjen et al. (1984)
	IVF-ET treatment for male infertility	Yovich et al. (1984)
	Gamete intrafallopian transfer by laparascopy	Asch et al. (1985)
1985	IVF-ET treatment in cases of pathological cervical factor	Hewett et al. (1985)
	Vaginal follicular aspiration under vaginal ultrasound control	Wikland et al. (1985)
1986	Pregnancy after cryopreservation of human oocytes	Chen et al. (1986)
	Direct intraperitoneal insemination	Forrler et al. (1986a,b)
	Pregnancy after translaparoscopic zygote intrafallopian transfer	Devroey et al. (1986)
1987	Pregnancy after pronuclear-stage tubal transfer	Yovich et al. (1987)
	Embryo transfer after tubal catheterization through the vagina	Jansen and Anderson (1987)
1988	Pregnancy after insemination under the zona pellucida	Ng et al. (1988)
1989	Assisted hatching	Cohen et al. (1991)
1990	Cocultures	Bongso et al. (1992)
1992	Intracytoplasmic sperm injection (ICSI)	Ng et al. (1991

The approach through the vagina ensures a short distance to the follicles, does not cause skin injury, and can be carried out without general anesthesia in most patients. The rate of complications (perforation, intra-abdominal bleeding, peritonitis) is very low (Table 2). Since ultrasound-guided follicular aspiration has become common throughout the world, laparoscopic oocyte collection is now extremely rare.

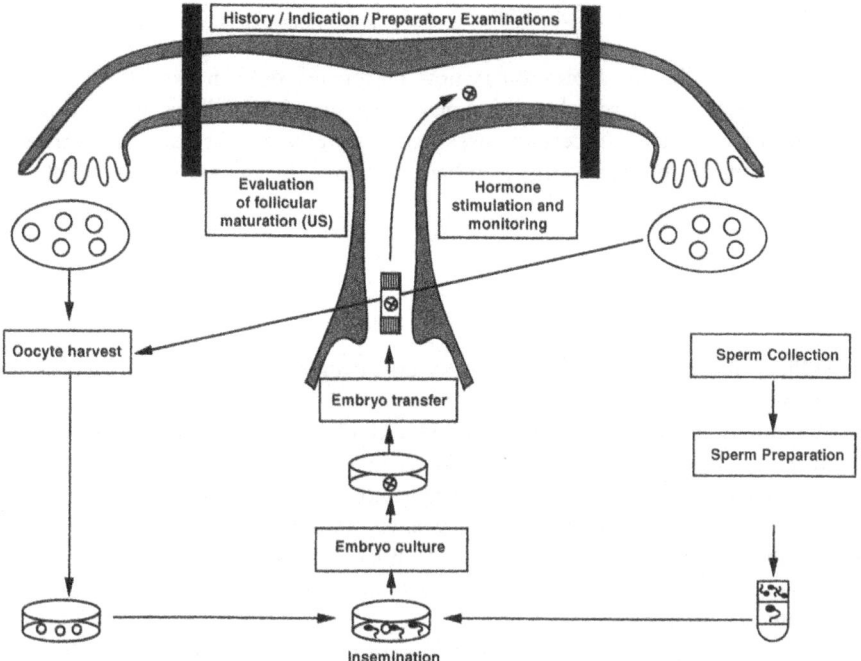

Fig. 1. In vitro fertilization: principle and procedure

Table 2. Complications after oocyte retrieval based on retrieval technique (from German Central IVF Register 1994)

Method	Cycles	Bleeding	Intestinal injury	Peritonitis	Other
Laparoscopic follicular aspiration	364	1	1	0	0
Transvesical aspiration/ abdominal ultrasound	28	0	0	0	0
Vaginal aspiration/vaginal ultrasound[a]	11 326	8	0	4	6
Other	37	1	0	0	0
Total	11 755	10	1	4	6

[a] No distinction between manual and automatic needle guidance is made.

Laparoscopic Follicular Aspiration

Laparoscopic follicular aspiration is now performed only in exceptional cases. When laparoscopy is scheduled for diagnostic reasons, follicles may be aspirated at the same time in certain cases (e.g., to evaluate a case of endometriosis or the prospects for microsurgical tubal correction, or as part of intratubal gamete transfer).

Advantages

- Follicles are punctured under direct view of the ovaries, reducing the risk of vascular or intestinal injury.
- Diagnostic exploration of the abdomen is possible: inferior portion of the liver (e.g., chlamydial infection, guitar string-like adhesions are typical of the Fitz-Hugh-Curtis syndrome), suspected hepatitis (it is important to detect a case of hepatitis to ensure laboratory safety and avoid infection!).
- Simultaneous adhesiolysis can be performed laparoscopically.
- If necessary, simultaneous electro- or laser coagulation of endometrial implants can be done.
- Further possibilities for endoscopic operations, e.g., for sactosalpinx.

Disadvantages

- Intraoperative risks:
  - General anesthesia and subsequent temporary patient monitoring are required.
  - Risk of vascular and intestinal injury, especially after multiple laparotomy; laparotomy with longitudinal incision may be necessary (risk of hysterectomy due to uncontrollable bleeding is below 1:1000).
- Postoperative risks:
  - Bleeding from incision sites
  - Infection in the small pelvis (postoperative risk below 1%).

Patient Preparation

- The abdominal wall is disinfected and the Verres needle checked for patency.
- The Verres needle is introduced into the abdominal cavity by incision of the umbilical fossa.
- A CO peritoneum is created by insufflating about 3 l gas using an insufflator.
- The Verres needle is replaced with the trocar of the surgical laparoscope (Karl Stortz, Tuttlingen, Germany; external diameter 10 mm, internal diameter 5 mm).

- The ovarian fixation forceps is introduced through an additional suprasymphyseal incision (with the external tube of the trocar in place).

Preparation of the Aspiration Needle. The Teflon tube in the lumen of the needle is pushed forward slightly and cut off flush at the front.

Surgical Laparoscope with a Straight Optical System. The aspiration needle is introduced with the Teflon tube through a third incision in the lower abdomen (either directly through the abdominal wall or through the trocar tube).

Surgical Laparoscope with an Angular Optical System. The aspiration needle is introduced with the Teflon tube through the operating channel of the laparoscope.

Follicular Aspiration

The ovaries are held with a forceps to restrict mobility during puncture. The follicles around the top ovarian pole are punctured first. The preovarian follicle is punctured preferably at an avascular site at the top to avoid leakage.

Follicular fluid is aspirated at a vacuum of 150 mmHg. If the follicles rupture prematurely or during aspiration, the contents of the pouch of Douglas must also be aspirated. If necessary, flush the pouch of Douglas and aspirate the contents.

After Follicular Aspiration

Reexplore the internal genital area, especially for signs of postoperative bleeding. After a final exploration of the upper abdomen, retract surgical instruments, release the pneumoperitoneum, and remove the trocar tube. Close incisions with interrupted sutures and apply a sterile plaster.

Postoperative Care

The patient must be monitored in hospital for 6–24 h. Care must be taken to detect any signs of vascular complications and bleeding. After 6–24 h, the patient is discharged with instructions about her inability to drive, the possibility of circulatory complications or of infection, and the continued risk of overstimulation (her liquid uptake should be more than 3 l/day). She must come back immediately if there are any complaints, especially abdominal tension, breathing difficulties, first signs of thrombosis, circulatory disorders, or fever.

Ultrasound-Guided Follicular Aspiration with a Transabdominal Transducer

The following methods of aspiration under transabdominal ultrasound control are of merely historical significance:

1. Transvesical follicular aspiration under transabdominal ultrasound guidance. In 1981 percutaneous transvesical follicular aspiration was described by Lenz et al. (1981). Several Scandinavian groups reported the successful use of this method (Hamberger et al. 1982, Lenz and Lauritzen 1982). The drawbacks are that the bladder wall, which is punctured in this operation, does not become completely painless under local anesthesia, and that the patient must maintain a full bladder for a considerable length of time.
2. Periurethral follicular aspiration with transabdominal ultrasound guidance. In this method follicles were aspirated free-hand through the urethra under transabdominal ultrasound guidance (Parsons et al. 1985).
3. Transvaginal follicular aspiration under transabdominal ultrasound guidance. The transvaginal route under transabdominal ultrasound guidance was first described by Dellenbach et al. (1984). This method also requires a full bladder as a sound window, with the associated strain on the patient and frequent problems visualizing the follicles.

Ultrasound-Guided Follicular Aspiration with a Vaginal Transducer

Principle

The follicles are punctured with a needle connected to the vaginal transducer with a guide. The ultrasound system displays a beam on the ultrasound screen corresponding to the selected direction of the needle (Fig. 2). The method was described by Wikland et al. in 1985, and the advantages of this method have been confirmed by several groups (Feichtinger and Kemeter 1986, Cohen et al. 1986, Lenz et al. 1987). Because of its clear advantages compared with the other techniques described above, transvaginal follicular aspiration is currently considered the method of choice for in vitro fertilization.

Advantages

- The risk of injury is low.
- Follicles can be localized accurately because of their short distance from the transducer.
- No hospitalization is required.
- No operating theater is required.
- Fewer staff are required.
- Ultrasound aspiration is possible even in cases of severe adhesions in the small pelvis, if the ovaries can be visualized close to the vaginal pole with no interposed vessels or intestinal loops.

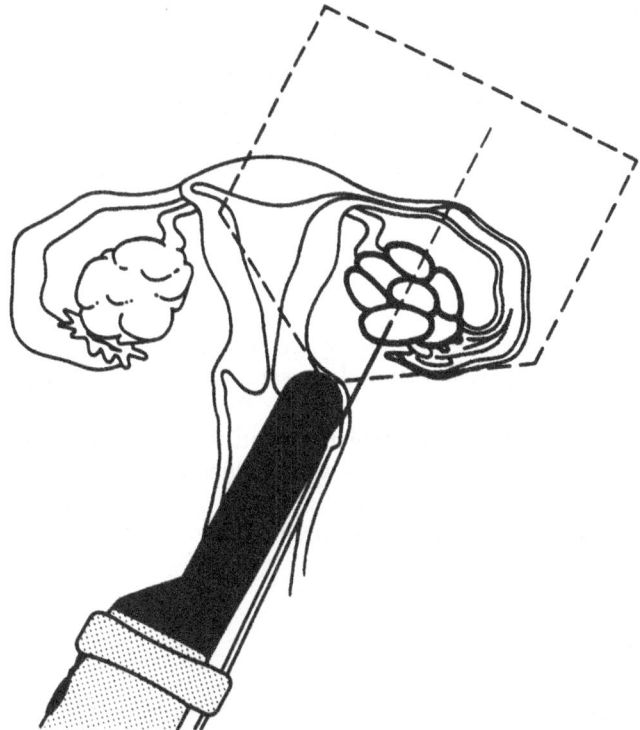

Fig. 2. Transvaginal ultrasound aspiration of follicles. To aspirate the oocyte with the follicular fluid the upper vaginal fornix and the follicular wall are punctured by the needle

- The procedure can be learned easily and quickly.
- Costs are lower than with laparoscopic oocyte retrieval.

Disadvantages, Risks

- Risk of vascular and intestinal injury; laparotomy with longitudinal incision may be required
- Risk of hysterectomy in cases of uncontrollable bleeding (below 1:1000)
- No adhesiolysis or additional evaluation of the abdomen possible as in laparoscopy
- Risk of postoperative inflammation of the small pelvis (<1%).

Automated Transvaginal Follicular Aspiration under Vaginal Ultrasound Guidance

The method described above can be improved by using an automatic aspiration system attached to the vaginal transducer (automatic aspiration system, Labotect, Göttingen, Germany).

Principle

Using a spring mechanism, the needle is projected quickly and accurately into the target follicle after the device has been set for a desired penetration depth. Little pain is caused. The penetration depth is determined by a guide beam displayed on the ultrasound screen by a program integrated in the ultrasound system.

Advantages

- The user can learn quickly how to operate the system.
- The ovary is not moved forward, due to the sharp needle profile and the high-speed mechanism.
- Accurate needle placement prevents follicles from being pierced through.
- It is possible to aspirate small follicles (< 1 cm diameter), which may well contain mature oocytes.
- The complication rate is extremely low.

Disadvantages

- Investment and maintenance costs are higher.
- Manual adjustment of penetration depth prolongs the puncturing procedure. It is further possible to insert a metal sleeve (guide sleeve) into the peritoneum after the initial entry of the needle, which means that several follicles can be aspirated without having to perforate the peritoneum each time the needle is retracted. However, the guide sleeve may get in the way when remote follicles are being punctured, which means that the vaginal wall and the peritoneum must be penetrated several times.

Equipment

Ultrasound Systems

Ultrasound devices with the appropriate puncturing programs and vaginal transducers for vaginal follicular aspiration are now available from nearly all ultrasound system manufacturers. The following is a selection of manufacturers:
- Kontron Instruments, Werner-von-Siemens-Straße 1, 85375 Neufarn, Germany
- Kranzbuehler Medizinische Systeme, Beethovenstraße 239, 52665 Solingen, Germany
- Kretztechnik, Tiefenbach 15, 4871 Zipf, Austria
- Siemens

- Toshiba Corporation Medical Systems Division, 1-1, Shibaura, 1-Chome, Minato-Ku, Tokyo 105, Japan; near-focus, can be switched to 5.0 MHz remote-focus.

Vaginal Transducers

There are certain requirements for transducers used for aspiration:
- Slim shape for painless introduction into the vagina with instruments attached
- Possibility to attach the needle guide or the aspiration mechanism
- Visual field > 115°
- 5–7.5 MHz
- Penetration depth 10 cm
  Electronic transducers produce a better image than mechanical ones.

Aspiration with Manual Needle Guide (see above, "Ultrasound Systems")

Aspiration with Automatic Needle Guide

The automatic aspiration mechanism can be connected to the vaginal transducers by an automatic needle guide. This is produced by:
- Siemens, Erlangen, Germany
- Kretztechnik, Tiefenbach 15, 4871 Zipf, Austria.

Puncturing Needles

Various types of puncturing needles are available from several manufacturers. We use single-lumen stainless-steel needles. The tip comprises a sound field and can be visualized by ultrasound; it must be extremely sharp and must therefore be ground regularly (Fig. 3).

Some manufacturers of puncturing needles are:
- William A. Cook Australia PTY LTD, 12 Electronics Street, Brisbane Technology Park, Eight Mile Plains, Queensland 4113, Australia
- Labotec, Labor-Technik-Göttingen, Industriestraße 20, 37085 Göttingen, Germany
- Rocket of London, Imperial Way, Watford Herts, WD2 4XX, UK
- SWEMED Lab, Fullriggareg 12B, 421 74 V. Frölunda, Sweden.

Automatic Aspiration Mechanism

The aspiration mechanism is a patented mechanical precision instrument based on a spring allowing for accurate, quick, and low-pain placement of the needle

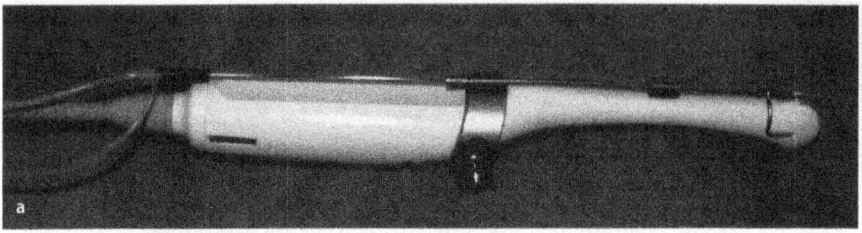

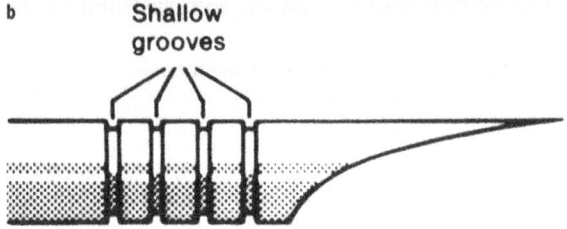

Fig. 3. a Puncturing needle connected to the vaginal transducer. **b** Needle tip (*diagram*): the sharp needle tip comprises ridges which appear as a shadow on ultrasound. This makes it possible to locate the needle tip by ultrasound

and for continuously adjustable penetration depth. For use, cleaning, and sterilization of the instrument, the instructions of the manufacturer (Labotect, Labor-Technik-Göttingen, Industriestraße 20, 37085 Göttingen, Germany) must be followed.

Aspiration and Washing Systems

The follicles can be aspirated and, if necessary, washed with various systems. There is a choice of mechanical or electrical equipment. The electrical devices (Fig. 4) can operate at a defined vacuum, but they are more expensive and require more maintenance than simple mechanical devices. It has been shown that the oocyte retrieval rate can be improved significantly from 70% to 96% per follicle by washing (Mettler 1995), and it is therefore recommended especially in cases of male infertility.

Some manufacturers of washing systems are:

- William A. Cook Australia PTY LTD, 12 Electronics Street, Brisbane Technology Park Eight Mile Plains, Queensland 4113, Australia
- Labotec, Labor-Technik-Göttingen, Industriestraße 20, 37085 Göttingen, Germany
- Rocket of London, Imperial Way, Watford Herts, WD2 4XX, UK
- SWEMED Lab, Fullriggareg 12B, 421 74 V. Frölunda, Sweden.

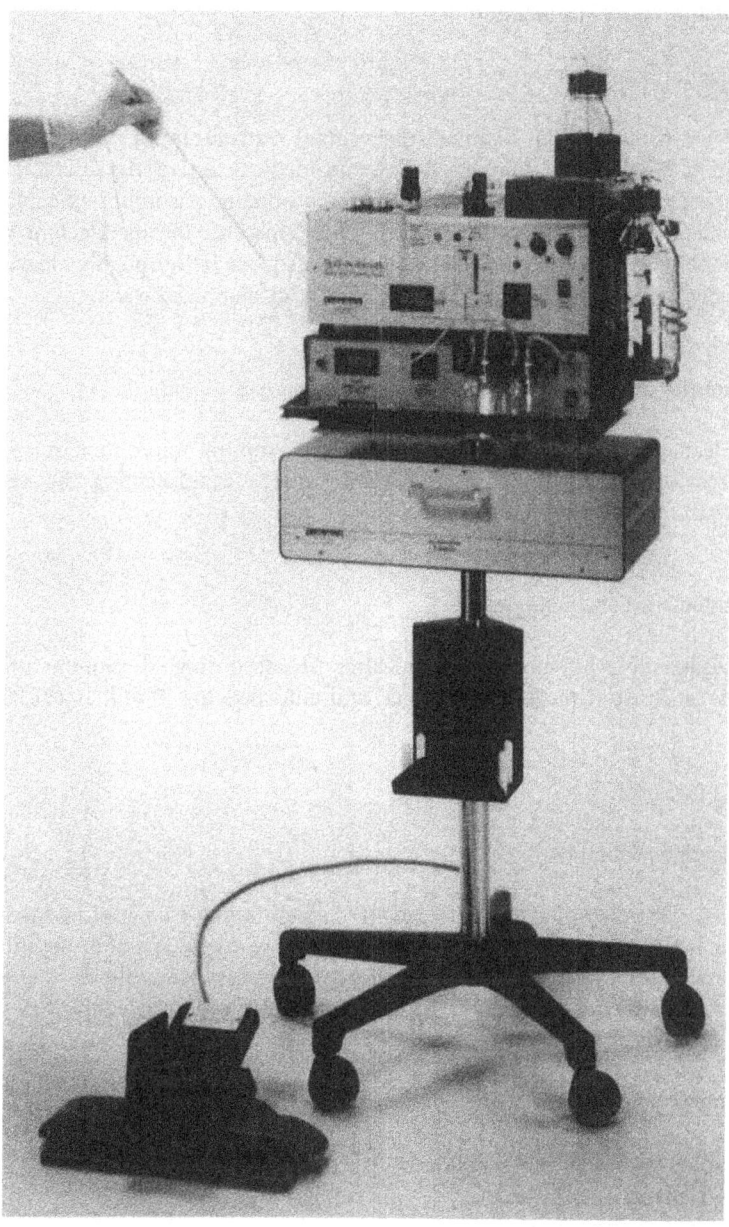

Fig. 4. Automatic flushing system and aspiration pump with stand (Labotect, Göttingen, Germany)

Disinfection/Sterilization

Vaginal Transducer

Prior to aspiration, disinfect the vaginal transducer for 15 min (Cidex Instrument Disinfection, Johnson & Johnson Medical; active ingredient: 2.5 g glutaraldehyde; activator: sodium hydrogen carbonate, trisodium phosphate, sodium salt of oxymethane sulfinic acid). Then rinse off the disinfectant residue with distilled water. After use the vaginal transducer is thoroughly cleaned mechanically under running water, then rinsed with deionized water.

Needles

Clean needles thoroughly after use under running water, then rinse with deionized water, and autoclave for 30 min at 121 °C, protecting the needle with a swab.

Automatic Puncturing System

Disassemble puncturing system after use according to manufacturer's instructions. Rinse with deionized water, and autoclave for 30 min at 121 °C.

Anesthesia

Routine Medication

Premedication includes 20 drops of Tramal (50 mg tramadol hydrochloride) and ½ tablet Dormicum 7.5 (3.75 mg midazolam hydrochloride) 30 min before the procedure. *Intraoperative medication*, if necessary, consists of ½ ampule Tramal i.v. (50–100 mg tramadol hydrochloride) during the procedure.

Further Analgesia

Futher analgesia may include:
- General anesthesia
- Intravenous short-term anesthesia
- Local anesthesia
- Other measures, e.g., acupuncture.
  Table 3 shows the role of various anesthetic procedures for ultrasound aspiration in IVF patients according to the German IVF Register 1994.

Table 3. Anesthesia and IVF (from Central IVF Register 1994)

Anesthesia	IVF/n	IVF/%
None	1428	8.8
Sedation	4800	29.7
Local anesthesia	1390	8.6
General anesthesia	7844	48.5
Neuroleptanesthesia	712	4.4
Epi-/peridural anesthesia	0	0
Other	1	0.01

Procedure of Transvaginal Follicular Aspiration Under Vaginal Ultrasound Guidance

Preparation

Administer 20 drops Tramal (50 mg tramadol hydrochloride) and ½ tablet Dormicum 7.5 (3.75 mg midazolam hydrochloride) 0.5 h before the operation. The patient should be fasting to allow for safe intubation if complications occur. Place a venous, indwelling cannula for intravenous administration of Ringer's lactate (500–1000 ml) and analgesics (½ ampule of Tramal i.v. = 50–100 mg tramadol hydrochloride).

The patient has emptied her bladder and is punctured in the lithotomy position. Wash the vagina with physiological saline.

Select the ultrasound program after connecting the transducer according to the manufacturer's instructions. Check the direction of the guide beam.

Manual Placement of the Needle

The puncturing needle is connected to an aspirating/flushing apparatus attached by a fixation ring to the front and rear ends of the vaginal transducer, thereby defining the direction of puncture corresponding to the guide beam on the ultrasound image. The aspirating/washing apparatus is checked using test tubes.

Automatic Puncturing System

The automatic puncturing system connected to the needle and aspirating/flushing system is fixed at the vaginal transducer. The spring mechanism of the automatic puncturing system is checked, and the aspirating/washing system is checked using test tubes.

Finding the Follicles

The transducer is dipped in 0.9% saline and cautiously introduced into the vagina. The uterus, both ovaries, and the iliac vessels are identified by visualization in both planes. The distance between the upper pole of the vagina and the ovaries is closely evaluated (care is taken to avoid vascular or intestinal interposition).

Repositioning of the patient may become necessary in order to permit depth localization of the closest accessible follicle (distance from the upper vaginal pole to the center of the follicle).

Aspiration with Manual Needle Placement

If the patient is conscious, she is briefly informed that the puncture is imminent. The needle is pushed forcefully forward to the center of the follicle. Needle tip ridges are shown in the ultrasound image. While the needle is kept in place, the adjacent follicles are punctured; the needle is not retracted from the abdominal cavity between aspirations.

Automatic Puncturing

The needle penetration depth is selected. The aspiration apparatus must be unlocked. If the patient is conscious, she is briefly informed that the aspiration is imminent.

By triggering a spring mechanism, the needle (external diameter 1.4 mm, internal diameter 1.1 mm), the tip of which can be seen in the ultrasound image due to a sound field, is propelled into the center of the follicle quickly and accurately, causing relatively little pain.

Follicle Aspiration

The contents of the follicle are aspirated by an automatic suction apparatus (vacuum level as defined by manufacturer's instructions) or mechanically, using a syringe. The aspirated follicular fluid is assessed (color: e.g., serous, bloody tinge, bloody, blood, endometrial fluid; quantity: 0.5–10 ml).

Flushing

If necessary, the follicle is flushed using an automatic flushing device or a syringe. The tube with the follicular fluid is closed, stored in a heating block or passed on to a biologist, if one is available. If necessary, the follicles may be flushed repeatedly. Care should be taken not to expand the follicle beyond its original size, to avoid unnecessary pain.

After Aspiration

Ultrasound monitoring should be performed for any intra-abdominal bleeding, for example, accumulation of liquid in the pouch of Douglas (up to 100 ml is normal, since flushing liquid may enter the pouch of Douglas during aspiration). A speculum is introduced into the external os to evaluate any bleeding from the posterior vaginal fornix. If necessary, a vaginal tampon is applied for 5 min.

Follow-up

The patient is monitored for 2 h (risk of circulatory complications, bleeding). After this period, she is discharged with the following instructions:
• She should not drive.
• Circulatory complications are possible.
• Postoperative bleeding is possible.
• There is a continued risk of hyperstimulation (she should drink more than 3 l/day).
  She should come back immediately if she has any complaints, especially abdominal tension, breathing difficulties, signs of beginning thrombosis, circulatory disorders.

Laboratory

An embryological laboratory is used to isolate the oocytes, process the sperm, fertilize the oocytes, and incubate the embryos (Fig. 5). Sterile techniques are used to avoid infection of the cell cultures and negative consequences for embryonic development. After more than a decade of global IVF practice the procedure has now become routine. There are many successful variations (Table 4). The IVF methods described here, which range from oocyte search to embryo transfer, correspond to the standards established by the IVF Standards Commission, the Working Group on Reproductive Medicine of the German Society for Gynecology and Obstetrics, and the Safety and Standards Committee of the European Society of Human Reproduction and Embryology.

Facilities

Transport Routes

The laboratory rooms should be located inside the IVF unit to ensure short distances and direct communication (Fig. 6). To keep the transport routes for oocytes or embryos as short as possible, follicle aspiration and embryo transfer should be performed in rooms immediately adjacent to the laboratory unit.

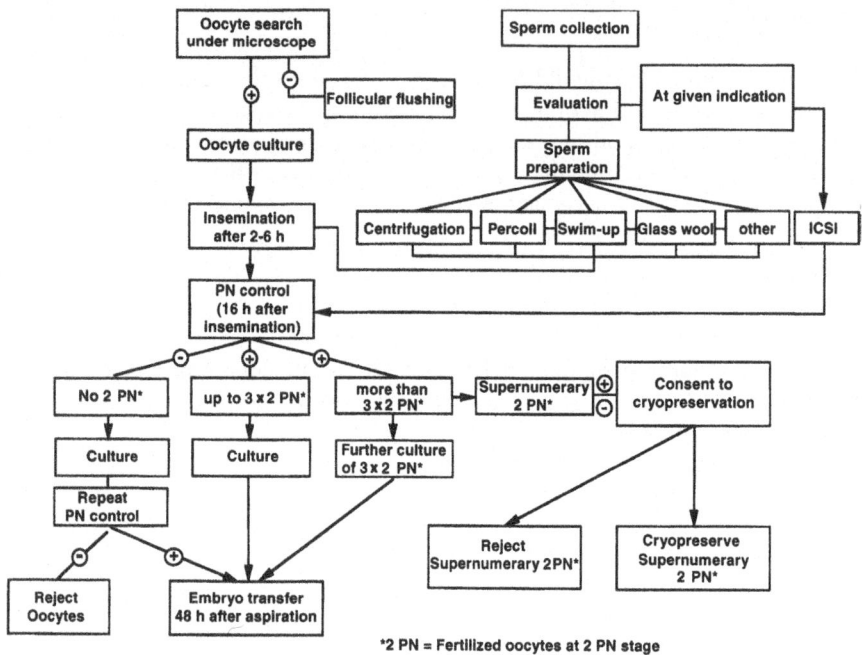

Fig. 5. Flow diagram of biological activities during IVF

Only a short period should pass between aspirating the oocyte, taking it into culture, and placing it into the incubator.

If the distance between the aspiration room and the laboratory is too great, the collection tubes for the follicular fluid are closed tightly and put into intermediate storage at 37 °C. If the fluid is contaminated with blood, it should be diluted with enough medium to avoid coagulation. The oocyte search then starts after the aspiration operation has been completed.

Air Conditioning

Depending on the geographic location of the laboratory, air conditioning with controlled air filters for the laboratory may be indispensable to reduce airborne contamination and to keep the temperature in the laboratory within a range ensuring the reliable operation of the incubators. (Many incubators have no cooling system, so that their internal temperature may rise above 37.5 °C at very high ambient temperatures, for example, due to direct sunlight. In this case, the incubators must no longer be used for oocyte and embryo culture). If the laboratory is located inside the operating area, the air-conditioning system must be separate from the system for the operating rooms to avoid the toxic effects of anesthetic gases and disinfectants on oocytes and embryos. Care must be taken not to draw in contaminated air (e.g., exhausts from the hospital or busy roads).

Table 4. Common laboratory methods for IVF (from Seifert-Krauss et al. 1994)

Workplace
 Laboratory table
 Laminar-flow hood
 Laminar-flow hood with integrated table heating
Lighting
 Daylight
 Blinds drawn
 Green filter
Clothing
 Laboratory gown
 ±gloves (unpowdered), mouth cover, head cover
 Operating gown
Incubation vessels
 Microwell plates
 Culture tubes
 Culture dishes with oil cover
Incubation atmosphere
 5% CO_2, 5% O_2, 90% N_2
 5% CO_2, ambient air
Sperm preparation
 Centrifugation
Percoll technique
 Swim-up
 Glass-wool filter
 Pentoxifylline or equivalent
Common culture media
 Hams F 10
 Human tubal fluid
 Wittingsham's
 Menezo (serum-free)
 Medicult Universal IVF Medium (serum-free)
Serum added
 Patient serum (homologous serum)
 Pooled cord blood
 None

Building Materials

Materials discharging embryotoxic substances into the environment must not be used for the construction of laboratories. Solvent residues in paints (walls, etc.), wood (furniture), and floor covering (PVC) must be avoided. Building materials suggested for use are:

- Nontoxic paints
- Floor tiles/stone floor
- Tiled walls
- No curtains
- Metal shutters or whitewashed windows.

Resting room after aspiration	Follicular aspiration/ embryo transfer	Embryo-logical Laboratory	ICSI	Sperm preparation room	Office	Sperm collection	Cryo-Preser-vation

Corridor

Secretariat/ registration	Waiting room	Blood collection	Consulting room	Ultrasound and gyneco-logical examina-tion	toilettes

a

b

Workplace

The following elements should be considered for the workplace:
- A laboratory table of stainless steel, for example, in the operating room or in the laboratory for cell and tissue culture
- A laminar flow hood (vertical or horizontal flow) if the working environment cannot be kept clean.

  Many groups use a laminar flow hood (Fig. 7a,b) when handling oocytes and embryos to ensure sterile conditions. The inevitable disadvantages are faster degassing of CO_2-buffered media and pH changes. Working under the laminar flow hood is not considered necessary by the Standards Commission of the Working Group of the German Society for Gynecology and Obstetrics, unless the laboratory is located in a nonsterile environment, such as a corridor. It is suggested that preparatory work (preparing media, aliquoting, adding antibiotics, filling dishes) be performed under the laminar flow hood. Oocytes and embryos should be handled at the lab table or on a special heated table (Henning Knudson, Denmark).

Before each operation all surfaces are cleaned with water. Once weekly, all surfaces and the equipment in the laboratory are thoroughly cleaned with a phosphate-free 1% detergent which is not toxic to tissue cultures (7X-PF Laboratory Detergent by ICN Pharmaceuticals), wiped down with water, and rubbed dry. Alcohol should not be used.

Clothing

A distinction must be made between clothing for the protection of staff (infection risk) and clothing to ensure sterility. Clothing requirements during the handling of oocytes range from simple laboratory gowns to gloves and mouth cover and on to a complete set of operating-room clothes with sterile gowns, gloves, hair, and mouth covers. Gloves must not contain any tissue-toxic powder (Biogel, LRC Products, Hygiene Gloves, Beiersdorf, Hamburg, Germany). It is suggested that for the oocyte search a laboratory gown, nonpowdered gloves, and hair and mouth covers be used. A laboratory gown should also be used for other procedures and, optionally, nonpowdered gloves.

Fig. 6. Example of an IVF ward layout. The laboratory for oocyte and embryo culture is located in the center of the ward, next to the operating theater, where the follicles are aspirated. The laboratory is linked by a corridor to the adjacent rooms for microinjection, sperm preparation, medium preparation, and cryopreservation. These rooms are connected by a clean corridor with the rest of the ward, where a research laboratory, rest and changing rooms, and storage facilities may be arranged

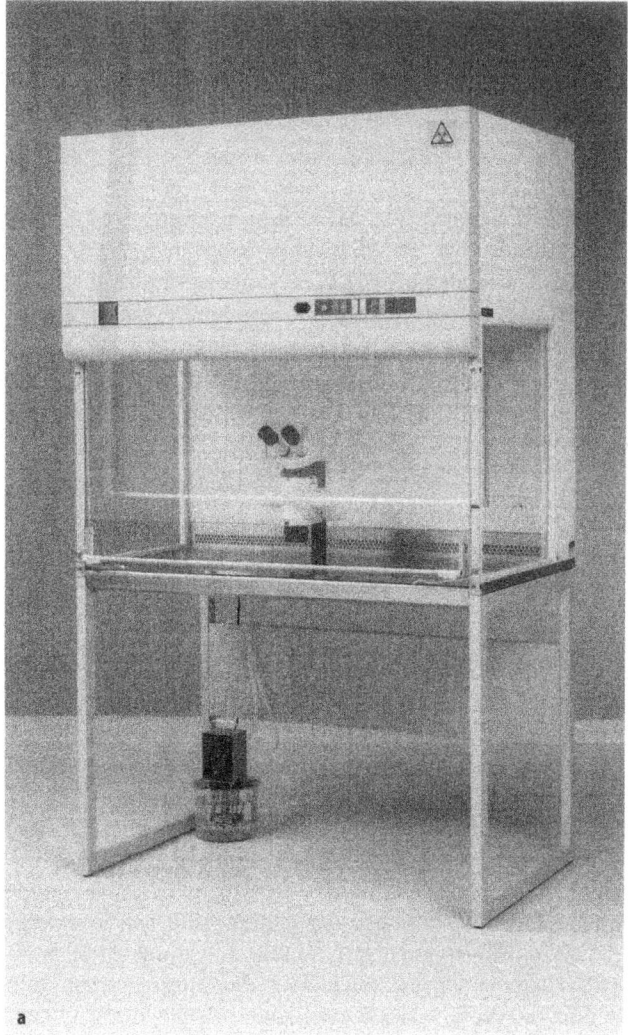

Fig. 7a. Work station with operator and product protection. N-24W with built-in stereo microscope and split flow window (K-System, Henning Knudsen Engineering A/S, Denmark)

Incubators

Requirements

Tissue culture requires reliable incubators maintaining a set gas concentration at a constant temperature of 37 °C and high humidity and restoring it quickly after having been opened (Fig. 8). Some working groups (Vienna, Norfolk) use ambient air enriched with 5% CO_2 for culture. Most groups work with a gas concentration of 5% CO_2, 5% O_2, and 90% N_2.

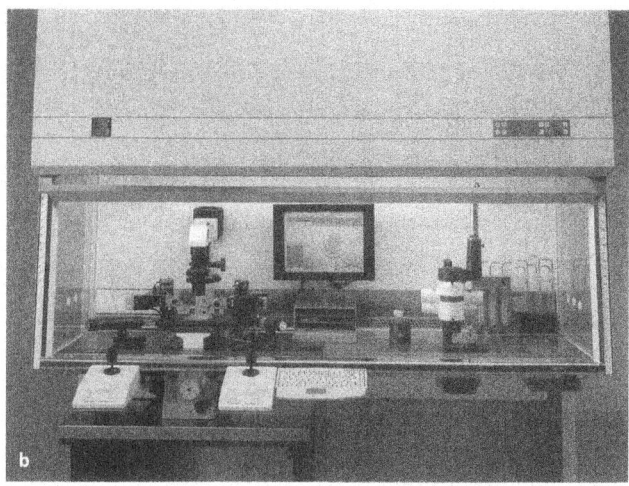

Fig. 7b. Multi-purpose work station: K-System providing aseptic conditions when performing IVF, IVM, ICSI, and PGD. The K-Systems MP work station consists of: built-in Computer Generated Image System, a heated area built into the table plate itself, built-in stereo microscope with heated stage, gassing facilities, built-in mini CO_2 incubator, built-in inverted microscope for ICSI and biopsies, built-in anti-vibration table for the inverted microscope, product and operator protection (K-System, Henning Knudsen Engineering A/S, Denmark)

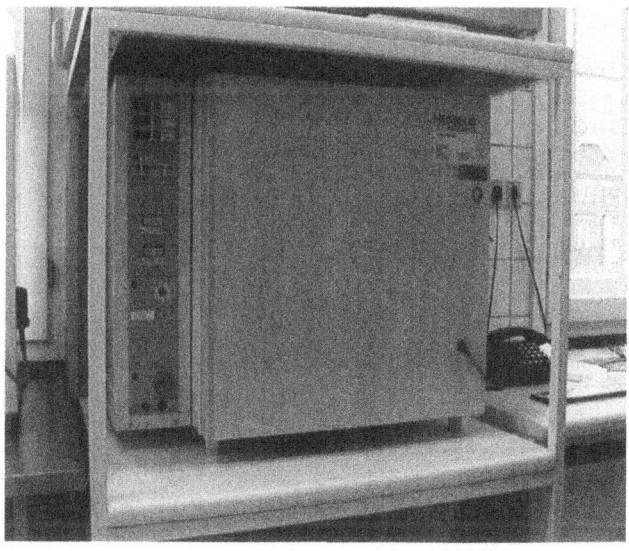

Fig. 8. Incubator for oocyte and embryo culture (Heraeus Cytoperm 8088). A glass front comprising six separate doors makes it possible to open different sections separately

An analysis of current data failed to show any significant improvements in human IVF results by using 5% CO_2, 5% O_2, and 90% N_2 compared with a mixture of 5% CO_2 and atmospheric air, which is less expensive. However, based on the data reported in the literature on the toxic effects of high levels of oxygen on cells and embryos, it appears useful to protect human embryos from oxidative stress during in vitro culture (Dumoulin et al. 1995).

Gases of the highest grade purity should be used (e.g., Sauerstoffwerk Friedrich Guttroff):

- CO2: >99.7% by volume; further components:
  - Air (N+O) >500 vpm
  - Hydrocarbons ≤:5 vpm
  - Humidity ≤50 vpm
- N2: >99.999% by volume; further components:
  - Oxygen ≤3 vpm
  - Hydrocarbons ≤0.2 vpm
  - Humidity ≤5 vpm

Each gas is fed centrally to the laboratory through two copper pipes (with a shuttle valve). There must be a gas connection with a reducing valve to 0.5–1.5 bars.

To remove any dirt particles entrained from the gas cylinders, the gas may be passed through ultrapure water before entering the incubator. Pollutants in ambient air may impair the incubation conditions. If this is the case, processed gases should be used exclusively in the incubator.

If the ambient temperature is too high, the incubator temperature may rise so as to damage the oocytes and embryos irreversibly. For a laboratory with small, poorly vented rooms an air-conditioning system is recommended.

Maintenance and Cleaning

Incubators should be cleaned and sterilized regularly according to the manufacturer's instructions. Temperature and CO_2 concentrations should be controlled regularly using instruments not connected to the incubator display. A thermometer should be put inside the incubator permanently in a glass filled with distilled water to check the temperature. The principle of CO_2 measurement with a Fyrete device (CO_2 indicator Fyrete by Bacharach, Pittsburgh, Pa., USA) is the expansion of a calibrated fluid depending on the CO_2 content when a gas mix is fed into it. The manufacturer's instructions concerning constant high air humidity must be strictly adhered to.

Frequent opening of the incubator leads to changes in the sensitive incubator environment, compromising the development of oocytes and embryos. The following measures are therefore recommended:

- Use incubators with separate doors for the different shelves.
- Use several incubators for the different procedures to cause the least possible disruption of the incubation environment for oocytes and embryos by opening incubator doors.

• Put trays (melamine trays) inside the incubator which are easier to clean than the incubator itself.

Culture Dishes and Tools

Sterilized material suitable for tissue culture should be used when handling oocytes, embryos, and semen. Normal catheters and syringes may contain substances toxic to tissue (e.g., lubricants). If such materials are used (e.g., insulin syringes for embryo transfer), they are first washed thoroughly with distilled water or medium. Material which has been sterilized with ethylene oxide must be allowed to degas for 10–14 days to ensure that no residual tissue-toxic gas remains on it.

The oocyte search is carried out in preheated tissue culture dishes (Falcon 3003/Becton-Dickinson). The oocytes are inseminated and the embryos cultured in microwell culture dishes (Nunclon, Nunc, Denmark), which are highly suitable for this purpose.

Outside the incubator, the pH, humidity, and temperature must be kept constant. Therefore it is indispensable to work quickly on heated plates or on a specially heated table.

Oocytes and embryos are transferred with disposable micropipettes (Blau Brand intraMark) linked to pipette aids (Brandt; Fig. 13). Prior to transfer the embryos are picked up with an embryo transfer catheter (T.D.T Set, Laboratoire C.C.D. 60, Rue Pierre Charon 75008 Paris, France) linked to an insulin syringe (Braun, Melsungen, Germany; Fig. 25).

Glassware and Other Sterilization Tools

After use, glassware and other sterilization tools should be thoroughly cleaned under running water, carefully rinsed with deionized water, dried, and autoclaved at 121 °C for 30 min in stainless steel boxes (Desktop autoclave, Webeco, Germany, A40 DS202). Glassware should be cleaned with a special machine (Mielab Corp., Mich.) using special detergents (Newdisher A8), then dried and sterilized. Needles, puncturing guides, etc. are placed in heat-sealed bags before sterilization (Impulssiegelgerät, Hawo-Gerätebau, 74821 Mosbach, Germany).

Prior to use all instruments which come into contact with oocytes, embryos, or semen, such as follicle aspiration kits, are thoroughly rinsed with medium or PBS. Newly bought equipment should be cleaned thoroughly with distilled water to remove any oil, dust and other contaminants resulting from the manufacturing process.

Water

Water of different purity levels is used for preparing culture media and for washing the material which must be sterilized. Ultrapure water is used to prepare culture media (Seromed, Biochrom, Berlin, Germany). The equipment which must be sterilized is precleaned with tap water, thoroughly rinsed with deionized water produced by a deionizer (Behropur, Behr Labortechnik, Düsseldorf, Germany), and finally rinsed with distilled water, or Analar Water (Corp. Paesel, Frankfurt, Germany).

If large quantities of water of a certain purity are required regularly, it is useful to integrate the appropriate purification system into the laboratory. Water purification equipment must be checked regularly for micro-organisms and other contaminants such as proteins according to the manufacturer's instructions, to ensure constant water quality.

Ultrapure Water. The distillate of processed ultrapure water must be pyrogen free. It must have a conductivity of 0.06–0.08 µS/cm.

Purification by Biochrom is a multistage process: Precleaning is done with activated carbon and an anion/cation exchanger. Final cleaning takes place in a cyclone: all entrained bubbles below 0.5 mm from the steam are removed by acceleration to 500 µg.

Purification by fivefold distillation through a quartz column is possible if no multidistillation water is available.

Deionized Water. Deionized water must have a conductivity of less than 10 µS/cm. The purification system is manufactured by Behr Labortechnik. Water is passed through a cartridge filled with ion-exchange resins, which remove all salts as well as silicic and hydrochloric acid. A conductivity meter indicates when the cartridge must be replaced.

Media

Successful in vitro fertilization has been performed with many different culture media, and no single medium has so far been proven superior by reliable studies in terms of oocyte fertilization, embryonic development, and pregnancy rates (Table 5). The media can be made in the laboratory or bought from commercial suppliers. The purchase of commercial media simplifies laboratory operations significantly, the disadvantage being that quality assurance is outside the control of the laboratory manager.

Table 5. Culture media for IVF (mg/l)

	Medicult Universal Medium[a]	Ham's F10[b]	Menezo's BZ[c]	Earle's olution[d]	Whitting-hams's T6[e]	Human tubal fluid[e]
NaCl	6800	7400	6100	6800	5719	5939
KCL	400	285	–	400	106	350
$CaCl_2$ $2H_2O$	265	44.1	–	265	262	300
$MgCl_2$ $6H_2O$	–	–	–	–	96	–
$NaHCO_3$	2200	1200	1800	2200	2101	2101
SSR 2/A (buffer)	1	–	–	–	–	–
SSR2/B (insulin)	0.5	–	–	–	–	–
$MgSO_4$	100	152.8 ($\times 7H_2O$)	200 ($\times 7H_2O$)	100	–	49 ($\times 7H_2O$)
KH_2PO_4	–83	60	–	–	50	
Na_2HPO_4	125	290 ($\times 7H_2O$)	154 ($\times 12H_2O$)	125	51	–
Na acetate	–	–	50	–	–	–
Na lactate	–	–	–	–	4.65 ml/l (60% ig)	2399
Ca lactate	–	–	50	–	–	–
Na pyruvate	0.8 mM	110	250	–	52	36
$CuSO_4$ $5H_2O$	–	0.0025	–	–	–	–
$FeSO_4$ $7H_2O$	–	0.834	–	–	–	–
$ZnSO_4$ $7H_2O$	–	0.0288	–	–	–	–
Serum albumin	10000 (human)	–	10000 (human)	–	–	–
Glucose	1000	1100	1200	1000	1000	500
Streptomycin	50	–	40	–	50	50
Vitamin C	–	–	50	–	–	–
Cholesterol	–	–	25	–	–	–
Lipoic acid	–	0.2	–	–	–	–
Phenol red	11	1.2	15	11	10	10
Thymidine	–	0.7	–	–	–	–
Hypoxanthine	–	4	–	–	–	–
pH	7.2–7.4	7.4	7.4	7.4±0.2	7.4	ND
H_2O (mosmol/kg)	280	300	280	280±5%	280	ND

[a] Holst and Berteussen (1990).
[b] Lopata et al. (1980).
[c] Testart et al. (1982).
[d] Purdy (1982).
[e] Quinn et al. (1985).

Requirements

The manufacture of a culture medium requires ultrapure water and chemicals. It is based on a balanced buffered culture medium combined with energy substrates such as glucose and sodium pyruvate.

Antibiotics may be present in the starting medium or added before use (e.g., penicillin/streptomycin by Biochrom, Berlin, Germany; concentration of the original solution 10000/10000 µg/ml). To avoid the adhesion of oocytes or embryos to the walls of containers or catheters, protein, for example, in the form of human albumin, must be added.

The osmolarity of the medium must be in the range of 275–290 mosmol/kg and the pH after equilibration with CO_2 in the range of 7.35–7.45. Complex media may also contain amino acids, nucleotides, hormones and growth factors, adhesion factors, and transport proteins.

Quality Assurance

Quality assurance of the final medium should exclude endotoxins (limulus test by Scanmedical, external LAL ELISA test), as well as bacteria or viruses. It should ascertain the survival of:

- Spermatozoa (incubation of a defined number of normal sperm in 1 ml medium, documentation of survival time: motile sperm should still be present in the medium after 5 days)
- Single or two-cell mouse embryos
- Defined cell lines (hybridoma cell line 1E6, Hybritest, Medikult Linaris; determination of the growth rate of hybridoma cell line 1E6 in serum-free medium. Cell growth is compared with a known standard microscopically and with a Coulter Counter after 96 h)

After preparation, the medium is passed through sterile filters and divided into convenient portions (Schleicher & Schuell, FP 030/0, disposable filter holder Rotrand; pore size: 0.2 μm sterile, pyrogen free). Media that are bought ready-made are sterile and must only be aliquoted. Depending on the type and manufacturer, they can be stored for 14 days to 5 weeks. Prior to use the pH of the medium is adjusted in the CO_2 incubator (equilibration of the medium overnight).

Preparation of Ham's F10

Preparatory Work

- Switch on and calibrate analytical balance (Sartorius, Analytic) and osmometer.
- Switch on laminar-flow hood, clean it thoroughly with alcohol, and keep it running for at least 30 min.
- Prepare starting substances, solutions, and disposable materials:
  - Ham's F10 dry medium with L-glutamine and 1.2 mg/ml phenol red but no $NaHCO_3$ (for 1 l water; Biochrom)
  - Penicillin G powder, embryo tested (Sigma)
  - Streptomycin sulfate powder, embryo-tested (Sigma)
  - Calcium lactate 5 H_2O, soluble, ultrapure (Merck)
  - Sodium bicarbonate solution 7.5% (Gibco)
  - Ultrapure water 1 l, sterile, to make up the medium (Biochrom)

- Ultrapure water, sterile, to wash the filter and the syringe and to adjust the osmolarity
- Two sterile 100-ml sample beakers with lids (Becton Dickinson)
- Sterile round-bottom tubes, 6 ml (Falcon 2003)
- 50-ml tissue culture flasks (Becton Dickinson)
- Sterile disposable syringes (20 ml), prewashed with ultrapure water (Becton Dickinson)
- Sterile filters 0.2-μm pore size, pyrogen free (Schleicher & Schuell)
- Pipettes, etc.

Starting Substances

- Put 50 mg penicillin G into a tube.
- Put 50 mg streptomycin sulfate into a tube.
- Put 308 mg calcium lactate into a tube.

Mixing the Medium Under the Laminar-Flow Hood

- Put 80 ml ultrapure water from the 1-l bottle into each of the two 100-ml sample beakers.
- Put Ham's F10 powder and the other weighed substances into one beaker.
- Close the beaker, shake until all crystals are dissolved (= concentrate).
- Place sterile filter on a 20-ml syringe and rinse with ultrapure water (reject filtrate).
- Using the syringe, sterile-filtrate concentrate through the prerinsed filter back into the 1-l bottle (if filter becomes clogged, replace with a new prerinsed filter).
- Mix contents of the bottle well.
- Sample a small quantity of medium from the bottle and adjust osmolarity to 245 mosmol/kg using ultrapure water.
- Check: If 666 μl 7.5% sodium bicarbonate solution is added to 22 ml medium, the resulting osmolarity should be 280 mosmol/kg.
- Check: After equilibration in the incubator, the pH of the medium (including sodium bicarbonate) should be in the range of 7.35–7.45.
- Aliquot the remaining medium (not containing sodium bicarbonate) into sterile 50-ml culture flasks (22 ml/flask) with a sterile 10-ml pipette.

Quality Control

- Have an aliquot of the medium tested for sterility (after incubating it for a few days to allow the growth of any bacteria).
- Sperm survival test (incubation of a defined number of normal sperm/ml medium; documentation of survival time: after 5 days, there should still be motile sperm present).

- Medicult Hybritest (Medicult Linaris supplies a test kit and evaluates the test when it is returned to them).
- Exact documentation of medium formulation (batch numbers of the chemicals) in the laboratory manual.
- Storage of the 22-ml aliquots at −20 °C for a maximum of 3 months
- Immediately after thawing at room temperature and before use, sodium bicarbonate is added to the medium:
  - 666 µl 7.5% sodium bicarbonate solution is pipetted into a flask containing 22 ml medium; the sodium bicarbonate concentration is equivalent to 2.2 g/l.
  - When sodium bicarbonate is added, the color changes: the medium turns pink (the color indicates a pH shift: yellow = too acid; purple = too alkaline).
  - Add the exact quantity, since any deviation would significantly change osmolarity.

Addition of Serum

Serum is added to culture media in order to improve the culture conditions.

Advantages

Serum contains nutrients, hormones, growth hormones, enzymes, protease inhibitors, and proteins which neutralize toxins. It also prevents nonspecific absorption and modulates pH, viscosity, and surface tension.

Disadvantages

Due to its complex composition, serum contains unknown factors in variable concentrations. It is not a physiological culture medium and may contain toxic and infectious components (hepatitis B, HIV, cytomegalovirus, slow virus infections, etc.).

Serum collection means more time and effort required from patients and staff compared with culture media with serum replacements.

Due to the infection risk to embryos, the addition of serum is the subject of current dispute. Using patient serum minimizes the infection risk; the disruptive influence of, for example, steroid hormones and growth factors cannot be ruled out. Thus, prior to IVF treatment the patient's serum must be tested for hepatitis, HIV, cytomegalovirus, etc. The serum is then heat-inactivated, filter-sterilized, and deep-frozen.

Collection and Processing of Patient (Homologous)Serum for the IVF Program

The blood should be sampled between day 7 of the cycle and 1 day before aspiration. It is collected using disposable, sterile 10-ml syringes rinsed several times with sterile ultrapure water to remove tissue-toxic lubricants.

The samples are filled into sterile centrifuge tubes (Becton Dickinson, 14 ml). They are processed within 2–3 h of sampling (or stored at 4 °C) by centrifugation at 2000 µg for 30 min (possibly less); 4–5 ml serum is aspirated with a sterile 10-ml pipette (avoid entraining blood!) and filled into a second labeled centrifugation tube and the lid closed tightly. Recentrifugation is done at 2000 µg for 10 min. Then the serum is aspirated with a fresh sterile 10-ml pipette and filled into a third sterile tube.

Note: If serum has an orange hue, it is hemolytic and must be recentrifuged. If it is opaque, it is lipemic and must be recentrifuged.

Inactivation and Filter Sterilization of Patient Serum

The serum is inactivated at 56 °C in the heating block for 30 min. (Preheat heating block, control temperature, set time.) To prepare for filter sterilization, switch on the laminar-flow hood, clean it thoroughly with alcohol, and keep the hood switched on for at least 30 min. Then lay out the following tools on the hood table:
- Centrifugation tube with heat-inactivated serum
- Three sterile tubes with lids (Becton Dickinson, Falcon 2003) for:
  1. Sperm preparation
  2. Oocyte and embryo culture
  3. Embryo transfer
- One sterile 5-ml syringe (Becton Dickinson, F 38241), rinsed three times with ultrapure water
- One sterile disposable injection cannula (Braun Melsungen, Sterican 0.9& 70 mm/20 G × $2^{4/5}$), placed on the rinsed syringe
- Sterile filter, pyrogen-free, pore size 0.2 µm (Schleicher & Schuell FP 030/3).

To sterilize the filter, open the serum tube and place the lid on the table with the opening pointing upwards. Aspirate serum into a syringe through a cannula, then draw in some air. Hold up the syringe, pull off the cannula, and place a filter on the syringe using a sterile technique.

Reject the first drops filtered. Filter 1 ml serum into each of the tubes, and close the tubes tightly. Freeze at –20 °C. Thaw only the tubes that are to be used on the same day.

Cocultures

For the purposes of IVF, coculture means embryo culture in the presence of heterologous cell lines. It is based on the finding made by cell culture researchers that cells tend to grow and multiply better in the presence of other cells. It is the goal of embryo coculture to achieve the best possible embryo development to blastocyst stage and to transfer the embryo into the uterus between day 5 and day 7 after aspiration, i.e., at the time of physiological implantation.

Advantages associated with coculture are higher implantation rates and the in vitro selection of embryos with high cleavage rates. The disadvantages are that much more laboratory equipment and work are required; there is possible infection of the embryo by the cocultured cells, and the cocultured cells may have a tumorigenic effect.

Experience with cocultures of human embryos with vero cells so far shows that under these conditions embryo development continues to the blastocyst stage, and that the intrauterine embryo transfer can proceed between days 5 and 7 after follicular aspiration. The pregnancy rate per embryo transfer rises with the stage of extrauterine embryo development.

Coculture is not yet used routinely by most groups because of the much higher complexity of the procedure than that of conventional culture and owing to concerns about possible contamination and infection of the embryo.

Table 6. Examples for the use of serum-free medium (A) and medium requiring the addition of serum (B) in IVF

	A	B
Follicular washing with PBS+pen/strep+heparin	–	–
Oocyte handling		
Washing medium	Medicult Universal IVF medium	Ham's F10
Insemination of oocytes	Medicult Universal IVF medium	9/10 Ham's F10 1/10 homologous serum
Culture medium from PN control onwards	Medicult Universal IVF medium	9/10 Ham's F10 1/10 homologous serum
Sperm preparation		
Percoll (40/80%)	–	–
Washing medium	Medicult Universal IVF medium	9/10 PBS 1/10 homologous serum
Insemination medium	Medicult Universal IVF medium	9/10 Ham's F10 1/10 homologous serum
Swim-up		
Washing medium	Medicult Universal IVF medium	9/10 PBS 1/10 homologous serum
Insemination medium	Medicult Universal IVF medium	9/10 Ham's F10 1/10 homologous serum
Transfer medium	Medicult Universal IVF medium	7/10 Ham's F10 3/10 homologous serum

Media for IVF Operations

The complex procedure of preparing the media and the above-mentioned disadvantages of serum as an additive to the medium have caused the replacement of Ham's F10 by commercial medium containing synthetic surrogate serum and human albumin as the protein component (Medicult Universal Medium, Medicult a/s Lerso Parkalle 42, 2100 Copenhagen, Denmark). The medium is divided into sterile aliquots (50-ml cell culture flasks/Greiner Labortechnik) and may then be used for the following 4 weeks. The laboratory procedures involve the use of Medicult Universal Medium, but they may also be carried out using serum-containing media, such as Ham's F10 (Table 6, Fig. 9a–c).

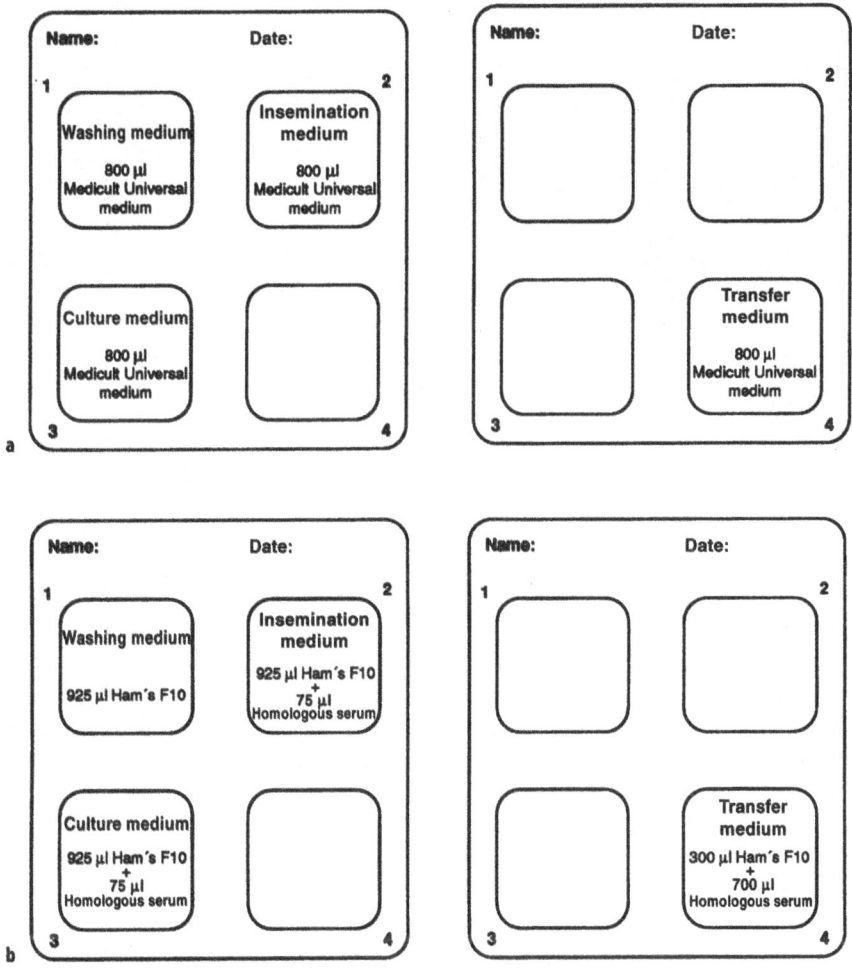

Fig. 9a, b. Filling sequence for the culture dishes in the different steps of IVF. **a** Using Medicult Universal Medium. **b** Using Ham's F10 and homologous serum.

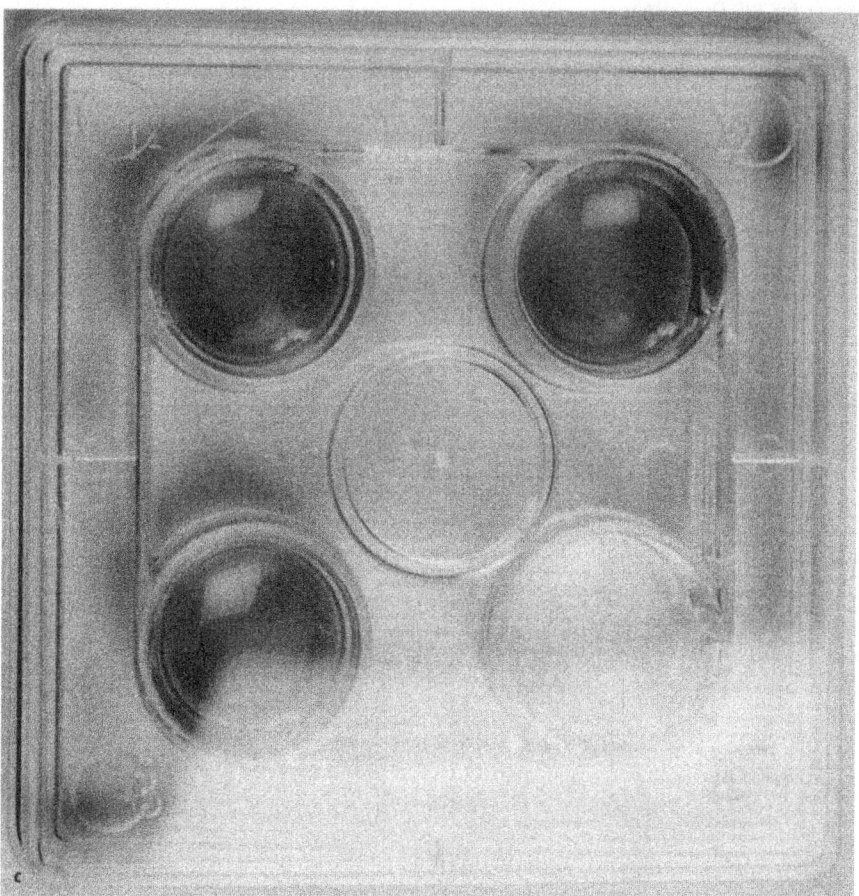

Fig. 9c. Tissue culture dish for the cultivation of oocytes and embryos. Wells 1–3 contain culture medium

Oocyte Search

The oocytes can be located in parallel with follicular aspiration. To maintain the vitality of oocytes, all procedures must be sterile and quick. Unnecessary distance from one workplace to the next should therefore be avoided, and the biologist's workplace should be arranged close to the aspiration room.

Method

The follicular aspirate is collected in tubes using a sterile technique (26 ml; Sarstedt, Nuernbrecht, Germany) and passed on to the biologist as soon as possible. The follicular fluid is distributed over several culture dishes for oocyte localization. The typical striae of the cumulus oophorus can be seen with the naked eye. The cumulus is evaluated under the microscope at × 40–125 magnification (Fig. 10a–c).

The polar body (Fig. 11a,b) is an unambiguous indicator of oocyte maturity. However, it may not be visible if the cumulus is too dense. The degree of oocyte maturity can also be assessed on the basis of cumulus cell density and the appearance of the corona radiata around the oocytes (Fig. 12).

The cumulus and the oocyte are transferred into the first well of a microwell dish containing medium, using a glass capillary connected to a pipette aid (Fig. 13); they are freed of erythrocytes, immediately transferred into fresh medium (second well), and cultured in an incubator.

Preparation

Six labeled microwell dishes (Nunclon, Nunc Denmark) are filled with 800 µl culture medium per well and equilibrated overnight in the incubator (e.g., Heraeus Cytoperm 8088; Fig. 8). A warm plate (Medax) is heated to 37 °C (monitor temperature). A sterile 200-µl glass capillary (Brand, Intramark) is connected to a pipette aid, and mouth cover, head cover, and nonpowdered gloves are donned.

As aspiration proceeds, follicular fluid is distributed over several preheated tissue culture dishes and these are shaken gently so that the cumulus surround-

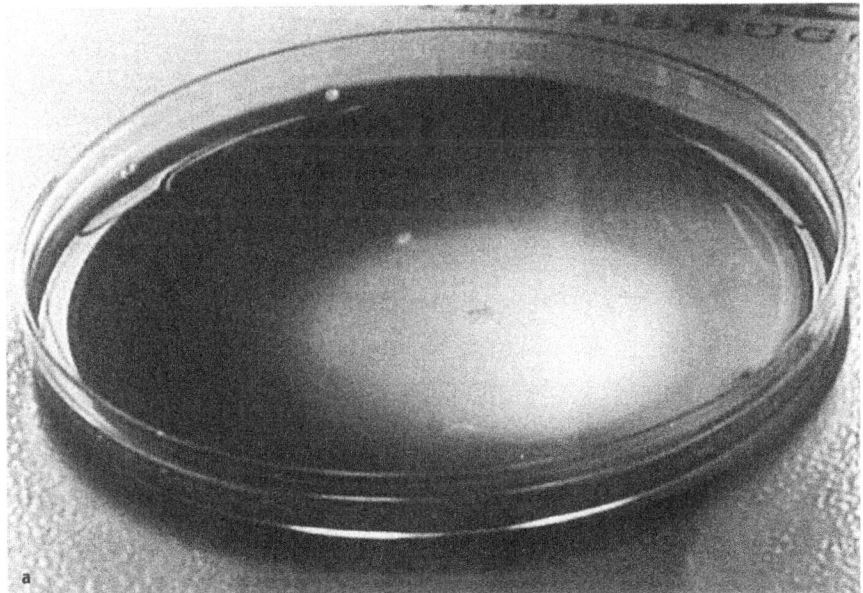

Fig. 10a. Human oocytes surrounded by cumulus cells in a Petri dish immediately after aspiration (natural size)

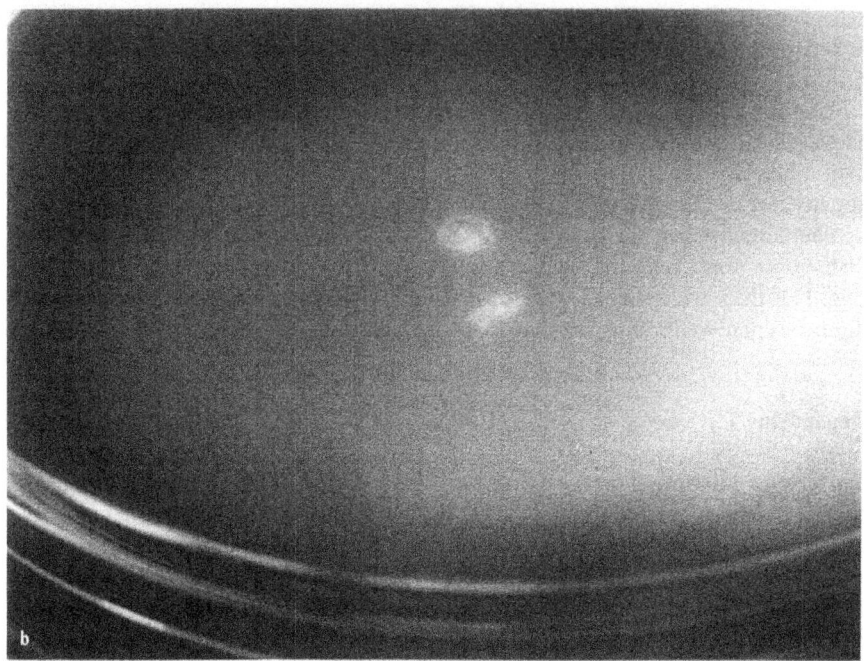

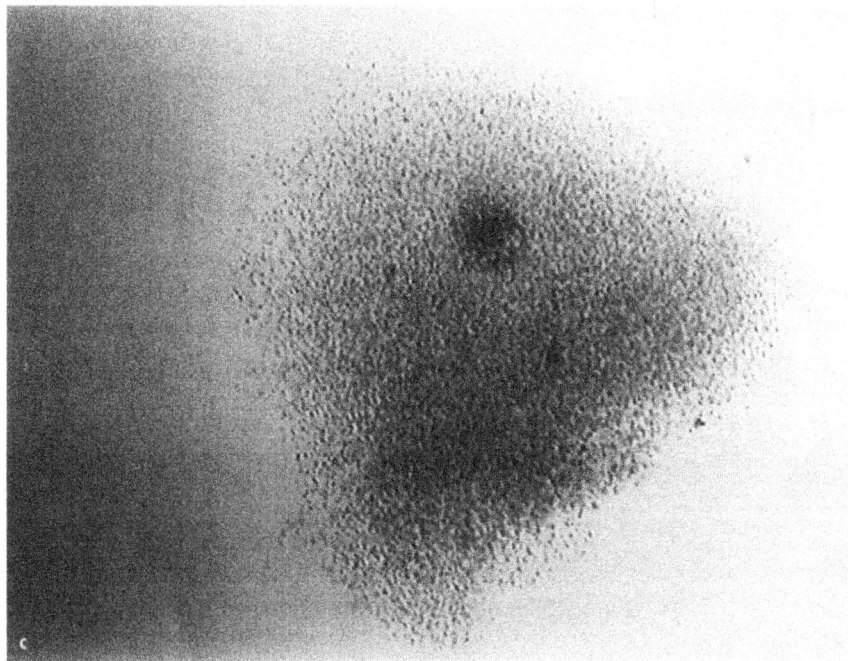

Fig. 10 b, c. b Human oocytes surrounded by cumulus cells. **c** Human oocyte surroundet by
cumulus × 100

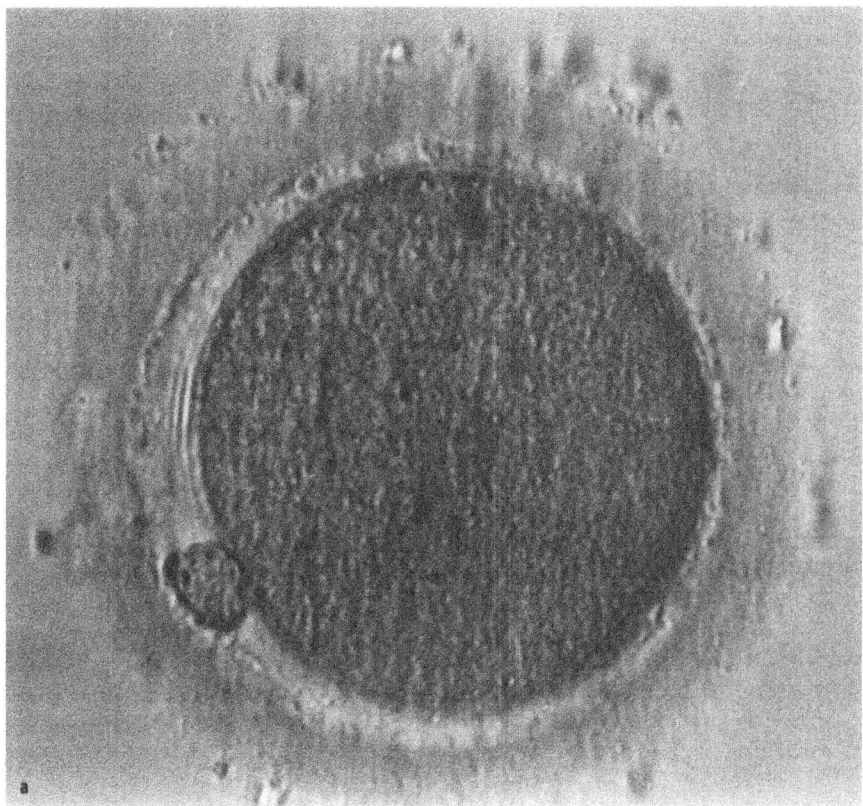

Fig. 11a. Mature oocyte with expelled polar body; metaphase II of meiosis. × 400

ing the oocyte is spread out. Try to spot the oocyte with the naked eye: the cumulus appears as a transparent stria reminiscent of egg white; the oocyte with the corona radiata normally appears as a minute, white spot in the cumulus. Next, evaluate oocyte maturity under the microscope (Leitz/Fluovert) at lowest (× 40) and second-lowest (× 125) magnifications.

Take the prepared dish out of the incubator and remove the lid. Briefly rinse the glass capillary in well no. 1: aspirate some liquid and release, then aspirate some liquid again. Place the capillary above the oocyte and aspirate the oocyte. Drop the oocyte into well no. 1 (no microscope is required).

Wash the oocyte: rinse the capillary in well no. 1 (to remove follicular fluid), pick up some medium from well no. 2, pick up the oocyte again and drop it into well no. 2 (no microscope required). Remove the remaining fluid from the capillary. Close the culture dish and place it into the incubator.

Use several incubators and organize the procedure in such a way as to have as long intervals as possible between incubator openings. Carry out the entire operation as quickly as possible. Do not speak or cough, etc., over the oocyte. Make sure that as little liquid as possible is entrained into the next well.

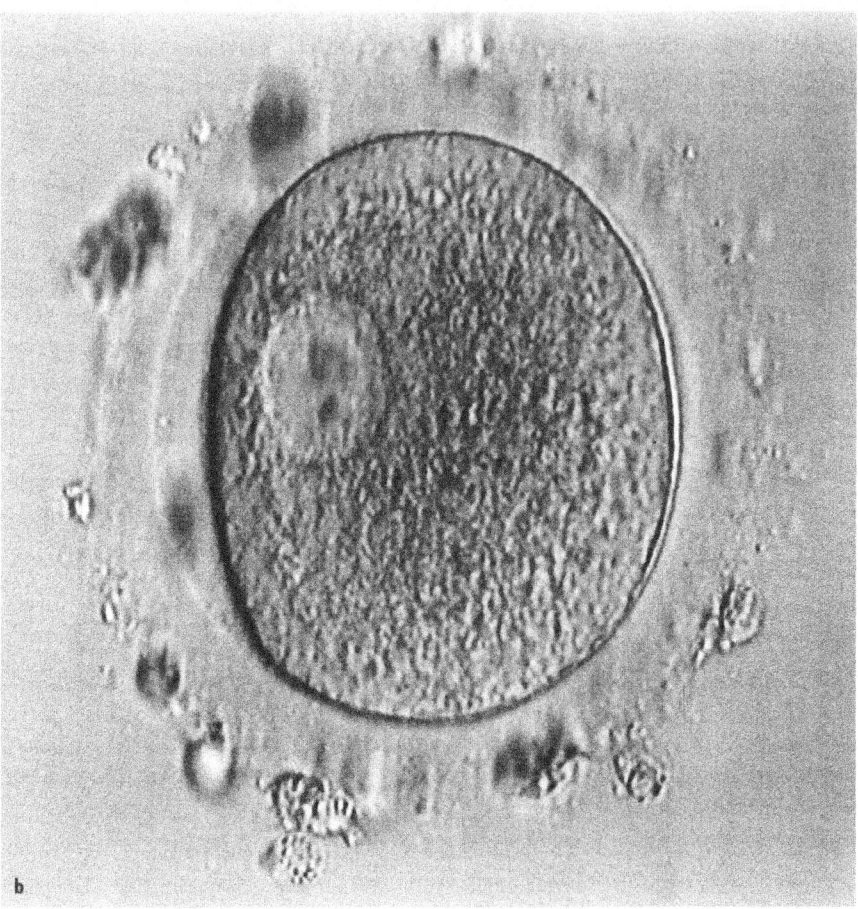

Fig. 11b. For comparison: immature oocyte with clearly visible germinal vesicle; prophase I of meiosis. × 400

Record the oocyte data on a form, optionally adding cumulus size. Then process the other aspirates as described. When each culture dish contains one oocyte, add a second one per dish, then a third, etc.

Sperm Collection and Preparation

Since the introduction of IVF a wide variety of sperm preparation methods have been used worldwide. Various methods have been developed by different laboratories (Table 7), but improved techniques have failed to significantly increase the fertilization rate if the semen sample is of poor quality. A survey among German IVF laboratories in 1993 showed that sperm preparation is by

Schematic diagram of the oocyte and its environment	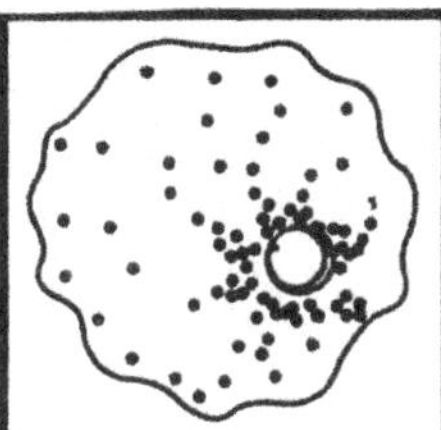	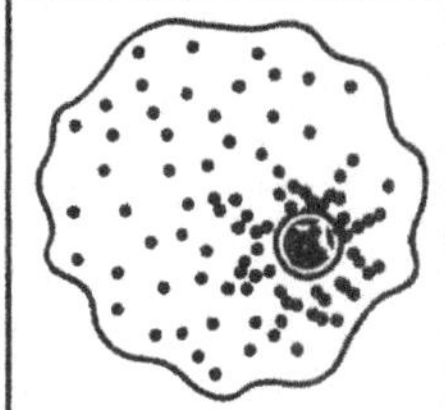	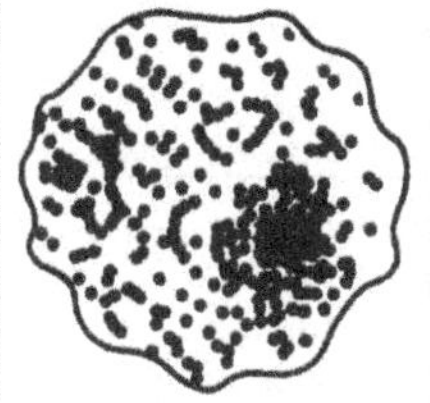
Maturational status	mature (+++)	intermediate maturity (++)	immature (+)
Oocyte	round clear cytoplasm, first polar body may be visible	cytoplasm and zona pellucida barely visible	invisible oocyte
Cumulus oophorus	low cell density, expanded silvery-white sticky	relatively high cell density	very high cell density, additional cell aggregates present in most cases
Corona radiata	relatively low cell density, may be radiate	high cell density	very high cell density

Fig. 12. Morphological evaluation of the maturity of oocyte-cumulus complexes (Veeck et al. 1983)

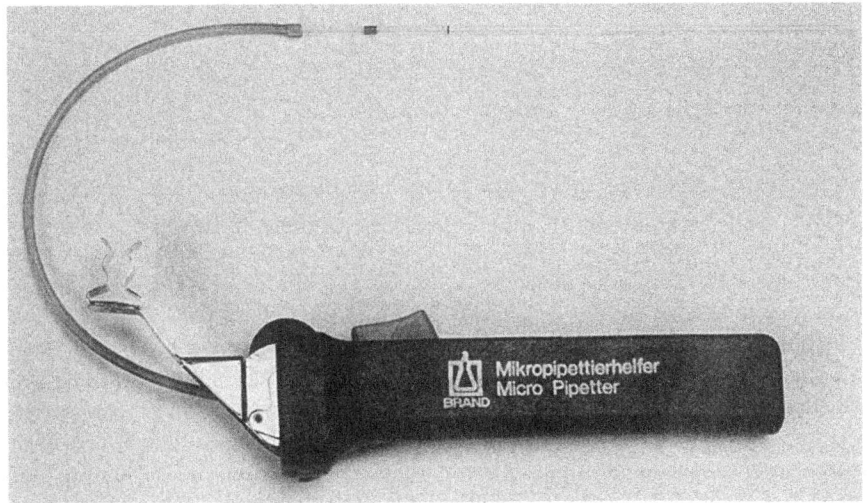

Fig. 13. Pipette aid (Brand) with connected glass capillary to pick up the oocytes

Table 7. Sperm preparation for IVF (from German Central IVF Register 1995)

Method	Cycles	Transfers	Fertilization rate (%)	Polyploid PN/oocytes	Pregnancies	Preg/ET
Percoll filter	4176	2999	51.6	3.8	933	31.1
Swim-up	5087	3875	50.1	2.9	926	23.9
Centrifuge	1315	1008	50.9	1.5	166	16.5
Glass-wool filter	178	149	49.1	6.4	24	16.1
Pentoxifylline or equivalent	285	218	57.4	4.9	49	22

Table 8. Semen quality

a: Normal semen parameters according to WHO (1992)	
Volume	2.0 ml or more
pH	7.2–8.0
Sperm count	20×10^6/ml or more
Total sperm count	40×10^6 per ejaculate or more
Motility	≥50% with progressive motility (i.e., category "a" and "b") or ≥25% with fast linear motility (i.e., category "a" within 60 min after collection)
Morphology	≥30% of normal shape

b: Nomenclature of some semen parameters	
Normozoospermia	Normal semen quality as defined above
Oligozoospermia	Sperm count below 20×10^6/ml
Asthenozoospermia	<50% sperm with progressive motility (categories "a" and "b") or <25% sperm with fast linear motility (category "a")
Teratozoospermia	<30% sperm with normal morphology
Oligo-astheno-terato-zoospermia	All three variables are impaired
Azoospermia	No sperm in ejaculate
Aspermia	No ejaculate

far the least established procedure: nearly half of all IVF centers polled had changed their technique in the preceding 3 years (Seifert-Klauss et al. 1994).

The aims of sperm preparation are (a) to remove seminal plasm, which prevents capacitation and fertilization of the oocyte, (b) to concentrate progressively motile sperm, and (c) to remove detritus and contaminants.

If possible, the man delivers his semen about 2 h before the scheduled insemination by masturbating into a sterile beaker after at least 2 days of sexual abstinence. In exceptional cases cryosperm is used. Some centers recommend keeping a frozen semen sample in reserve in case the man is unable to deliver sperm at the scheduled time. After a liquefaction period of 15–30 min, the sperm are evaluated (according to the 1992 WHO criteria; Table 8). They are counted in a Makler chamber under the microscope and classified as follows:

- Quick progressive motility
- Slow or sluggish progressive motility
- Nonprogressive motility
- Immobility.

Percoll Gradient Technique

Because they have a higher density, centrifugation causes the motile sperm to accumulate at the bottom of a medium with discontinuous density gradients (Fig. 14). Percoll is pipetted into tubes in declining concentrations; liquefied seminal plasm is overlaid and centrifuged. The pellet with motile sperm located in the higher density layer is retrieved, resuspended in culture medium, recentrifuged, and resuspended again. The Percoll gradient method reduces the amount of cellular detritus, especially leukocytes (Bolton et al. 1986), and significantly increases the percentage of motile sperm (Pousette et al. 1986).

Sperm preparation steps using Percoll are as follows:

- After collection allow 15–30 min for the semen to liquefy at room temperature.
- Count 10 µl of the liquid semen into a Makler chamber (Sefi Medical Instruments (Fig. 15a–c).
- Prepare two Percoll gradients (40/80%) in conical 15-ml centrifuge tubes (Becton Dickinson).
- Pipette 1 ml 80% Percoll medium (Medicult Linaris) into the first centrifuge tube and carefully overlay it with 1 ml 40% Percoll medium. Prepare a second gradient in the same way.
- Layer equal portions of liquefied semen over both Percoll gradients.

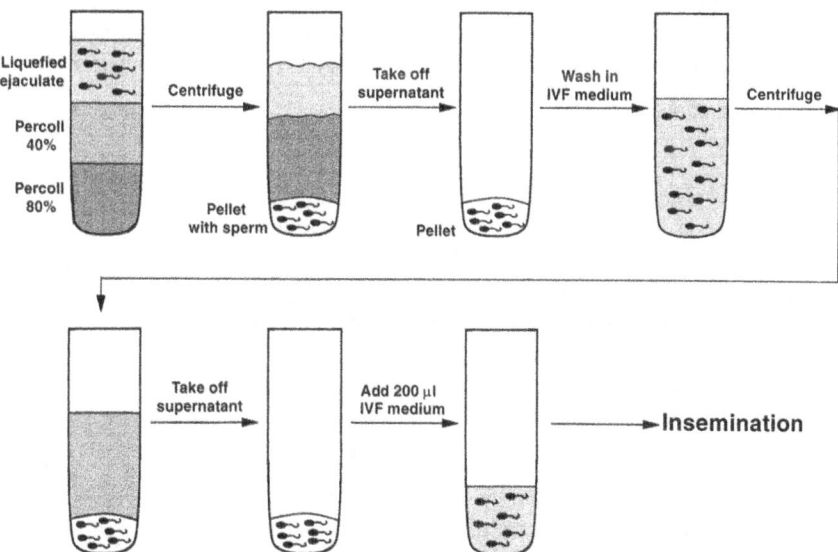

Fig. 14. Sperm preparation with the Percoll technique

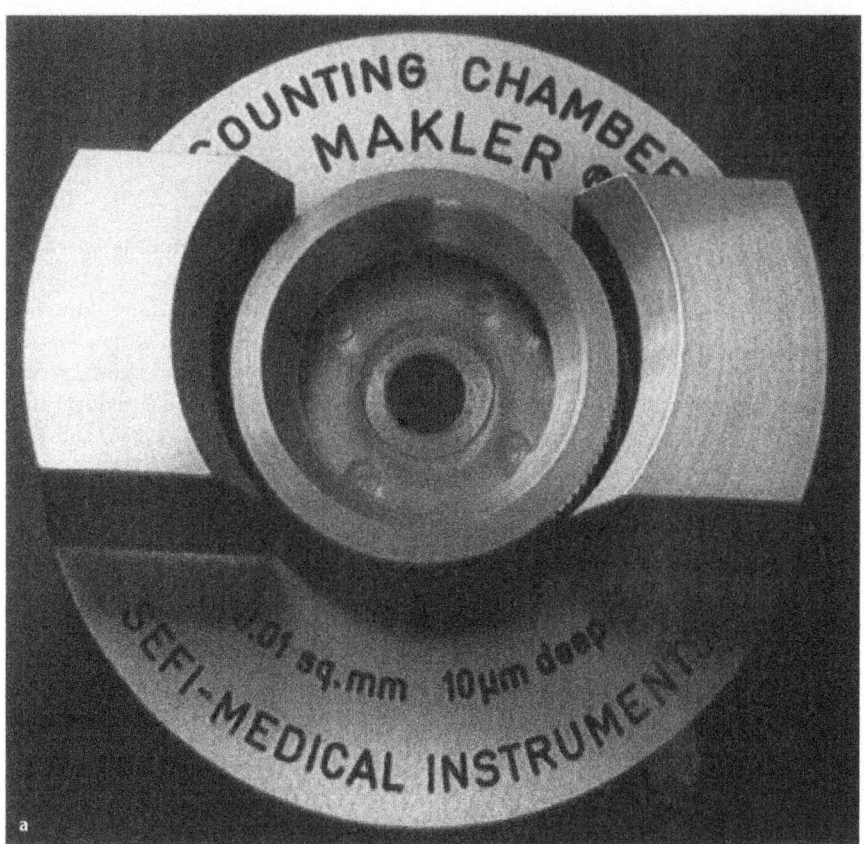

Fig. 15a–c. a Makler chamber for counting sperm (Sefi Medical Instruments, Haifa, Israel). b Counting grid in the cover plate of the Makler chamber (the number of sperm in ten squares of the grid equals the sperm concentration in millions per milliliter). c Makler chamber with sperm and counting grid. × 400

- If sperm volume is less than 1 ml, use only one gradient.
- Centrifuge at 300 µg for 20–30 min (e.g., Megafuge 1.0, Heraeus Sepatech).
- Reject supernatant and resuspend the sperm pellets accumulated at the bottom of the two centrifuge tubes in 1.5 ml of Universal IVF Medium (Medicult Linaris) each, then unite the contents of both tubes.
- Centrifuge at 550 µg for 10 min.
- Resuspend the pellet in 0.2 ml Universal IVF Medium; count 10 µl sperm suspension into the Makler chamber (Fig. 15a–c) and use the rest for insemination (50000–100000 sperm of good motility per chamber).

In Germany, Percoll is no longer recommended for human IVF because it is not a product of pharmaceutical quality. As a substitute for Percoll another system of gradient solutions can be used for sperm preparation, e.g., Sil Select (H. Janssen, Hamburg). The Sil Select gradient solutions consist of silane-covered

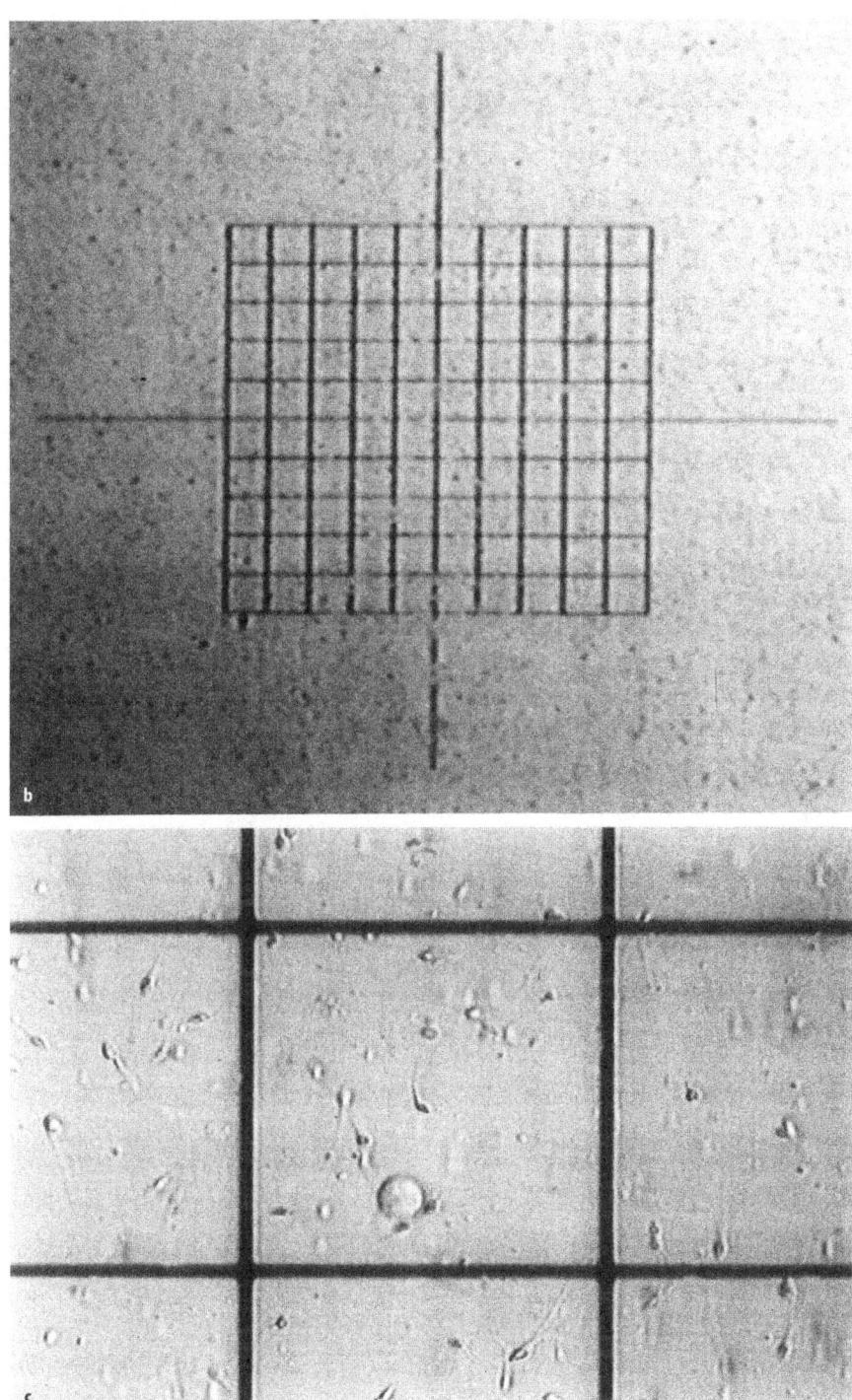

silicate particles diluted in HEPES-buffered EBSS (Earle's buffered salt solution) and are offered as 45% and 90% solutions. Sperm preparation is performed analogous to the Percoll technique described above.

Swim-Up Technique

After centrifugation the progressively motile sperm actively migrate (i.e., swim up) from the pellet to the fresh medium, so that they can be selected for insemination (Fig. 16). The ejaculate is mixed with culture medium and centrifuged. The supernatant containing seminal plasm is rejected, while the sperm-containing pellet is carefully overlaid with fresh culture medium. During subsequent incubation (5–60 min) the motile sperm migrate into the medium. Part of the supernatant is aspirated with a pipette and used for insemination.

Sperm preparation steps using the swim-up technique are as follows:

- Allow semen to stand at room temperature for 15–30 min after collection until it has liquefied.
- Pipette liquid semen into a round-bottom tube (Becton Dickinson, Falcon 2001), add an equal volume of Universal IVF Medium, and mix well.
- Measure 10 µl dilute semen into the Makler chamber (Fig. 15a–c), bearing in mind the dilution factor.
- Meanwhile, centrifuge the sperm at 550 µg for 10 min, then reject the supernatant and resuspend the sperm accumulated at the bottom of the tube (pellet) in approximately 3 ml Universal Medium.
- Centrifuge at 550 µg for 10 min, and reject the supernatant.
- Carefully overlay the pellet with 1 ml Universal IVF Medium and place the tube into the CO_2 incubator (e.g., Labotec Gasboy 40 °C).

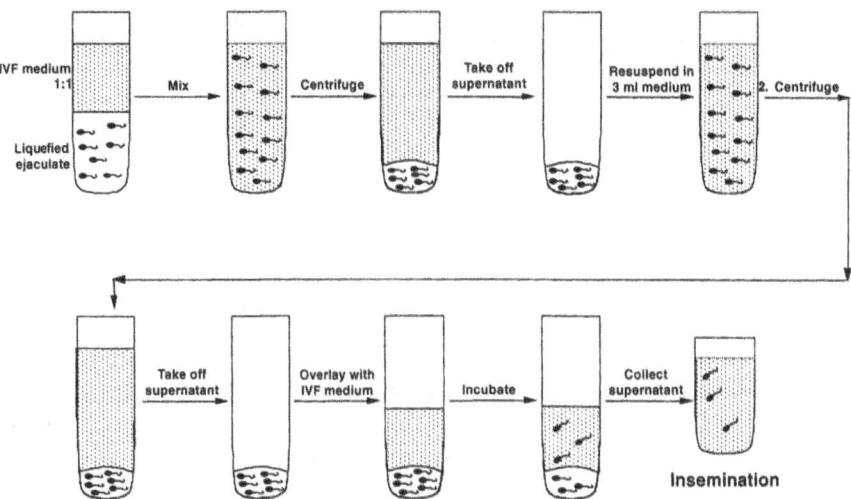

Fig. 16. Sperm preparation using the swim-up technique

- When the sperm migrating from the pellet turn the overlaid medium opaque (after about 5–60 min), 200 ml is pipetted off from the surface of the overlaid medium and transferred into a smaller tube (Becton Dickinson, Falcon 2003).
- Count 10 µl of the sperm suspension into the Makler chamber (Fig. 15a–c).
- Inseminate with 50000–200000 sperm per chamber.

Further Sperm Preparation Methods

Mini-Swim-Up Technique (Al-Hasani et al. 1995)

The principle of the mini swim-up technique is to concentrate motile sperm in the smallest possible volume of medium in cases of oligo-astheno-teratozoo-spermia of varying severity. The procedure is as follows:

- After sperm preparation according to the Percoll or swim-up techniques (see above), resuspend the pellet obtained after the last centrifugation in 1 ml Universal IVF Medium and transfer it into an Eppendorf reaction tube.
- Centrifuge at 550 µg for 2–3 min.
- Carefully lift off supernatant with an Eppendorf pipette.
- Overlay pellet with 5–10 µl universal IVF medium.
- Incubate for a few minutes to several hours.
- Use part or all of the supernatant for insemination or injection (for intracytoplasmic sperm injection) (Fig. 17).

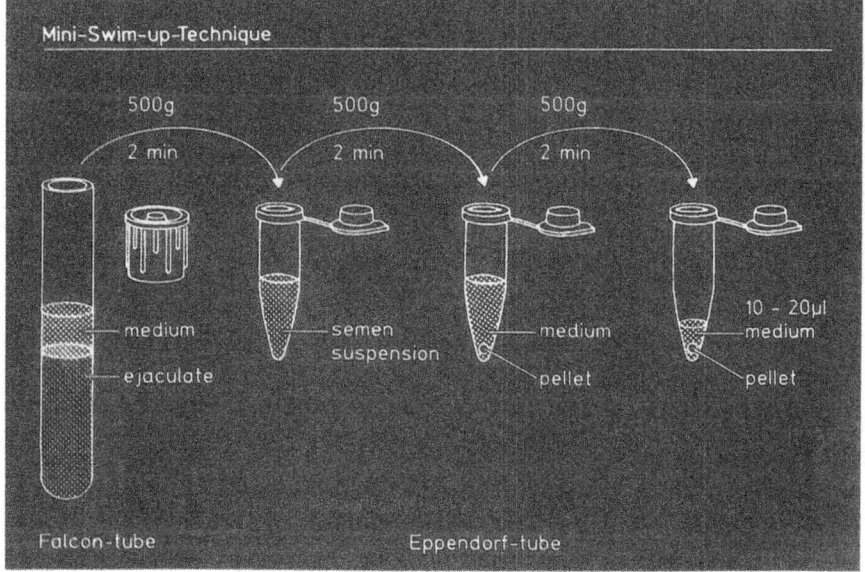

Fig. 17. Mini-swim-up technique

Centrifugation

The principle of centrifugation is to separate cellular (sperm, round cells, etc.) and acellular (seminal plasm) semen components. The semen is mixed with medium and centrifuged once or repeatedly at 250–550 µg. The sperm-containing pellet is resuspended and used for insemination.

Glass-Wool Filtration (Al-Hasani et al. 1996)

The principle of glass-wool filtration is to separate dead sperm or sperm with surface defects (morphologically defective sperm), which adhere to the glass wool, from motile sperm passing the filter (Fig. 18). First, 15–20 mg of glass wool (code 112, John Manville, Oak Brook II, Denver, Col., USA) is pressed into the bottom of each insulin syringe. Next, the glass-wool filter is rinsed with a few milliters of medium. Then the semen is added and passes the glass-wool filter via gravitation.

Pentoxfylline and 2-Deoxyadenosine

Both pentoxifylline and 2-deoxyadenosine are used to improve sperm motility. Since they have been associated with alterations of intracellular mechanisms, for example, changes in intracellular calcium transport and RNA transcription, pentoxifylline and 2-deoxyadenosine cannot be recommended at present (Tournaye et al. 1994).

Preparation of Testicular Sperm

Enzymatic Method

Prepare a stock solution of collagenase (collagenase type IA, cell-culture tested) using Universal IVF Medium as a solvent (concentration of the collagenase: e.g., 600 IU/0.1 ml). Aliquots of the stock solution can be stored at –20 °C for

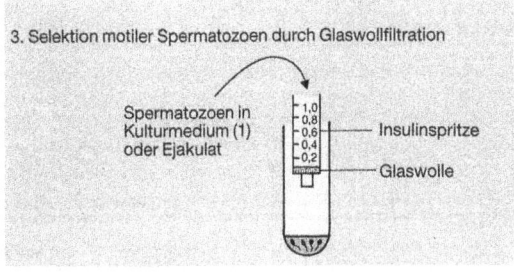

Fig. 18. Glass-wool-filtration

further usage. Now add the collagenase solution to Universal IVF Medium. The final concentration of the enzyme should be 400 IU/ml; e.g., use a cell culture dish containing 1.4 ml Universal IVF Medium and add 0.1 ml of the stock solution containing 600 IU collagenase. Next prepare a water bath of 37 °C.

Now place the tube with the frozen testicular biopsy into the 37 °C water bath for 3 min to thaw it. Transfer the thawed testicular biopsy into the culture dish containing Universal IVF Medium with collagenase. Use a sterile pair of forceps to transfer the biopsy into the IVF medium. Put the culture dish into an incubator (5% CO_2, 37 °C) for approximately 2–4 h, depending on the size of the biopsy.

Suspend the tissue using a sterile pipette tip, and centrifuge the suspension (550 µg, 10 min). Discard the supernatant. Resuspend the pellet with Universal IVF Medium and centrifuge again (550 µg, 5 min). Discard the supernatant, and use the pellet for intracytoplasmic sperm injection.

Mechanical Method

After being placed into a Petri dish (Falcon 3037) containing Ham's F 10 medium, the tissue is minced using sterile scissors and a scalpel to gently tear apart the individual tubuli seminiferi. Then the tissue is incubated for another 3–5 h in Ham's F 10 medium. The supernatant is put into 2-ml Eppendorf tubes and centrifuged at 500 µg for 1 min. The pellet is resuspended using 3–5 µl Ham's F 10, and 1 µl of this suspension is transferred into a Petri dish containing a droplet of Ham's F 10 medium.

Microinjection Procedure (Al-Hasani et al. 1995)

The choice of apparatus and the manufacturing of the pipettes has been described previously (Al-Hasani et al. 1995). The inverted microscope with an OIC contrast objective, hydraulic micromanipulators, and injection devices are manufactured by the Narishige company, Tokyo. The microelectrode puller for the borosilicate glass capillary tubes used in the manufacturing process of the pipettes is supplied by the Sutter Company, Novato, Calif., USA. The injection pipettes, which need to be manufactured in the laboratory before the procedure, should measure 3–4 µm in inner diameter (Fig. 19).

The ICSI procedure is carried out on a heated stage at 37 °C, where 5 microdroplets of medium containing the ova and one containing the sperm are placed in a Petri dish. These droplets are covered with about 3.5 ml of lightweight paraffin oil. At a magnification of × 200, a single spermatozoon is immobilized by gentle depression of the injection pipette on its middle section until motion ceases. The single most immobile spermatozoon is then aspirated tail-first into the tip of the injection pipette. Care is taken to avoid curling of the tail in the pipette. The injection pipette now containing the spermatozoon is advanced towards the microdroplet containing the oocyte. The oocyte is rotated

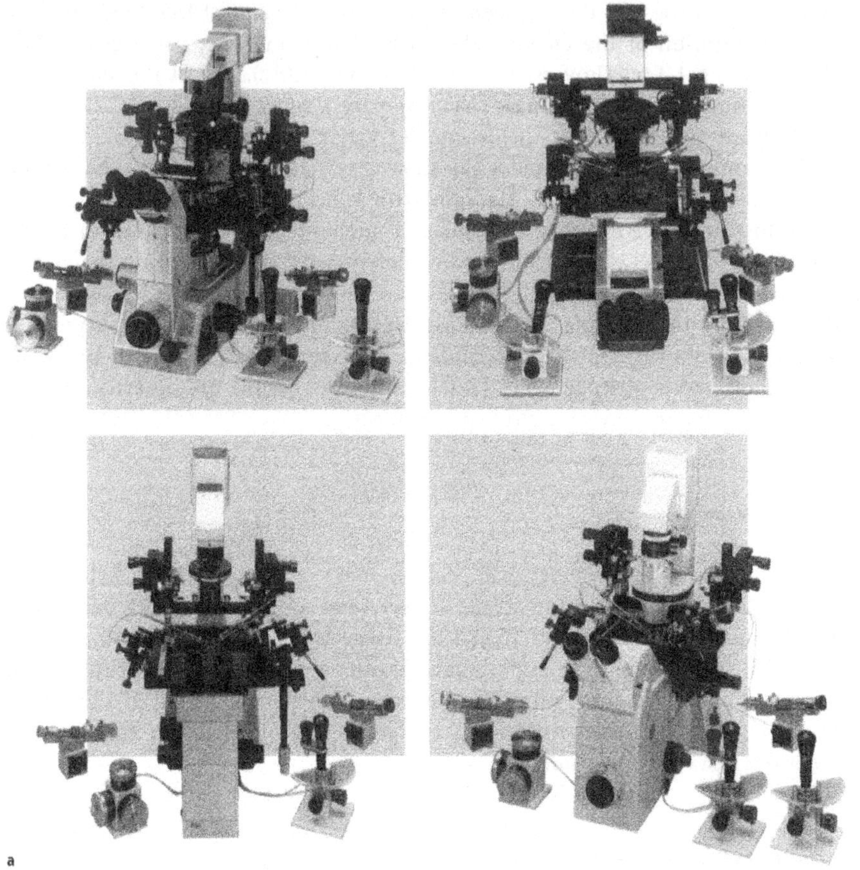

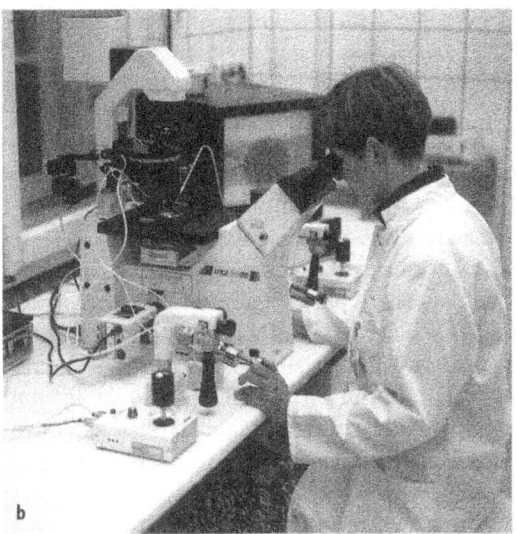

Fig. 19. Microinjection system for ICSI (intracytoplasmic sperm injection). **a** Technical equipment: reverse microscope and Narishigi micromanipulator. **b** Leica microscope and Narishigi micromanipulator as used at the University Women's Hospital in Heidelberg (Narishigi Europe Ltd., Unit 7, Willow Business Park, Willow Way, London SE26 4QP, UK)

at 100-fold magnification until the polar body comes to rest at the 12 o'clock or the 6 o'clock position and is kept in this position with the holding pipette, measuring 20 μm i.d. Then the oocyte and the pipette are brought into focus, and after the sperm is advanced towards the tip of the injection pipette, the latter is advanced to penetrate the oolemma at 3 o'clock. The pipette is advanced towards the center of the oocyte to ensure easy and atraumatic puncture of the oolemma. After the head of the sperm has left the injection pipette, the latter is withdrawn to stop PVP solution or medium from entering the cytoplasm of the oocyte. As a rule, three to four oocytes are injected and then suspended in Ham's F-10 medium. If more oocytes are available, these are injected at a later stage. At 16–18 h after injection, oocytes are examined for the presence of two or more pronuclei. If more than three oocytes have been fertilized, these are cryopreserved. The embryos are transferred into the uterine cavity after an additional 24 h.

Insemination of Oocytes

Method

After aspiration the oocytes are cultured for a few hours in the CO_2 incubator before they are inseminated in microwell dishes. Approximately 100 000 motile sperm of the category "a" (see Table 8) are added to the culture medium containing the oocytes. In case of poor sperm quality, up to 500 000 sperm of good motility may be added to each well. However, the oocytes should then be transferred to fresh medium earlier, as the nutrients in the medium are metabolized quicker by more sperm.

The time of insemination is normally 4–6 h after aspiration. However, no differences in terms of fertilization and pregnancy rates have been found when the oocytes were inseminated 3–20 h after oocyte harvest (Fisch et al. 1989), and insemination is possible even 24 h after aspiration. Oocytes which have not been fertilized may also receive an intracytoplasmic sperm injection 24 h later.

Insemination begins 4–6 h after follicular aspiration. (If the Percoll technique is used for sperm preparation, insemination should follow immediately.) Prepare the pipette (Varipette/Eppendorf) and sterile pipette syringe (Pipettentips/Eppendorf). Loosen the lid of the tube containing sperm.

Take the culture dishes with the oocytes from the incubator and place them on a warm plate. Quickly inseminate one dish after the other. Open the lid and add the calculated sperm quantity to the oocyte(s) in well no. 2. Dip the pipette tip some distance into the medium, steering clear of the cumulus, which could adhere to the tip. Close the lid.

Inspect one dish under the microscope to check whether enough sperm have been added. Put the dishes back into the incubator.

Oocyte and Embryo Culture

After insemination the oocytes are cultured for another 16–20 h. By this time most cumulus cells have been dispersed by the activity of the sperm (Fig. 20). The granulosa cells which remain attached to the oocytes and prevent their evaluation are removed so that any pronuclei (PN) become clearly visible (Fig. 21).

Oocytes with an aberrant number of pronuclei (Fig. 22) are not unusual after in vitro fertilization; according to the literature, the incidence varies between 1% and 25%. After the first cleavage, these embryos are indistinguishable from those with a normal set of chromosomes. It is therefore crucial to determine the number of pronuclei before fusion takes place (Veeck 1991). Oocytes with an aberrant number of pronuclei are not suitable for embryo transfer.

Up to three oocytes at the pronuclear stage (2 PN) are cultured in the incubator for another 24–30 h. By then they will have reached the four- to eight-cell stage and can be transferred to the patient. Any remaining oocytes are cryopreserved or rejected, as the couple desires.

PN monitoring proceeds as follows:

- Use inspection pipette with mouth tube (oocyte pipette/International Medical; Fig. 23).

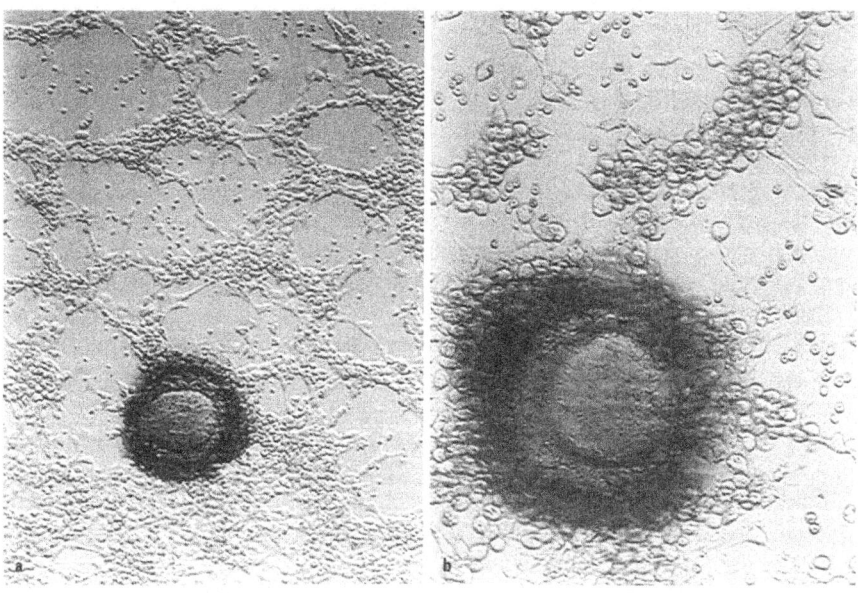

Fig. 20. a Human oocyte, dispersed cumulus; pronuclei cannot be evaluated (about 18 h after insemination). × 200 **b** Human oocyte with dispersed cumulus. The granulosa cells adhering to the bottom of the culture dish can be readily distinguished from erythrocytes entrained into the culture medium along with follicular fluid; pronuclei cannot be evaluated. × 400

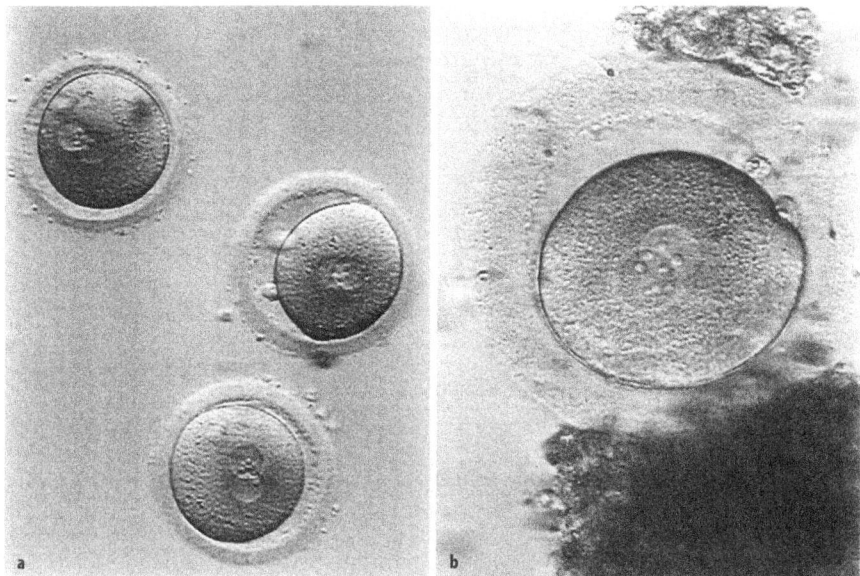

Fig. 21. a Three human oocytes at the pronuclear stage. The granulosa cells have been removed, two pronuclei can be seen at the center of each ooplasm (approx. 18 h after insemination). × 200 **b** Human oocyte. Most granulosa cells have been removed; two pronuclei are located at the center of the ooplasm (approx. 18 h after insemination). × 400

- Switch on microscope (Leitz/Fluovert) at minimum light intensity.
- Take microwell dishes out of incubator one after the other. First evaluate oocyte under the microscope while keeping lid on dish (× 100; low light intensity). At the same time, check for sperm motility (× 250).
- Lift lid, briefly rinse capillary in medium, and reject rinsing liquid.
- After taking in fresh medium, aspirate oocyte under the microscope (× 40) and place into fresh medium (well no. 3).
- Wash oocyte using a pipette (repeated aspiration and release) until the oocyte is practically free of granulosa cells. Close lid.
- Evaluate pronuclei at × 40–250 magnification, place culture dish into incubator.
- Record number of pronuclei and oocyte morphology.
- Continue with the other culture dishes as described above.
- Once all oocytes have been freed of their granulosa cells, select three oocytes at the pronuclear stage for transfer and place into a well together.

Oocytes are selected on the basis of (a) oocyte morphology (cytoplasm, fragmentation), duration of the granulosa cell removal step, and (c) thickness of the zona pellucida.

Now the time for the transfer is arranged with the physicians and the patient. The patient is asked to come with a full bladder, which normally facilitates introduction of the embryo transfer catheter.

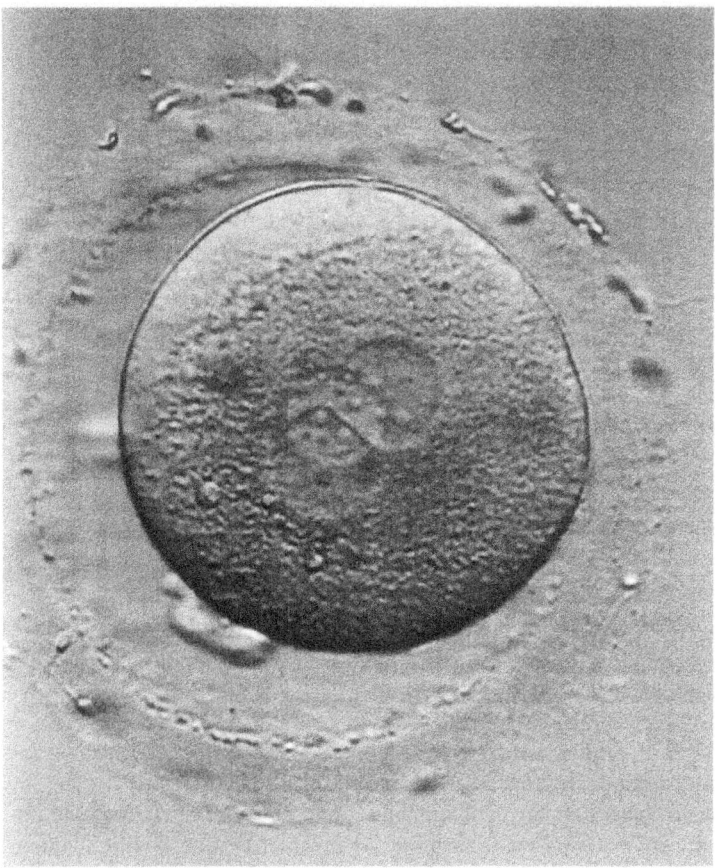

Fig. 22. Human oocyte with three pronuclei (approx. 18 h after insemination). × 400

Embryo Transfer

About 48 h after insemination the embryos are transferred to the uterus of the patient. At this time they have reached the two- to eight-cell stage (Fig. 24a–c). The oocytes may have divided equally (blastomeres of equal size), or they may be more or less highly fragmented (Fig. 24d). Occasionally, oocytes do not start dividing but degenerate instead (Fig. 24e).

The embryos are normally picked up in a small volume (< 75 µl) of culture medium by means of a rigid polyfluoroethylene catheter (i.d. 0.8–1 mm) connected to an insulin syringe. The catheter is advanced into the uterus through the cervical canal until its tip is close to the fundus. The full bladder of the patient facilitates catheterization. If the cervical canal proves difficult to pass, a metal guide catheter may also be used, and the embryos are transferred through a second catheter pushed into the guide catheter (see below). The embryos may be transferred with the patient in the lithotomy position.

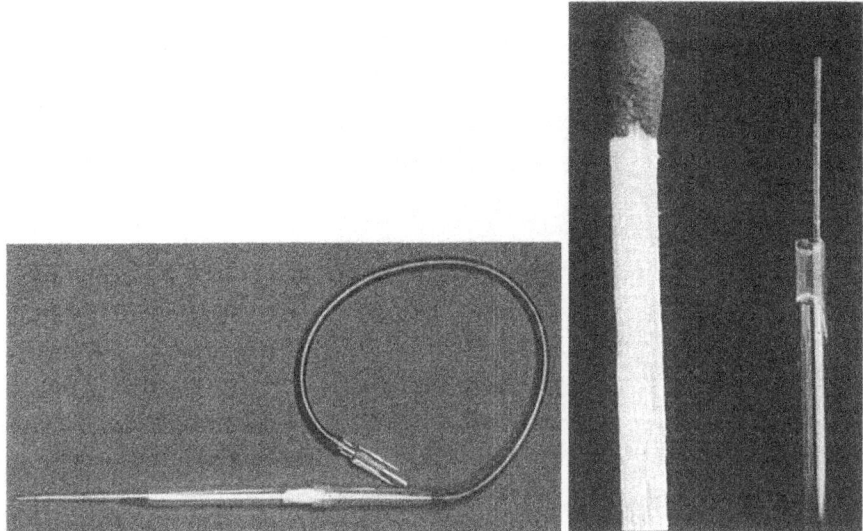

Fig. 23. a Inspection pipette (oocyte pipette/International Medical) with mouth tube for PN control. **b** Tip of inspection pipette compared with a match

Analgesia or anesthesia is not required in most cases. If necessary, mild general anesthesia (induction with thiopental, maintenance with O_2/N_2O/halothane) may be considered.

In order to reduce the risk of multiple pregnancy, not more than three embryos may be transferred, according to a statutory stipulation in Germany. However, some countries allow the transfer of more than three embryos.

Many centers ask their patients to remain in the position of transfer for a period of several minutes to several hours. There are no reliable studies on the strengths and weaknesses of this practice, but it is perceived as a pleasant experience by many patients.

The embryos are transferred in the lithotomy position without medication using a disposable embryo transfer catheter kit (T.D.T. Set, Laboratoire C.C.D., Paris, France; Fig. 25). Sterile unpowdered gloves should be worn (Hygiene-handschuh, Beiersdorf, Hamburg).

A sterile insulin syringe (Braun Melsungen) is rinsed three times with PBS buffer (Biochrom) to remove lubricant, while the syringe is kept sterile. Universal IVF Medium is taken into the syringe and air bubbles are removed.

The filled insulin syringe is firmly attached to the sterile transfer catheter and the catheter is rinsed with Universal IVF Medium. The syringe should be filled only to a certain self-selected level, say 0.5 ml, which must be sufficient for the medium to emerge from the catheter tip (the volume of the catheter is 0.2 ml). The catheter so prepared is set aside using a sterile technique.

The guide catheter is handed to the physician using a sterile technique. Meanwhile the physician has introduced the speculum into the external os and swabbed it carefully with physiological saline.

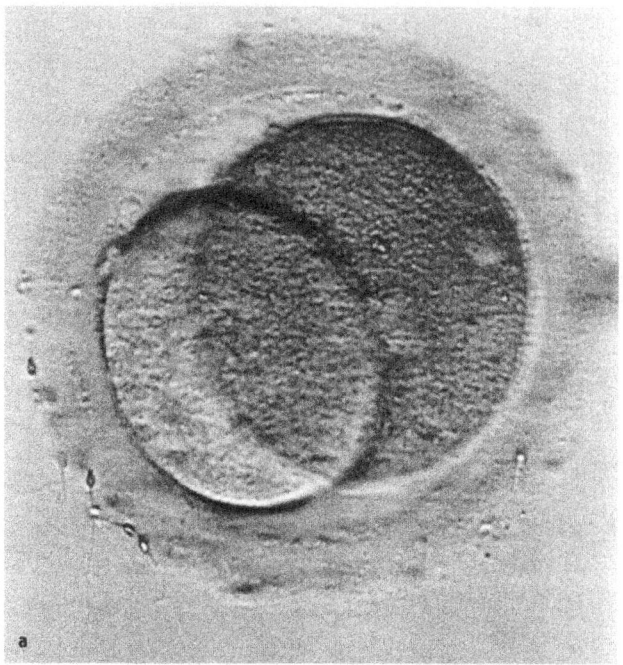

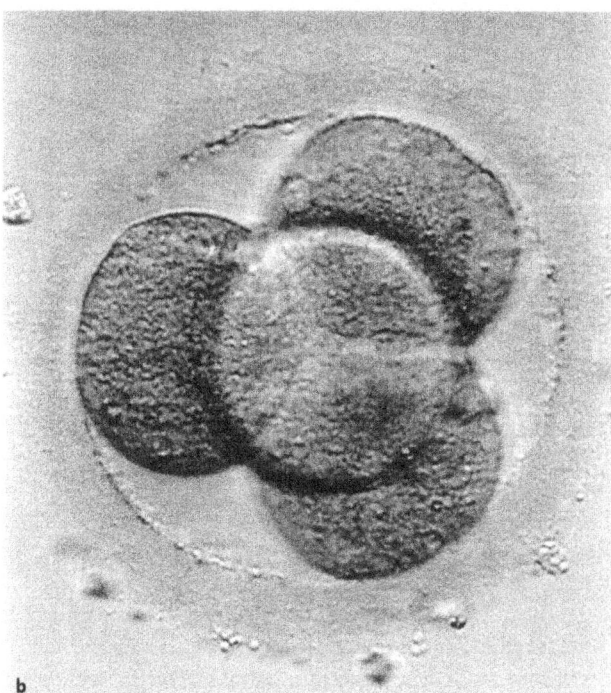

Fig. 24. a Human embryo at two-cell stage (approx. 48 h after insemination). × 400 **b** Human embryo at four-cell stage (approx. 48 h after insemination). × 400

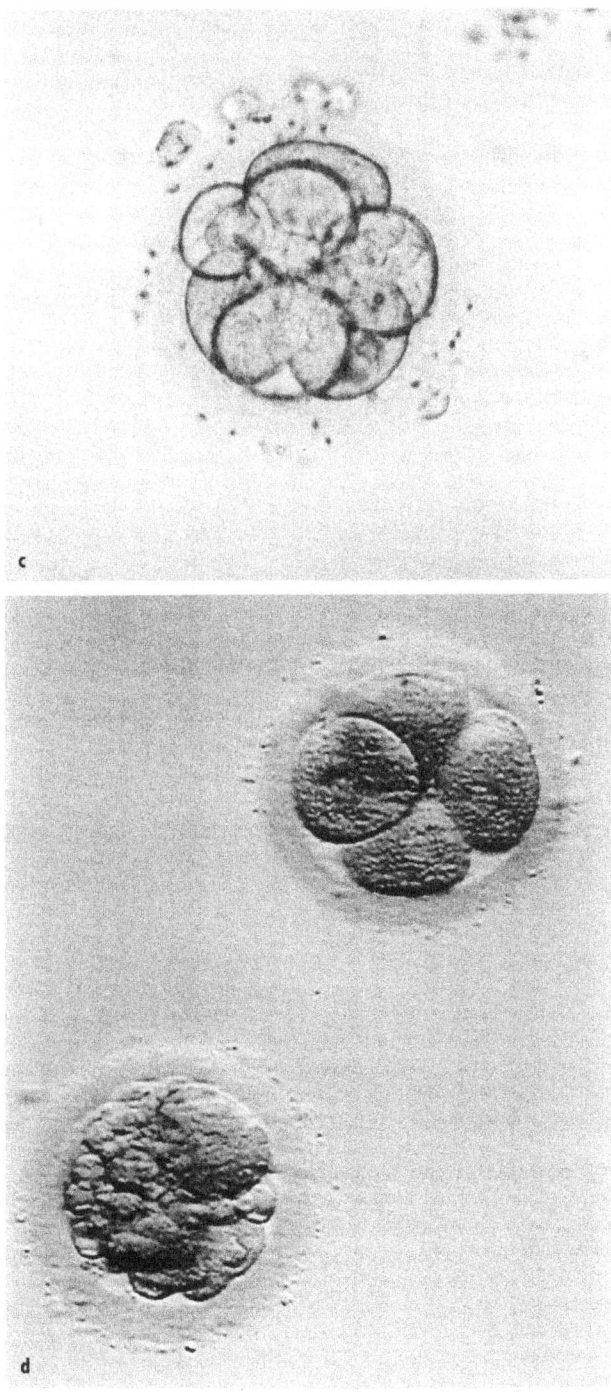

Fig. 24. c Human embryo at eight-cell stage (approx. 48 h after insemination). × 125 **d** Two human embryos about 48 h after insemination: right, an equally divided embryo at the four-cell stage, left, a highly fragmented embryo. × 200

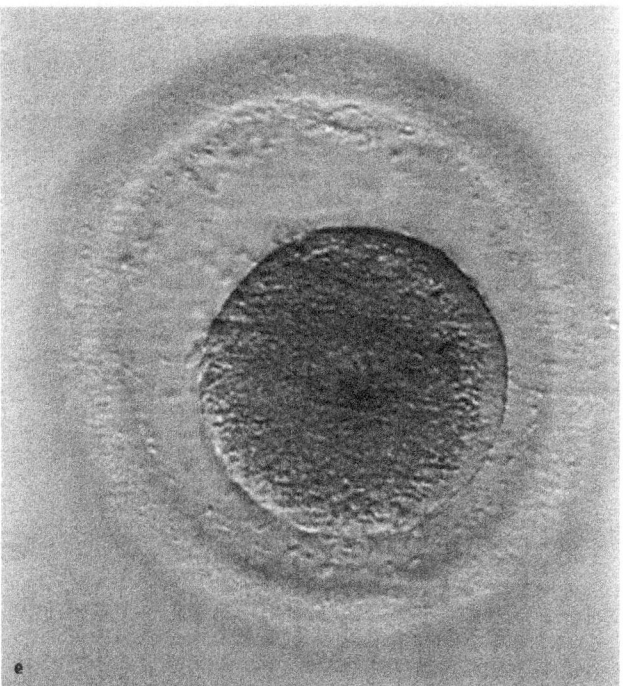

Fig. 24. e Fertilized human oocyte which has failed to develop into an embryo. Both pronu-clei are still visible inside the degenerate oocyte. × 400

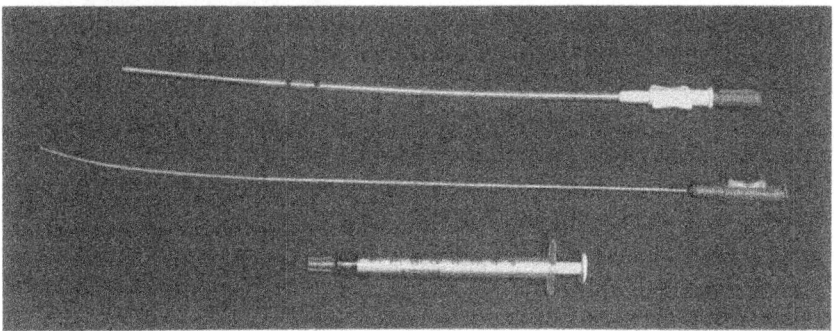

Fig. 25. Embryo transfer catheter kit T.D.T. Set, Laboratoire C.C.D., Paris, France. *Catheter no. 1:* guide catheter, Standard Fryman Catheter, with flexible, distal segment (4.5 cm) and plastic-coated metal guide to catheterize the uterus. *Catheter no. 2:* ultrathin Teflon catheter for embryo injection

Fig. 26. Principle of embryo pick-up into transfer catheter

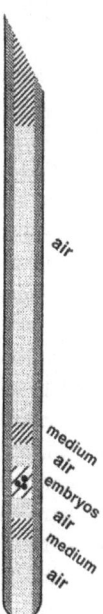

The guide catheter is passed atraumatically through the external os to a depth of at least 7 cm, preferably 7.5 cm. If possible, instruments to extend the uterus should not be used. The tip of the catheter should be placed adjacent to the uterine fundus.

Following placement of the guide catheter, the culture dish containing the embryos is taken out of the incubator. Under the microscope (minimum light intensity) the embryos are taken from the culture dish (well no. 3) into the transfer catheter in a specific sequence (Fig. 26), using a sterile technique.

The front part of the catheter is kept warm and protected from light by holding it between finger and thumb. The syringe on the other end of the catheter is held with the other hand and carried to the patient.

The transfer catheter is introduced into the guide catheter and advanced to at least the first mark of the guide catheter (7 cm). No resistance should be felt. The guide catheter is retracted slightly without moving the transfer catheter.

The embryos are injected slowly into the uterus. Do not inject more liquid (culture medium) than has entered the catheter when taking in the embryos (approx. 20 µl). The self-selected mark on the syringe (see above) helps in assessing the volume to be injected: If the catheter and the syringe are filled with medium to a level of 0.5 ml before taking in the embryos, the amount injected equals the additional amount present in the catheter and the syringe after taking in the embryos.

Both catheters are cautiously retracted. The liquid left in the catheter system after transfer is checked for any remaining embryos under the microscope. Should any embryos have adhered to the catheter, they are immediately transferred into fresh medium, placed into the incubator, and the embryo transfer is repeated.

The patient is asked to remain in her position for a few minutes. The success of IVF with embryo transfer (ET), expressed as pregnancies per transfer, is currently about 25% according to data provided by German-speaking working groups (Table 9).

The success of IVF-ET depends on many factors, including the indication for the procedure and the quality of the embryos transferred. The best results with IVF-ET have been achieved in cases of tubal infertility. In cases of male subfertility, endometriosis, and unexplained infertility results have been less positive. With regard to the embryos, it is difficult to assess their quality based on morphological and biochemical criteria. Morphologically intact embryos are considered to have a good chance of continued development. The quality of the embryo probably depends on oocyte development and culture conditions:

- *Number of embryos transferred*: The pregnancy rate rises with the number of embryos transferred. On the other hand, the risks related to multiple pregnancy must be considered.
- *Patient age*: The pregnancy rate per embryo transfer declines significantly after the age of 40. The cause of this reduced fertility is declining ovarian function rather than poor uterine/endometrial quality.
- *Uterine anomalies*: Uterine septi and other congenital deformities, adenomyomas, intrauterine infections, adhesions (for example, after an abortion), may compromise implantation.
- *Readiness of the endometrium for implantation*: It is difficult to assess the significance of endometrial status for implantation and maintenance of pregnancy. The following factors seem to play a role:
  - Asynchrony between embryo development and endometrial maturation. The embryos are transferred approximately 48 h after follicular aspiration, while the embryos of oocytes fertilized in vivo implant in the uterine cavity after 5–7 days.
  - Adequate endocrine function during the luteal phase.
  - Endometrial secretion proteins/leukotrienes and immunological factors may also play a role in embryo development.

Table 9. IVF results (from German Central IVF Register 1994)

Working groups	$n=43$
Cycles with follicular aspiration	$n=9214$
Fertilization rate (Ooc.)	52.1%
Cycles with embryo transfer	$n=6336$
Mean number of embryos	$d=2.5$
Pregnancies	$n=1737$
Pregnancies per aspiration	18.8
Pregnancies per transfer	27.4
Abortions	$n=334$
Term pregnancies	$n=1204$
Term pregnancies per ET	19

- Technique of embryo transfer: Embryos should be transferred nontraumatically. If they are transferred through the cervical canal, bacterial contamination of the uterus cannot be ruled out completely. The ultrasound guidance of embryo transfer has not yielded an improved success rate.
The transfer of embryos by the surgical route, i.e., uterine puncture, has not become common practice.

References

Acosta AA, Swanson RJ, Ackerman SB, Kruger TF, van Zyl JA, Menkveld R (1990) Human spermatozoa in assisted reproduction. Williams and Wilkins, Baltimore

Al-Hasani S, Küpker W, Baschat AA, Sturm R, Bauer O, Diedrich C, Diedrich K (1995) Mini-swim up: a new technique of sperm preparation for intracytoplasmic sperm injection. J Assist Reprod Genet 12:428

Al-Hasani S, Alpüstün S, Ludwig M, Diedrich K, Bauer O, Küpker W, Wolff A, Krebs D (1996) The combination of two semen preparation techniques (glass wool filtration and swim-up) and their effect on the morphology of recovered spermatozoa and outcome of IVF-ET. Int J Androl 19:55–60

Asch RH, Ellsworth LR, Balmaceda JP, Wong PC (1985) Gamete intrafallopian transfer (GIFT): a new treatment for infertility. Int J Fertil 30:41–46

Beier HM, Lindner HR (1983) Fertilization of the human egg in vitro. Springer, Heidelberg New York Tokyo

Bettendorf G, Breckwoldt M (1989) Reproduktionsmedizin. Fischer, Stuttgart

Bolton VN, Warren RE, Braude PR (1986) Removal of bacterial contaminants from semen for in vitro fertilisation or artificial insemination by the use of buoyant density centrifugation. Fertil Steril 46:1128–1132

Bongso A, Ng SC, Fong CY, Anandakumar C, Marshall B, Edirisinghe R, Ratnam S (1992) Improved pregnancy rate after transfer of embryos grown in human fallopian cell co-culture. Fertil Steril 58:569–574

Chen C et al (1986) Pregnancy after human oocyte cryopreservation. Lancet 1:884–886

Cohen J, Debacte C, Pez JP, Junca AM, Cohen-Bacrie P (1986) Transvaginal sonographically controlled follicle puncture for oocyte retrieval for IVF. J In Vitro Fertil Embryo Transf 3:309–313

Cohen J, Alikani M, Malter H, Adler A, Talansky BE, Rosenwaks Z (1991) Partial zona dissection or subzonal sperm insertion: microsurgical fertilization alternatives based on evaluation of sperm and embryo morphology. Fertil Steril 56:696–706

Craft I et al (1982) Birth following oocyte and sperm transfer to the uterus. Lancet 2:773

de Kretzer D, Dennis P, Hudson B (1973) Transfer of a human zygote. Lancet 2:729

Dellenbach P, Nisband I, Moreau L et al (1984) Transvaginal sonographically controlled ovarian follicle puncture for egg retrieval. Lancet 1:1467

Devroey P, Braeckmans P, Smitz J et al (1986) Pregnancy after translaparoscopic zygote intrafallopian transfer in a patient with sperm antibodies. Lancet 1:1329

Dumoulin JCM, Vanvuchelen RMT, Land JA, Pieters MH, Geraedts JPM, Evers JLH (1995) Effect of oxygen concentration on in vitro fertilization and embryo culture in the human and the mouse. Fertil Steril 1:115–119

Edwards RG, Brody SA (1995) Principles and practice of assisted human reproduction. Saunders, Philadelphia

Edwards RG, Livingstone C (1990) Assisted human conception. British Medical Bulletin. In: Edwards RG (ed) Churchill Livingstone, London

Feichtinger W, Kemeter P (1986) Transvaginal sector scan sonography for needle-guided transvaginal follicle aspiration and other applications in gynecologic routine and research. Fertil Steril 45:722–725

Fisch B et al (1989) The effect of preinsemination interval upon fertilization of human oocytes in vitro. Human Reprod 4:954–956

Fischl H (ed) (1995) Kinderwunsch. Krause und Pacherrnegg, Purkersdorf

Fishel S (1986) In vitro fertilisation. Symonds Press Limited, Oxford

Forrler A, Dellenbach P, Nidsand I, Moreau L (1986a) Direct intraperitoneal insemination in
unexplained infertility and cervical infertility. Lancet 1:916–917

Forrler A, Dellenbach P, Nidsand I, Moreau L (1986b) Direct intraperitoneal insemination:
first results confined. Lancet 2:1468

Hamberger L, Wickland M, Nilsson L, Janson PO, Sjogren A, Hillensjo T (1982) Methods of
aspiration of human oocytes by various techniques. Acta Med Rom 20:370–378

Hard AD (1909) Artificial impregnation. Med World 27:163–164

Heape W (1980) Preliminary note on the transimplantation and growth of mammalian ova
within a uterine foster mother. Proc Royal Soc 48:457–458

Hewett J et al (1985) Treatment of idiopathic infertility, cervical mucus hostility and male
infertility. Artificial insemination with husband's semen or in vitro fertilization? Fertil
Steril 44:350–355

Hinrichsen KV (1990) Humanembryologie. Springer, Berlin Heidelberg New York

Holst N, Berteussen K (1990) Optimizing and simplification of culture conditions in human
in vitro fertilization and preembryo replacement by serum-free media. J In Vitro Fertil
Embryo Transf 1

Jansen RPS, Anderson LC (1987) Catheterisation of the fallopian tubes from the vagina.
Lancet 2:309–310

Jones HW, Jones GS, Hodgen GD, Rosenwaks Z (1986) In vitro fertilization. Williams and
Wilkins, Baltimore

Kerin JFP et al (1984) Improved conception rate after intrauterine insemination of washed
spermatozoa from men with poor-quality semen. Lancet 1:533–535

Krebs D, Al-Hasani (1984) Eizellgewinnung. In: Krebs D (ed) Praktikum der extrakorpora-
len Befruchtung. Urban and Schwarzenberg, Munich

Lenz S, Lauritzen J (1982) Ultrasonically guided percutaneous aspiration of human follicles
under local anesthesia: a new method of collecting oocytes for in vitro fertilisation. Fertil Steril 38:673–677

Lenz S, Lauritzen JG, Kjellow M (1981) Collecting of human oocytes for in vitro fertilisation by ultrasonically guided follicular puncture. Lancet 1:1163

Lenz S, Leeton J, Renou P (1987) Transvaginal recovery of oocytes for IVF using vaginal ultrasound. J In Vitro Fertil Embryo Transf 4:51–55

Lopata A et al (1980) Pregnancy following intrauterine implantation of an embryo obtained
by in vitro fertilization of a preovulatory egg. Fertil Steril 33:117–120

Ludwig H, Tauber PF (1978) Human fertilization. Thieme, Stuttgart

Lutjen P et al (1984) The establishment and maintenance of pregnancy using in vitro fertilization and embryo donation in patient with primary ovarian failure. Nature 307:174–175

Mahadevan M, Trounson AO, Leeton JF (1983) The relationship of tubal blockage, infertility
of unknown cause, suspected male infertility and endometriosis to success of in vitro
fertilisation and embryo transfer. Fertil Steril 40:755–762

Mettler L (1995) Die IVF als etablierte Therapie. In: Fischl FH (ed) (1995) Kinderwunsch.
Krause and Pachernegg, Purkersdorf, pp 173–186

Ng SC et al (1988) Pregnancy after transfer of multiple sperm under the zona. Lancet 2:790

Ng SC, Bongso A, Ratnam SS (1991) Microinjection of human oocytes: a technique for severe oligoasthenoteratozoospermia. Fertil Steril 56:1117–1123

Parsons J, Booker M, Goswamy R et al (1985) Oocyte retrieval for in vitro fertilisation by
ultrasonically guided needle aspiration via the urethra. Lancet 1:1076

Pousette A, Akerlof E, Rosenborg L, Fredericsson B (1986) Increase of progressive motility
and improved morphology of human spermatozoa following their migration through
Percoll gradients. Int J Androl 9:1–13

Purdy JM (1982) Methods for fertilization and embryo culture in-vitro. In: Edwards RG,
Purdy JM (ed) Human conception in-vitro. Academic, London, pp 135–156

Quinn P, Kerin JF, Warnes GM (1985) Improved pregnancy rate in human in vitro fertilization, with the use of medium based on the composition of human tubal fluid. Fertil Steril 44:493–498

Rabe T, Runnebaum (1994) Fortpflanzungsmedizin. Springer, Berlin Heidelberg New York

Rock J, Menkin MF (1944) In vitro fertilisation and cleavage of human eggs. Science 100:105–107

Schenk SL (1878) Das Saugetier künstlich befruchtet ausserhalb des Muttertieres. Mitteilungen aus dem embryologischen Institut der K. und K. Universität Wien 2:107

Schill W, Bollmann W (1986) Spermakonservierung, Insemination, In-vitro-Fertilisation. Urban and Schwarzenberg, Munich

Seifert-Klauss V, Tescher A, Lauritzen C, Stützle R, Berg FD (1994) Laboratory routine in IVF: state of the art in Germany. Fertilitat 10:229–233

Steptoe PC, Edwards RG (1970) Laparoscopic recovery of preovulatory human oocytes after priming of ovaries with gonadotropins. Lancet 2:683–689

Steptoe PC, Edwards RG (1976) Reimplantation of a human embryo with subsequent tubal pregnancy. Lancet 1:880

Steptoe PC, Edwards RG (1978) Birth after the reimplantation of human embryo. Lancet 2:366

Testart J et al (1982) In vitro fertilization. Success of IVF in spontaneous and stimulated cycles and technical procedures used. In: Rolland R et al (eds) Proceedings of the 4th Reinier de Graaf Symposium. Excerpta Medica, Amsterdam, pp 352–358

Tournaye H, Van der Linden M, Van den Abeel E, Devroey P, Van Steirteghem AC (1994) Mouse in vitro fertilisation using sperm treated with pentoxifylline and 2-desoxyadenosine. Fertil Steril 62:644–647

Trounson AO, Leeton JF, Wood EC, Webb J, Wood J (1981) Pregnancies of humans by fertilisation in vitro and embryo transfer in the controlled ovulatory cycle. Science 212:681–682

Veeck LL (1987) Atlas of the human oocyte and early conceptus. Williams and Wilkins, Baltimore

Veeck LL (1991) Atlas of the human oocyte and early conceptus, vol 2. Williams and Wilkins, Baltimore

Veeck LL, Wortham JWE, Wittmeyer J (1983) Maturation and fertilisation of morphologically immature human oocytes in a program of in vitro fertilisation. Fertil Steril 39:594–602

Wikland M, Enk L, Hamberger L (1985) Transvesical and transvaginal approaches for the aspiration of follicles by the use of ultrasound. Ann NY Acad Sci 442:184–194

Wood C, Trounson A (1989) Clinical in vitro fertilisation. Springer, Berlin Heidelberg New York

World Health Organization (1992) Recent advances in medically assisted conception. WHO Technical Report Series, WHO, Geneva

World Health Organization (1993) WHO-Laborhandbuch zur Untersuchung des menschlichen Ejakulates und der Spermien-Zervikal-Schleim-Interaktion. Springer, Berlin Heidelberg New York

Yovich JL et al (1984) Treatment of male infertility by in-vitro fertilisation. Lancet 2

Yovich JL et al (1987) Pregnancies after pronuclear stage tubal transfer. Fertil Steril 48:851–857

Evolution of Pregnancies and Initial Follow-up of Newborns Delivered after Intracytoplasmic Sperm Injection

G. D. Palermo, Q. V. Neri, R. Raffaelli, O. K. Davis, Z. Rosenwaks

Introduction

Intracytoplasmic sperm injection (ICSI) represents a major breakthrough in assisted reproductive technology (ART) [1–3], because of its ability to achieve fertilization regardless of semen parameters or dysfunctional spermatozoa. ICSI has essentially eliminated the use of in vitro insemination with donor sperm, since the outcome of ICSI with compromised semen is comparable in couples with normal semen undergoing in vitro fertilization (IVF). Even with immature (epididymal and testicular) spermatozoa, ICSI has produced results comparable to those achieved with freshly ejaculated semen, further broadening the application of this treatment [4, 5]. Its safety has been demonstrated in many ART programs worldwide [6–9] and in case series from 35 different programs published in a European survey [7]. Nevertheless, there is still some concern that this treatment may carry risks [10–15].

This chapter concerns the first and largest case series on ICSI in the United States. We report on the in vivo development of embryos and conceptuses with data compiled on the in utero growth and subsequent delivery of offspring; the frequency of chromosomal abnormalities in embryos and fetuses; and the method of delivery. We compare the frequency of congenital defects observed in ICSI offspring with that following standard IVF treatment at our institution. In addition, we examine the impact of maternal age, semen origin, and other semen parameters on fertilization and pregnancy outcome.

Methods

This study includes the pregnancies obtained in all 1835 couples treated in 2607 cycles of assisted fertilization with ICSI, performed between September 1993 and December 1997 at The Center for Reproductive Medicine and Infertility, The New York Presbyterian Hospital-Weill Medical College of Cornell Medical Center University. The ICSI technique was reviewed and approved by the Committee on Human Rights in Research of the New York Presbyterian Hospital-Weill Medical College of Cornell University. All couples were counseled about ICSI as a new assisted reproduction technique and were informed of the many unknown aspects of this treatment, and written consent was obtained from all participants.

In 2165 cycles semen parameters were compromised and thus were consider-ed unsuitable for successful IVF [16–18], and in 311 cycles surgical retrieval of sperm from either the epididymis or testis was required, leaving ICSI as the only therapeutic option. An additional 131 cycles followed previous fertilization with standard IVF despite normal semen parameters. The mean maternal age was 35.7±5 years. Of the total number of couples, 1296 underwent a single ICSI treatment; 385 experienced the procedure twice, 104 couples three times, 34 couples four times, and 12 five times; three were treated six times, and one couple had seven treatments. All men requiring epididymal aspiration because of congenital absence of the vas deferens were counseled regarding the risks of mutations of the cystic fibrosis transmembrane-conductance regulator (CFTR) gene and the risks of transmission, and it was recommended that both partners undergo CFTR gene mutation testing.

Semen collection methods for ejaculated, epididymal, and testicular samples, as well as semen analysis for ICSI, have been reported previously [2, 19], as have the preparation of oocytes and the microinjection technique [1, 2, 19–21]. About 12–17 h following ICSI, integrity of the oocyte cytoplasm was assessed and the number and size of pronuclei were noted; cleavage was evaluated 24 and 48 h after injection, and assisted hatching with eventual fragment removal was performed on selected embryos [22]. Morphologically good quality em-bryos were transferred approximately 72 h after ICSI, the number being depen-dent upon maternal age [19]. Corticosteroids, prophylactic antibiotics, and pro-gesterone supplementation were administered until pregnancy assessment [13].

Serum βhCG was measured 10 days after embryo transfer, with a "biochemical pregnancy" defined as a significant increase in hCG levels (> 10 mIU/ml) between days 10 and 20 after the luteinizing hormone (LH) surge. Delayed menstruation was not considered to be a criterion of pregnancy. Clinical pregnancy was de-fined as the presence of a gestational sac as well as at least one viable fetal heart at ultrasonographic screening on day 49. Prenatal diagnosis was performed via amniocentesis. In cases of miscarriage, pathological and genetic assessments were carried out on the expelled embryonic/trophoblastic material. All the preg-nancies included in this study have been followed to term. For children born else-where, gynecologists and pediatricians provided reports which included a detailed morphological examination on approximately 20% of ICSI neonates born at our institution. A detailed physical examination was performed at birth.

The following nomenclature was employed for congenital malformations: ma-jor malformations included those with either surgical and/or functional conse-quences and minor malformations were those with no surgical or functional importance. A minor anomaly was distinguished from a normal variation if it occurred in ≤4% of the infants in the same racial group. Anomaly and malfor-mations were considered synonymous with a structural abnormality [23, 24].

Statistical analysis was performed with SAS (Statistical Analysis System, Cary, NC, USA). Statistical procedures were carried out with one-tailed χ^2 tests using a 5% level of significance to evaluate all hypotheses. Where appropriate, Fisher-type adjustments were made to assure no violations owing to small cell counts in χ^2 procedures.

We compared the frequency of congenital malformations among neonates conceived after ICSI with malformations among neonates conceived after IVF at our institution. We examined the effect of maternal age, semen origin, and sperm count on outcomes of fertilization and pregnancy.

Results

Among 2607 ICSI cycles there were 211 biochemical pregnancies, and 90 were very early miscarriages (blighted ova), while 1180 pregnancies developed a viable heartbeat. Subsequently, 124 patients miscarried and seven patients had an ectopic pregnancy, resulting in a delivery rate of 40.0% (Table 1).

A total of 1564 neonates were born from 1042 deliveries. The gender distribution of the offspring included 785 females and 779 males (ratio 1.01:1), with an overall frequency of multiple pregnancies of 41.4% (431/1042): 363 twins (34.8%), 67 triplets (6.4%), and one quadruplet (0.09%).

The evolution and outcome of the implanted embryos are depicted in Table 2, showing an implantation rate of 25.9% sacs and 23.2% sacs with a positive fetal heartbeat. An additional 17.3% of the embryos were lost (329/1906), as detailed in Table 2. The frequency of high-order gestations diagnosed by transvaginal ultrasonography at 6 weeks was 45.8% (541/1180): 383 twins (32.5%), 134 triplets (11.3%), and 22 quadruplets (1.9%).

Of the 109 miscarriages, cytogenetic information was available in 31 cases (Table 3). The karyotypes indicate that all trisomies occurred in women >35 years old. Furthermore, among 15 patients >36 years of age (mean 37.6±3), pregnancies were therapeutically terminated after prenatal diagnosis in five because of trisomy 21, in two for trisomy 18, in one for chromosome 18 translocation, and in one case of Klinefelter's syndrome. Other reasons for cessation of pregnancy were neural tube defect ($n=1$), physical accident ($n=1$), elective termination ($n=2$), and unknown ($n=2$).

In 52.6% ($n=548$) of cases newborns were delivered vaginally, with seven requiring instrumental assistance: forceps ($n=3$) and vacuum ($n=4$). The indications for delivery by cesarean section (47.4%; $n=494$) are listed in Table 4. For

Table 1. Pregnancy outcome of 2607 cycles of intracytoplasmic sperm injection[a]. (*ICSI* intracytoplasmic sperm injection, *ellipses* indicate data not applicable, *hCG* human chorionic gonadotropin)

	No. (%)	No. of negative outcomes
ICSI cycles	2607 (...)	...
Embryo transfer	2487 (...)	...
Positive hCG test results	1481 (56.8)	211 biochemical pregnancies; 90 blighted ova
Positive fetal heartbeats	1180 (45.3)	124 miscarriages and therapeutic abortions; 7 ectopic pregnancies
Deliveries	1042 (40.0)	...

[a] Percentages are proportions of ICSI cycles.

Table 2. In vivo evolution and pregnancy outcome of embryos generated by intracytoplasmic sperm injection[a]. (*Ellipses* data not applicable)

	No. (%)	No. of complications in pregnancy evolution
Embryos replaced	8231	
Embryonic sacs implanted	2134 (25.9)	99 anembryonic sacs
Implanted embryos displaying a fetal heartbeat	1906 (23.2)	111 vanishing, 7 ectopics, 129 miscarriages, 64 selective reductions, 18 therapeutic abortions
Remaining fetal heartbeats at 20 weeks gestation	1577 (19.1)	13 fetal deaths
Live offspring delivered	1564 (19.0)	14 neonatal deaths
Surviving offspring	1550 (18.8)	...

[a] Percentages indicate proportion of embryos.

Table 3. Chromosomal assessment in patients with miscarriages

Karyotype	No. of cases	Mean maternal age (years)	Gestation type	
			Singleton	Twin
Trisomy 9	1	42.0	1	–
Trisomy 13	2	39.0	2	–
Trisomy 15	1	39.0	1	–
Trisomy 16	3	38.3	3	–
Trisomy 21	2	39.5	2	–
Trisomy 22	6	41.0	6	–
Trisomy 9; trisomy 16	2	35.0	–	2
Trisomy 7; trisomy 16	2	40.0	–	2
Double trisomy (18; 21)	1	40.0	1	–
Euploidy	7	36.4	6	1
Euploidy; trisomy 6	1	37.0	–	1
Euploidy; trisomy 13	1	36.0	–	1
Euploidy; trisomy 14	1	40.0	1	–
Euploidy; euploidy/trisomy 16	1	35.0	–	1

118 cases no data were available. The mean gestational age was 36.3 weeks for singletons, 33.9 weeks for twin gestations, and 31.9 weeks for triplets. Premature deliveries (before 37 weeks of gestation from the first day of the last menstrual period) occurred in 620/1042 cases (59.5%), the majority being multiple pregnancies (56.3%; $n = 349$). The mean birth weight was 3282 g for single pregnancies, 2539 g for twins, and 1960 g for triplets.

Only 27 of the 1564 newborns (1.7%) exhibited congenital abnormalities: 16 were major and 11 were minor (Table 5). As indicated, 20 (73.3%) of the malformations occurred in the multifetal gestations. Nonetheless, ICSI newborns experienced a lower rate of congenital malformations than that seen with standard IVF ($p < 0.0196$; Table 6).

Table 4. Indications for cesarean section in 1042 deliveries after ICSI (n=494)

Indication	No. of cases
Multiple pregnancy	273
Intrapartum fetal distress	20
Breech presentation	15
Preeclampsia	12
Placenta previa	8
Premature rupture of membranes with failed induction	5
Failure to progress due to cephalo-pelvic disproportion	10
Failure of second fetus to progress (first fetus delivered vaginally)	6
Transverse lie	3
Active herpes virus	4
Abruptio placentae	2
Failure to progress due to fibroid	2
Failed induction	4
Macrosomatia	4
Preeclampsia and transverse lie	1
Breech presentation and placenta previa	2
Oligohydramnios	4
Chorion amnionitis	1
Indications unavailable, not clear, or not identified	118
Total	

Table 5. Relationship of congenital malformation or chromosomal defect with pregnancy order

Category/abnormality	Gestation Type	
	Singleton	Multiple[a]
Major		
Cardiovascular	2	1
Chromosomal	2	1
Facial	0	2
Gastrointestinal	2	2
Neurological	1	2
Urological	0	1
Minor		
Cardiovascular	0	2
Neurological	1	0
Skeletal	1	0
Urogenital	3	4

[a] Multiple gestations: ten sets of twins, five sets of triplets.

To evaluate the effect of maternal age on pregnancy outcome after ICSI, three age-groups were considered: ≤35 years, 36–39 years, and ≥40 years (Table 7). For each category, implantation characteristics were examined, as well as pregnancy outcome and delivery rate. Among women ≤35 years old, the pregnancy wastage was only 2.8%, whereas among women 36–39 years old, pregnancy loss increased significantly to 4.5% and among those at least 40 years old to 6.5%

Table 6. Incidence of congenital abnormality in relation to the insemination technique

	Technique, n (%)	
	ICSI	IVF
Cycles	2607	2881
Offspring delivered	1564	1601
Newborns with major malformations	16 (1.0)	30 (1.9)
Newborns with minor malformations	11 (0.7)	24 (1.5)
Total malformations	27 (1.7)[a]	54 (3.4)[a]

a χ^2, 2 × 2, 1 df; Difference in congenital malformations between ICSI and IVF, $p < 0.01$.

Table 7. Pregnancy outcome and congenital abnormality rates according to maternal age

Maternal age (years)	No. of cycles	Pregnancies with		
		Positive fetal heartbeat (% of cycles)	Deliveries (% of cycles)	Abnormalities (% of deliveries)
≤35	1203	667 (55.4)[a]	626 (52.0)[b]	12 (1.7)
36–39	804	337 (41.9)[a]	288 (35.8)[b]	6 (0.7)
≥40	600	176 (29.3)[a]	128 (21.3)[b]	1 (0.2)
Total	2607	1180 (45.3)	1042 (40.0)	27 (1.0)

a χ^2, 2 × 3, 2 df; Difference in clinical pregnancy rate by maternal age, $p = 0.0001$.
b χ^2, 2 × 3, 2 df; Difference in delivery rate by maternal age, $p = 0.0001$.

($p < 0.001$). Similarly, the number of clinical pregnancies and subsequent deliveries appears markedly diminished for women 36–39 and at least 40 years of age ($p < 0.001$).

No differences were found in the miscarriage rate ($p = 0.965$) or in the frequency of congenital malformations as a function of spermatozoal maturity ($p = 0.97$; Table 8). For example, 45 of 70 patients whose cases involved testicular spermatozoa presented with a positive hCG titer; three of these pregnancies subsequently aborted. One such baby exhibited a ventricular septal defect.

For the purpose of examining any potential relationship between congenital abnormalities and severely compromised semen parameters, couples were divided into three groups:

1. Cryptozoospermic (i.e., sperm present only after processing)
2. Oligozoospermic ($\leq 1 \times 10^6$ spermatozoa in the ejaculate)
3. Those with no morphologically normal spermatozoa.

Our evidence indicates no correlation between congenital anomalies and any abnormal semen parameter (data not shown). In fact, there were no statistical differences in the frequency of congenital malformations between couples considered in these three groups and the remaining couples with less severely compromised semen.

Table 8. Pregnancy outcome in relation to semen origin. (*FHB* fetal heartbeat, *hCG* human chorionic gonadotropin)

Cycles	Ejaculated sperm ($n = 2296$)	Epididymal sperm ($n = 241$)	Testicular sperm ($n = 70$)
Positive hCGs	1279	157	45
Positive fetal heartbeats (% of cycles)	1010 (44.0)	134 (55.6)	36 (51.4)
Miscarriages (% of+FHB)	93 (9.2)	13 (9.7)	3 (8.3)
Ectopic pregnancies (% of+FHB)	6 (0.6)	0 (0.0)	1 (2.8)
Therapeutic abortions (% of+FHB)	13 (1.3)	1 (0.7)	1 (2.8)
Deliveries (% of cycles)	891 (69.7)	120 (76.4)	31 (44.3)
Deliveries with malformations (% of deliveries)	23 (2.6)	3 (2.5)	1 (3.2)

[a] Data not applicable.
[b] Pearson χ^2, with 2 *df*.

Discussion

A viable fetal heart developed in over 45% of the 2607 ICSI cycles in this study, with almost 39% resulting in the birth of live offspring. Pregnancy wastage was similar to that observed with conventional in vitro insemination, and to that seen at other centers where ICSI is performed [25, 26]. Cytogenetic information was obtained on 31 of the 109 patients who experienced a pregnancy loss, revealing that a chromosomal trisomy was responsible for 24 cases of arrested embryo growth. It is noteworthy that in this cohort of patients the mean maternal age was 38.4 years (range: 31-43). Similarly, in seven patients with a mean maternal age of 39.1 years, pregnancies were terminated due to chromosomal abnormalities (mainly trisomies) evidenced at prenatal diagnosis, which further supports the premise that aneuploidy increases with advancing maternal age [27-32]. Due to this more frequent occurrence of chromosomal abnormalities associated with increasing age, the rate of pregnancy loss was nearly three times higher in women ≥40 years than in those ≤35 years of age; in addition, clinical pregnancies and delivery rate were drastically diminished among patients older than 36 years.

A recent report of ICSI pregnancies described that a sex chromosomal abnormality was present in 27% of 15 cases [10]. However, these findings have not been confirmed by other centers that have reported an occurrence of sex chromosomal abnormalities ranging between 0.8% and 7.3% [33-36]. In the present study we encountered one sex chromosomal abnormality (Klinefelter's syndrome [37]; 47, XXY), representing a frequency of 0.17% (1/578); as such, it has not been clearly demonstrated that any specific genetic aberration is directly associated with the performance of ICSI [31, 32, 37].

When analyzing the phenotype of ICSI offspring, we encountered a 1.0% frequency of major malformations. This frequency was low compared with the 1.9% major malformations observed in our IVF population. It is also lower, however, than the 3.7% seen in the normal fertile population of the state of New York

[38]. These findings were supported by a previous study [39] that described a 3.8% major malformation rate in neonates born after treatment by ICSI, which corresponded to the frequency observed after standard IVF treatment (4.6%). An updated report by the same group [33] demonstrated that among an even greater number of ICSI newborns only 2.6% presented with congenital anomalies (23/877).

When the occurrence of congenital abnormalities following treatment by assisted reproduction is evaluated, the following factors must be considered: maternal age, infertility etiology and medical history, medications and/or drugs used for treatment, ovulation induction, and luteal phase support [8, 40–42]. Furthermore, microsurgical fertilization employs chemical compounds such as hyaluronidase, to digest the cumulus-corona cells, and polyvinylpyrrolidone, a medium used to decelerate spermatozoa prior to injection, not to mention the physical perforation of the zona pellucida, should be evaluated [17]. It was suggested that differences in the execution of the technique (e.g., the amount of cytoplasm aspirated during oocyte activation) might be responsible for the occurrence of zygote abnormalities [43]. Temperature fluctuations in the culture setting, as well as the possibly more vulnerable state of ICSI-generated zygotes/ embryos, which are sensitive to suboptimal or toxic culture conditions, should be also considered. All these elements may result in damage to the cytoskeleton and mitotic spindle of the fertilized oocyte, impairing subsequent embryo development and implantation. Thus the occurrence of congenital malformations after ICSI might be related to the specific setting and/or expertise of the team performing the procedure.

In this study we found that the highest frequency of congenital malformations was observed in neonates born from mothers in the most fertile age-group (i.e., ≤35 years). This is most likely due to the higher frequency of multiple gestations in this cohort of women. We reported a 45.8% frequency of multiple gestations, which is comparable to the 44.61% observed in our IVF series. Since the number of embryos replaced at our center was comparable to the average number replaced nationally [44], the higher occurrence of multiple pregnancies observed in this study appears to be related more to implantation efficiency rather than to the number of embryos replaced. The more frequent occurrence of congenital malformations in multifetal pregnancies compared with singleton gestations (3.0% and 2.3%, respectively) is similar to that other studies reporting on pregnancies resulting from assisted reproduction [45–47]. In fact, since there are inherent risks associated with high-order gestations, which account for nearly 46% of the pregnancies at our center, we are considering reducing the number of embryos replaced in selected couples for whom this reduction would not jeopardize their chances for a successful outcome.

To investigate whether a correlation exists between spermatozoal maturity and the frequency of malformations following assisted fertilization by ICSI, we compared the pregnancy outcome in cycles using freshly ejaculated, epididymal, and testicular spermatozoa. We observed only one abnormality (0.6%) in the 157 pregnancies resulting from the use of epididymal sperm. One malformation (2.2%) was reported in the 45 pregnancies with sperm from a testicular biopsy, which allows us to infer that the ICSI procedure is a relatively safe technique

[8]. The majority of the malformations occurred when freshly ejaculated semen was utilized ($n = 23$; 85.2%). When the fresh samples were severely oligo- or teratospermic, no remarkable differences were found in the occurrence of congenital abnormalities (2.3% and 2.5%, respectively) compared with couples who had less severely compromised semen parameters ($n = 1169$). In these couples, 12 of 457 deliveries included a malformation (2.6%). These data would seem to illustrate that no clear correlation can be established between suboptimal semen and frequency of congenital anomalies in ICSI offspring.

A theoretical concern regarding the use of suboptimal spermatozoa in ICSI is the potential for transmitting the genetic abnormalities responsible for male infertility [17, 19, 31, 32, 37, 48–50]. Despite this concern, ICSI is accepted as the only therapeutic option for patients with congenital absence of the vas deferens, a male genital tract abnormality associated with a gene deletion labeling these individuals as carriers of cystic fibrosis [51, 52]. Similarly, patients afflicted with Kartagener's syndrome or other ciliary dyskinesia may transmit the disease and their infertility to their offspring. In these cases, genetic screening and patient counseling are crucial, and preimplantation genetic testing as well as prenatal evaluation should be considered.

In summary, recent evidence demonstrates that the evolution of pregnancies and the occurrence of congenital malformations following treatment by ICSI are similar to the outcomes of other assisted reproduction procedures. As found in the more recent studies [7, 8, 36, 53–56], the outcome for these offspring is in the normal range and any frequency of congenital anomalies thus far reported seems to be nongenetic in nature and not clearly linked to sperm defects as presently classified. Nonetheless, genetic screening, including preimplantation and prenatal diagnosis, as well as genetic counseling should be offered to these patients, particularly those undergoing ICSI with immature gametes. Careful monitoring of the technique, together with continued, meticulous obstetric and pediatric follow-up, will certainly help to alleviate any concerns.

Acknowledgements. We thank the clinical and scientific staff of The Center for Reproductive Medicine and Infertility for their expert assistance.

References

1. Palermo G, Joris H, Devroey P, Van Steirteghem AC (1992) Pregnancies after intracytoplasmic injection of single spermatozoon into an oocyte. Lancet 340:17–18
2. Palermo G, Joris H, Derde MP, Camus M, Devroey P, Van Steirteghem AC (1993) Sperm characteristics and outcome of human assisted fertilization by subzonal insemination and intracytoplasmic sperm injection. Fertil Steril 59:826–835
3. Van Steirteghem AC, Liu J, Joris H, Nagy Z, Janssenwillen C, Tournaye H et al (1993) Higher success rate by intracytoplasmic sperm injection than by subzonal insemination. Report of a second series of 300 consecutive treatment cycles. Hum Reprod 8:1055–1060
4. Silber SJ, Nagy ZP, Liu J, Godoy H, Devroey P, Van Steirteghem AC (1994) Conventional IVF versus intracytoplasmic sperm injection for patients requiring microsurgical sperm aspiration. Hum Reprod 9:1705–1709

5. Schoysman R, Vanderzwalmen P, Nijs M, Segal L, Segal-Bertin G, Geerts L et al (1994) Pregnancy obtained with human testicular spermatozoa in an in vitro fertilisation program. J Androl 15 [Suppl]:10–3S

6. Bonduelle M, Desmyttere S, Buysse A, Van Assche E, Schietecatte J, Devroey P et al (1994) Prospective follow-up study of 55 children born after subzonal insemination and intracytoplasmic sperm injection. Hum Reprod 9:1765–1769

7. Bonduelle M, Hamberger L, Joris H, Tarlatzis BC, Van Steirteghem AC (1995) Assisted reproduction by intracytoplasmic sperm injection: an ESHRE survey of clinical experiences until December 1993. Hum Reprod Update 1:3, CD-ROM

8. Palermo GD, Colombero LT, Schattman GL, Davis OK, Rosenwaks Z (1996) Evolution of pregnancies and initial follow-up of newborns delivered after intracytoplasmic sperm injection. JAMA 276:1893–1897

9. Mitchell AA (1997) Intracytoplasmic sperm injection: offering hope for a term pregnancy and a healthy child? BMJ 315:13–14

10 In't Veld P, Brandenburg H, Verhoeff A, Dhont A, Los F (1995) Sex chromosomal abnormalities and intracytoplasmic sperm injection. Lancet 336:773

11. De Jonge C, Pierce J (1995) Intracytoplasmic sperm injection – what kind of reproduction is being assisted? Hum Reprod 10:2518–2520

12. Patrizio P (1995) Intracytoplasmic sperm injection (ICSI): potential genetic concerns. Hum Reprod 10:2520–2523

13. Kurinczuk JJ, Bower C (1997) Birth defects in infants conceived by intracytoplasmic sperm injection: an alternative interpretation. Br Med J 315:6–15

14. Bonduelle M, Devroey P, Liebaers I, Van Steirteghem A (1997) Major defects are overestimated. BMJ 315:11–12

15. Van Opstal D, Los FJ, Ramlakhan S, Van Hemel JO, Van Den Ouweland AMW, Brandenburg H, Pieters MHEC, Verhoeff A, Vermeer MCS, Dhont M, In't Veld PA (1997) Determination of the parent of origin in nine cases of prenatally detected chromosome aberrations found after intracytoplasmic sperm injection. Hum Reprod 12:682–686

16. Palermo G, Rosenwaks Z (1995) Assisted fertilization for male-factor infertility. Semin Reprod Endocr 13:39–52

17. Palermo GD, Cohen J, Rosenwaks Z (1996) Intracytoplasmic sperm injection: a powerful tool to overcome fertilization failure. Fertil Steril 65:899–908

18. Schlegel PN, Palermo GD, Goldstein M, et al (1997) Testicular sperm extraction with intracytoplasmic sperm injection for non-obstructive azoospermia. Urology 49:435–440

19. Palermo GD, Cohen J, Alikani M, Adler A, Rosenwaks Z (1995) Intracytoplasmic sperm injection:a novel treatment for all forms of male factor infertility. Fertil Steril 63:1231–1240

20. Palermo GD, Alikani M, Bertoli M, Colombero LT, Moy F, Cohen J, Rosenwaks Z (1996) Oolemma characteristics in relation to survival and fertilization patterns of oocytes treated by ICSI. Hum Reprod 11:172–176

21. Takeuchi T, Ergun B, Huang TH, Rosenwaks Z, Palermo GD (1999) A reliable technique of nuclear transplantation for immature mammalian oocytes. Hum Reprod 14:1312–1317

22. Cohen J, Alikani M, Adler A, Berkeley A, Davis O, Ferrara T et al (1992) Microsurgical fertilization procedures: absence of stringent criteria for a patient selection. J Assist Reprod Gen 9:197–206

23. Smith DW (1975) Classification, nomenclature and naming of morphological defects. J Pediatr 87:162–164

24. Holmes LB (1976) Congenital malformations. N Engl J Med 295:204–207

25. Medical Research International (MRI), Society for Assisted Reproductive Technology (SART), The American Fertility Society (1992) In-vitro fertilization-embryo transfer (IVF-ET) in the United States: 1990 results from the IVF-ET Registry. Fertil Steril 57:15–24

26. Wisanto A, Magnus M, Bonduelle M, Liu J, Camus M, Tournaye H et al (1995) Obstetric outcome of 424 pregnancies after intracytoplasmic sperm injection. Hum Reprod 10:2713–2718

27. Hassold T, Chiu D (1985) Maternal age-specific rates of numerical chromosome abnormalities with special reference to trisomy. Hum Genet 70:11–17
28. Warburton D, Kline J, Stein Z, Strobino B (1986) Cytogenetic abnormalities in spontaneous abortions of recognized conceptions. In: Porter IH, Willey A (eds) Perinatal genetics: diagnosis and treatment. Academic, New York, pp 133–148
29. Munné S, Dailey T, Sultan KM, Grifo J, Cohen J (1995) The use of first polar bodies for preconception diagnosis of aneuploidy. Hum Reprod 10:1014–1020
30. Munné S, Alikani M, Tomkin G, Grifo J, Cohen J (1995) Embryo morphology, developmental rates and maternal age are correlated with chromosomal abnormalities. Fertil Steril 64:382–391
31. Colombero LT, Hariprashad JJ, Tsai MC, Rosenwaks Z, Palermo GD (1999) Incidence of sperm aneuploidy in relation to semen characteristics and assisted reproductive outcome. Fertil Steril 72:90–96
32. Palermo, GD, Schlegel PN, Hariprashad JJ, Ergun B, Mielnik A, Zaninovic N, Veeck LL, Rosenwaks Z (1999) Fertilization and pregnancy outcome with intracytoplasmic sperm injection for azoospermic men. Hum Reprod 14:741–748
33. Liebaers I, Bonduelle M, Van Assche E, Devroey P, Van Steirteghem A (1995) Sex chromosomal abnormalities after intracytoplasmic sperm injection (letter). Lancet 346:1095
34. Govaerts I, Englert Y, Vamos E, Rodesch F (1995) Sex chromosomal abnormalities after intracytoplasmic sperm injection (letter). Lancet 346:1096
35. Aytoz A, Camus M, Tournaye H, Bonduelle M, Van Steirteghem A, Devroey P (1998) Outcome of pregnancies after intracytoplasmic sperm injection and the effect of sperm origin and quality on this outcome. Fertil Steril 70:500–505
36. Bonduelle M, Aytoz A, Van Assche E, Devroey P, Liebaers I, Van Steirteghem A (1998) Incidence of chromosomal aberrations in children born after assisted reproduction through intracytoplasmic sperm injection. Hum Reprod 13:781–782
37. Palermo GD, Schlegel PN, Sills ES, Veeck LL, Zaninovic N, Menendez S, Rosenwaks Z (1998) Births after intracytoplasmic injection of sperm obtained by testicular extraction from men with nonmosaic Klinefelter's syndrome. N Engl J Med 338:588–590
38. New York State Department of Health (1990) Congenital malformations registry: annual report. Albany, New York
39. Bonduelle M, Legein J, Buysse A, Devroey P, Van Steirteghem AC, Liebaers I (1994) Comparative follow-up study of 130 children born after ICSI and 130 children born after ICSI and 130 children born after IVF. Proc 10th Ann Meeting of the European Society of Human Reproduction and Embryology, 1994. Hum Reprod 9 [Suppl 4]:38
40. Sclesselmann JJ (1979) How does one assess the risk of abnormalities from human invitro fertilization? Am J Obstet Gynecol 135:135–148
41. Biggers JD (1981) In vitro fertilization and embryo transfer in human beings. N Engl J Med 304:336–342
42. Lancaster P (1987) Congenital malformations after in-vitro fertilization. Lancet 2:1511
43. Tesarik J (1995) Sex chromosomal abnormalities after intracytoplasmic sperm injection (letter). Lancet 346:1096
44. Svendsen TO, Jones D, Butler L, Muasher SJ (1996) The incidence of multiple gestations after in vitro fertilization is dependent on the number of embryos transferred and maternal age. Fertil Steril 65:561–565
45. Cohen J, Mayaux MJ, Guihard-Moscato ML (1988) Pregnancy outcomes after in vitro fertilization. Ann N Y Acad Sci 541:1–6
46. Doyle PE, Beral V, Botting B, Wale CJ (1990) Congenital malformations in twins in England and Wales. J Epidemiol Community Health 45:43–48
47. Aytoz A, De Catte L, Camus M, Bonduelle M, Van Assche E, Liebaers I, Van Steirteghem A, Devroey P (1998) Obstetrics outcome after prenatal diagnosis in pregnancies obtained after intracytoplasmic sperm injection. Hum Reprod 13:2958–2961
48. Ma K, Inglis JD, Sharkey A, Bickmore WA, Hill RE, Prosser EJ et al (1993) A Y-chromosome gene family with RNA-binding protein homology: candidates for the azoospermia factor AZF controlling human spermatogenesis. Cell 75:1287–1295

49. Kobayashi K, Mizuno K, Hida A, Komaki R, Tomita K, Matsushita L et al (1994) PCR analysis of the Y-chromosome long arm in azoospermic patients: evidence for a second locus required for spermatogenesis. Hum Mol Genet 3:1965–1967
50. Brandell RA, Mielnik A, Liotta D, Ye Z, Veeck LL, Palermo GD, Schlegel PN (1998) AZFb deletions predict the absence of spermatozoa with testicular sperm extraction: preliminary report of a prognostic genetic test. Hum Reprod 13:2812–2815
51. Patrizio P, Asch RH, Handelin B, Silber SJ (1993) Aetiology of congenital absence of the vas deferens: genetic study of three generations. Hum Reprod 8:215–220
52. Schlegel PN, Cohen J, Goldstein M, et al (1995) Cystic fibrosis gene mutations do not affect sperm function during in vitro fertilization with micromanipulation for men with bilateral congenital absence of the vas deferens. Fertil Steril 64:421–426
53. Bonduelle M, Joris H, Hofmans K, Liebaers I, Van Steirteghem A (1998) Mental development of 201 ICSI children at 2 years of age. Lancet 22:1553–1554
54. Baron L, Basso G, Blanco L, Valzacchi R (1998) Psychological follow-up of children born after intracytoplasmic sperm injection (ICSI). Proc 16th Ann Meeting of The American Society of Reproductive Medicine. Fertil Steril 70 [Suppl 1]:S29
55. ESHRE Task Force on Intracytoplasmic Sperm Injection (1998) Assisted reproduction by intracytoplasmic sperm injection: a survey on the clinical experience in 1994 and the children born after ICSI, carried out until 31 December 1993. Hum Reprod 13:1737–1746
56. Sutcliffe AG, Taylor B, Li J, Thornton S, Grudzinskas JG, Lieberman BA (1999) Children born after intracytoplasmic sperm injection: population control study. Br Med J 318:704–705

Outcome of Children Born after In Vitro Fertilization (IVF) and Intracytoplasmic Sperm Injection (ICSI)*

M. Ludwig, K. Diedrich

In Vitro Fertilization and Intracytoplasmic Sperm Injection

Is There a Health Risk for the Children?

When the first child was born after in vitro fertilization (IVF) in 1978, a new treatment option became available for previously infertile couples [49]. Tubal obstruction no longer meant that the couple had to go without children of their own. Major statistical evaluations suggest that up to 60% of all couples conceive after up to four IVF attempts.

In 1992, Palermo et al. [36] reported the first births after a method they called intracytoplasmic sperm injection (ICSI): They had succeeded in injecting individual sperms into oocytes. Further studies revealed that it was now possible to achieve oocyte fertilization and pregnancy even in severe cases of male subfertility [54, 55]. A few years later, there were reports about the success of this treatment in men with azoospermia when epididymal [47] or testicular aspirates [16] were used. The aspiration of sperm from the epididymides (MESA, microsurgical epididymal sperm aspiration) and from the testes (TESE, testicular sperm extraction) and their use in ICSI have now become well-established procedures worldwide. Conservative estimates suggest that more than 300000 children have been born after this type of treatment.

Are There Any Risks for the Children?

The health of children born after IVF and ICSI has been under critical review for some time now. Some argued that the expectations pinned on a "imaginary child" born after "cold" conception could influence the "warm parent-child relationship"; others feared that the expectations could not be met by the "real" child actually born, and that this would result in developmental problems in early childhood [24]. Colpin et al. [13], finally, criticized that the physician

---

* This paper was previously published in German as: Ludwig M, Diedrich K (1999) In vitro Fertilisation und intrazytoplasmatische Spermieninjektion: Gibt es ein Gesundheitsrisiko für die geborenen Kinder? Dtsch Arztebl 96:A-2892–2901. The paper has been changed and updated.

could disrupt the parent-child relationship as a "third parent". In particular, there were concerns about whether these "unnatural" techniques could provoke an increased incidence of malformation.

Critics believed that ICSI might be associated with additional genetic risks such as increased chromosomal aberrations, mutations of the cystic fibrosis gene (CFTR), and Y-chromosomal deletions in subfertile men. These risks were recently summarized and critically discussed in a review [18]. For this reason, we have set out to investigate the following questions:

- What data are available on the development of children born after conventional IVF treatment?
- Is there any influence of cryopreservation on the incidence of abnormalities in childbirth and postnatal development?
- Is there an increased health risk for children conceived by ICSI?

Postnatal Development of Children after In Vitro Fertilization

Large volumes of data concerning the rate of malformations in children after IVF treatment have been published in the past 20 years. Not a single publication has demonstrated a difference in the malformation rate of IVF children.

Quality of Parenting

In contrast to the above-described expectation of an abnormally negative family structure, no difference emerged in the various publications between spontaneously conceived children and those born after hormonal stimulation [13, 41]. Kentenich and Stauber [25] found no difference in breast-feeding behavior between IVF mothers and the mothers of spontaneously conceived children.

Other authors did describe differences between the two groups of children, but these differences were rather in favor of the new reproductive techniques: Weaver et al. [57] found a tendency to increased caring for the child (overprotection), and Golombok et al. [20] observed a more emotional way of treating the children as well as increased involvement of the father in the parent-child relationship. In another publication, these authors found that the parent-child relationship is of a higher quality in IVF families [19]. A recent study looked at the situation in families with IVF twins. In a very small study population of only 14 families, the authors found a higher stress level among the parents and saw this as a reflection of the high demands the parents put on the quality of parenting. However, it cannot be ruled out that these differences will even out if the relatively small population is increased and that other factors, such as the much higher proportion of multiparae in the control population may have caused the difference [14], since multiparae are known to be under less stress from parenting.

In a retrospective-prospective study, Braverman et al. [10] recently tried to collect data about the development of pregnancy, but also about parenthood after IVF. It emerged that the parents had a positive attitude both to pregnancy and to parenthood as such; they did not consider the IVF parents to be more cautious than non-IVF parents in dealing with their children and saw no difference with respect to medical or emotional problems.

None of the references was able to show any abnormal development for these children (Tables 1–3). However, various authors pointed out that, naturally, the multiple pregnancy rate and the consequently higher rate of prematurity affects the overall morbidity of the children. Therefore, reducing the multiple pregnancy rate is one of the foremost goals of modern infertility therapy and has been included in the new revised Guidelines for Assisted Reproduction issued by the Federal Chamber of Physicians in Germany [61].

Cryopreservation of Embryos

In Germany, only fertilized oocytes, but no zygotes (embryos), may be cryopreserved. However, some experience with the cryopreservation of embryos has accumulated in other countries.

The first study concerning the health of 283 children born after embryo cryopreservation, thawing, and transfer showed no difference in malformation rate and perinatal data when compared with 253 children born after embryo transfer, but without cryopreservation [57].

Sutcliffe et al. [50] published the data of 91 children born after embryo cryopreservation with an average age of 2 years (25.08±12.86 months). The Griffith scale, which is used to assess mental development, showed normal results.

Salat-Baroux et al. [44] studied 84 children with an average age of 5.2±1.0 years. They found a normal malformation rate of 4.7%. The other data about these children were also in the expected range.

Table 1. Postnatal development of children after IVF, aged between 9 and 14 months[a]

Reference	No.	Age (months)	Test/criterion	Result
[63][b]	20	12	Griffith scale	Better and faster development in some cases
[40][c]	37	9	Psychomotor development	Normal
[43][b]	1411	~12	Physical development	Normal (but effect of higher prematurity rate!)
			Diseases	
			Malformations	
[8][c]	84	13	Bayley Scale	
			Malformations	Normal

[a] No study showed any abnormal development. The only remarkable finding is the higher rate of prematurity, which is due to the higher multiple pregnancy rate in the study population.
[b] Study not controlled.
[c] Study controlled.

Finally, Olivennes et al. [34] studied a population of 89 children aged between 1 and 9 years after cryopreservation at the embryonic stage. No developmental difference was found compared with an age-matched normal population.

Although the data available are limited, the conclusion at this stage can only be that an assumption of differences with respect to malformation rate and postpartum development after cryopreservation is not warranted.

Table 2. Postnatal development of children after IVF, aged between 1 and 7 years [a]

Reference	No.	Age (months)	Test	Design	Results
[33]	33	12–37	Bayley Scale	Noncontrolled	Normal
[32]	83	13–30	Bayley Scale	Controlled	Normal (higher values for mental and psycho-motor development)
[15]	173	12–43	–	Noncontrolled	Normal
[9]	31	30–45	Standford-Binet Intelligence Scale	Controlled, blind, matching	Normal
[9]	85	12–30	Bayley Scale	Controlled, blind, matching	Normal
[41]	30	≥28	General Cognitive Index	Controlled, blind	Normal
[45]	314	22.5–25.5	Physical development	Controlled	Normal
[11]	99	33–85	Griffith Scale, Achenbach Child Behavior Check-list	Controlled	Normal
[6]	131	22–26	Bayley Scale	Controlled	Normal

[a] Most studies used a measuring system to assess mental development (Bayley, Standford-Binet, and Griffith Scales) and were at least controlled studies. In two studies, clear matching criteria were possible. In these cases, the examiner did not know whether the child came from the IVF or the control population. No indications for any abnormal mental development were found.

Table 3. School performance of IVF children, aged 6–13 years [a] (from [27])

Performance level	No.	Percentage
Gifted	8	2.2
≥1 year ahead	24	6.5
<1 year ahead	180	48.6
Average	129	34.9
<1 year behind	14	3.8
≥1 year behind	14	3.8
Special school	1	0.2

[a] Study concerned school performance compared with the expected performance of spontaneously conceived peers. More than 90% of the IVF children either showed average performance or were ahead of their non-IVF peers. One child attended a special school because of mental retardation (Down's syndrome).

Intracytoplasmic Sperm Injection

Prenatal Diagnosis

Table 4 provides an overview of the prenatal chromosome analysis data. Apart from the three studies discussed below, the results match those known from normal pregnancies. In't Veld et al. [24] reported a 33% increase in chromosomal abnormalities after ICSI, but the study group comprised only 15 cases. As a human geneticist, In't Veld does not have any cases of his own but was referring to diagnostic findings made available to him, so that a high degree of selection must be assumed. However, this letter to *The Lancet* raised serious concerns about the safety of ICSI. A similar assessment must be made of the findings of van Opstal et al. [54], who reported nine chromosomal abnormalities among 71 fetuses which had undergone invasive prenatal diagnosis. Again, the patient group had been preselected instead of representing the total number of findings of a single center. A further interesting factor is that, according to the authors, 25 of the 71 prenatal examinations were carried out because of the mothers' age, two because of abnormalities on prenatal ultrasound, and two due to previous pregnancies resulting in children with congenital abnormalities. No details are given as to which group the abnormal cases originated from. Palermo et al. [38], too, report an abnormality rate of 7.3%, but, again, there seems to be considerable selection involved. In only 9.8% of a total of 1105 pregnancies was prenatal diagnosis performed.

The most comprehensive information about this aspect has been provided by a group working with van Steirteghem [7]. They performed 1082 prenatal diag-

Table 4. Chromosomal abnormalities after ICSI[a]

Reference	Type	Number	Percentage
[24]	De novo	5/15	33.3
	Inherited	0/15	–
ICSI Task Force 1994 [3]	–	8/361	2.2
[53]	De novo	0/108	–
	Inherited	5/7	71.4
[54]	De novo	9/71	12.7
[5]	De novo	2/70	2.9
[31]	Inherited	3/18	16.7
[7]	De novo	18/1082	1.7
	Inherited	10/1082	0.9
[29]	De novo	0/74	–
	Inherited	2/4	50
ICSI Task Force 1995 [28]	–	15/666	2.3
[38]	–	11/150	7.3

[a] Incidence of chromosomal abnormalities found on invasive prenatal diagnosis after ICSI. The table lists the incidence (if known) of de novo and inherited abnormalities. In most cases, the incidence of de novo abnormalities is on the same level as is usual for spontaneous pregnancies. The high incidences found by In't Veld et al. [24], Van Opstal et al. [54], and Palermo et al. [38] are due to selection of the pregnant women.

nostic examinations with 28 findings of genetic abnormality. Ten cases involved inherited abnormalities which can be traced to the increased rate of chromosomal abnormality in men with a reduced sperm count. In Germany, these men have for many years been advised to undergo chromosomal analysis, a principle included recently in the Guidelines for Assisted Reproduction (see comment on Article 3.2.13), which means it has become part of the Professional Medical Code (Scientific Board of the Federal Chamber of Physicians, 1998 [61]. This is to ensure that the couples are given balanced genetic advice before ICSI is carried out.

Thus, the data provided by Bonduelle et al. [7] suggest a de novo abnormality rate of about 1.7%. There were nine cases of gonosomal disorders, five findings of autosomal trisomy, and four of structural aberration. Although the rate of gonosomal abnormalities seems to be marginally increased, it should be borne in mind that, while it does call for further investigation, nine in 1082 cases is a low rate.

Nevertheless, it has rightly been concluded from these data that couples must be informed of this situation prior to undergoing ICSI. Additionally, it should be considered that many of the aberrations described rarely lead to aberrations at birth and sometimes become known only later in life, e.g., when the person concerned wants to start a family. On the other hand, against this background, the decision to undergo ICSI should be left completely up to the couple concerned. We can report that, in our experience, not a single couple has decided against treatment because of this risk. Although we inform each couple about the risks involved, only 35% of the couples want invasive prenatal diagnosis to be performed.

Malformations

The malformation rate found with some consistency after ICSI is 3–5% (Table 5). This corresponds to the rate given by major international malformation registers. It should therefore be fair to assume that the malformation rate at birth is not increased by ICSI. However, various skeptics have challenged this assumption. One reason is a publication by the Australian authors Kurinczuk and Bower [26], reviewing the data published by the Brussels working group. Using the Australian malformation catalogue, they calculated a malformation rate of more than 7%. The reason was that the Brussels group had used their own, nonrecognized malformation score, which distinguishes only between "major" and "minor" malformations. According to this score, the criterion for a "major" malformation is a physical handicap of the child or a necessary operation. The Australians compared this rate of more than 7% with the results of their own perinatal statistics based on more than 100 000 children showing a malformation rate of 2–3%, i.e., significantly less. They concluded that the malformation rate is increased by ICSI. The problem with this finding is that the malformation rates compared are based on different statistical criteria. The Brussels data were collected by human geneticists on a prospective and stan-

Table 5. Incidence of major malformations after ICSI

Reference	No. of severe malformations as a ratio of children born (%)
[2]	6/273 (2.2)
[3]	23/848 (2.7)
[21]	3/76 (3.9)
[37]	9/578 (1.6)
[4]	23/877 (2.6)
[59]	2/210 (1.0)
[3]	18/763 (2.3)
[28]	127/6692 (1.9)
[17]	18/662 (2.7)
[17a]	48/2665 (1.8)
[22]	4/143 (2.8)
[8]	4/89 (4.5)
[7]	4/164 (2.4)
[6]	57/1987 (2.9)
Danish Fertility Society [27]	17/730 (2.2)
[38]	23/1131 (2.0)
[30]	9/267 (3.4)
[60]	47/1192 (3.9)
FIVNAT [42]	65/2332 (2.8)
[52]	9/207 (4.3)
[48]	2/100 (2.0)
[1]	13/206 (6.3)[b]
[62]	1/76 (1.3)

[a] Incidence of major malformations found at birth in ICSI children. The malformation rates range between 1% and 6%. This corresponds to the incidence to be expected after spontaneous conception. The table covers more than 17 000 children from various national studies (Australia, Belgium, Denmark, Egypt, France, Germany, Great Britain, The Netherlands, Sweden, Switzerland, Turkey, USA) and from the global statistics of the ESHRE (European Society of Human Reproduction and Embryology) Task Force on ICSI.
[b] In this study from 934 pregnancies only 161 could be followed up (lost to follow-up rate: 83%). Therefore, a preselection may explain this slightly higher malformation rate. In the control group of this study from the same hospital, however, the malformation rate was also in the same range.

dardized basis including laboratory procedures, whereas the Australian perinatal analysis is a nonstandardized passive survey. This methodological shortcoming is confirmed by the data from other groups who have examined spontaneously conceived children for several years in a standardized way similar to the one used by the Brussels group. For example, Queißer-Luft and Spranger [39] published the data of 20 248 children from the German region of Mainz analyzed in a prospective, standardized malformation register called the Mainz model. There, too, the malformation rate is 7.3%. If the Brussels working group had included a control group in their study, Kurinczuk's and Bower's observation [26] would probably not have been made.

Therefore, a prospective, controlled study including a standardized examination of the children as well as the use of a standardized code of malformations is required in order to arrive at a reliable malformation rate after ICSI; the control group must consist of children born after spontaneous conception in the same period. Such a nation-wide multicenter study was launched in August 1998 and will produce reliable findings about the malformation rate after ICSI by mid 2001. The question is how to assess the malformation risk after ICSI until then. So far, there is no study without methodological shortcomings which shows an increased malformation risk after ICSI. The revised Guidelines on Assisted Reproduction issued by the Federal Chamber of Physicians unambiguously conclude that there is an "indication for ICSI if it is highly unlikely to achieve pregnancy because of severe male infertility or other reasons...".

Postnatal Development

Bowen et al. [8] published a study of 89 children born after ICSI, 84 children born after IVF, and 80 spontaneously conceived children. It looked at the developmental status of the children who had an average age of 13 months. The authors used the Bayley Score and measured not just the mental developmental index (MDI) but also the physical developmental index (PDI). The latter showed no significant differences between the three groups in any respect, while the MDI of boys born after ICSI was significantly lower than those for the two other groups. In the same edition of *The Lancet*, Bonduelle et al. [6] reported on 201 children born after ICSI and 131 children born after IVF and aged between 22 and 26 months. Using the same examination procedure, they found no MDI difference between ICSI and IVF children. Compared with the reference group, these children tended to be 1–3 months ahead of what could be expected at their age. This was true for both girls and boys.

When assessing these conflicting findings critically, it should be borne in mind that the children of the Bowen et al. study [8] are younger than those examined by Bonduelle et al. [6]. The population in the latter study is more than twice as large, so Bonduelle's findings should be considered more meaningful since the same examination methods were used. Looking more closely at the social background of the ICSI children examined by Bowen et al. [8], we observe that there are significant differences in the level of education and the number of foreigners among the ICSI parents compared with the other two groups.

It is also interesting, against this background, to note that the head of the Bowen et al. working group [6], Professor Saunders from Australia, has distanced himself from his own findings due to similar arguments made in another publication [45].

The inconspicuous results of the children were confirmed in a recent study by Sutcliffe et al. [51, 52] including 207 children born after ICSI who were compared with a matched control group. The results of this study were published in two parts with a smaller series first [51] and a larger one later [52]. In the larger series no differences were found between the two groups; these results were presented during the 15th annual meeting of the European Society of Human

Reproduction and Embryology. A total of 220 children born after ICSI were compared with 221 born after natural conception, after matching for several factors. In all, 22 IVF centers in the United Kingdom were involved in the recruitment of these children. The ICSI and control groups were comparable regarding all matching criteria; however, the maternal age, which was not a matching criterion, was significantly higher in the ICSI compared with the control population (mean: 33.56 vs. 30.42 years). The Griffith scale, which was used to measure the mental development at 1.5 years of age in both groups was not significantly different (mean: 98.1 vs. 98.7). In this final analysis all subscales were also comparable. In the first analysis [51] there was a significantly lower score for the eye-hand coordination ($p < 0.05$). However, this was discussed as having no impact for the further development of these children, and the difference was no longer present in the final analysis. Even if these data are interpreted with less caution, the practical conclusion can only be that more data on the development of ICSI children need to be gathered.

Conclusion

For several years now, the health of children born after IVF and ICSI treatment has been under critical review. Neither conventional IVF treatment nor cryopreservation was associated with an increased risk for the children with respect to abnormal family structures, malformations, or abnormalities in their further postnatal development.

The data regarding ICSI are not conclusive because the studies have failed to produce complete clarity owing to design errors. The least we can say is that the data currently available do not meet the demands of evidence-based medicine. There is no evidence of an increased risk of malformation at birth or abnormal postnatal development if the available information is analyzed critically. The views of German reproductive scientists are in line with international scientific opinion: ICSI is one of the established methods of assisted reproduction; it is the only effective treatment for severe male subfertility and is apparently not associated with an increased risk for the children born. Nevertheless, considering the importance of the issue, further studies are required both in Germany and internationally in order to corroborate the safety of ICSI.

References

1. Aboulgar MA, Mansour RT, Serour GI, Amin Y (1999) A prospective study of 206 babies born after intracytoplasmic sperm injection (ICSI). Fertil Steril 72 [Suppl 1]:7
2. Bonduelle M, Hanberger L, Joris H (1995) Assisted reproduction by ICSI: an ESHRE survey of clinical experiences until 3 December 1993. Hum Reprod Update 1:CD-ROM
3. Bonduelle M, Legein J, Wilkins A et al (1995) Follow-up study of children born after intracytoplasmic sperm injection. Hum Reprod 10:52–54
4. Bonduelle M, Legein J, Buysse A et al (1996) Prospective follow-up study of 423 children born after intracytoplasmic sperm injection. Hum Reprod 11:1558–1564

5. Bonduelle M, Aytoz A, Wilikens A et al (1998) Prospective follow-up study of 1987 children bom after intracytoplasmic sperm injection (ICSI). In: Filicori M, Falmigni C (eds) Treatment of infertility: the new frontiers. Communications Media for Education, Inc., New Jersey, pp 446–460

6. Bonduelle M, Joris H, Hofmans K et al (1998) Mental development of 201 ICSI children at 2 years of age. Lancet 351:1553

7. Bonduelle M, Willkens A, Buysse A, et al (1998) A follow-up study of children born after intracytoplasmic sperm injection (ICSI) with epididymal and testicular spermatozoa and after replacement of cryopreserved embryos obtained after ICSI. Hum Reprod 13 [Suppl 1]:196–207

8. Bowen JR, Gibson FL, Leslie Gl, Saunders DM (1998) Medical and developmental outcome at 1 year for children conceived by intracytoplasmic sperm injection. Lancet 351:1529–1534

9. Brandes JM, Scher A, Itzkovits J et al (1992) Growth and development of children conceived by in vitro fertilization. Pediatrics 90:424–429

10. Braverman AM, Boxer AS, Corson SL, et al (1998) Characteristics and attitudes of parents of children born with the use of assisted reproductive technology. Fertil Steril 70:860–865

11. Cederblad M, Friberg B, Ploman F et al (1996) Intelligence and behaviour in children born after in-vitro fertilization treatment. Hum Reprod 11:2052–2057

12. Coetsier T, Dhont M (1998) Avoiding multiple pregnancies in in-vitro fertillzation: who's afraid of single embryo transfer? Hum Reprod 13:2663–2664

13. Colpin H, Demyttenaere K, Vandemeulebroecke L (1995) New reproductive technology and the family: the parent-child relationship following in vitro fertilisation. J Child Psychol Psychiatry 36:1429–1441

14. Cook R, Bradley S, Golorribok S (1998) A preliminary study of parental stress and child behaviour in families with twins conceived by in-vitro fertilization. Hum Reprod 13:3244–3246

15. De Vos M, Alberda AT (1991) Follow-up of children born after IVF-treatment. 7th world congress on IVF and assisted procreation. Paris

16. Devroey P, Liu J, Nagy Z et al (1994) Normal fertilization of human oocytes after testicular sperm extraction and intracytoplasmic sperm injection. Fertil Steril 62:639–641

17. D.I.R. (1996) Deutsches IVF-Register

17a. D.I.R. (1998) Deutsches IVF-Register

18. Engel W, Schmid M, Pauer H-U (1998) Genetik und mikroassistierte Reproduktion durch intrazytoplasmatische Spermieninjektion. Dtsch Arztebl 95:1548–1553

19. Golombok S, Cook R, Bish A, Murray C (1994) New techniques in assisted contraception. Parents and their children happy with assisted conception. Br Med J 308:658–659

20. Golombok S, Brewaeys A, Cook R et al (1996) The European study of assisted reproduction families: family functioning and child development. Hum Reprod 11:2324–2331

21. Govaerts 1, Englert Y, Vamos E, Rodesch F (1995) Sex chromosome abnormalities after intracytoplasmic sperm injection. Lancet 346:1095–1096

22. Govaerts 1, Devreker F, Koenig I et al (1998) Comparison of pregnancy outcome after intracytoplasmic sperm injection and in-vitro fertilization. Hum Reprod 13:1514–1518

23. Hammer-Burns L (1987) Infertility as a boundary ambiguity: one theoretical perspective. Fam Process 26:359–372

24. In't Veld P, Brandenburg H, Verhoeff A et al (1995) Sex cromosomal abnormalities and intracytoplasmic sperm injection. Lancet 346:773

25. Kentenich H, Stauber M (1992) Schwangerschaft, Geburt und Partnerschaft in einer Familie mit "Retortenbaby". Psychother Psychosom Med Psychol 42:228–235

26. Kudnczuk JJ, Bower C (1997) Birth defects in infants conceived by intracytoplasmic sperm injection: an alternative interpretation. Br Med J 315:1260–1266

27. Loft A, Ejdrup B, Pedersen K et al (1998) Outcome after intracytoplasmic sperm injection (ICSI) – a Danish national cohort of 506 infants. Fertil Steril 70 [Suppl 1]:350

28. Ludwig M, Küpker W, Al-Hasani, Diedrich K (1996) Die intracytoplasmatische Spermatozoeninjektion (ICSI): Überblick über die aktuelle Situation. Frauenarzt 37:1624–1634

29. Ludwig M, Al-Hasani S, Ghasemi M, Gizycki U, Küpker W, Diedrich K (1999) Intrazy-toplasmatische Spermatozoeninjektion – ICSI (II). Geburt und Gesundheit von 267 Kindern. Geburtsh Frauenheilkd 59:395–401

30. Ludwig M, Geipel A, Küpker W, Al-Hasani S, Ghasemi M, Gizycki U, Diedrich K (1999) Intrazytoplasmatische Spermieninjektion – ICSI (I). Verlauf von 310 Schwan-gerschaften und Ergebnisse der Pränataldiagnostik. Geburtsh Frauenheilkd 59:387–394

31. Meschede D, Lemcke B, Stüssel J et al (1998) Strong preference for non-invasive prena-tal diagnosis in women pregnant through intracytoplasmic sperm injection (ICSI). Pre-nat Diag 18:700–705

32. Morin NC, Wirth FH, Johnson DH et al (1989) Congenital malformations and psycho-social development in children conceived by in vitro fertilization. J Pediatr 115:222–227

33. Mushin DN, Barreda-Hanson MC, Spensley JC (1986) In vitro fertilization children: early psychosocial development. J InVitro Fertil Embryo Transf 3:247–252

34. Olivennes F, Schneider Z, Remy V, et al (1996) Perinatal outcome and follow-up of 82 children aged 1–9 years old conceived from cryopreserved embryos. Hum Reprod 11:1565–1568

35. Olivennes F, Kerbrat V, Rufat P, et al (1997) Follow-up of a cohort of 422 children aged 6 to 13 years conceived by in vitro fertilization. Fertil Steril 67:284–289

36. Palermo G, Joris H, Devroey H, Van Steirteghem AC (1992) Pregnancies after intracy-toplasmic sperm injection of single spermatozoon into an oocyte. Lancet 340:17–18

37. Palermo G, Colombero RT, Schattman GL, Davis OK, Rosenwaks Z (1996) Evolution of pregnancies and initial follow-up of newborns delivered after intracytoplasmic sperm injection. JAMA 276:1893–1897

38. Palermo GD, Ergun B, Takeuchi T, Sills ES, Alonson L, Rosenwaks Z (1998) Maternal age as a factor in the embryonic and fetal abnormalities that occur following ICSI. In: Filicori M, Flamigni C (eds) Treatment of infertility: the new frontiers. Communica-tions Media for Education. Inc., New Jersey, pp 429–434

39. Queißer-Luft A, Spranger J (1997) Fehlbildungen bei Neugeborenen: Mainzer Modell. Kinderarzt 3764:1–6

40. Raoul-Duval A, Bertrand-Servais M, Frydman R (1990) Etude prospective et compara-tive du devenir des enfants nes par fecondation in vitro et de leumere. J Gynecol Ob-stet Biol Reprod 19:203–208

41. Ron-EL R, Lahat E, Golan A et al (1994) Development of children born after ovarian superovulation induced by long-acting gonadotropin-releasing hormone agonist and menotropins, and by in vitro fertilization. J Pediatr 125:734–737

42. Rossin-Amar B, Safi A, Pouly JL, Mouzon J (1999) Analysis of babies conceived by ICSI. Comparison with babies born after conventional in-vitro fertilization or natural conception. Hum Reprod 14:79–80

43. Rufat P, Olivennes F, de Mouzon J et al (1994) Task force report on the outcome of pregnancies and children conceived by in vitro fertilization (France: 1987 to 1989). Fer-til Steril 61:324–330

44. Salat-Baroux J, Mandelbaum J, Junca AM et al (1996) Cryopreservation of human em-bryos after in vitro fertilization: immediate and long-term results. Bull Acad Natl Med 180:83–91

45. Saunders D (1998) Follow-up of ICSI children. Access 5:9–10

46. Saunders K, Spensely J, Munro J, Halasz G (1996) Growth and physical outcome of chil-dren conceived by in vitro fertilization: Pediatrics 97:688–692

47. Silber SJ, Nagy Z, Liu J et al (1995) The use of epididymal and testicular spermatozoa for intracytoplasmic sperm injection: the genetic implications for male infertility. Hum Reprod 10:2031–2043

48. Singh L, Senn A, De Grandi P, Germond M (1999) Follow-up of 100 children, aged 1 and 2 years, born after intracytoplasmic sperm injection. Hum Reprod 14 (Abstract book): 58

49. Steptoe PC, Edwards RG (1978) Birth after the reimplantation of a human embryo. Lancet 2:366

50. Sutcliffe AG, D'Souza SW, Cadman J et al (1995) Outcome in children from cryopreserved embryos. Arch Dis Child 72:290–293
51. Sutcliffe AG, Taylor B, Li J, Thornton S, Grudzinskas JG, Lieberman BA (1999) Children born after intracytoplasmic sperm injection: population control study. Br Med J 318:704–705
52. Sutcliffe AG, Taylor B, Li J, Thornton S, Grudzinskas JG, Lieberman BA (1999) United Kingdom study of children born after intracytoplasmic sperm injection. Hum Reprod 14 (Abstract book):10
53. Tesarik J (1995) Sex chromosome abnormalities after intracytoplasmic sperm injection. Lancet 346:1096
54. Van Opstal D, Los FJ, Ramlakhan S et al (1997) Determination of the parent of origin in nine cases of prenatally detected chromosome aberrations found after intracytoplasmic sperm injection. Hum Reprod 12:682–686
55. Van Steirteghem AC, Liu J, Joris H et al (1993) Higher success rate by intracytoplasmic sperm injection than by subzonal insemination. Report of a second series of 300 consecutive treatment cycles. Hum Reprod 8:1055–1060
56. Van Steirteghem AC, Nagy Z, Joris H et al (1993) High fertilization and implantation rates after intracytoplasmic sperm injection. Hum Reprod 8:1061–1066
57. Wada I, Macnamee MC, Wick K, et al (1994) Birth characteristics and perinatal outcome of babies conceived from cryopreserved embryos. Hum Reprod 9:543–546
58. Weaver SM, Clifford E, Gordon AG et al (1993) A follow-up study of "successful"? IVF/GIFT couples: social-emotional well-being and adjustment to parenthood. J Psychosom Obstet Gynaecol 14:5–16
59. Wennerholm UB, Bergh C, Hamberger L et al (1996) Obstetric and perinatal outcome of pregnancies following intracytoplasmic sperm injection. Hum Reprod 11:1113–1119
60. Wennerholm UB, Bergh C, Hamberger L, Nilsson L, Wikland M (1999) Obstetric and perinatal outcome of pregnancies following intracytoplasmic sperm injection. Hum Reprod 14 (Abstract book):57–58
61. Wissenschaftlicher Beirat der Bundesärztekammer (1998) Richtlinien zur Durchführung der assistierten Reproduktion. Dtsch Arztebl 95:A3166–A3177
62. Yarah H, Demirol A, Bükülmez O, Gürgan T (1999) Obstetric outcome of singleton pregnancies achieved by in vitro fertilization (IVF) and intracytoplasmic sperm injection (ICSI). Fertil Steril 72 [Suppl 1]:110–111
63. Yovich JL, Parry TS, French NP, Grauaug AA (1986) Developmental assessment of twenty in vitro fertilization (IVF) infants at their first birthday. J In Vitro Fertil Embryo Transf 3:253–257

Laser in Assisted Reproduction

M. Montag, K. Rink, G. Delacrétaz, H. van der Ven

Introduction

Lasers were initially used for the treatment of male subfertility. The aim was to overcome fertilization failures in patients with severe oligoasthenoteratozoospermia (OAT). In these patients, the zona pellucida was found to be an obstacle which the low number of slowly moving spermatozoa present in OAT patients were unable to overcome. One approach was to create an artificial opening into the zona pellucida which should allow sperm cells to gain access to the perivitelline space and to fertilize the oocyte. Several methods for opening the zona pellucida have been proposed, based on mechanical or chemical methods. Mechanical zona opening involves the use of a sharp glass capillary mainly to cut or dissect the zona (zona cutting, Tsunoda et al. 1986; partial zona dissection, Malter and Cohen 1989). The chemical opening of the zona is achieved with acidic Tyrode's solution (Gordon and Talansky 1987). The use of these techniques have been described in detail in the literature (Depypere et al. 1988, Cohen 1992).

In contrast to mechanical and chemical zona opening, several groups investigated the use of lasers for the creation of openings into the zona pellucida, and both contact as well as noncontact laser systems were proposed. Efficient zona drilling was reported by Palanker et al (1991) using an argon fluoride excimer laser (ArF) emitting at 193 nm. This laser system required using air-filled pipettes for laser delivery due to the high absorption of the radiation by the culture medium, and this in turn required the use of micromanipulation equipment. Because the laser radiation has to be delivered directly to the zona, these types of lasers were termed contact lasers. Another contact laser, known as the erbium:yttrium-aluminum-garnet (Er:YAG) laser was introduced by Strohmer and Feichtinger (1992). This laser was used in combination with subzonal sperm insertion (SUZI) and allowed significantly higher fertilization rates in patients with OAT (Obruca et al. 1994).

In contrast to contact lasers, noncontact lasers allow for direct delivery of the laser beam through the objective. Tadir and co-workers investigated the use of pulsed lasers in the ultraviolet and visible spectrum with various wavelengths (266, 355, and 532 nm) using a neodymium:yttrium-aluminum-garnet Nd:YAG) laser system (Tadir et al. 1989a, 1991); however, the control of the operating procedure and the consistency of the system were not guaranteed. Neev et al. (1992a,b) used a pulsed 308-nm xenon chloride (XeCl) excimer laser. A major drawback of this system was the necessity of hundreds of laser shots to achieve a complete opening of the zona pellucida. In experimental studies, this laser proved to enhance fertilization rates by spermatozoa from long-term vasectomized mice after laser drilling of the zona of oocytes (El-Danasouri et al. 1993). Another, very similar system worked at a wavelength of 337 nm (Schütze et al. 1994), and zona drilling of openings with a width of 1 μm was accomplished within 10–20 s. This system was used in combination with a laser-based optical trap, which allowed for manipulation of living cells (Ashkin and Dziedzic 1987, Ashkin et al. 1987) including spermatozoa (Tadir et al. 1989b, Colon et al. 1992). Optical trapping was achieved by a focused laser beam working in the near infrared. Although it was initially applied for studies on sperm motility (Westphal et al. 1993, Araujo et al. 1994, Dantas et al. 1995, König et al. 1996), the combined approach of zona drilling and insertion of spermatozoa into the perivitelline space using the optical trap gained much attention (Schütze et al. 1994, Enginsu et al. 1995, Clement-Sengewald et al. 1996). However, this method, also called laser-SUZI, did not succeed in human IVF, first because potential mutagenic and cytotoxic effects of the ultraviolet laser for cutting (Kochevar 1989) and of the optical trap (Neev et al. 1993, König et al. 1996) could be not excluded. Second, the UV wavelength required immersion objectives and special culture dishes. Third, the SUZI technique itself did not succeed, because the introduction of intracytoplasmic sperm injection (ICSI; Palermo et al. 1992) proved to be far more efficient.

More recently, an indium-gallium-arsenic-phosphorus (InGaAsp) 1.48-μm diode laser was introduced (Rink et al. 1994). Although this laser system was initially developed for laser-SUZI, wasthe first to have an impact on assisted reproduction, mainly in the field of assisted hatching. The laser can be fitted to every inverted microscope (Fig. 1). The unique characteristic of the diode laser to absorb

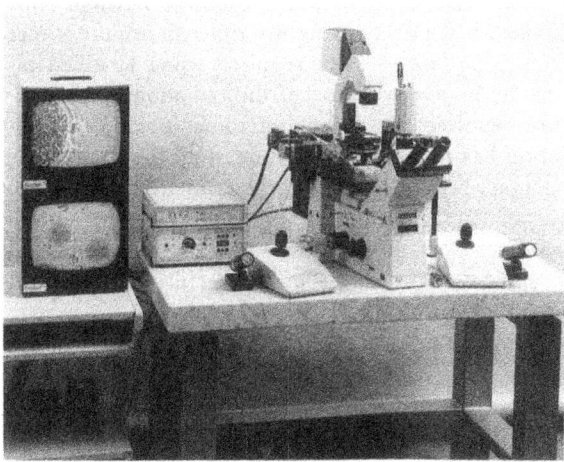

Fig. 1. A complete microscopic working station equipped with the 1.48-μm diode laser system (Fertilase, MTM Medical Technologies Montreux, Clarens, Switzerland) and micromanipulators for biopsy purposes

Fig. 2. Coupling of the 1.48-µm diode laser to an inverted microscope system. The laser beam is focused through the objective and hits the object in a tangential working mode. A reference laser working at 670 nm in the visible range of light is used for adjustment of the 1.48-µm diode laser

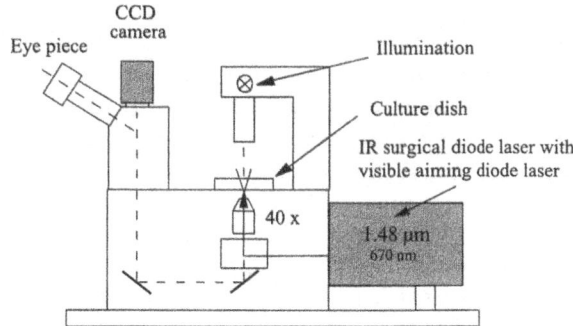

water and culture medium allow its use in combination with standard culture dishes (Rink et al. 1996). The continuous-wave operation enables zona drilling with a single laser irradiation using a pulse length of 5–20 ms (Fig. 2), where the variation in the irradiation time directly controls the size of a drilled opening. The safety and efficacy of the system were first demonstrated in mouse experiments (Germond et al. 1995, 1996). This laser was applied in human IVF for assisted hatching, and in 1995 the first baby made possible by this method was born in Switzerland. Subsequently, a variety of applications have been developed for the diode laser technique, and these are reviewed in the following sections.

Assisted Hatching

During early embryonic development, the embryo is surrounded by the zona pellucida. At the blastocyst stage the embryo must escape the zona prior to implantation. This process is known as hatching. The process of hatching in vivo is not yet fully understood, but in vitro studies show that blastocyst expansion and probably the presence of uterine lysins in vivo promote hatching (Cole 1967, McLaren 1968, Wright et al. 1978, Schiewe et al. 1995). The possibility has been discussed that an impairment of the hatching process may be the underlying reason for failed implantation in human IVF (Cohen 1991). A failure in hatching does prevent a pregnancy. Hatching deficiencies can result from zona hardening, which might occur after in vitro culture of human embryos (DeFelici and Siracusa 1982, Downs et al. 1986) or after cryopreservation (Tucker et al. 1991, Check et al. 1996). Further, some patients present with an unusually thick zona pellucida (>20 µm) and the corresponding embryos possess a reduced implantation potential (Cohen et al. 1992).

Several methods have been proposed to assist the hatching process (zona cutting: Tsunoda et al. 1986; zona drilling: Gordon and Talansky 1987; partial zona dissection: Malter and Cohen 1989). However, mechanical as well as chemical methods are difficult to apply and require some experience. These methods do not allow for the reproducible drilling of standardized openings, and the use of acidic Tyrode's solution can have an embryotoxic effect (Malter and Cohen 1989).

Strohmer and Feichtinger (1992) used the Er:YAG laser for assisted hatching. Although they reported good results, this type of contact laser did not succeed because the laser required additional micromanipulation equipment and disposable pipettes for laser delivery to the target. Antinori et al. (1996a) used the UV-laser system for assisted hatching, but due to its possible mutagenic effects (see above) this system did not attract much interest.

The introduction of the 1.48-μm diode laser system made it possible for the first time to meet all the requirements of assisted hatching. The ease of laser application and the proven efficiency and safety of this system made it the ideal tool for assisted hatching (Fig. 3). With the diode laser drill openings can be drilled into the zona pellucida which are identical in size. This reproducibility was the basis for the initiation of a multicenter study to clarify the potential benefit of assisted hatching. Preliminary data were presented in 1998 (Germond et al. 1998). So far, all available published data on laser-assisted hatching confirm the fact that assisted hatching is a successful treatment therapy for selected patients. This includes women over 35–37 years of age and patients with previous implantation failures (Antinori et al. 1996a, b, Germond et al. 1998, Montag and van der Ven 1999).

A main criticism in regard to assisted hatching is the argument that the large number of published studies, prospective as well as retrospective, are highly controversial. Whereas some authors clearly find a significant rise in the pregnancy rate for selected patient groups (Cohen et al. 1992, Liu et al. 1993, Schoolcraft et al. 1994, Stein et al. 1995), others report the opposite (Hellebault et al. 1996, Tucker et al. 1996, Bider et al. 1997, Lanzendorf et al. 1998, Magli et al. 1998). In the majority of these studies acidic Tyrode's solution was employed for zona drilling. We think that the use of acidic Tyrode's solution does not allow for the reliable drilling of equally sized openings. Most published studies do not comment on the size of the drilled opening and therefore cannot be compared with each other. However, Cohen and Feldberg showed that the size of a chemically drilled zona opening is of great importance for hatching efficiency (1991), and the same applies for laser-drilled openings (Montag and van der Ven 1999). The possible benefit of assisted hatching can be assessed only when all the parameters affecting hatching efficiency are considered properly, and ongoing studies on laser-assisted hatching will answer this question in the near future.

Biopsy Techniques

Several methods of assisted reproduction require the use of microcapillaries to penetrate the zona pellucida and to get access to the perivitelline space. This is a prerequisite for preimplantation genetic diagnosis, in order to allow for biopsy of polar bodies or blastomeres (Grifo 1992). It is also applied for the removal of cellular embryonic fragments, a technique which may enhance the implantation potential of the embryo (Cohen 1992).

Fig. 3 a, b. Human four-cell stage embryo before (**a**) and after (**b**) laser drilling of the zona pellucida for assisted hatching. The opening was drilled with a single laser irradiation at 18 ms pulse length. The sharp border of the opening can be seen clearly (*arrows*). The embryo was transferred back into the uterus immediately after laser drilling. *Bar*=12 μm. (Reprinted by permission from Springer-Verlag GmbH & Co. KG: Reproduktionsmedizin 1999; 15:45–54)

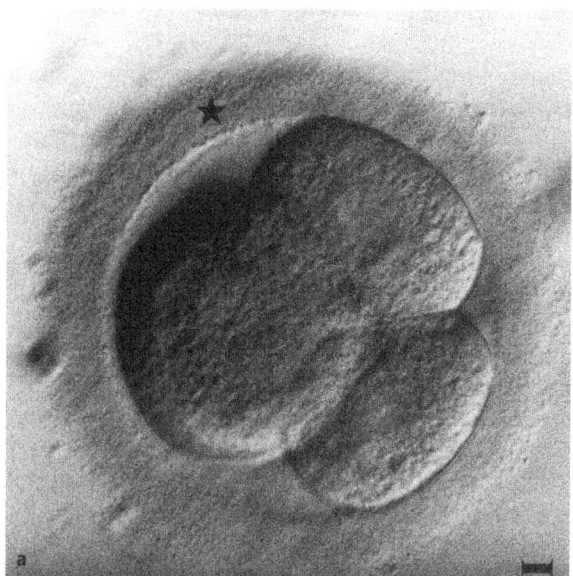

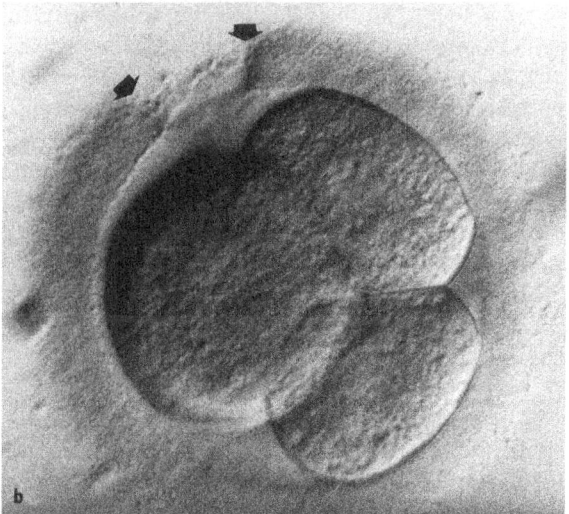

Usually, these biopsy methods have been used in combination with zona drilling with acidic Tyrode's solution or sharp capillaries. The advantages of the 1.48-μm diode laser overacidic Tyrode's solution have been already discussed in the previous section. Obviously, the diode laser is a valuable tool for any biopsy technique.

Polar Body Biopsy

Biopsy of the first and/or second polar body is applied for the diagnosis of maternal aneuploidies, which may result from nondisjunction during the first or second meiotic division (Verlinsky et al. 1990, Munné et al. 1995, Verlinsky and Kuliev 1996). The information derived from this investigation is of the uttmost importance for the patients. Therefore, the biopsy itself should be performed with great care, and possible damage to the polar body or the oocyte should be avoided. It has been estimated that 28% of all biopsied cells cannot be reliably diagnosed owing to technical problems that arise during the biopsy procedure or the subsequent cytogenetic analysis (Reubinoff and Shushan 1996). In particular, the use of sharp capillaries to open the zona and aspirate the polar body may cause damage to the polar body or the oocyte, which consequently may lead to loss of the genetic material.

We have developed a laser-based biopsy procedure which allows for fast and efficient removal of polar bodies (Montag et al. 1998; Fig. 4). The zygote is affixed to the holding capillary and the polar body is orientated in a way which allows immediate access with an aspiration needle. The zona pellucida is opened with a single laser irradiation applied to an area of the zona close to the polar body. Through this opening a blunt-ended, flame-polished aspiration capillary can be pushed towards the polar body, which is then gently aspirated. After the capillary has been withdrawn, the isolated polar body can be expelled and used for cytogenetic analysis. The main advantage of this approach is that blunt-ended capillaries can be used and this greatly reduces the risk of damage to the polar body or the oocyte. Experimental studies in the mouse have shown that the procedure does not affect further embryonic development. We have combined this technique with cytogenetic analysis by primed in situ hybridization and were able to arrive at a diagnosis in less than 2 h (Montag et al. 1997)

Blastomere Biopsy

In principle, the technique which we presented for polar body biopsy can be applied to blastomere biopsy as well, and the feasibility of this has been shown by Boada et al. (1998). So far, most centers still perform blastomere biopsy with the help of acidic Tyrode's solution (Handyside et al. 1990). This technique requires immediate washing of the embryos in order to remove the acidic solution prior to subsequent biopsy. Additional steps during the handling of the embryos enhance the potential risk of contamination, and this has to be considered if further molecular genetic analysis needs to be performed by polymerase chain reaction (PCR). The laser technique allows for a one-step procedure. Further, the size of the opening required for blastomere biopsy can be easily adapted online to the diameter of the blastomere or the aspiration capillary. The extensive use of acidic Tyrode's solution may have a negative impact on further embryonic development due to a possible loss of blastomeres through the large openings created by chemical zona drilling.

Fig. 4a–d. Laser-assisted polar body biopsy of the second polar body of a mouse zygote. The setup is identical to that used for blastomere biopsy. The zygote is orientated (**a**) and a laser-drilled opening is created close to the polar body in the zona pellucida (**b**). The polar body can be easily aspirated with the aspiration capillary (**c**) and remains intact after isolation (**d**). *Bar* = 10 μm for **a–d**. (Reprinted by permission from the American Society for Reproductive Medicine. Fertil Steril 1998; 69:539–542)

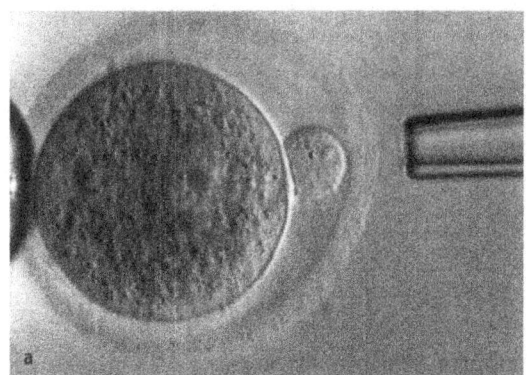

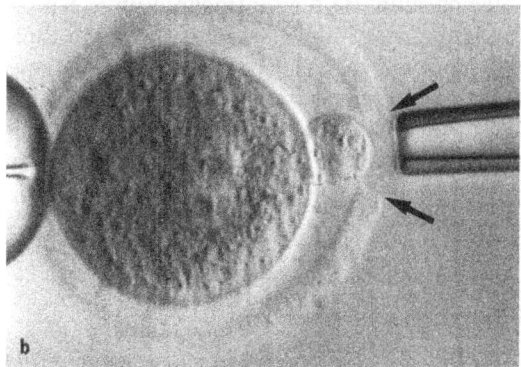

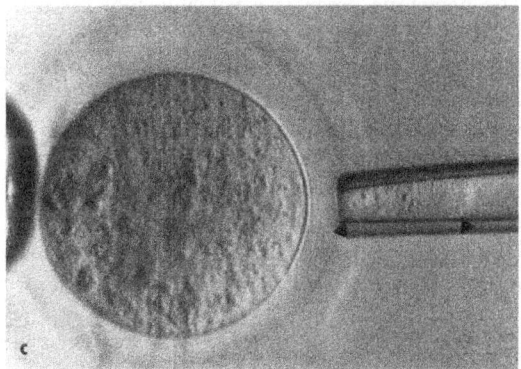

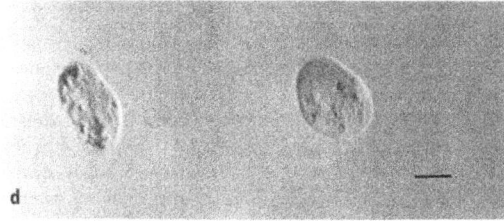

Cryopreservation of Single Spermatozoa in Empty Zona Pellucida

Since the introduction of ICSI (Palermo et al. 1992), men who have only a few spermatozoa in their ejaculate or in whom spermatozoa are retrievable from the epididymis (Tournaye et al. 1994) or the testis (Schoysman et al. 1993) can be successfully treated. For those cases where spermatozoa are present in numbers too low for conventional cryopreservation, an alternate method has been proposed by Cohen et al. (1997), whereby single spermatozoa are frozen in empty zona pellucida. We have improved this method by using the laser to produce empty zonae and for sperm immobilization (see below). In our approach we first drilled an opening into the zona of a degenerated oocyte and aspirated the ooplasm through this opening into a suction capillary (Fig. 5). Through the same opening, we then introduced up to ten spermatozoa and closed the opening with an oil droplet expelled from the capillary during its withdrawal. Not only does the oil droplet serve to close the opening, it also allows for easy detection of the empty zonae during subsequent freezing and thawing procedures. We further investigated the possibility of temporarily immobilizing spermatozoa prior to insertion into the empty zona. This approach resulted in reduced loss of spermatozoa prior to freezing and in higher recovery rates (Montag et al. 1999a).

Production of Hemizonae

The hemizona assay is a valuable tool for testing sperm function, e.g., sperm binding to human zona pellucida (Burkman et al. 1988), and it even makes it possible to predict the fertilization ability of spermatozoa (Gamzu et al. 1994). However, the accuracy of the hemizona assay is dependent on the availability of equal-sized hemizonae, as differences in the zona surface will influence the number of sperm which can bind. So far, the production of hemizonae has been performed with a microblade affixed to a micromanipulator (Burkman et al. 1988) or by manual bisection (Sanchez et al. 1995). We have used the diode laser to cut hemizonae. The principle of this application is the complete removal of the outer rim of the zona pellucida of an oocyte. This is best achieved

---

Fig. 5 a–h. Cryopreservation of single human spermatozoa in empty zona pellucida. The ooplasm of a degenerated human oocyte (**a**) was removed after laser-drilling of a single opening in the zona pellucida (**b, c**). Into the empty zona (**d**) either motile (**e**) or immobilized (**f**) spermatozoa were deposited. Motile spermatozoa dispersed throughout the empty zona (**e**), whereas immobilized spermatozoa remained at the site where they were deposited (**f**). The laser-drilled opening was closed with an oil droplet expelled from the capillary during withdrawal (**f**). Following freezing and thawing, spermatozoa were still viable, as shown by a hypo-osmotic swelling test (**g**) and were able to activate mouse oocytes after injection (**h**). *Bar*=15 µm for **a–g**. (Reprinted by permission from Blackwell Wissenschafts-Verlag GmbH, Andrologia 1999; 32:49–53)

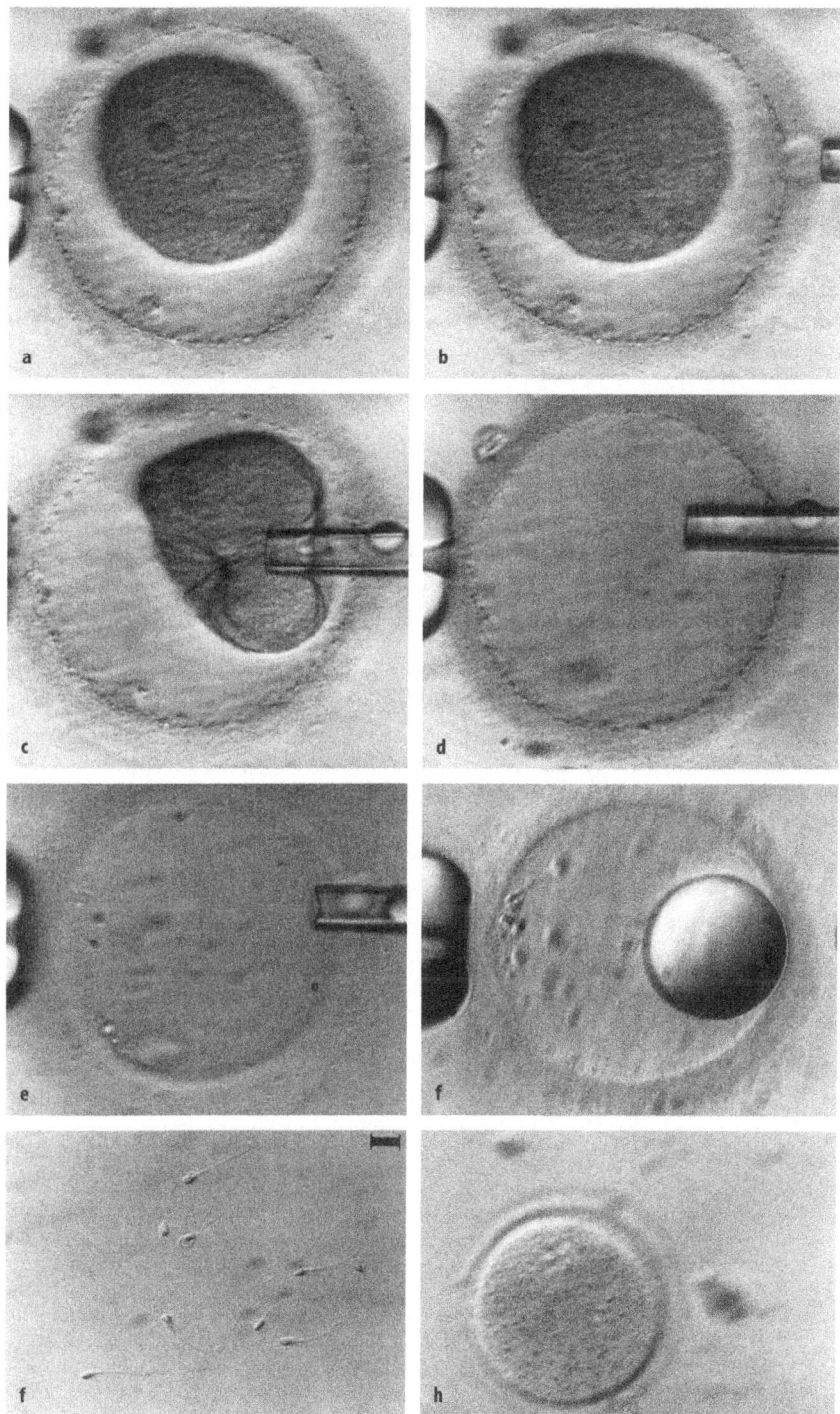

when the oocyte is affixed to a holding capillary and consecutive openings are drilled beside one another into the zona. Finally, the oocyte is turned by 90° and the two hemizonae can be separated using two holding capillaries, one attached to each side. Ooplasmic remnants can be removed from the inner parts of the hemizonae with the holding capillaries. We have compared this method of zona production with the manual bisection method and found no difference in the binding capacity of spermatozoa from that of control patients (Montag et al. 1999b). In our hands, laser-based bisection was much more practicable than manual bisection, especially because corresponding hemizonae were identical in size and all hemizonae could be used in the hemizona assay. This is of great advantage, as the number of human oocytes which are available for hemizona studies is usually limited.

Immobilization of Spermatozoa and Permeabilization of the Sperm Membrane

All aforementioned applications of the diode laser were aimed at the creation of openings in the zona pellucida. The thermal effect of laser drilling can be applied for other purposes as well. We have found that it is possible to use the laser for controlled immobilization of spermatozoa (Montag et al. 1999c) by applying a single laser shot which is aimed next to the sperm tail (Fig. 6). Our studies showed that the laser energy required for sperm immobilization is dependent on the progressive motility (Table 1). Fast-moving sperm are immobilized by a higher energy than slower ones. Above a certain energy threshold, a single laser shot immobilizes the spermatozoon and in addition leads to a permeabilization of the sperm membrane. We have further developed this method by the invention of a double laser shot technique, where a first laser shot aimed beside the sperm tail is used for immobilization and a second laser shot aimed directly at the tail is used for reliable permeabilization. This technique allows

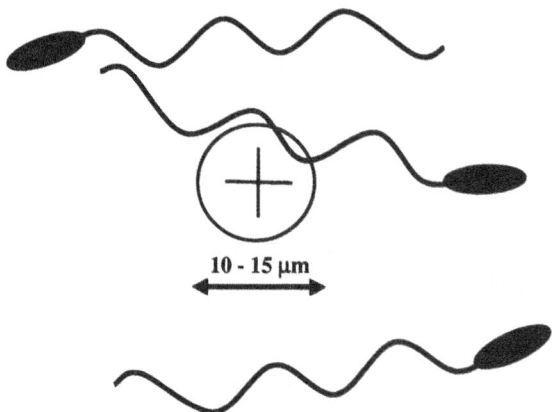

10 - 15 μm

Fig. 6. Laser-immobilization of human spermatozoa by a single laser shot aimed aside the middle of the sperm tail. Only the spermatozoon within the laser-interaction arc is affected. Depending on the amount of energy applied, immobilization is either temporary or permanent

Table 1. Laser energy necessary to cause motility arrest (either permanent or temporary) of all treated spermatozoa in different media following a single laser shot

Class of spermatozoa	Culture medium with 10% PVP	Culture medium without PVP
WHO A	0.5 mJ	2.0 mJ
WHO B	0.5 mJ	1.5 mJ
WHO C	0.5 mJ	0.5 mJ

for the treatment of spermatozoa prior to ICSI. It may be advantageous as sperm immobilization can be easily performed in culture medium. This approach may help to avoid the use of polyvinylpyrrolidone (PVP) for ICSI, as PVP is another toxic substance (Feichtinger et al. 1995, Jean et al. 1996, 1997, McDermott and Ray 1996, Strehler et al. 1998).

Measuring of Zona Hardening

The size of the opening in the zona pellucida is an indirect measure of zona hardness. This principle is based on the observation that under constant conditions (temperature of the medium and the heated microscope stage, culture dishes, laser energy, optical setup, culture medium) several drilled openings in the zona have the same size, because the same amount of energy is always directed at the zona. Consequently, different sizes of drilled openings are indicative of a difference in the structure or hardness of the zona. In their first publication on laser-assisted hatching, Germond et al. (1995) reported that the size of a laser-drilled opening in the zona of an oocyte differed from that in the zona of a zygote. This finding confirmed fertilization-induced zona hardening, which had already been detected by chemical means as early as 1976 (Inoue and Wolf 1976).

We investigated the sizes of laser-drilled openings in zonae pellucidae from mouse embryos grown either in vitro or in vivo. Up to the morula stage we found no differences; however, in early blastocysts the size of a laser-drilled opening in embryos grown in vitro was significantly smaller than that in an embryo grown in vivo (Montag et al. 1999d). These data show that in vitro, zona hardening occurs presumably due to blastocyst expansion, whereas in vivo the zona becomes softer due to the effect of uterine lysins, which promote global zona lysis prior to implantation.

Conclusions

The use of a 1.48-μm diode laser system in assisted reproduction offers an efficient and reliable means for drilling openings into the zona pellucida. This technique will help to clarify the potential benefit of assisted hatching in human reproduction. In addition, all techniques which require the instantaneous opening of the zona pellucida, such as polar body biopsy and blastomere biopsy, can be performed quickly and safely with the diode laser. New applications have been developed; the use of the laser facilitates the production of hemizonae, the generation of empty zona pellucida for cryopreservation of single spermatozoa, and the immobilization of spermatozoa. The precise control of the laser and the ease of application will stimulate further research and the development of new techniques in assisted reproduction.

Acknowledgements. The authors thank the staff of the IVF unit at the University of Bonn, Mrs. Przybilka for the photographic art work, and Laurent Descloux for stimulating discussions.

References

Antinori S, Selman HA, Caffa B et al (1996a) Zona opening of human embryos using a non-contact UV laser for assisted hatching in patients with poor prognosis of pregnancy. Hum Reprod 11:2488–2492

Antinori S, Panci C, Selman HA et al (1996b) Zona thinning with the use of laser: a new approach to assisted hatching in humans. Hum Reprod 11:590–594

Araujo E, Tadir Y, Patrizio P et al (1994) Relative force of human epididymal sperm. Fertil Steril 62:585–590

Ashkin A, Dziedzic JM (1987) Optical trapping and manipulation of viruses and bacteria. Science 235:1517–1520

Ashkin A, Dziedzic JM, Yamane T (1987) Optical trapping and manipulation of single cells using infrared laser beams. Nature 330:769–771

Bider D, Livshits A, Yonish M et al (1997) Assisted hatching by zona drilling of human embryos in women of advanced age. Hum Reprod 12:317–320

Boada M, Carrera M, De La Iglesia C et al (1997) Successful use of a laser for human embryo biopsy in preimplantation genetic diagnosis: report of two cases. J Assist Reprod Genet 15:301–305

Burkman LJ, Coddington CC, Franken DR, Kruger TF, Rosenwaks Z, Hodgen GD (1988) The hemizona assay (HZA): development of a diagnostic test for the binding of human spermatozoa to the human hemizona pellucida to predict fertilization potential. Fertil Steril 49:688–697

Check JH, Hoover L, Nazari A, O'Shaughnessy A, Summers D (1996) The effect of assisted hatching on pregnancy rates after frozen embryo transfer. Fertil Steril 65:254–257

Clement-Sengewald A, Schütze K, Ashkin A et al (1996) Fertilization of bovine oocytes induced solely with combined laser microbeam and optical tweezers. J Assist Reprod Genet 13:259–265

Cohen J (1991) Assisted hatching of human embryos. J In Vitro Fertil Embryo Transf 8:179–190

Cohen J (1992) Zona pellucida micromanipulation and consequences for embryonic development and implantation. In: Cohen J, Malter HE, Talansky BE, Grifo J (eds) Micromanipulation of human gametes and embryos. Raven, New York, pp 191–222

Cohen J, Feldberg D (1991) Effects of the size and number of zona pellucida openings on hatching and trophoblast outgrowth in the mouse embryo. Mol Reprod Dev 30:70–78

Cohen J, Alikani M, Trowbridge J, Rosenwaks Z (1992) Implantation enhancement by selective assisted hatching using zona drilling of human embryos with poor prognosis. Hum Reprod 7:685–691

Cohen J, Garrisi GJ, Congedo-Ferrara TA et al (1997) Cryopreservation of single human spermatozoa. Hum Reprod 12:994–1001

Cole RJ (1967) Cinemicrographic observation on the trophoblast and zona pellucida of the mouse blastocyst. J Embryol Exp Morphol 17:481–490

Colon JM, Sarosi P, McGovern PG et al (1992) Controlled micromanipulation of human sperm in three dimensions with an infrared laser optical trap: effect on sperm velocity. Fertil Steril 57:695–698

Dantas ZN, Araujo E, Tadir Y et al (1995) Effect of freezing on the relative escape force of sperm as measured by a laser optical trap. Fertil Steril 63:185–188

DeFelici M, Siracusa G (1982) Spontaneous hardening of the zona pellucida of mouse oocytes during in vitro culture. Gamete Res 6:107–113

Depypere HAT, McLaughlin KJ, Seamark RF et al (1988) Zona cutting and zona drilling for assisted fertilization in the mouse. J Reprod Fertil 84:205–211

Downs SM, Schroeder AC, Eppig JJ (1986) Serum maintains the fertilizability of mouse oocytes matured in vitro by preventing hardening of the zona pellucida. Gamete Res 15:115–122

El-Danasouri I, Westphal LM, Neev Y et al (1993) Zona opening with 308 nm XeCl excimer laser improves fertilization by spermatozoa from long-term vasectomized mice. Hum Reprod 8:464–466

Enginsu ME, Schütze K, Bellanca S et al (1995) Micromanipulation of mouse gametes with laser microbeam and optical tweezers. Hum Reprod 10:1761–1764

Feichtinger W, Obruca A, Brunner M (1995) Sex chromosomal abnormalities and intracytoplasmic injection. Lancet 346:1566

Gamzu R, Yogev L, Amit A et al (1994) The hemizona assay is of good prognostic value for the ability of sperm to fertilize oocytes in vitro. Fertil Steril 62:1056–1059

Germond M, Nocera D, Senn A, Rink K, Delacrétaz G, Fakan S (1995) Microdissection of mouse and human zona pellucida using a 1.48-μm diode laser beam: efficacy and safety of the procedure. Fertil Steril 25:604–611

Germond M, Nocera D, Senn A et al (1996) Improved fertilization and implantation rates after non-touch zona pellucida microdrilling of mouse oocytes with a 1.48-μm diode laser beam. Hum Reprod 11:1043–1048

Germond M, Primi MP, Senn A et al (1998) Diode laser for assisted hatching: preliminary results of a multicentric prospective randomized study. Hum Reprod 13 Abstract Book 1:84–85

Gordon JW, Talansky BE (1987) Assisted fertilization by zona drilling: a mouse model for correction of oligospermia. J Exp Zool 239:347–381

Grifo J (1992) Preconception and preimplantation genetic diagnosis: polar body, blastomere, and trophectoderm biopsy. In: Cohen J, Malter HE, Talansky BE, Grifo J (eds) Micromanipulation of human gametes and embryos. Raven, New York, pp 191–222

Handyside A, Kontogianni E, Hardy K, Winston RML (1990) Pregnancies from biopsied human preimplantation embryos sexed with a Y-specific DNA amplification. Nature 344:768–780

Hellebault S, De Sutter P, Dozortsev D et al (1996) Does assisted hatching improve implantation rates after in vitro fertilization or intracytoplasmic sperm injection in all patients? A prospective randomized study. J Assist Reprod Genet 13:19–22

Inoue M, Wolf DP (1976) Comparative solubility properties of the zonae pellucidae of unfertilized and fertilized mouse ova. Biol Reprod 11:558–565

Jean M, Barriere P, Mirallie S (1996) Intracytoplasmic sperm injection without polyvinylpyrrolidone: an essential precaution? Hum Reprod 11:2332

Jean M, Barriere P, Mirallie S (1997) Development of a successful ICSI programme without the use of PVP. Hum Reprod 12:1115–1116

Kochevar IE (1989) Cytotoxicity and mutagenicity of excimer laser radiation. Lasers Surg Med 9:440–445

König K, Tadir Y, Patrizio P et al (1996) Effects of ultraviolet exposure and near infrared laser tweezers on human spermatozoa. Hum Reprod 11:2162–2164

Lanzendorf SE, Nehchiri F, Mayer JF et al (1998) A prospective, randomized, double-blind study for the evaluation of assisted hatching in patients with advanced maternal age. Hum Reprod 13:409–413

Liu HC, Cohen J, Alikani M et al (1993) Assisted hatching facilitates earlier implantation. Fertil Steril 60:871–875

Magli MC, Gianaroli L, Ferraretti AP et al (1998) Rescue of implantation potential in embryos with poor prognosis by assisted hatching. Hum Reprod 13:1331–1335

Malter HE, Cohen J (1989) Partial zona dissection of the human oocytes: a non-traumatic method using a micromanipulation to assist zona pellucida penetration. Fertil Steril 51:139–148

McDermott A, Ray B (1996) Intracytoplasmic sperm injection without polyvinylpyrrolidone: an essential precaution? Hum Reprod 11:2332

McLaren (1968) A study of blastocysts during delay and subsequent implantation in lactating mice. J Endocrinol 42:453–463

Montag M, van der Ven H (1999) Laser assisted hatching in assisted reproduction. Croatian Med J 40:398–403

Montag M, van der Ven K, Delacrétaz G, Rink K, van der Ven H (1997) Efficient preimplantation genetic diagnosis using laser assisted microdissection of the zona pellucida for polar body biopsy followed by primed in situ labeling (PRINS). J Assist Reprod Genet 14:476

Montag M, van der Ven K, Delacrétaz G, Rink K, van der Ven H (1998) Laser-assisted microdissection of zona pellucida facilitates polar body biopsy. Fertil Steril 69:539–542

Montag M, Dieckmann U, Rink K et al (1999a) Laser-assisted cryopreservation of single human spermatozoa in cell-free zona pellucida. Andrologia 32:49–53

Montag M, Lemola R, van der Ven H (1999b) Fast and efficient production of equally sized hemizonae using a 1.48-µm diode laser system and their use in the hemizona assay. Hum Reprod 14 (Abstract book 1):144

Montag M, Rink K, Descloux L et al (1999c) The use of a 1.48-µm diode laser system in assisted reproduction: laser-drilling of the zona pellucida and laser-assisted immobilization of spermatozoa. Assist Reprod Rev 9:205–213

Montag M, Rink K, Delacrétaz G, van der Ven H (1999d) Hardness of the zona pellucida at different stages of mouse embryonic development in vitro and in vivo as measured indirectly by a 1.48-µm diode laser. Hum Reprod 14 (Abstract book 1):168

Munné S, Dailey T, Sultan KM et al (1995) The use of first polar bodies for preimplantation diagnosis of aneuploidy. Mol Hum Reprod 10:1014–1020

Neev J, Tadir Y, Asch R et al (1992a) Laser zona dissection using short power UV lasers. Proc Soc Photo-optical Instrumentation (SPIE) 1650:62–69

Neev J, Tadir Y, Ho P et al (1992b) Microscope delivered ultraviolet laser zona dissection: principles and practices. J Assist Reprod Genet 9:513–523

Neev J, Gonzalez A, Licciardi F et al (1993) Opening of the mouse zona pellucida by laser without a micromanipulator. Hum Reprod 8:939–944

Obruca A, Strohmer H, Sakkas D et al (1994) Use of lasers in assisted fertilization and hatching. Hum Reprod 9:1723–1726

Palanker D, Ohad S, Lewis A et al (1991) Technique for cellular microsurgery using the 193-nm excimer laser. Lasers Surg Med 11:580–586

Palermo G, Joris H, Devroey P, Van Steirteghem A (1992) Pregnancies after intracytoplasmic sperm injection of a single spermatozoon into an oocyte. Lancet 340:17–18

Reubinoff BE, Shushan A (1996) Preimplantation diagnosis in older patients: to biopsy or not to biopsy. Hum Reprod 11:2071–2075

Rink K, Delacrétaz G, Salathé RP et al (1994) 1.48-µm diode laser microdissection of the zona pellucida of mouse zygotes. Proc SPIE 213A:412–422

Rink K, Delacrétaz G, Salathé RP et al (1996) Non-contact microdrilling of mouse zona pellucida with an objective-delivered 1.48-µm diode laser. Lasers Surg Med 18:52–62

Sanchez R, Finkenzeller C, Schill WB, Miska W (1995) Comparison of two methods to obtain hemizonae pellucidae for sperm function tests. Hum Reprod 10:2945–2947

Schiewe MC, Hazeleger NL, Sclimenti C, Balmaceda JP (1995) Physiological characterization of blastocyst hatching mechanisms by use of a mouse antihatching model. Fertil Steril 63:288–294

Schoolcraft WB, Schlenker T, Gee M et al (1994) Assisted hatching in the treatment of poor prognosis in vitro fertilization candidates. Fertil Steril 62:551–554

Schoysman R, Vanderzwalmen P, Segal-Bertin G, van de Casseye M (1993) Successful fertilization by testicular spermatozoa in an in-vitro fertilization programme. Hum Reprod 8:1339–1340

Schütze K, Clement-Sengewald A, Ashkin A (1994) Zona drilling and sperm insertion with combined laser microbeam and optical tweezers. Fertil Steril 61:783–786

Stein A, Rufas O, Amit S et al (1995) Assisted hatching by partial zona dissection of human pre-embryos in patients with recurrent implantation failure after in-vitro fertilization. Fertil Steril 63:838–841

Strehler E, Baccetti B, Sterzik K et al (1998) Detrimental effects of polyvinylpyrrolidone on the ultrastructure of spermatozoa (Notulae seminologicae 13). Hum Reprod 13:120–123

Strohmer H, Feichtinger W (1992) Successful clinical application of laser for micromanipulation in an in vitro fertilization program. Fertil Steril 58:212–214

Tadir Y, Wright W, Berns M (1989a) Cell micromanipulation with laser beams. In: Capitanio GL, Asch RH, De Cecco L et al (eds) G.I.F.T. from basics to clinics. Raven, New York, pp 359–368

Tadir Y, Wright WH, Vafa O et al (1989b) Micromanipulation of sperm by a laser generated optical trap. Fertil Steril 52:870–873

Tadir Y, Wright W, Vafa O et al (1991) Micromanipulation of gametes using laser micro beams. Hum Reprod 6:1011–1016

Tournaye H, Devroey P, Liu J et al (1994) Microsurgical epididymal sperm aspiration and intracytoplasmic injection: a new effective approach to infertility as a result of congenital bilateral absence of the vas deferens. Fertil Steril 61:1045–1051

Tsunoda Y, Yasiu T, Nakamura K et al (1986) Effect of cutting the zona pellucida on the pronuclear transplantation in the mouse. J Exp Zool 240:119–125

Tucker MJ, Cohen J, Massey JB et al (1991) Partial zona dissection of the zona pellucida of frozen thawed human embryos may enhance blastocyst hatching, implantation, and pregnancy rates. Am J Obstet Gynecol 165:341–345

Tucker MJ, Morton PC, Wright G et al (1996) Enhancement of outcome from intracytoplasmic sperm injection: does co-culture or assisted hatching improve implantation rates? Hum Reprod 11:2434–2437

Verlinsky Y, Ginsberg N, Lifchez A et al (1990) Analysis of the first polar body: preconception genetic diagnosis. Hum Reprod 5:826–829

Verlinsky Y, Kuliev A (1996) Preimplantation diagnosis of common aneuploidies in infertile couples of advanced maternal age. Hum Reprod 11:2076–2077

Westphal LM, ElDanasouri I, Shimizu S et al (1993) Exposure of human spermatozoa to the cumulus-oophorus results in increased relative force as measured by a 760-nm laser optical trap. Hum Reprod 8:1083–1086

Wright RW, Watson JG, Chaykin S (1978) Factors influencing the in vitro hatching of mouse blastocysts. Anim Reprod Sci 1:181–188

Assisting Reproduction with the Use of Donor Eggs

J. A. Schnorr, J. P. Toner

Introduction

For many years, sperm donation for artificial insemination has been available for the treatment of male-factor infertility. With the development of assisted reproduction technologies (ART) during the 1980s, new therapeutic options became available for the treatment of infertility. One such development is the use of donated eggs with in vitro fertilization (IVF) in women with decreased ovarian reserve, premature ovarian failure, heritable genetic abnormalities, and those who have previously undergone multiple unsuccessful IVF attempts.

Human pregnancies following donor-egg IVF were first reported in 1984 [1]. Today, 222 programs in the United States offer donor-egg IVF to couples who might otherwise never achieve pregnancy without this intervention. According to the 1996 Assisted Reproductive Technology Success Rate, published by the Centers for Disease Control, donor eggs were used in approximately 8% of all ART cycles, or 5162 cycles, in 1996. Usage increases with the woman's age, with donor egg cycles accounting for fewer than 5% of ART cycles in women younger than 38 years of age but over 70% in women older than 46 years of age [2].

The live birth rate per fresh transfer for women using donated eggs was 39.3% (in 534 cycles) in women younger than 35 years of age, 39.2% (in 816 cycles) in women 35–39, and 38.9% (in 2472 cycles) in women older than 39. These pregnancy rates compare very favorably to the 1996 live birth rate per transfer in nondonor egg ART, which was 33.6% in women under 35, 26.8% in women 35–39, and 12.4% in women older than 39 years of age (Fig. 1) [2]. This has led to the realization that the decline in pregnancy rates in conventional IVF has much more to do with the age of the egg than the age of the uterus, though both play some role. Consequently, it has been very gratifying to many women that the use of donor eggs can overcome their own difficulties in conceiving, even when their age is relatively advanced.

In the most common contemporary approach, a known or anonymous volunteer first undergoes controlled ovarian hyperstimulation so that multiple eggs are produced. The eggs are transvaginally retrieved and fertilized with the sperm of the recipient's partner using either standard IVF or intracytoplasmic sperm injection (ICSI) techniques. A limited number of the resultant embryos are then transferred to the recipient, who has been hormonally synchronized during the same cycle (or the embryos may be cryopreserved for transfer at a later time). In one

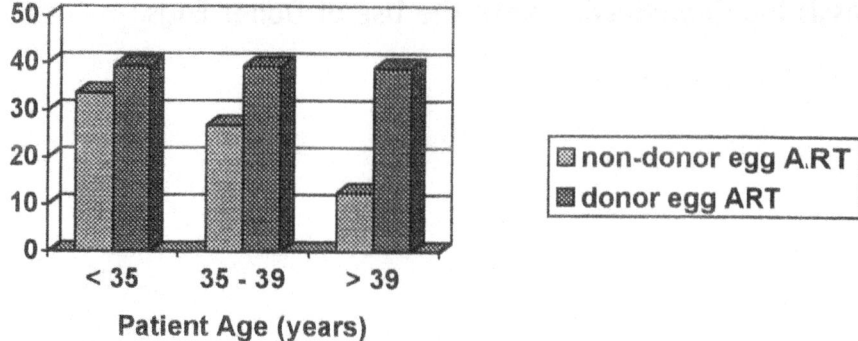

Fig. 1. Live births per 100 transfers, 1996

variation of the basic approach, the egg donor is herself infertile, and her eggs are divided between her and a recipient couple once they are retrieved.

Since this book is designed to be more of a practical manual of how ART is practiced than a compendium review of the historical background, scientific deductions, and variations in practice patterns, we have tried to be concise and practical in our remarks on the management of a donor-egg program. We begin by considering current indications for the use of donated eggs, then discuss our view of an appropriate evaluation and screening of potential egg recipients, and what risks may be imposed upon the recipient by this form of ART. Next we consider the selection of egg donors, their screening, and the potential risks they face. The matching process, a synchronization protocol, and post-transfer management are described. The chapter concludes with a consideration of some features of the donor-egg program at the Jones Institute.

Donor Egg Recipients

Indications

A primary indication for the use of donor eggs is premature ovarian failure (POF), defined as hypergonadotropic hypogonadism occurring before the age of 40 years. It is estimated that POF affects approximately 1% of the female population [3]. The etiology of POF is idiopathic in approximately 50% of cases, while in 45% the cause is immunological and in 2.5% chromosomal [4]. Other causes of POF are iatrogenic and include bilateral oophorectomy, irradiation, and chemotherapy, especially with alkylating agents. Abnormalities of the X-chromosome (e.g., Turner's syndrome), congenital thymic aplasia, galactosemia, and the resistant ovary syndrome (Savage syndrome) are also causes of POF, though rare [5].

Incipient ovarian failure is a second indication for the use of donated oocytes. Egg donation has been successfully utilized in the infertility treatment of these women of advanced reproductive age who demonstrate an elevated early follicular-phase FSH level, suggestive of poor ovarian reserve. These women exhibit a poor response to hyperstimulation and have markedly decreased pregnancy rates after IVF, even when young. The use of donor eggs offers these patients a much greater chance of achieving a pregnancy. Similarly, women in their middle to late 40s have very poor pregnancy rates with IVF, even when their egg production is ample, and should thus be offered donor eggs as primary therapy.

The use of donor eggs is also indicated when a patient would like to avoid the transmission of a genetic abnormality such as an autosomal dominant disorder or sex-linked recessive disorder. A patient with a balanced translocation would also benefit from use of donor eggs. Utilization of donor eggs for these indications may decrease in the future, as specific gene probes are developed and preimplantation genetic techniques are refined [5].

Finally, women who have undergone multiple previous unsuccessful IVF attempts are candidates for egg donation. This is particularly relevant when poor egg quality is suspected to be the fundamental problem.

Evaluation and Screening

The goal of the evaluation and screening of the recipient is to ensure that she is in good physical and mental health to undergo the rigors of donor-egg IVF and hopefully a consequent pregnancy. The American Society for Reproductive Medicine (ASRM) states in their guidelines for egg donation:

> In view of the lack of knowledge about the physiological effects and risks of establishing pregnancy in women of advanced reproductive age, it is recommended that potential recipients over the age of 40 undergo a thorough evaluation including psychological assessments, cardiovascular screening, and high-risk obstetrical consultation before being approved to receive donated oocytes [6].

The initial evaluation includes a full discussion of the donor-egg IVF process. During this discussion, the potential stresses, risks, and costs, as well as reasonable expectations for success are reviewed. A complete physical examination is performed to detect potential uterine abnormalities as well as to screen for other physical abnormalities. Table 1 lists the required screening tests for egg recipients at our clinic.

Risks to Recipients of Donor Eggs

Patients undergoing donor-egg IVF are subjected to additional risks beyond those usually attributed to IVF (the risk of multiple gestation and the inherent risks of the procedure). On average, pregnancies are more apt to be complicated as the age of the pregnant woman increases. While healthy older women without overt medical disease are at somewhat decreased risk for complicated pregnancies, the level of risk is clearly still above that seen at younger ages.

Table 1. Screening of egg recipients

Test/consultation	When needed
Hysterosalpingogram, saline hysterosonography or hysteroscopy	Within 3 years
Pap smear	Within 1 year
Mammogram	Within 5 years if recipient is between ages 35 and 40, within 2 years if she is between ages 41 and 50, and within 1 year if she is 51 years or older
Fasting glucose level	Within 3 years if anyone in recipient's immediate family or two or more people among her relatives have diabetes, if she is obese, or if she has had diabetes while pregnant
Electrocardiogram	Within the year if recipient is aged 40 years or more
Total cholesterol level	Within the year if a parent or sibling of the recipient has/had a total > 240 mg/dl, if members of her family developed premature (< 55 years) cardiovascular disease, if she has diabetes, or if she smokes
Fecal occult blood screening	Within the year if the recipient is aged > 50 years, or has/had first-degree relatives with colorectal cancer, or has had endometrial, ovarian, or breast cancer herself, or has had inflammatory bowel disease, adenomatous polyps, or colorectal cancer herself, or has family members with polyposis coli or cancer family syndrome
Preconceptual counseling	If recipient is age 35 years or more, with an obstetrician, to review risks of pregnancy
General medical screening	If recipient is age 45 years or more, or gets short of breath, has a heart murmur, or has an abnormal electrocardiogram, a high total cholesterol, or blood in her stools
Psychological counseling	Recommended for all, but not required

Some of this increase is due to the higher proportion of women at these advanced ages who already have known medical problems such as high blood pressure, diabetes, and obesity. For example, the incidence of chronic hypertension in pregnant women aged 40 or greater has been reported to be 16% and is significantly elevated when compared with the approximately 2% incidence in the general population [7]. Kirz and colleagues observed a threefold increase in the incidence of diabetes when more than 1000 women older than 35 were compared with nearly 5350 control women aged 20–25 [8]. The incidence of abruptio placentae and placenta previa are similarly increased [9, 10]. Finally, older women are more likely to have an instrument-assisted vaginal delivery (OR 7.5) or cesarean section (OR 7.3) [11, 12].

Although the actual risk is unknown and egg donors are screened for sexually transmitted diseases (STD), a potential risk of transmission of infection through egg donation remains. To date, embryo cryopreservation after egg donation is not required. However, the ASRM recommends that patients be given the choice to cryopreserve all embryos for 6 or more months after donor STD screening or to accept the unknown risk of STD transmission associated with the transfer of fresh embryos.

Egg Donors

Screening and Selection

The ASRM has published guidelines for the recruitment and screening of egg donors [6]. These guidelines propose that prospective egg donors undergo selection and screening procedures which are similar to those recommended for sperm donors. Egg donors should be young (<35), in overall good health, and not have, or be a carrier of, any known genetic disorders transmitted by traditional mendelian inheritance that pose "serious functional or cosmetic handicaps." Similarly, the donors should neither have any malformations acquired because of multifactorial/polygenic inheritance nor be a carrier of a balanced translocation which may become unbalanced in subsequent offspring.

In our program, potential donors undergo a series of screening phases. By dividing the screening process into these phases, the cost of screening potential donors is minimized, while the ultimate quality of donors is assured. In our clinic, only about 20% of women who call us to become egg donors end up being qualified.

Phase 1 is detailed in Table 2. The information required to complete this phase can be obtained in a telephone interview, thus eliminating potential donors who do not meet the above requirements prior to an office visit.

Phase 2 of donor screening consists of a questionnaire and measurement of serum basal hormone levels to determine ovarian reserve. The medical and family history of a potential donor can be ascertained initially with this questionnaire, which asks for a thorough accounting of the patient's past medical history and the past medical history of her family. Serum follicle-stimulating hormone (FSH), serum luteinizing hormone (LH), and serum estradiol levels are obtained on day 3 of the donor's menstrual cycle. Phase 2 also includes a psychological evaluation of whether the donor has adequately addressed the potential medical, legal, ethical, and emotional ramifications associated with egg donation. This is particularly important in nonanonymous donation in which a recipient couple chooses their own donor, usually a close relative. Phase 2 is outlined in Table 3.

The third and final phase of egg-donor screening consists of an interview, a physical examination, and screening tests for STDs. The purpose of the interview is to review the donor's medical history and to clarify any remaining issues or questions that the potential donor may have regarding the process of

---

Table 2. Screening of egg donors: phase 1

Donor age between 21 and 34
Both ovaries present
Not overweight
Nonsmoker
Off hormonal contraception for >2 months
Not adopted
If donor meets above criteria, then proceed to phase 2

Table 3. Screening of egg donors: phase 2

Review questionnaire:
  Eliminate those with serious functional or cosmetic handicaps or unknown family background
  Eliminate those with high-risk behavior for STDs
If OK: evaluate basal FSH, LH, and estradiol
If OK: review psychological evaluation
If OK: donor should come to clinic for phase 3

Table 4. Screening of egg donors: phase 3

Physical examination
Cervical cultures
  Gonorrhea
  Mycoplasma (ureaplasma)
  Herpes
  Chlamydia
Blood tests
  Syphilis serology
  HIV-1 and HIV-2 (antigen and antibody tests)
  Hepatitis B and C
  Thalassemia (in Greeks, Italians, and Asians)
  Cystic fibrosis (in all Caucasians)
  Sickle-cell (in African-Americans)
  Tay-Sachs (in European Jews)
  Type and Rh

egg donation. Phase 3 is outlined in Table 4. Once a donor has passed all screening tests and evaluations, the matching of the recipient with the proposed donor is begun.

Potential Risks to Egg Donors

The potential risks to egg donors are similar to those experienced by patients undergoing controlled ovarian hyperstimulation and IVF. These risks include ovarian hyperstimulation, infection, hemorrhage, injury to adjacent structures during egg retrieval, and complications of anesthesia.

· Epidemiological studies have reported an association between the use of ovulation-inducing medications and an increased incidence of ovarian cancer [13–15]. While the data are acknowledged even by their authors as being inconclusive, the relationship is biologically plausible. As a consequence, we limit our egg donors to no more than five "lifetime" cycles of egg donation, whether or not they were all performed by us. Additionally, due to the recent studies indicating a lower incidence of ovarian cancer with past oral contraceptive use, we further recommend the use of oral contraceptives [16].

The Matching Process

Recipients are matched with donors based upon shared physical features such as height, body build, skin, eye, and hair color. Matching of blood type is not necessary, but it is desirable in the case of an Rh-negative recipient or for couples who wish their child to be compatible with their own blood types so that the child will not "accidentally" discover that he or she resulted from egg donation. Recipient couples often add other constraints to their request for a donor, most commonly a certain level of education. Once the staff of the Donor Egg Program makes a tentative match, a summary of the donor's characteristics is provided to the recipient couple. This couple is also given information regarding the donor's previous pregnancy outcomes, medical and surgical conditions, and educational and work histories.

Synchronization of Recipient and Donor

If a transfer of "fresh" (never cryopreserved) embryos is planned, careful synchronization of the recipient and donor is critical to a successful outcome. Adequate endometrial development with exogenous steroids is essential. Accordingly, while the donor undergoes superovulation and egg retrieval, the recipient receives exogenous estrogen and progesterone to prepare the endometrium for implantation. Various markers of adequate endometrial development have been proposed including serum estradiol levels, endometrial thickness as measured by ultrasoonography, and late luteal phase endometrial biopsy in a test cycle.

In 1997, Remohi et al. prospectively evaluated serum estradiol concentrations and ultrasound measurements of endometrial thickness in 465 donor egg cycles. They demonstrated that endometrial thickness was significantly greater when serum estradiol concentrations were greater than 400 pg/ml as compared with those less than 100 pg/ml. There was a positive correlation ($p = 0.0044$) between endometrial thickness and implantation, although none of the parameters examined was able to predict the outcome of ovum donation [17].

Also in 1997, Potter et al. evaluated the role of endometrial biopsy during hormone replacement cycles in donor-oocyte recipients. Thirty-six concurrent recipients underwent test cycles with endometrial biopsy. Recipients more than 40 years of age received 100 mg of i.m. progesterone in oil daily and those less than 40 years of age received 50 mg of i.m. progesterone. Despite the increased dosage, late luteal phase endometrial biopsies indicated that five of the 20 patients older than 40 years had out-of-phase endometrial biopsies (greater than 2 days). All of the 16 patients younger than 40 had in-phase biopsies. All out-of-phase biopsies were subsequently corrected with higher doses of progesterone. Pregnancy rates did not differ between the two age-groups [18].

Within our clinic, we request test cycle endometrial biopsies during the late luteal phase of a hormone replacement cycle from women who are considered to be at high risk for having an "out-of-phase" biopsy. This includes women over the age of 40 or those with a history of an endometrial disorder such as Asherman's syndrome or poor endometrial development during ovarian stimulation.

Many protocols for preparation of the recipient have been described, and most seem to be sufficient to the task. Estrogens may be administered orally, transdermally, or parenterally. There is some evidence that the supraphysiologic estradiol concentrations associated with oral administration of micronized estradiol may be associated with a lag in endometrial development based upon histology and beta-3-integrin expression [19]. It is now clear that the artificial "follicular" phase of these cycles can be shortened or lengthened to a remarkable degree to accommodate synchronization without any ill effects on the chance for pregnancy.

Conventional progesterone replacement with the daily administration of i.m. progesterone in oil has been the mainstay of therapy over the past decade. The options for progesterone replacement have expanded in recent years with the introduction of vaginally administered micronized progesterone, which offers convenience and ease of administration. Crinone 8% (90 mg), administered daily and twice daily, has been prospectively evaluated in donor egg cycles at the Jones Institute for Reproductive Medicine [20, 21]. Recently, 86 women undergoing donor egg cycles with either crinone 8% (90 mg) administered daily or 100 mg i.m. progesterone once daily were compared. Serum progesterone concentrations were consistently lower in the crinone group than in the i.m. progesterone group. However, 42 of the 42 endometrial biopsies were in phase in the crinone group, compared with 42 of 44 in the i.m. progesterone group. Clinical pregnancy, ongoing pregnancy, implantation, and miscarriage rates were not statistically different between the two groups [20].

One successful protocol implemented at our clinic uses transdermal estradiol patches and crinone 8% (90 mg) administered daily. Occasionally, GnRH agonists are used in the recipient cycle for synchronization; however, the vast majority of our recipient cycles involve the administration of estradiol patches on day 1 of the menstrual cycle. The dose of estradiol is increased until the day of the donor egg retrieval (see Table 5). Also on the day of retrieval, progesterone therapy is initiated and continued until the luteoplacental shift in pregnancy.

Once the eggs are retrieved, they are inseminated with sperm from the recipient's partner after a preincubation interval of 2-8 h. The resulting embryos are either cryopreserved or transferred to the synchronized recipient 3-5 days later. In an effort to reduce the number of multiple pregnancies, we are transferring

Table 5. Synchronization protocol

Donor	Recipient
Days 1–4 of stimulation	1–0.1 mg estradiol patch QOD
Days 5–8 of stimulation	2–0.1 mg estradiol patches QOD
Day 9 through the day prior to retrieval	4–0.1 mg estradiol patches QOD
Day of retrieval and continuing for 30 days	2–0.1 mg estradiol patches QOD; progesterone administration (i.m., or crinone)
Next 30 days	No estradiol supplements; progesterone administration (i.m., or crinone) then stop

embryos to an increasing number of patients at the blastocyst stage; two or three blastocysts are transferred, depending on grade. If a day-3 transfer is performed, the best three of six embryos are being transferred.

Post-Transfer Management

After embryo transfer, the recipient is taken to the recovery room, where she will remain for 1 h of bed rest before being discharged to home. Estrogen and progesterone replacement is continued, as described in Table 5. Serial serum estradiol and progesterone levels are measured on days 14 and 16 following transfer to be sure that the hormone replacement is adequate. A serum pregnancy test (β-hCG) run on the same samples determines whether pregnancy has occurred. If the pregnancy test is negative, then hormone replacement is discontinued and a menses will subsequently begin. If the cycle has been successful, then the hormone replacement therapy is continued, with monitoring of the peripheral estradiol and progesterone concentrations at 6 and 10 weeks after transfer. Replacement therapy is presently being discontinued 60 days after embryo transfer.

Results of the Jones Institute Donor Egg Program

In order to provide some insight into what variables are important to the outcome of a donor egg program, we present the following data based on our own program.

Overall Results in One Program

The recent results of the Jones Institute Donor Egg Program are summarized in Tables 6 and 7. Recent changes in the program seem to have increased the implantation rate significantly. These have included:
- Use of a Wallace rather than a Jones catheter for transfer
- Use of pure FSH medication rather than an FSH/LH blend

Table 6. Results of fresh transfers (in percent)

	1998	1997	1996	1995	1994	1993
No. of recipients	119	106	148	78	68	45
Implantation rate (sacs/embryo transferred)	13	22	26	19	18	18
Clinical pregnancy rate (/transfer)	36	47	43.2	52	40	42
Delivery rate (/transfer)	26	33	36	32	34	29

Table 7. Results of cryotransfers (in percent)

	1998	1997	1996	1995	1994	1993
No. of recipients	56	49	55	14	31	25
Implantation rate (sacs/embryo)	13	15	10	10	9	13
Clinical pregnancy rate (/transfer)	28	20	27	36	23	44
Delivery rate (/transfer)	16	12	18	29	16	32

Table 8. Results of implantation based on patient age (in percent)

	Recipient age		
	<34	35–39	40+
No. of recipients	62	120	325
Implantation rate (sacs/embryo transferred)	25	15	20
Clinical pregnancy rate (sac/transfer)	46	38	43
Delivery rate (/transfer)	42	25	32

- Selection of the best available embryos for transfer from a number twice that intended for transfer, rather than a policy involving no selection of the morphologically better embryos.
  Our initial experience with blastocyst culture and transfer has demonstrated increased implantation and pregnancy rates.

Effect of Recipient's Age on Outcome

As mentioned earlier, the use of donor eggs seems to overcome the primary hurdle that older women face, i.e., declining egg quality. However, there may be a decline in uterine receptivity with aging as well. Our own data on this issue, shown in Table 8, are from 1995 through 1998. It may be important to mention that only a few of the women in our program were older than 50 years at the time of their embryo transfer, so our data may understate the negative effect of advanced female age.

Effect of Donor's Age on Outcome

It is clearly important to also establish the effect of the egg donor's age on outcome, and these data are shown in Table 9. It appears that donors over the age of 30 are less likely to produce a pregnancy than those who are younger. Nonetheless, we still accept a donor up to the age of 34 if she is known or related to the recipient.

Table 9. Results of implantation based on donor's age (in percent)

Age (years)	Clinical pregnancy rate (sac/transfer), n/total (%)	Ongoing pregnancy rate (delivery or pregnancy ongoing >20 weeks/ transfer), n/total (%)
<26	68/162 (42)	53/162 (33)
26–28	53/123 (43)	39/123 (32)
29–30	124/308 (40)	96/308 (31)
31–32	23/74 (31)	17/74 (23)
33–34	19/65 (29)	13/65 (20)
All	254/674 (38)	191/674 (28)

Table 10. Effect of embryo quality on outcome

Grade of best embryo	Chance for pregnancy/fresh transfer (%)	Chance for delivery/ fresh transfer (%)
1 (best)	102/190 (53)	80/190 (42)
2	68/166 (41)	51/166 (31)
3	9/33 (27)	9/33 (27)
4 (worst)	3/9 (33)	2/9 (22)

Effect of Embryo Quality on Outcome

It is apparent that many human embryos are chromosomally abnormal, and that some of these abnormal embryos display poor growth in culture. We have assessed the effect of embryo quality on pregnancy outcome when donor eggs are employed, in order to gauge the importance of this factor (see Table 10). We have concluded that (a) for embryos resulting from donor eggs the relationship between embryo quality and pregnancy outcome is very significant, but that (b) even poor-quality embryos have a reasonable potential for producing pregnancy (we discount the few grade-5 embryos because of small sample size).

Endometrial Pattern and Thickness Do not Influence Pregnancy Rates in Unstimulated Recipients of Donor Eggs

Prior reports on IVF patients linking endometrial thickness and pattern to pregnancy potential are confounded by the degree of ovarian hyperstimulation. To control for this factor, endometrial pattern and thickness were correlated with pregnancy rates in donor-egg recipients. Transvaginal ultrasonography was performed on the morning of progesterone supplementation to evaluate both the bilaminar thickness in the upper fundus (Table 11) and the endometrial pattern (A: homogeneous, hyperechogenic; B: outer hyperechogenic and inner hypoechogenic layer; Table 12). As shown in the tables, neither thickness

Table 11. Effect of endometrial thickness on outcome

Thickness (mm)	Clinical pregnancy rate/transfer (%)	Ongoing pregnancy rate/transfer (%)
4–7	5/23 (22)	4/23 (17.0)
8–9	21/75 (28)	14/75 (19)
10–11	26/81 (32)	21/81 (26)
12–13	17/49 (35)	15/49 (31)

Table 12. Effect of endometrial pattern on outcome

Pattern	Clinical pregnancy rate/transfer (%)	Ongoing pregnancy rate/transfer (%)
A	6/29 (21)	5/29 (17)
B	74/206 (36)	57/206 (27)

($\chi^2 = 1.23$, $p = 0.27$) nor pattern influenced pregnancy rates ($\chi^2 = 2.62$, $p = 0.10$), though trends favor the thicker and trilaminar types.

Summary

Donor eggs have proven to be a valuable means of achieving pregnancy in many cases in which the wife's own egg quality and/or quantity is substantially diminished. The technique is complex to perform properly, but the high pregnancy rates bring great rewards, both to the patients and to the staff involved in providing the service. Although the use of donor eggs is a simple form of substitution therapy that does not directly "fix" the underlying problem, the donor egg approach will undoubtedly remain an important facet of assisted reproduction until basic scientific work provides clinicians with a means to repair eggs of poor quality or limited quantity. In the meantime, this technique permits many couples to realize their dream of having and raising children, which was out of reach even a decade ago. As such, donor egg programs provide an indispensable service to the patients themselves and society at large, now at the close of the second millennium.

References

1. Lutjen P, Trounson A, Leeton J, Findlay J, Wood C, Renou P (1984) The establishment and maintenance of pregnancy using in vitro fertilization and embryo donation in a patient with primary ovarian failure. Nature 307:174–175
2. Control CfD (1996) 1996 Assisted reproductive technology success rates.
3. Coulam CB (1982) Premature gonadal failure. Fertil Steril 38:645–655

4. Falsetti L, Scalchi S, Villani MT, Bugari G (1999) Premature ovarian failure. Gynecol Endocrinol 13:189–195
5. Moomjy MCI, Owen D, Applegarth L, Rosenwaks Z (1995) Donor Oocytes in assisted reproduction – an overview. Semin Reprod Endocrinol 13:173–186
6. The American Society for Reproductive Medicine (1998) Guidelines for gamete and embryo donation. Fertil Steril 70 [Suppl 1]:5S
7. Yasin SY, Beydoun SN (1988) Pregnancy outcome at greater than or equal to 20 weeks' gestation in women in their 40s. A case-control study. J Reprod Med 33:209–213
8. Kirz DS, Dorchester W, Freeman RK (1985) Advanced maternal age: the mature gravida. Am J Obstet Gynecol 152:7–12
9. Mestman JH (1980) Outcome of diabetes screening in pregnancy and perinatal morbidity in infants of mothers with mild impairment in glucose tolerance. Diabetes Care 3:447–452
10. Hansen JP (1986) Older maternal age and pregnancy outcome: a review of the literature. Obstet Gynecol Surv 41:726–742
11. Dulitzki M, Soriano D, Schiff E, Chetrit A, Mashiach S, Seidman DS (1998) Effect of very advanced maternal age on pregnancy outcome and rate of cesarean delivery. Obstet Gynecol 92:935–939
12. Tuck SM, Yudkin PL, Turnbull AC (1988) Pregnancy outcome in elderly primigravidae with and without a history of infertility. Br J Obstet Gynaecol 95:230–237
13. Mosgaard BJ, Lidegaard O, Kjaer SK, Schou G, Andersen AN (1997) Infertility, fertility drugs, and invasive ovarian cancer: a case-control study [see comments]. Fertil Steril 67:1005–1012
14. Rossing MA, Daling JR, Weiss NS, Moore DE, Self SG (1994) Ovarian tumors in a cohort of infertile women [see comments]. N Engl J Med 331:771–776
15. Whittemore AS, Harris R, Itnyre J (1992) Characteristics relating to ovarian cancer risk: collaborative analysis of 12 US case-control studies. IV. The pathogenesis of epithelial ovarian cancer. Collaborative Ovarian Cancer Group. Am J Epidemiol 136:1212–1220
16. La Vecchia C, Franceschi S (1999) Oral contraceptives and ovarian cancer. Eur J Cancer Prev 8:297–304
17. Remohi J, Ardiles G, Garcia-Velasco JA, Gaitan P, Simon C, Pellicer A (1997) Endometrial thickness and serum oestradiol concentrations as predictors of outcome in oocyte donation. Hum Reprod 12:2271–2276
18. Potter DA, Witz CA, Burns WN, Brzyski RG, Schenken RS (1998) Endometrial biopsy during hormone replacement cycle in donor oocyte recipients before in vitro fertilization-embryo transfer. Fertil Steril 70:219–221
19. Krasnow JS, Lessey BA, Naus G, Hall LL, Guzick DS, Berga SL (1996) Comparison of transdermal versus oral estradiol on endometrial receptivity. Fertil Steril 65:332–336
20. Jobanputra K, Toner JP, Denoncourt R, Gibbons WE (1999) Crinone 8% (90 mg) given once daily for progesterone replacement therapy in donor egg cycles. Fertil Steril 72:980–984
21. Gibbons WE, Toner JP, Hamacher P, Kolm P (1998) Experience with a novel vaginal progesterone preparation in a donor oocyte program. Fertil Steril 69:96–101

Oocyte Maturation In Vivo and In Vitro: Principles of Regulation

W. Küpker, K. Diedrich

Development of Oocytes

Oogenesis begins early in fetal development. Germ cells can already be detected in 24-day-old embryos. Primordial germ cells move from an extragonadal site and enter the cortex of the differentiating gonad. Ovarian development starts. Primordial germ cells are precursors of actively dividing oogonia, which begin a high frequency of mitotic activity to reach the first meiotic prophase as oocytes. Germ cells in this stage are present within the first 4 months of fetal development and are estimated to number 5–6 million. The phase of multiplication of oogonia ends in the fifth month of fetal life [1]. The maturing oocyte is a direct derivative of the primary germ cell. After having finished the mitotic phase of multiplication, oogonia – now known as oocytes – are encompassed by follicular or granulosa cells. The oocyte enters the first stage of meiotic prophase, the leptotene having passed the preleptotene. It is during preleptotene, i.e., the interphase of the last mitotic division, that final DNA replication takes place in preparation for meiosis and signals the transformation of oogonia into oocytes. The oocyte remains in prophase for a long time. In prophase, oocytes progress through four different stages. After up to 6 h, as confirmed by studies on mouse oocytes, they change to zygotene. During zygotene, homologous chromosomes pair and synapse to form what appear to be single chromosomes, but are actually bivalents composed of four chromatids. It takes up to 40 h to complete zygotene. In the following stage, the pachytene, genetic crossing over and recombination takes place. It takes approximately 4 days before oocytes enter the final stage of diplotene, with chromosomes displaying chiasmata as a result of crossing over. Oocytes remain in diplotene stage, also called the dictyate stage, until ovulation. The oocyte has formed a characteristic nucleus called the germinal vesicle. Prior to birth almost all fetal oocytes have reached the final stage of dictyate. The human ovary provides approximately 2 million oocytes at the time of birth. Merely 5%, i.e., 300 000 oocytes survive the following 7 years and form the pool of unfertilized eggs in the sexually mature adult [2].

Maturation of Oocytes – Basic Considerations

Oocyte maturation is defined as the reinitiation and completion of the first meiotic division, subsequent progression to metaphase II, and the nuclear and cytoplasmic processes which become essential for fertilization and early embryo development. Oocytes are arrested in prophase I of meiosis during the fetal period. Completion of the first meiotic division takes place when oocytes have undergone extensive growth in cellular interaction with the granulosa and theca cells. The oocyte undergoes asymmetric cytokinesis and extrudes the first polar body containing a haploid chromosome complement. The first meiotic division is completed, the second meiotic division is initiated, but oocytes remain arrested in metaphase II until contact is made with a spermatozoon. The initiation of maturation in fully grown oocytes which are present in antral follicles is based on the mid-cyclic onset of the luteinizing hormone (LH) surge or the external administration of human chorionic gonadotropin (hCG). Mechanisms of oocyte maturation in vivo and in vitro are still under investigation. In vitro animal models provided insight into the importance of substances affecting oocyte maturation and its inhibition, such as cAMP, calcium, cell-cycle proteins, growth factors, GnRH, gonadotropins, purines, and steroids.

Structural Changes during Oocyte Maturation

Germinal Vesicle Breakdown

The nucleus of an oocyte is the germinal vesicle (GV) (Fig. 1). The most striking event of the reinitiation of meiosis is the disappearance or breakdown of

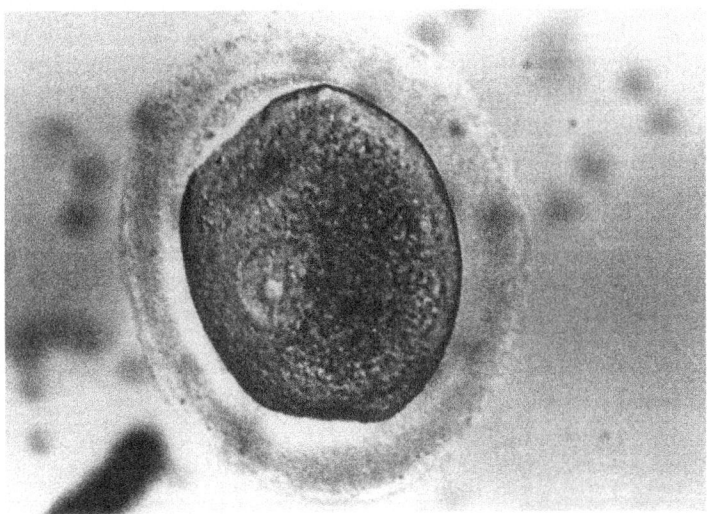

Fig. 1. Germinal vesicle

the GV (GVB). The acquisition of competence to undergo GVB is a multistep process. GVB is initiated in human and animal oocytes in vivo by the LH surge or atretic degeneration of follicles, but when they are removed from their antral follicles or after removal of the entire oocyte-cumulus cell complex, spontaneous gonadotropin-independent maturation may occur in culture media as well. Within a few hours of culture in vitro fully grown oocytes undergo complete GVB [3, 4]. GVB begins with undulations of the nuclear envelope (Fig. 2) which continues for approximately 1–2 h. These undulations may be correlated to the onset of chromosome condensation. Breaks in the nuclear envelope can be detected within 2 h, and after approximately 3 h the nuclear envelope has completely disappeared in rabbit, rat, and mouse oocytes; it is likely to be involved later in formation of the pronuclear membrane. In human beings this process initiating chromosome condensation takes 20–24 h.

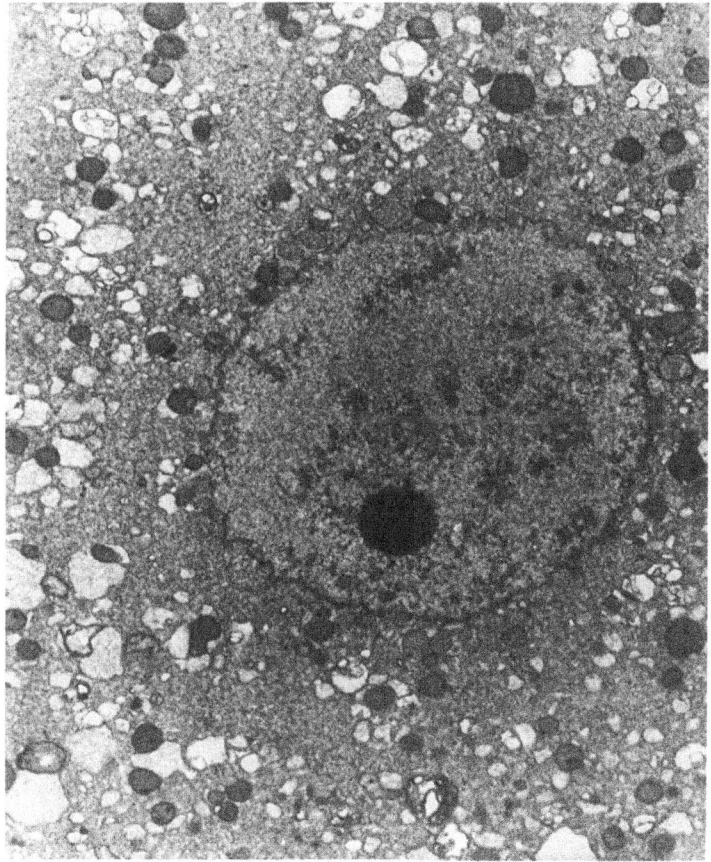

Fig. 2. Germinal vesicle with undulating nuclear envelope and onset of chromosome condensation

Meiotic Maturation and Chromosome Formation

Chromosome condensation and spindle formation are the following steps in the scheduled program of the maturing oocyte to complete meiosis. Directly subsequent to GVB – when the nuclear envelope and its inner lining, the fibrillar network of laminae, start to dissolve – chromosomes have moved from the center of the nucleus towards the undulating membranes, where condensation takes place. Chiasmata move to the ends of the chromosomes and chromatin becomes heterochromatic. After completion of condensation the chromosomal bivalents appear V-shaped and telocentric. They are often attached to fragments of the nuclear envelope. Being highly condensed, chromosomes become arranged in the center of the oocyte, waiting to line up on the metaphase spindle. During GVB and chromosome condensation, kinetochores and the microtubule system appear to organize the spindle formation. The spindle does not display centrioles as is typical for mitotic cells; rather, it derives from so-called pericentriolar material which forms the spindle poles during prometaphase. The spindle apparatus increases in size and moves to the periphery of the oocyte. The barrel-shaped spindle is surrounded by mitochondria, vacuoles, and granules. Metaphase I (Fig. 3) lasts for a few hours and leads to anaphase I, when chromosomal bivalents move towards the opposite ends of the spindle and the whole spindle rotates 90°. During telophase I the extrusion of the first polar body is prepared. Homologous chromosomes become separated, and one half is extruded with cytoplasmic material such as mitochondria, ribosomes, and cortical granules into the perivitelline space (Fig. 4). This takes place in late telophase. The oocyte has reached metaphase II (Fig. 5). Progressive maturation beyond metaphase II marks the beginning of fertilization or indicates parthenogenetic activation of the oocyte.

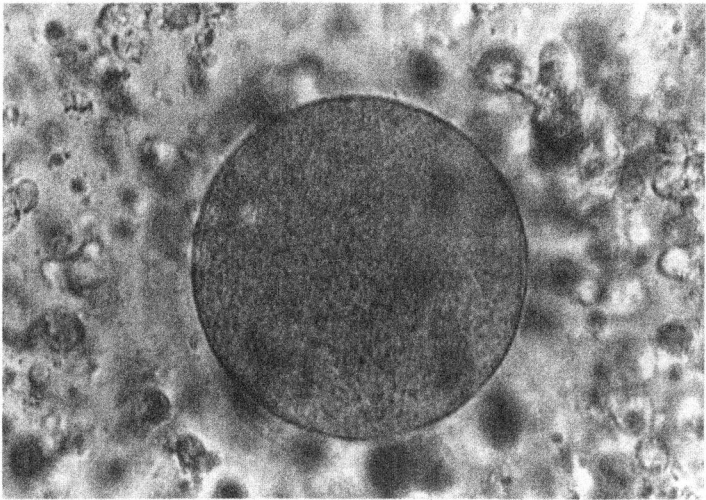

Fig. 3. Metaphase-I oocyte

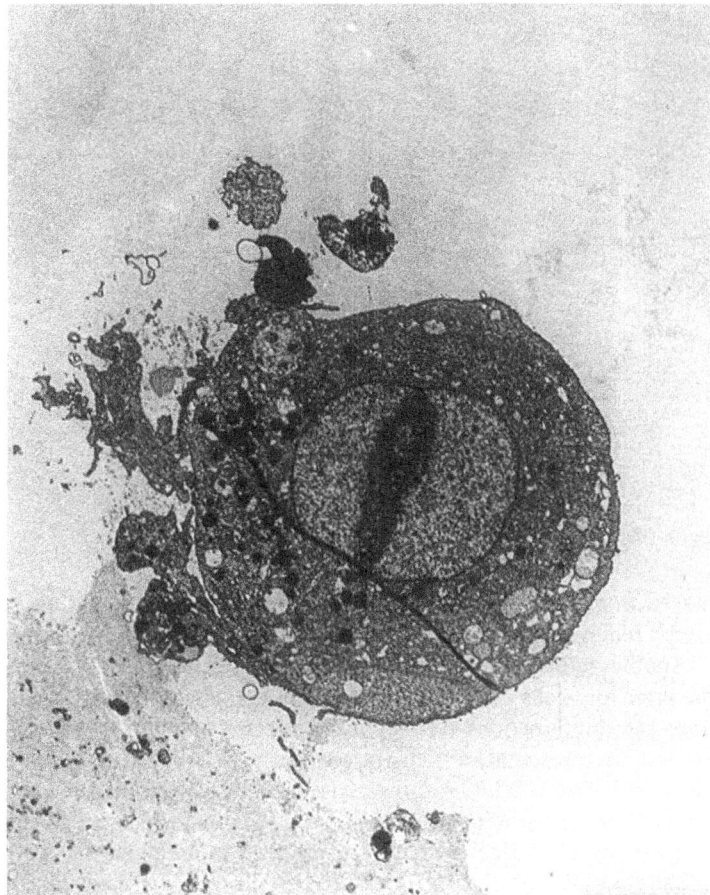

Fig. 4. First polar body with cortical granules and chromosomes

Regulation of Oocyte Maturation

Gonadotropins and Intercellular Communication

In human and animal oocytes the preovulatory LH surge or the administration of human chorionic gonadotropin (hCG) induces GVB in vivo or when follicles are placed in culture. But there are no receptors for LH on the oocytes. There-fore, it is hypothesized that LH probably induces GVB indirectly by the action of granulosa cells [5]. LH apparently induces a block of intrafollicular commu-nication and reduces the transfer of maturation-arresting substances to the oo-cyte. According to this hypothesis, LH-induced GVB is initiated the same way as spontaneous GVB when oocytes have lost their contact to cumulus and gran-ulosa cells. It is known that oocytes enclosed in an antral follicle, when re-

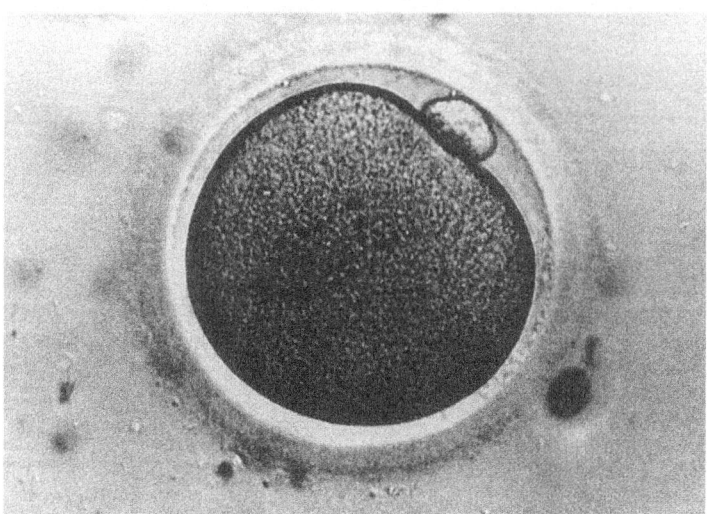

Fig. 5. Metaphase-II oocyte

moved from their environment, do not resume meiosis. But adding gonadotropin or removing the oocyte from the follicle results in resumption of meiosis.

Another hypothesis is that LH triggers production of a GVB-inducing signal in the granulosa cells being transmitted into the oocyte through so-called gap junctions [6]. Gap junctions are regions of physical continuity between cellular membranes. They resemble a network connecting granulosa cells, cumulus cells, and the oocyte. The cells are metabolically and ionically coupled through the gap junctions. They consist of proteins called connections, which act as channels permitting the rapid passage of small molecules. It is assumed that LH-induced GVB, transferred through the gap-junction system, may be mediated by calcium. LH induces an increase of free inositol 1,4,5-triphosphate (IP3) [7] and calcium in the granulosa cell. Both substances are transferred via gap junctions to the oocyte. The role of calcium will be discussed later. Follicle-stimulating hormone (FSH) is assumed to promote signals for GVB induction to a much greater extent in cumulus-enclosed oocytes than in cumulus-denuded oocytes. This would mean that maintenance of gap-junction communication between cumulus cells and the oocyte is essential for FSH stimulation of maturation [8].

The Role of Cyclic Adenosine Monophosphate (cAMP)

Cyclic AMP, which is present in the oocyte, appears to be a candidate involved in maintenance of meiotic arrest (Fig. 6), since the mode of cAMP action is known. Cyclic AMP activates a cAMP-dependent protein kinase (PK-A). An inhibitory basal level of cAMP within the oocyte activates PK-A. The active form of the heterotetramer PK-A is the catalytic subunits after binding of cAMP to the inhibitory subunits of the PK-A complex. PK-A phosphorylates oocyte pro-

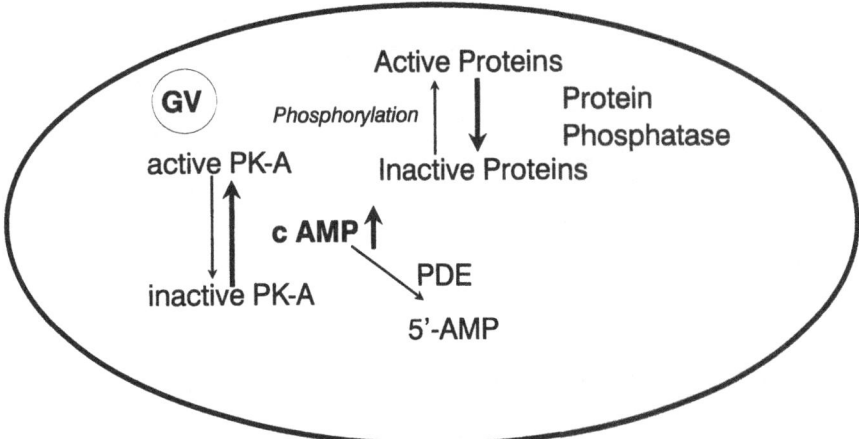

Fig. 6. Maintenance of meiotic arrest

teins which are necessary for GVB. Continuous phosphorylation of proteins maintains the meiotic arrest. Resumption of meiosis, on the other hand, is triggered by a decrease in the inhibitory level of oocyte cAMP mediated through the action of cAMP phosphodiesterase (PDE) (Fig. 7). cAMP phosphodiesterase promotes the reassociation of the active catalytic subunits of PK-A with its regulatory subunits, which prevents PK-A from carrying on with phosphorylation. Oocyte proteins become dephosphorylated and meiotic maturation will be initiated. Some experiments indicate the involvement of different substances in regulating the oocyte cAMP levels. Spontaneous maturation of mouse oocytes does not occur in vitro in the presence of cAMP analogues such as dbcAMP or 8bcAMP or phosphodiesterase inhibitors such as isobutyl methylxanthine (IBMX) and theophylline [9, 10]. Forskolin maintains oocytes in meiotic arrest via direct stimulation of adenylate cyclase to increase the cAMP level [11, 12]. Phosphodiesterase activity to increase or decrease cAMP levels in the oocyte is responsible for the onset or arrest of maturation and is modulated itself by calmodulin. The origin of active cAMP is still unclear. Cumulus cell-free oocytes produce cAMP on stimulation by forskolin [13], but forskolin treatment produces only a delay of GVB. Thus, higher amounts of cAMP are needed to maintain meiotic arrest. It is still unclear if sufficient cAMP is created by the oocyte itself or originates in granulosa cells. As mentioned above, oocytes are coupled to granulosa and cumulus cells by gap junctions. Gap junctions allow diffusion of small molecules from one cell to another, so cAMP may possibly diffuse from granulosa cells to the oocyte. Another theory is that stimulated granulosa cells promote the oocyte to produce cAMP itself.

Furthermore, it is suggested that other types of protein kinases (PK) may be involved in the regulation of oocyte maturation. Stimulation of the PK-C system with phorbol esters and diacylglycerol also results in a transient inhibition of GVB [4].

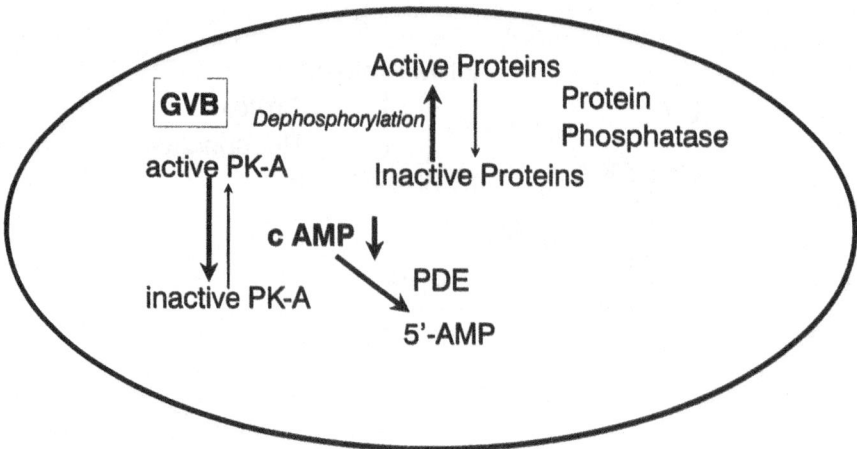

Fig. 7. Resumption of meiotic maturation

Purines

Although cAMP seems to play a major role in oocyte maturation and meiotic arrest, other substances present in the follicle are also likely to participate in meiotic arrest. Hypoxanthine and adenosine were detected in mouse oocytes and follicular fluid [14, 15]. Hypoxanthine inhibits GVB when applied to denuded mouse oocytes. Moreover, the inhibitory effect of purines is increased in cumulus cell-enclosed oocytes. This observation suggests that the intercellular gap-junction pathway to the oocyte provides regulation of uptake and metabolism of those putative granulosa cell-generated substances. Adenosine displays a transiently inhibitory effect on GVB similar to that of forskolin in culture, but when augmented by hypoxanthine the inhibitory effect persists. Direct injection of adenosine into the oocyte does not show any effect. The theory is that hypoxanthine inhibits cAMP phosphodiesterase and therefore prevents hydrolysis of oocyte cAMP. Adenosine promotes the cAMP formation, acting at the oocyte surface by stimulating the adenylate cyclase [16]. Purines may also be involved, to regulate the suppressive effects of guanyl compounds on oocyte maturation. Guanosine monophosphate (GMP), a product of the conversion of inosine monophosphate (IMP), plays an essential role in the maintenance of meiotic arrest. GMP is itself converted to guanosine triphosphate (GTP), which interacts subsequently with G-proteins present on the oolemma and membranes of the cumulus cells. GTP is able to suppress GVB as well, as binding to G-proteins mediates an increase of cAMP levels within the oocyte.

Maturation-Promoting Factor

Maturation-promoting factor (MPF) is a cytoplasmic factor and was detected in both mitotic and meiotic cells. Another name for this substance is M-phase promoting factor, owing to its ability to promote a G2- to an M-phase transition [17]. MPF apparently regulates chromosome condensation and nuclear envelope breakdown. MPF was initially demonstrated by injection of cytoplasm from progesterone-treated oocytes into untreated recipients, which resulted in maturation of the untreated oocytes [18]. It should be noted that progesterone plays a key role in the onset of oocyte maturation in amphibians. The formation of MPF seems to be independent of nuclear activity. It was demonstrated that treating enucleated *Xenopus* oocytes with progesterone and injecting their cytoplasm into nucleated non-progesterone-treated oocytes resulted in MPF activity in these cells, with subsequent maturation [18]. Protein synthesis is necessary for the initial production of MPF, but it is not required for further maturation-promoting activity. Cycloheximide fails to prevent the autocatalytic amplification of MPF as well as treatment with cytochalasin does [19]. These findings suggest that oocytes contain a store of inactive MPF. Protein synthesis is merely essential to activate it. Small amounts of active MPF are able to amplify MPF activity without any further protein synthesis. MPF is a protein kinase consisting of two components, cyclin B and p34^{cdc2}. The small subunit which is called p34 is a protein homologue of the cdc2+ gene product of fission yeast necessary for the G2-M transition. Cdc2 homologues have been detected in cells of a variety of organisms, including mammals [20]. The kinase activity of p34 remains high during M phase, resulting in the phosphorylation of diverse proteins. Histone H1 is one target for p34 kinase [21]. Phosphorylation of histone H1 is suspected to be involved in the condensation process of chromatin that takes place during M phase [22]. Another substrate for p34 are the laminae forming the fibrillar network of the inner surface of the nuclear envelope. Phosphorylation of the laminae is assumed to be responsible for the nuclear envelope breakdown. Moreover, p34 is likely to interact with the microtubular system and enhances maturation by organizing the spindle apparatus through phosphorylation.

The other subunit of MPF is cyclin B, a protein representing the group of cyclins which accumulate during interphase and are destroyed by proteolysis after mitosis during each cell cycle [23]. The role of cyclin B is to activate p34 kinase when they complex with p34. Cyclins, like p34, also seem to be universal cell-cycle regulators in eukaryotes. Cyclins are homologues to the gene product of cdc13 in fission yeast. While p34 requires dephosphorylation for activation, cyclin B has to be phosphorylated to become active when preexisting in complexes with p34, whereas it forms directly active MPF when synthesized de novo. c-MOS (p39 mos), which is a product of the c-mos proto-oncogene, apparently triggers cyclin B activation. C-MOS is a kinase that is necessary for induction of maturation. Studies on *Xenopus* showed that injecting c-MOS mRNA into the oocyte induces maturation, while inhibiting c-MOS prevents maturation [24]. c-MOS phosphorylates cyclin B in vitro. Briefly, c-MOS activates cy-

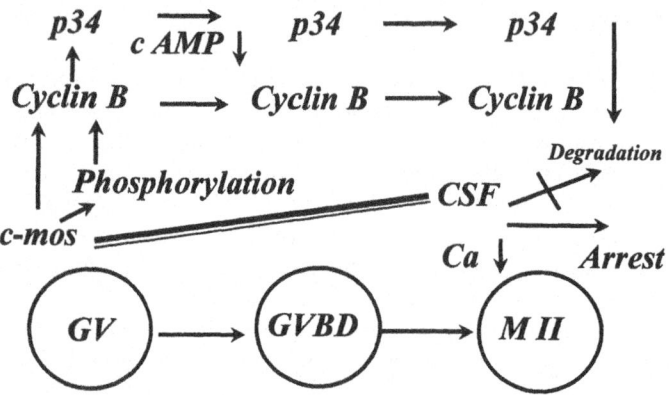

Fig. 8. Maturation-promoting factor and meiotic arrest

clin, which in turn activates p34. There is some question regarding how MPF activity is controlled in the oocyte. There are some good reasons for assuming that active p34 is directly controlled by PKA activity resulting from a decreased concentration of cAMP in the oocyte. Elevation of cAMP inhibits the formation of p34/cyclic B complex and p34 remains inactive. MPF exhibits its activity as long as cyclins are present. Degradation of cyclins at the end of the M phase inactivates MPF, allowing the cell cycle to continue. Arrest of the mature oocyte at metaphase II is probably due to a cytostatic factor (CSF) present in the cytoplasm which stabilizes MPF by blocking cyclin degradation (Fig. 8). It is assumed that CSF exhibits its function in the absence of calcium. Application of the calcium chelator EGTA retains the CSF-mediated arrest. There is evidence that CSF is actually c-MOS protein [25]. It remains to be clarified why c-MOS has different functions, activating maturation and promoting metaphase arrest.

Growth Factors, GnRH, and Steroids

There is some evidence that growth factors are involved in oocyte maturation. Epidermal growth factor (EGF) and transforming growth factor (TGF) α and β seem to promote resumption of meiosis in follicle-enclosed oocytes, but the mechanisms of inducing GVB are still unclear to date. The activation of phosphatidyl inositol and calcium pathways is associated with the action of angiotensin II, which is likely to be regulated by TGFβ. GnRH induces maturation of oocytes, but much more slowly than LH. A possible mode of action for GnRH is to activate PK-C. The effective role of steroids for oocyte maturation remains unclear. Nonphysiological high concentrations of testosterone, progesterone, and pregnenolone seem to inhibit oocyte maturation either alone or in conjunction with agents increasing the cAMP level. Estradiol, on the other hand, seems to improve induction of maturation.

Calcium

As it is known that calcium inhibitors such as verapamil transiently prevent GVB by elevating cAMP levels within the oocyte, a most striking role of calcium in the initiation of oocyte maturation must be considered. Calcium is essential in culture medium to sustain completion of meiosis in maturing oocytes. Activation of calcium within the oocyte starts via the phosphoinositide (IP43) pathway. Calcium may be released by the granulosa cells through gap junctions to the oocyte responding to the LH surge. GVB is mediated by calcium. IP3 induces the mobilization of calcium stores within the oocyte. Free calcium activates cAMP phosphodiesterase, resulting in a decrease of cAMP concentration below the threshold needed to maintain meiotic arrest, and initiates GVB.

Oocyte Maturation In Vitro – Clinical Considerations

Animal studies in vivo and in vitro revealed biochemical pathways that are assumed to be involved in oocyte maturation. As more was learned about these mechanisms, it turned out that in vitro maturation might be possible under specific culture conditions. Actually, mammalian follicular oocytes are able to mature in vitro when they are isolated from follicles and placed in appropriate culture medium. This was first demonstrated in the rabbit [26] and has been confirmed in man [27] and various other animals. The apparently normal fertilization and development of rodent oocytes grown inside cultured follicles are encouraging [28]. Progress in techniques of in vitro maturation could provide a demonstration of complete developmental competence in mice [29]. Nevertheless, questions remain about which nutritional environment is required for culturing human oocytes to provide normal fertilization and embryo development in women. What hormones and growth factors are important? What are the mechanisms of oocyte-specific gene expression? What are the major steps in the signal transduction system of the granulosa cell-oocyte complex [30]? Do the size and the stage of the retrieved oocytes play a role in their further development?

There are some papers in the literature reporting successful oocyte maturation in vitro [31] leading to subsequent pregnancies in human beings. In one study oocytes were aspirated from small follicles (2–5 mm in diameter) taken from the ovarian tissue of woman undergoing surgery for ectopic pregnancy or ovarian cysts. Oocytes were cultured in either follicular fluid (FF), which had been obtained from women attending an IVF program and added to Ham's F-10, or Ham's F-10 with 20% fetal cord serum (FCS). Oocytes were cultured for 32–48 h to reach metaphase II stage as a sign of full maturation. The maturation and fertilization rate was much higher using the follicular fluid containing medium than the FCS containing medium. One triplet pregnancy was achieved [32]. In another study small oocytes ranging between 2 and 10 mm in diameter were retrieved by transvaginal ultrasound-guided aspiration in unstimulated cycles of woman with polycystic ovary syndrome (PCOS). Patients had received hCG prior to oocyte retrieval to induce luteinization. Oocytes were matured in vitro for 36–48 h, followed by intracytoplasmic sperm injection and assisted hatching. Culture medium consisted of recombinant human follicle-stimulating hormone (rFSH) and human chorionic gonadotropin (hCG). The maturation rate in the treatment cycle without a leading follicle was 55% and the fertilization rate 45%. In the treatment cycle with a leading follicle 18 mm in diameter, which was left intact to potentially enhance uterine and embryo synchrony, the maturation rate was 77% and the fertilization rate 80%. Five embryos resulted from this cycle, with a subsequent singleton pregnancy [33]. Nevertheless, the impact of the presence of a leading follicle is still debatable. Tucker et al. [34] report the birth of a healthy child after cryopreservation of immature oocytes with subsequent in vitro maturation, while Beckers' group [35] noted a fertilization rate of 10% with no subsequent transfer.

In summary, up to now the clinical results of in vitro maturation of immature oocytes are basically disappointing and reports on live-born children are not more than anecdotal. It was shown that immature oocytes retrieved in the mid-follicular phase of a natural, unstimulated cycle may have the potential for maturation and fertilization, but pregnancy rates of 3% [36] are not sufficient to implement this procedure into standard ART programs; in contrast, the results of Cha et al. [37], with a pregnancy rate of 25% in a series of 72 PCOS patients, have to be taken into account.

These reports demonstrate that oocyte maturation with subsequent fertilization and pregnancy can be achieved in human beings, but many further studies are needed to evaluate culture conditions and to bring oocyte maturation in vitro to a clinical routine, which would mean a great improvement for the patients. They would not need to undergo ovarian stimulation with the potential risk of hyperstimulation syndrome and other inconveniences associated with the administration of fertility drugs. The essential components are optimal maturation media and a synchronized endometrium in which the transferred embryos can implant.

References

1. Blandau RJ, White BJ, Rumery RE (1963) Observation of the movements of the living primordial germ cells in the mouse. Fertil Steril 14:482
2. Tsafriri A, Bar-Ami S, Lindner HR (1983) Control of the development of meiotic competence and of oocyte maturation in mammals. In: Beier HM, Lindner HR (eds) Fertilization of the human egg in vitro. Springer, Berlin Heidelberg New York
3. Urner F, Schorderet-Slatkine S (1984) Inhibition of denuded mouse oocyte meiotic maturation by tumor promoting phorbol esters and its reversal by retinoids. Exp Cell Res 154:600
4. Bornslaeger EA, Poueymirou WT, Mattei P, Schultz RM (1986) Effects of protein kinase C activators on germinal vesicle breakdown and polar body emission of mouse oocytes. Exp Cell Res 165:507
5. Dekel N (1988) Spatial relationship of follicular cells in the control of meiosis. In: Haseltine FP, First NL (eds) Progress in clinical and biological research. Meiotic inhibition: molecular control of meiosis. Alan R. Liss, New York, p 87

6. Downs SM, Daniel SAJ, Eppig JJ (1988) Induction of maturation in cumulus cell-enclosed mouse oocytes by follicle-stimulating hormone and epidermal growth factor: evidence for a positive stimulus of somatic cell origin. J Exp Zool 245:86

7. Homa ST, Webster SD, Russell RK (1991) Phospholipid turnover and ultrastructural correlates during spontaneous germinal vesicle breakdown of the bovine oocyte: effects of a cyclic AMP phosphodiesterase inhibitor. Dev Biol 146:461

8. Fagbohun CF, Downs SM (1991) Metabolic coupling and ligand-stimulated meiotic maturation in the mouse oocyte-cumulus cell complex. Biol Reprod 45:851

9. Schultz RM, Montgomery R, Belanoff J (1983) Regulation of mouse oocyte maturation: implication of a decrease in oocyte c AMP and protein dephosphorylation in commitment to resume meiosis. Dev Biol 97:264

10. Warikoo PK, Bavister BD (1989) Hypoxanthine and cyclic adenosine 5'-monophosphate maintain meiotic arrest of rhesus monkey oocytes in vitro. Fertil Steril 51:886

11. Racowsky C (1984) Effect of forskolin on the spontaneous maturation and cyclic AMP content of rat oocyte-cumulus complex. J Reprod Fertil 72:107

12. Urner F, Herrmann WL, Baulieu EE, Schorderet-Slatkine S (1983) Inhibition of denuded mouse oocyte meiotic maturation by forskolin, an activator of adenylate cyclase. Endocrinology 113:1170

13. Bornslaeger EA, Schultz RM (1985) Adenylate cyclase activity in zona-free mouse oocytes. Exp Cell Res 156:277

14. Downs SM, Coleman DL, Ward-Bailey PF, Eppig JJ (1985) Hypoxanthine is the principal inhibitor of murine oocyte maturation in low molecular weight fraction of porcine follicular fluid. Proc Nat Acad Sci U S A 82:454

15. Eppig JJ, Ward-Bailey PF, Coleman DL (1985) Hypoxanthine and adenosine in murine ovarian follicular fluid: concentrations and activity in maintaining oocyte meiotic arrest. Biol Reprod 33:1041

16. Salustri A, Petrungaro S, Conti M, Siracusa G (1988) Adenosine potentiates forskolin-induced delay of meiotic resumption by mouse denuded oocytes: evidence for an oocyte surface site of adenosine action. Gamete Res 21:157

17. Kishimoto T (1988) Regulation of metaphase by a maturation-promoting factor. Dev Growth Differ 30:105

18. Masui Y, Markert CL (1971) Cytoplasmic control of nuclear behavior during meiotic maturation of frog oocytes. J Exp Zool 177:129

19. Wasserman WJ, Masui Y (1975) Effects of cycloheximide on cytoplasmic factor initiating meiotic maturation in Xenopus oocytes. Exp Cell Res 91:381

20. Draetta G (1987) Identification of p34 and p13, human homologs of the cell cycle regulators of fission yeast encoded by cdc2+ and suc1+. Cell 50:319

21. Arion D (1988) cdc2 is a component of the M phase-specific histone H1 kinase: Evidence for identity with MPF. Cell 55:371

22. Matsumoto YI (1980) Evidence for the involvement of H1 histone phosphorylation in chromosome condensation. Nature 284:181

23. Evans T, Rosenthal ET, Youngblom J (1983) Cyclin: A protein specified by maternal mRNA in sea urchin eggs that is destroyed at each cleavage division. Cell 33:389

24. Roy L, Singh B, Gauthier J, Arlinghaus R, Nordeen S, Maller J (1990) The cyclin B2 component of MPF is a substrate for the c-mos protooncogene product. Cell 61:825

25. Sagata N, Watanabe N, Vande Woude GF, Ikawa Y (1989) The c-mos proto-oncogene product is a cytostatic factor responsible for meiotic arrest in vertebrate eggs. Nature 342:512

26. Pincus G, Enzmann EV (1935) The comparative behavior of mammalian eggs in vivo and in vitro. J Exp Med 62:655

27. Edwards RG (1965) Maturation in vitro of mouse, sheep, cow, pig, rhesus monkey and human ovarian oocytes. Nature 208:349

28. Spears N (1994) In-vitro growth of ovarian oocytes. Hum Reprod 9:969

29. Schroeder AC, Eppig JJ (1984) The developmental capacity of mouse oocytes that matured spontaneously in vitro is normal. Dev Biol 102:493

30. Eppig JJ (1994) Further reflections on culture systems for the growth of oocytes in vitro. Hum Reprod 9:974

31. Trounson AO, Wood C, Kausche A (1994) In vitro maturation and the fertilization and developmental competence of oocytes recovered from untreated polycystic ovarian patients. Fertil Steril 62:353
32. Cha KY, Koo JJ, Choi DH, Han SY, Yoon TK (1991) Pregnancy after in vitro fertilization of human follicular oocytes collected from non-stimulated cycles, their culture in vitro and their transfer in a donor oocyte program. Fertil Steril 55:109
33. Barnes FL, Crombie A, Gardner DK, Kausche A, Lacham-Kaolan O, Suikkari AM, Tiglias J, Wood C, Trounson AO (1995) Blastocyst development and birth after in-vitro maturation of human primary oocytes, intracytoplasmic sperm injection and assisted hatching. Hum Reprod 10:3243
34. Tucker MU, Wright G, Morton PC, Massey JB (1998) Birth after cryopreservation of immature oocytes with subsequent in vitro maturation. Fertil Steril 70:578
35. Beckers BG, Pieters MH, Ramos L, Zeilmaker GH, Fauser BC, Braat DD (1999) Retrieval, maturation and fertilization of immature oocytes obtained from unstimulated patients with polycystic ovary syndrome. J Assist Reprod Genet 16:81
36. Thornton MH, Francis MM, Paulson RJ (1998) Immature oocyte retrieval: lessons from unstimulated IVF cycles. Fertil Steril 70:647
37. Cha KY, Chung HM, Han SY (1996) Successful in vitro maturation, fertilization and pregnancy by using immature follicular oocytes collected from unstimulated polycystic ovary syndrome patients. Proc Annu Meeting American Society of Reproductive Medicine, Abstract O-044

Preimplantation Diagnosis

I. Liebaers, W. Lissens, K. Sermon, E. Van Assche, C. Staessen, H. Joris,
A. Van Steirteghem

Introduction

The ability to hyperstimulate the ovaries, retrieve ova, and fertilize them has
made in vitro fertilization (IVF) a safe and effective treatment for infertility.
Several tens of thousands of children have been born to couples who were unable to conceive otherwise. IVF has opened the door to several reproductive advances such as oocyte donation, embryo freezing, and assisted fertilization procedures such as the recently introduced procedure of intracytoplasmic sperm
injection (ICSI) to alleviate severe male-factor infertility. IVF also made preimplantation genetic diagnosis possible as an option to couples at risk for serious
genetic disease. Rather than terminating a pregnancy after conventional prenatal diagnosis, embryo analysis permits selection of embryos without disease to
be replaced in the uterus.

Outline of Preimplantation Diagnosis

The outline of a preimplantation diagnostic procedure on an eight-cell human
embryo is illustrated in Fig. 1. Eight-cell embryos can be obtained about 70 h
after oocyte retrieval for IVF alone or for IVF combined with ICSI. There is
also a theoretical possibility that such embryos might be obtained after in vivo
conception and uterine lavage. One or two blastomeres can be biopsied from
this embryo by micromanipulation. The diagnostic procedure [polymerase
chain reaction (PCR) or fluorescent in situ hybridization (FISH) is carried out
on these isolated blastomeres. One may expect the result at the end of day three
after oocyte retrieval. Meanwhile, the biopsied embryo (containing six blastomeres) is kept in culture ($37\,^{\circ}$C, 5% O_2, 5% CO_2, and 90% N_2). If the diagnostic
procedure requires more than 1 day, it may be worth freezing the biopsied embryo, which can then be replaced after thawing in a subsequent cycle. Two or
maximum three disease-free embryos can be replaced into the uterus as soon
as the results are available, usually in the evening of day 3. If more disease-free
embryos are available than required for transfer, these supernumerary embryos
can also be frozen for later replacement. Affected embryos should be further
analyzed to confirm the diagnosis on the individual blastomeres of the biopsied
embryo as part of research experiments to improve the diagnostic procedures.

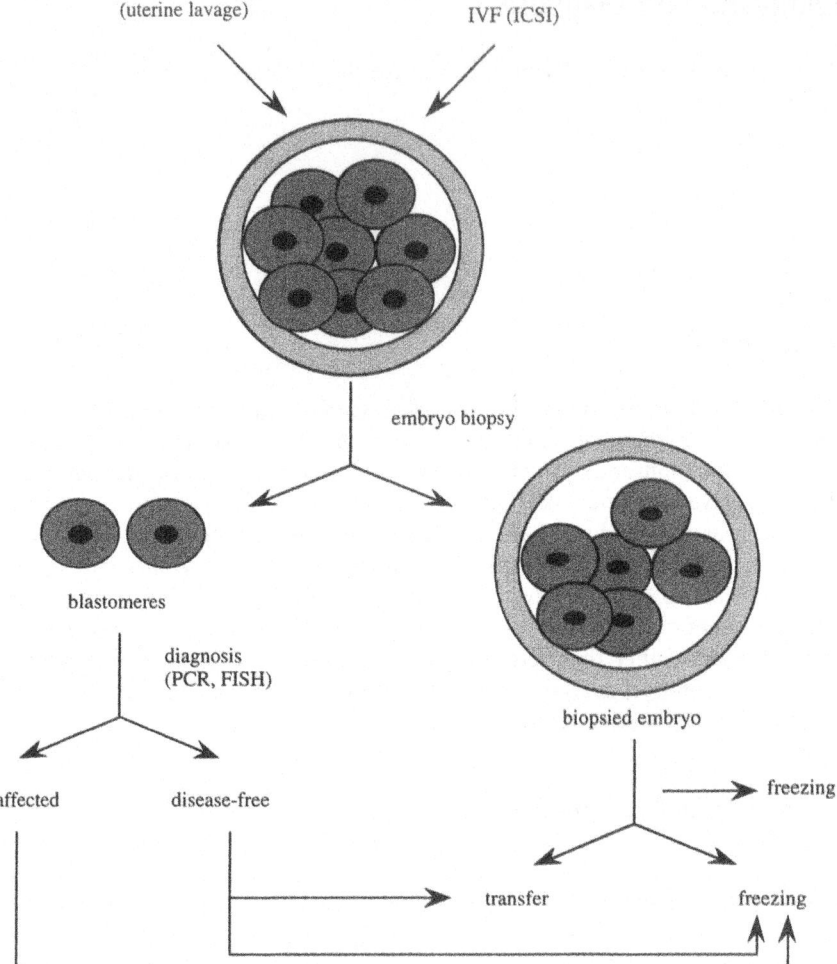

Fig. 1. Outline of preimplantation diagnosis

Indications for Preimplantation Diagnosis

The indications for preimplantation diagnosis are the same as those for conventional amniocentesis and chorionic villus sampling. Couples who may benefit are those at risk of (a) chromosomal disorders especially translocations, (b) monogenic X-linked, autosomal recessive or autosomal dominant disorders, and (c) mitochondrial diseases.

At present, couples who choose this novel procedure must be carefully counseled about the complex nature of preimplantation diagnosis, which requires a highly experienced team to carry out (a) IVF with or without assisted fertilization by ICSI, (b) the embryo biopsy procedure by micromanipulation, (c) the

PCR or FISH procedure on single cells, and (d) the possible cryopreservation of embryos.

Approaches to Preimplantation Diagnosis

There are three different approaches to preimplantation genetic diagnosis: (a) polar body biopsy, (b) biopsy of the trophectoderm, and (c) removal of one or two blastomeres from a cleaving preimplantation embryo.

Polar-body biopsy involves the removal of the nonfunctioning haploid set of chromosomes of the first meiotic division. Polar body diagnosis can be used for X-linked and autosomal recessive disorders as well as for autosomal dominant disorders or chromosomal aberrations in the women; only the genotype of the female partner is determined. Oocytes are retrieved from women in whom ovulation has been induced by gonadotropins. After removal of the surrounding cumulus and corona cells, the polar body becomes clearly visible and can be removed by micromanipulation. If a mutant allele for an autosomal recessive disorder is detected in the polar body, it may be concluded that the primary oocyte contains a normal allele. Normal oocytes can be fertilized in vitro and embryos can be replaced. If the polar body contains the normal allele, the primary oocyte has the mutant allele and is not inseminated. The polar body contains only one allele, but there are two copies because each chromosome consists of two sister chromatids. The primary oocyte and the first polar body may contain copies of the two alleles if cross-over has occurred between homologous chromosomes. In that case the genotype of the secondary oocytes cannot be predicted without further testing of the second polar body after fertilization. Polar body diagnosis, also called preconceptual diagnosis, has had limited application and success in clinical practice. This method also has the disadvantage that the removal of the first and possibly the second polar body is technically difficult [1–3].

Trophectoderm biopsy certainly has the advantage that more cells are available to carry out the diagnostic procedure. A human blastocyst contains about 200 cells. If a small opening is made in the zona pellucida, a small number of cells (10–30) herniate through the slit and can be excised [4]. Such a number of cells would make the further genetic analysis more easy. Blastocysts can be obtained after IVF and further in vitro culture but the number of 2-PN oocytes reaching the blastocyst stage has remained low, i.e., only 20–25% of the normally fertilized oocytes. It may be possible that better in vitro culture conditions, for example, using coculture systems, will increase the blastocyst formation rate. Another approach to obtaining blastocysts is uterine lavage after in vivo or in vitro fertilization [5]. In practice, lavage is practically possible only after superovulation, and so far very few embryos have been recovered. Both the mediocre yield of blastocysts after IVF and in vitro culture and the poor results after superovulation and uterine lavage have had as a consequence that trophectoderm biopsy has not been applied clinically [6].

Embryo biopsy at the cleavage stage is another approach which so far has been most often and most succesfully applied at the clinical level. IVF can be considered a well-established procedure to obtain preimplantation embryos with about eight blastomeres. Various steps are involved in IVF: (a) ovarian superovulation to obtain several preovulatory oocytes, (b) retrieval of the cumulus-oocyte complexes, (c) selection of motile spermatozoa from the partner's semen, (d) insemination of the cumulus-oocyte complexes, (e) in vitro culture in medium, (f) assessment of fertilization 16–18 h after juxtaposition with the spermatozoa, and (g) evaluation of further embryo development 24 h and 48 h later. Eight-cell embryos are usually present at about 72 h after oocyte retrieval. This can be planned to occur early in the morning of day 3 after oocyte pick-up [7–9]. It has been the experience of all groups performing IVF that oocytes may fail to become fertilized, especially in couples with severe male-factor infertility. Several procedures for assisted fertilization have been developed to overcome this problem. The intracytoplasmic injection procedure of a single spermatozoon (ICSI) especially, has been successful in alleviating infertility in patients with even extremely impaired semen [10]. In some situations, spermatozoa obtained after microsurgical sperm aspiration such as in congenital bilateral absence of the vas deferens (CBAVD) or even sperm obtained after testicular sperm extraction in obstructive and nonobstructive azoospermia can be used [11].

Biopsy Procedures at the Cleavage Stage

Embryo biopsy on an eight-cell embryo involves the removal by micromanipulation of one or two blastomeres. The requirements for a successful biopsy procedure are (a) that the removed blastomere be intact and suitable for the diagnostic procedure, (b) that the biopsied embryo retains its full developmental potential to implant into the uterine endometrium, and (c) if necessary, that the biopsied embryo can be successfully frozen and thawed. The number of blastomeres that are removed depends on the stage of embryo development in which the embryo biopsy is carried out. The more cells present in the embryo, the more cells can be removed. For eight-cell embryos two blastomeres can be biopsied. Hardy et al. reported in 1907 that the removal of one or two cells at the eight-cell stage reduced the cellular mass but did not affect preimplantation development in vitro to the blastocyst stage between days 5 and 6; many biopsied embryos hatched from the zona pellucida in vitro.

Different procedures have been reported for the removal of blastomeres. In our Center in earlier cases of pelvic inflammatory disease (PID) a hole was made in the zona pellucida using acid Tyrode's solution, followed by the insertion of a biopsy pipette and gentle aspiration of the blastomere in the pipette. The pipette was then removed and the blastomere expelled in the surrounding medium. Later, the blastomeres were removed by placing the hole in the zona pellucida at 12 h and extruding the blastomere through the hole by gentle pushing with a blunt pipette at 3 h [12]. The extrusion method is now preferred because the risk of lysing the blastomere is smaller and because the morphology of the blastomere is better preserved, which is important for FISH. The biopsy procedure was validated in a large experimental study investigating the in vitro and in vivo development of cryopreserved and noncryopreserved eight-cell mouse embryos, from which one to seven blastomeres were removed by micromanipulation. When up to three blastomeres were removed, there was no significant effect on the rate of in vitro blastocyst formation. Living young were found even after the biopsy of four blastomeres, and after biopsy of one or two blastomeres, the same percentage of living young was obtained as in the nonbiopsied control embryos. Survival after cryopreservation was excellent and no different from nonbiopsied embryos, independently of the number of blastomeres biopsied. Cryopreservation had no further impact on the in vitro and in vivo development of the biopsied embryos [13].

Diagnostic Procedures on Single Blastomeres

In conventional prenatal diagnosis the diagnostic analysis can be carried out on a few mg of chorionic tissue or on a few millions of amniocytes. In preimplantation diagnosis at the eight-cell cleavage stage embryo only one or two blastomeres are available for genetic analysis. Extremely sensitive techniques must be used, such as PCR and FISH.

Polymerase Chain Reaction

Initially described in 1985, PCR has been modified in recent years and is now a fully automatic procedure [14, 15]. PCR has many applications in science and medicine, in fundamental research, and in diagnostic methods.

The human haploid genome contains about 3×10^9 base pairs of DNA. Genetic disorders may be caused by several changes in DNA. These changes may involve a point mutation or the deletion or insertion of one or a few base pairs. Before PCR, complicated indirect methods were used to detect these small changes in the DNA. The cyclical process in PCR makes millions of copies of a small portion of DNA; in each PCR cycle the amount is doubled. It becomes easy to detect an error in the amplified portion of this DNA since millions of copies of DNA are present.

The principle of PCR is simple and mimics DNA replication in mitosis: each of the two daughter cells has the same amount of DNA as in the dividing cell. The two complimentary DNA strands become separated and an exact complimentary copy of the single-stranded DNA is made using the DNA building blocks present in the cell: the four deoxynucleotides dATP, dCTP, dGTP and dTTP. DNA synthesis occurs always in one direction, i.e., 5'-phosphate group of deoxyribose of the added deoxynucleotide is added to the 3'-phosphate group of the preceding deoxynucleotide. The enzyme polymerase requires as a starting point a small piece of double-stranded DNA. PCR mimics this process by mixing in a test tube the different components required for the synthesis: (a) double-stranded target DNA such as the DNA which is present in a single blastomere, (b) thermostable DNA polymerase, usually Taq polymerase from the thermophylic bacterium *Thermus aquaticus,* (c) the four deoxynucleotides and (d) two short single-stranded oligonucleotides or primers (20 or 30 base pairs usually). The two primers are synthesized in the laboratory and are selected in terms of the piece of DNA to be analyzed in the target DNA. They are complimentary to the end parts of the target DNA and are the starting points of the DNA synthesis by the polymerase enzyme. A PCR cycle usually consists of three steps: (a) heating at 94 °C to denature the target DNA and to make single-stranded DNA, (b) annealing at 50 °–60 °C to hybridize or bind the primers on to the target DNA, and (c) synthesis of new DNA from the primers by Taq polymerase at 72 °C, which is the optimal temperature for this thermophylic enzyme. In each cycle the piece of DNA located between the two primers is doubled. After 30 cycles 109 copies are made of the DNA fragment and after 50 cycles 1015 copies. A PCR apparatus preprogramed for the changes in temperature makes this an automated procedure. PCR is highly specific and sensitive and millions of copies of a piece of DNA can be made in 5–6 h.

An additional advantage of PCR is that it can be applied on each piece of DNA in the genome if the sequence of that piece is known to synthesize the two primers in the laboratory. Theoretically PCR allows preimplantation diagnosis of each genetic disease with a known molecular defect. In practice one must verify each time that the synthesis of the target sequence is specific and efficient. Target sequences with many repeats of, for example, a CA dinucleotide repeat may cause problems. There may also be problems of sensitivity when a target sequence from contaminating DNA from the operator, or from a previous PCR reaction gives a false-positive reaction. Special precautions are necessary to avoid such contamination.

Two examples will illustrate the use of PCR for preimplantation diagnosis on biopsied single blastomeres: (a) PCR for X- and Y-specific sequence for gender determination and (b) PCR for the detection of the DF508 deletion of cystic fibrosis transmembrane regulator gene in human embryos resulting from intracytoplasmic sperm injection with epididymal sperm.

Amplification of X- and Y-Chromosome Specific Regions from Single Human Blastomeres

A PCR assay is used for the simultaneous detection of X and Y chromosomes in human blastomeres [16]. The PCR mixtures are decontaminated by incubation with 2 U restriction enzyme *AluI* at 37 °C for 3 h. The restriction enzyme is then inactivated by incubation at 65 °C for 20 min. The mixture is added to heat-denatured blastomeres and blanks. In a first round of PCR both X- and Y-specific fragments are amplified with primers which are common to both chromosomes and are derived from the X-linked steroid sulfatase gene and the Y-linked pseudogene. In a second round of PCR, fragments specific to each chromosome are generated: both an X and a Y fragment in male embryos, only an X fragment in females. The efficiency and accuracy of this assay are high; it generates no false-positive amplification signals and allows sexing in about 6 h after embryo biopsy. In an example from our Center, 115 blastomeres were obtained from 23, two- to eight-cell embryos, after removal of the zona pellucida and incubation in Ca^{2+}- and Mg^{2+}-free medium. Of these 115 blastomeres, 11 (9.6%) did not show a clear nucleus after careful light microscopic examination and were not used for further analysis by PCR. In 88 out of 104 blastomeres (84.6%), X-specific (female blastomeres) or X- and Y-specific (male blastomeres) fragments were detected after amplification. The PCR results for different blastomeres from the same embryo were always concordant: all individual blastomeres were either typed as male or as female. As expected, all male embryos also always showed an X-chromosome-specific fragment. In contrast, 16 blastomeres (15.4%) showed neither X-specific nor Y-specific fragments after amplification. No amplification signals were detected in 104 blank samples. These results show that decontamination with AluI is very efficient. Of the 23 embryos, 9 were found to be male and 14 female. There is no statistical difference between the theoretical distribution (11.5 male and 11.5 female embryos) and the observed distribution by two analysis. This PCR assay is believed to be suitable for preimplantation diagnosis for couples at risk of X-linked genetic diseases.

Preimplantation Diagnosis of the Cystic Fibrosis DF508 Mutation by PCR in Human Embryos Resulting from ICSI with Epididymal Sperm

Men with congenital bilateral absence of the vas deferens have been regarded as presenting a mild form of cystic fibrosis. In our Center preimplantation diagnosis was carried out in an infertile couple in which both partners are carriers of the DF508 mutation and the male partner has CBAVD [17–19]. Microsurgical epididymal sperm aspiration was performed to obtain spermatozoa; 12 oocytes were retrieved after controlled ovarian stimulation and ovulation induction. ICSI was carried out on all 12 oocytes that had extruded the first polar body and 11 oocytes remained intact after injection. Five oocytes were fertilized normally and cleaved to the four- to eight-cell stage. One or two blastomeres were removed by micromanipulation. Single blastomeres were put into PCR tubes containing 20 µl of distilled water. Two consecutive PCRs with nested primers were performed. After PCR the results indicated that two embryos were affected (homozygous for the DF508 mutation) and three embryos were carriers of the DF508 mutation. In one blastomere, no DNA amplification was obtained by PCR. None of the six blanks showed any sign of false-positive amplification. The three carrier embryos were morphologically sound and were transferred into the uterus on day three after ICSI. The patient conceived and had an uneventful pregnancy. Amniocentesis was carried out at 16 weeks of pregnancy and the result showed (a) a normal 46, XY karyotype and (b) the heterozygous carrier status for the DF508 mutation. The patient delivered a healthy boy.

The use of PCR has also been applied for the diagnosis of Duchenne's muscular dystrophy [20] and more recently for Steinert's myotonic dystrophy [21, 22] by looking at the presence in the blastomeres of the unaffected allele of the affected parent because the expanded allele cannot be amplified by PCR.

Fluorescent In Situ Hybridization

Another approach to gender determination in an embryo consists of coloring the X and Y chromosomes by FISH [23-27]. DNA sequences specific to each human chromosome have been isolated in recent years. These sequences may correspond to one gene, a part of a gene or a DNA region which is present only once on a particular chromosome. In FISH one is mainly interested in repeat sequences which can be detected rapidly and easily. Such sequences are present in the centromeric regions of the chromosomes. Especially centromeric probes are used to detect specific chromosomes by FISH. Such probes can be labeled in vitro with fluorochrome dyes. This can be achieved by (a) direct incorporation of the fluorochrome couplet to a nucleotide or (a) indirectly by incorporation of a biotin-labeled nucleotide which can be visualized by an avidin-fluorochrome complex. The chromosomes in a blastomere are (a) fixed on a microscopic slide and (b) heated to make the chromosome and the labeled DNA probe single-stranded. Using appropriate conditions the probe can then hybridize on complimentary regions in the chromosomes. After washing out the unbound probe the fluorescence of the chromosomes can then be detected under the fluorescence microscope. Using different fluorochromes to label the X and Y chromosome with specific centromeric probes, it becomes possible to observe in a single blastomere two X chromosomes (female embryo) or one X and one Y chromosome (male embryo). FISH is suitable for preimplantation diagnosis on embryos because of its sensitivity and efficiency and because it takes about 6-8 h to carry out the whole procedure. Unlike PCR, contamination is not a problem when FISH is used. This procedure is now preferentially used for sex determination. By using supplementary and specifically labeled probes for chromosomes 21, 18, and 13, the most common aneuploidies can also be diagnosed [28]. Procedures are now worked out to diagnose unbalanced chromosomal translocations in embryos from balanced translocation carriers.

Clinical Experience with Preimplantation Genetic Diagnosis

The clinical experience is still limited. Around 40 children have been born so far, most of them at the Hammersmith Hospital in London where the team of Winston and Handyside started this novel procedure [29-31]. The pregnancy rate and take home baby rate seems to equal the results obtained in regular IVF. In our Center 17 cycles were started to perform preimplantation diagnosis for 11 patients. One cycle had to be canceled before oocyte retrieval. In two cycles, no cleavage stage embryos developed and in three others no embryos were available for transfer after preimplantation diagnosis. Three pregnancies occurred in 11 cycles in which embryos were replaced in the uterus. Two healthy babies were born and one is going to be born respectively to a couple at risk for cystic fibrosis, a couple at risk for Duchenne's muscular dystrophy and a couple at risk for hemophilia A (Table 1).

Table 1. PIDs carried out at the Brussels Free University

Cycles	Patients	Disease	PCR/FISH	Oocytes ≥2PN	Embryos ≥4-cell analyzed	Genotype			Transfer	Pregnancy	Birth
1.	1	CF(ΔF508)	PCR	8	7	2U	5C	0A	2U	0	0
2.	2	CF(ΔF508)	PCR	–	–	–	–	–	–	–	–
3.	3	CF(ΔF508) (CBAVD)	PCR	5	5	0U	3C	2A	3C	1	1 boy
4.	2	CF(ΔF508)	PCR	22	14	2U	5C	7A	2U	0	0
5.	4	CF(2183AA→G) (1717–1G→A) (CBAVD)	PCR	4	2	0U	2C	0A	0	0	0
6.	3	CF(ΔF508) (CBAVD)	PCR	8	6	4U	1C	1A	3U	0	0
7.	4	CF(2183AA→G) (1717–1G→A) (CBAVD)	PCR	2	0	–	–	–	0	0	0
8.	5	CF(ΔF508)	PCR	12	2	1U	0C	1A	1U	0	0
9.	5	CF(ΔF508)	PCR	6	2	0U	0C	2A	0	0	0
10.	3	CF(ΔF508) (CBAVD)	PCR	4	0	–	–	–	0	0	0
11.	6	CF(ΔF508) ? (CBAVD)	PCR	7	7	2U	3C	2A?	2U	0	0
12.	7	MD	PCR	11	8	5U	–	3A	3U	0	0
13.	8	DMD	PCR	14	4	1F	–	3M	1F	0	0
14.	8	DMD	PCR	11	6	4U	–	2A	3U	1	1 girl
15.	9	X-linked MR	PCR	9	5	2F	–	3M	2F	0	0
16.	10	DMD	FISH	12	9	5XY	–	3P	0	0	0
17.	11	HemA	FISH	5	5	2XX,1XY	–	1?	2XX	1	ongoing
Total	11								11	3	2 (1 ongoing)

CF, Cystic fibrosis; CBAVD, congenital absence of the vas deferens; MD, myotonic dystrophy; DMD, Duchenne's muscular dystrophy; MR, mental retardation; HemA, hemophilia A; U, unaffected; C, carrier; A, affected; F, female; M, male

Conclusion

So far it seems that preimplantation diagnosis is performed only in a limited number of couples at risk. However, before any firm conclusions can be drawn further evaluation is necessary both at the technical level and at the clinical application level.

References

1. Verlinsky Y, Ginsberg N, Lifchez A, Valle J, Moise J, Strom C (1990) Analysis of the first polar body: preconception genetic diagnosis. Hum Reprod 5:826–829
2. Strom C, Verlinsky Y, Milayeva S, Evskilov S, Cieslak J, Lifchez A, Valle J, Moise J, Ginsberg N, Applebaum M (1990) Preconception genetic diagnosis of cystic fibrosis. Lancet 336:306–307
3. Verlinsky Y, Rechitsky S, Evsikov S, White M, Cieslak J, Lifchez A, Valle J, Moise J, Strom C (1992) Preconception and preimplantation diagnosis for cystic fibrosis. Prenat Diagn 12:103–110
4. Dokras A, Sargent IL, Ross C, Gardner RL, Barlow DH (1990) Trophectoderm biopsy in human blastocysts. Hum Reprod 5:821–825
5. Buster JE, Bustillo M, Rodi IA, Cohen SW, Hamilton MH, Simon JA, Thorneycroft IH, Marshall JR (1985) Biologic and morphologic development of donated human ova recovered by nonsurgical uterine lavage. Am J Obstet Gynecol 153:211–217
6. Carson SA, Smith AL, Scoggan JL, Buster JE (1991) Superovulation fails to increase human blastocyst yield after uterine lavage. Prenat Diagn 11:513–522
7. Hardy K, Martin KL, Leese HJ, Winston RML, Handyside AH (1990) Human preimplantation development in vitro is not adversely affected by biopsy at the 8-cell stage. Hum Reprod 5:708–714
8. Handyside AH, Kontogianni EH, Hardy K, Winston RML (1990) Pregnancies from biopsied human preimplantation embryos sexed by Y-specific DNA amplification. Nature 344:768–770
9. Winston RML, Handyside AH (1993) New challenges in human in vitro fertilization. Science 260:932–936
10. Van Steirteghem A, Tournaye H, Van der Elst J, Verheyen G, Liebaers I, Devroey P (1995) Intractyoplasmic sperm injection three years after the birth of the first ICSI child. Hum Reprod 10:2527–2528
11. Nagy Z, Liu J, Janssenswillen C, Silber S, Devroey P, Van Steirteghem A (1995) Using ejaculated, fresh and frozen-thawed epididymal and testicular spermatozoa gives rise to comparable results after intracytoplasmic sperm injection. Fertil Steril 63:808–815
12. Tarin JJ, Handyside AH (1993) Embryo biopsy strategies for preimplantation diagnosis. Fertil Steril 59:943–952
13. Liu J, Van den Abbeel E, Van Steirteghem A (1993) The in-vitro and in-vivo developmental potential of frozen and non-frozen biopsied 8-cell mouse embryos. Hum Reprod 8:1481–1486
14. Saiki RK, Scharf S, Fallona F et al (1985) Enzymatic amplification of β-globin genomic sequences and restriction site analysis for diagnosis of sickle cell anemia. Science 230:1350–1354
15. Mullis KB (1990) The unusual origin of the polymerase chain reaction. Sci Am April 1990:36–43
16. Liu J, Lissens W, Devroey P, Van Steirteghem AC, Liebaers I (1994) Amplification of X- and Y-chromosome-specific regions from single human blastomeres by polymerase chain reaction for sexing of preimplantation embryos. Hum Reprod 9:716–720

17. Liu J, Lissens W, Devroey P, Van Steirteghem AC, Liebaers I (1992) Efficiency and accuracy of polymerase-chain-reaction assay for cystic fibrosis allele DF508 in single cell. Lancet 339:1190–1192

18. Liu J, Lissens W, Devroey P, Van Steirteghem AC, Liebaers I (1993) Polymerase chain reaction analysis of the cystic fibrosis DF508 mutation in human blastomeres following oocyte injection of a single sperm from a carrier. Prenat Diagn 13:873–880

19. Liu J, Lissens W, Silbern SJ, Devroey P, Liebaers I, Van Steirteghem A (1994) Birth after preimplantation diagnosis of the cystic fibrosis ΔF508 mutation by polymerase chain reaction in human embryos resulting from intracytoplasmic sperm injection with epididymal sperm. JAMA 272:1858–1860

20. Liu J, Lissens W, Van Broeckhoven C et al (1995) Normal pregnancy after preimplantation DNA diagnosis of a dystrophin gene deletion. Prenat Diagn 15:351–358

21. Brook JD, Mc Currach ME, Harley HG et al (1992) Molecular basis of myotonic dystrophy: expansion of a trinucleotide (CTG) repeat at the 3' end of a transcript encoding a protein kinase family member. Cell 68:799–808

22. Mahadevan M, Tsilfidis C, Sabourin L et al (1992) Myotonic dystrophy mutation: an unstable CTG repeat in the 3' untranslated region of the gene. Science 255:1253–1255

23. Griffin DK, Wilton LJ, Handyside A, Atkinson GHG, Winston R, Delhanty JDA (1993) Diagnosis of sex in preimplantation embryos by fluorescent in situ hybridisation. Br Med J 306:1382

24. Delhanty JDA, Griffin DK, Handyside AH, Harper J, Atkinson GHG, Pieters MHEC, Winston RML (1993) Detection of aneuploidy and chromosomal mosaicism in human embryos during preimplantation sex determination by fluorescent in situ hybridisation (FISH). Hum Mol Gen 2:1183–1185

25. Munné S, Weier HUG, Stein J, Grifo J, Cohen, JA (1993) A fast and efficient method for simultaneous X and Y in situ hybridization of human blastomeres. J Ass Reprod Gen 10:82–90

26. Coonen E, Dumoulin CM, Ramaekers FCS, Hopman AHN (1994) Optimal preparation of preimplantation embryo interphase nuclei for analysis by fluorescence in-situ hybridization. Hum Reprod 9:533–537

27. Harper J, Coonen E, Ramaekers F, Delhanty J, Handyside A, Winston R, Hopman A (1994) Identification of the sex of human preimplantation embryos in two hours using an improved spreading method and fluorescent in-situ hybridization (FISH) using directly labelled probes. Hum Reprod 9:721–724

28. Munné S, Lee A, Rosenwaks Z, Grifo J, Cohen J (1993) Diagnosis of major chromosome aneuploidies in human preimplantation embryos. Hum Reprod 8:2185–2191

29. Verlinsky Y, Handyside A, Simpson JL, Edwards R, Kuliev A, Muggleton-Harris A, Readhead C, Liebaers, I, Coonen E, Plachot M, Carson S, Strom C, Braude P, Van Steirteghem A, Monk M, Ginsberg N, Pieters M, De Sutter P, Gimenez C, Kontogianni E, Matthew C, Wilton L (1993) Current progress in preimplantation genetic diagnosis. J Ass Reprod Genet 10:353–360

30. Harper JC, Handyside AH (1994) The current status of preimplantation diagnosis. Current Obstet Gynaecol 4:143–149

31. Harper JC (1996) Preimplantation diagnosis of inherited disease by embryo biopsy: an update of the world figures. J Ass Reprod Genet 13:1–6

Genetics in Assisted Reproduction – Basic Aspects and Clinical Perspectives

M. Ludwig, K. Diedrich

Introduction

The new techniques of assisted reproduction, as introduced by Steptoe and Edwards (1978) with the first birth after a pregnancy following in vitro fertilization in the human being, have helped to fulfill the desire of several million couples worldwide for children. The development of more invasive techniques, especially the invention of intracytoplasmic sperm injection, has helped also to treat cases of severe male factor subfertility (Palermo et al. 1992).

Several genetic syndromes with a risk of inherited infertility are well known. Therefore, infertile couples as a whole have an increased risk of transmitting infertility to their offspring. However, with the treatment of men with severe impairment of semen quality, there were also new, until then unknown or disregarded problems of genetics. These problems will be discussed in this chapter.

Chromosome Abnormalities in Men with Male Factor Infertility

Among the first to show an increased risk of chromosome abnormalities in men with azoospermia were Ferguson-Smith et al. (1957). They described a Barr body in ten of 91 men with azoospermia. Two years later, Jacobs and Strong (1959) demonstrated that these men suffered from an abnormality which is called Klinefelter's syndrome (47, XXY), with one additional X-chromosome.

DeBraekeler and Dao (1991) reviewed 20 studies on chromosome abnormalities in men with male infertility; these results are summarized in Table 1. The most frequent abnormality was a Klinefelter's syndrome (4.6%), which is more than 40 times more frequent in this group than in the general population.

The high prevalence and correlation of balanced translocations (DeBraekeler and Dao 1991) and male infertility can be explained by a disturbance of chromosome pairing during meiosis. Translocations lead to abnormal chromosome pairing figures, since not just two chromosomes are paired but at least three (chromosome trivalent), in a synaptonemal complex. This leads to unpaired parts of the chromosomes which can disturb X-chromosome related genetic regulations during meiosis. It was shown by Johanisson et al. (1993) that a correlation exists between the increased frequency of the XY bivalent and the Robertsonian trivalent association and the extent of germ cell impairment.

Table 1. Chromosomal changes in men with azoospermia or oligozoospermia (from De Braekeleer and Dao 1991)

Condition n (%)	47,XXY	46,XY/ 47,XXY	Other numeric gonosomal aberrations	Y-chromosom- al structural aberrations	46,XX	Robertsonian translocations	Balanced translocations	Inversions	Additional chromosomes
Azoospermia: 1450 (15.5)	159 (11.6)	13 (0.9)	12 (0.9)	15 (1)	11 (0.8)	2 (0.1)	11 (0.8)	1 (0.1)	1 (0.1)
Oligozoosper- mia: 2105 (5.4)	12 (0.6)	9 (0.4)	14 (0.7)	9 (0.4)	–	32 (1.5)	20 (0.9)	10 (0.5)	8 (0.4)
Azoospermia or oligozoo spermia: 5652 (6.9)	253 (4.5)	6 (0.1)	25 (0.4)	24 (0.4)	6 (0.1)	38 (0.7)	26 (0.5)	3 (0.05)	8 (0.05)
Total: 9207 (7.9)	424 (4.6)	28 (0.3)	51 (0.5)	48 (0.5)	17 (0.2)	72 (0.8)	57 (0.6)	14 (0.2)	17 (0.2)

Table 2. Chromosomal aberrations in 1116 men undergoing ICSI (from Scholtes et al. 1998)

Aberration	Karyotype	No. of aberrations (%)
Autosomal		
Numerical		
-Marker chromosomes	47, XY, +mar (unknown origin)	1 (0.09)
	47, XY, +dic (15)(q11)	1 (0.09)
	47, XY, +i (13)(pter- > 10)	1 (0.09)
Structural		
-Translocations	-der (13; 14) (q10; q10)	8 (0.72)
	-der (14; 21) (q10; q10)	2 (0.18)
	-der (14; 15) (q10; q10)	1 (0.09)
	46, XY, t (1; 9)(q44; p11.2)	1 (0.09)
	46, XY, t (4; 11; 18)(p12; q15.1; q23)	1 (0.09)
	46, XY, t (3; 10)(p25; q26)	1 (0.09)
	46, XY, t (1; 3)(p36.5; q21)	1 (0.09)
	46, XY, t (8; 13)(q24.1; q22)	1 (0.09)
	46, XY, t (9; 14)(p22; q22)	1 (0.09)
	46, XY, t (X; 3)(q26; q23)	1 (0.09)
	46, XY, t (4; 19)(q34; q13.3)	1 (0.09)
	46, XY, t (6; 18)(q26; q23)	1 (0.09)
-Inversions	46, XY, inv(3)(q21; p25)	1 (0.09)
	Inv(9)qh	8 (0.72)
-Duplications	–	0
Sex chromosomal		
Numerical		
-Complete	47, XXY	3 (0.27)
	47, XYY	3 (0.27)
-Mosaicism	47, XXY/46, XY	2 (0.18)
	47, XYY/46, XY	3 (0.27)
	47, XYY/49, XYYYY/46, XY	1 (0.09)
	45, X/47, XYY	1 (0.09)
	45, X/46, XY	2 (0.18)
Structural		
-Complete	46, X, inv (y) (q11.2; q12)	1 (0.09)
	46, X, inv (y) (p11.2; q12)	1 (0.09)
-Mosaicism	–	0

It can be expected that chromosome abnormalities are at least ten times more frequent in men with male infertility (5.1%) than in the general population (0.38%) (Van Assche et al. 1996). Van Assche et al. (1996) reviewed the data from seven surveys of cytogenetics in infertile men and compared these data with those of more than 95 000 unselected newborn babies.

One of the largest single series has been published by Scholtes et al. (1998), who described chromosomal abnormalities in 4.48% of the 1116 men included. A list of anomalies found is given in Table 2.

Since chromosome abnormalities clearly correlate with the number of sperms in the ejaculate (Van Assche et al. 1996), all male partners with fewer than 20 million sperm/ml should be karyotyped prior to ICSI to give the couples the possibility of risk estimation before the procedure is started. This is important, since chromosome abnormalities – especially autosomal ones – carry a high risk of abortion and malformations in the offspring if carried to term.

Chromosome Abnormalities in Female Partners of Men with Male Factor Infertility

Interestingly, also female partners of men with severely impaired semen parameters who were planned for an ICSI procedure showed an increased risk of chromosome aberrations in several studies (Meschede et al. 1998a, Scholtes et al. 1998). Scholtes et al. (1998) published data from 1164 women whose partners had severe semen impairment and who planned to undergo an ICSI treatment. In this population 9.79% of abnormal karyotypes were found. In 27 women (2.32%) autosomal structural aberrations and in 87 (7.47%) numerical anomalies involving sex chromosomes were found. Even if most gonosomal aberrations and mosaics were excluded from analysis, since they may have no clinical relevance for the couples, the prevalence of anomalies remained increased.

Meschede et al. (1998a) reported on 477 couples who planned to undergo an ICSI procedure. In 436 women who were karyotyped, 24 abnormalities were described (5.5%). These authors also discussed the possibility that in cases of low-level sex chromosome mosaicism without signs of Turner's syndrome, there might be an increased risk of bearing an aneuploid child.

Although there is only little information on the fertility and pregnancy course of women with low-level mosaicism, there might be an infertility problem if these abnormalities in females were "combined" with severe male factor infertility. This may explain why in a cohort of couples who were planned for an ICSI treatment, a higher prevalence of chromosome abnormalities was observed also in the female partners.

Further studies have to be done, especially regarding the question of whether the hypothesized increased rate of gonosomal aberrations in fetuses following ICSI (Bonduelle et al. 1998a) must be attributed to the father or to the mother.

Treatment Outcome of Couples with Chromosome Abnormalities

Couples who are diagnosed to have either a male or a female chromosomal abnormality do not necessarily give up their plan to undergo an ICSI treatment, not even after genetic counseling. In a recently published Dutch multicenter follow-up study of 75 ICSI couples, of whom the male partners had a chromosome abnormality, 56% of the couples did not refrain from the ICSI treatment (Giltay et al. 1999). In all, 29 men with sex chromosome and 46 men with autosomal chromosome aberrations were included. In cases of sex chromosome abnormalities 59% and in cases of autosomal chromosome aberrations 54% proceeded with the ICSI treatment. Ten couples had not yet decided whether to proceed or not when the article was published. These numbers are interesting, especially since in cases of unbalanced autosomal chromosome aberrations the risk for the child to be affected is much higher compared with cases of sex chromosome aberrations.

The chance of conceiving under these circumstances is still a matter of debate. In the study by Giltay et al. (1999), 11 of 42 couples became pregnant (26%). However, in another study significantly lower fertilization, implantation, and pregnancy rates were found in those couples where either the male or the female partner was affected by a chromosome abnormality (Montag et al. 1997) (Table 3). This observation was made in cases of constitutional aberrations. In cases of low-level mosaicism in male and female partners there were a significantly reduced fertilization rate and transfer rate, but no differences in implantation and pregnancy rates. The abortion rate was high in cases where both partners were affected (40%).

These data are confirmed by Scholtes et al. (1998). They published data of couples with different chromosome abnormalities undergoing an ICSI treatment and described a significantly reduced implantation rate per embryo if male gonosomes were affected and a tendency towards a lower implantation rate if female gonosomes were affected (Table 4). The same held for the pregnancy rates in these two subgroups.

Another working group found no difference in the treatment outcome between those couples with and those without chromosome abnormalities (Testart et al. 1996). The results are summarized in Table 5. There was no difference neither in mean number of embryos transferred or in clinical pregnancy or implantation rates.

In our own study, we confirmed the results of Testart et al. (1996) and did not find any difference in couples with male constitutional chromosome abnormality compared with our general ICSI population (Ludwig et al. 1999a). Eight couples were studied, from 60 metaphase-II oocytes 37 were fertilized

Table 3. Results of ICSI treatment in couples where either the male or the female partner was affected by a chromosome abnormality (from Montag et al. 1997)

	Constitutional chromosome aberration			Control group	
	Total	Male partner affected	Female partner affected	Matched couples	Unaffected couples
No. of couples	16	8	8	16	322
Mean age of women (years)	34±4.6	33.5±6.2	34.2±3.4	33±4	34.2±4.3
No. of cycles	30	20	10	30	394
Fertilization rate (%)	93/252 (36.9)	61/156 (39.1)	32/96 (33.3)	125/251 (49.8)	2298/4016 (57.2)
Implantation rate per embryo transferred (%)	4/76 (5.3)	1/50 (2)	3/26 (7.7)	11/74 (14.9)	118/387 (10.6)
Ongoing pregnancy rate (%)	7.1	5.3	11.1	25	21

Table 4. Results of ICSI treatment in cases of autosomal or gonosomal aberrations in one of the partners (from Scholtes et al. 1998)

Aberration	No. of patients	Implantation rate per embryo (%)	No. of ongoing pregnancies/no. of births (%)
Male gonosomes	9	3.8[a]	0/1 (8.3)
Male autosomes	27	23.1[a]	0/9 (27.2)
Female gonosomes	54	9.4	2/7 (12.5)
Female autosomes	15	16.3	0/5 (25)

[a] Values are significantly different from each other ($p < 0.05$).

(61.7%); one triploid pronuclear stage was observed. Five pregnancies were achieved, but three ended in an abortion due to chromosome abnormalities in the fetuses. The others led to the birth of three healthy children with either normal or balanced karyotypes.

Our experience with such couples is still small. However, in each case there must be professional genetic counseling concerning the possible risks for the offspring and the possible lower probability of having fertilized oocytes and a pregnancy going to term. The couples should also be counseled to agree to the transfer of only two embryos, to minimize the risk of having one fetus with an unbalanced chromosome abnormality.

Mutations of the Cystic Fibrosis Transmembrane Conductance Receptor Gene in Infertile Men

Mutations of the cystic fibrosis transmembrane conductance regulator (CFTR) gene can lead to a wide spectrum of clinical presentations. The most severe forms of cystic fibrosis with chronic lung and pancreatic impairment and lethal complications in the first weeks of life are one end of the spectrum. At the other end is the congenital bilateral absence of the vas deferens (CBAVD), leading to obstructive azoospermia in an otherwise healthy male.

CFTR mutations have a frequency of about 1:25–1:30, and more than 700 mutations are known so far. The CFTR gene encodes a chloride channel, which is cAMP regulated. Histologically, there is a wide variety of pictures of spermatogenesis in patients suffering from cystic fibrosis. It ranges from normal spermatogenesis to different stages of maturation arrest with highly disturbed morphological differentiation problems in the remaining sperm (Gottlieb et al. 1991, Kaplan et al. 1968). Therefore, the CFTR gene seems to play a role in the embryonic development of the male genital tract and the regulation of spermatogenesis. This is supported by the observation of van der Ven et al. (1996), who described an increased rate of CFTR mutations even in men suffering from different grades of oligo-astheno-teratozoospermia. Patrizio et al. (1993a,b) showed a decreased fertilization capacity of sperm from men with CBAVD in conventional IVF. However, there is no impairment of the fertiliza-

Table 5. Results of ICSI treatment in couples with chromosome abnormalities (from Testart et al. 1996)

Chromosome abnormality	No. of couples transfers	No. of embryo	Transferred embryos		No. of pregnancies		No. of fetuses Total (%) of transfers
			Total	Mean ±standard deviation	Total	Clinical (% of transfers)	
In men	11	13	31	2.4±0.3	7	4 (30.8)	5 (16.1)
In women	3	5	16	3.2±0.7	1	1 (20.0)	2 (12.5)
None	247	272	680	2.5±0.1	102	78 (28.7)	108 (15.9)

tion process if ICSI is used for these patients. Therefore, a disturbance in zona penetration or capacitation is proposed to be the problem in these men (Silber et al. 1994).

Most patients who suffer from CBAVD are heterozygotes for CFTR mutations. Others are compound heterozygotes and have one severe and one mild mutation, and a third group show two mild mutations. The presence of two severe mutations will almost always lead to the full-blown picture of cystic fibrosis.

Some patients with CBAVD do not show any CFTR mutation. This can be due to several factors, which have to be ruled out to make sufficient genetic counseling possible.

One possibility is poly-T-polymorphisms in intron 8. Here, five, seven, or nine thymidines (5T, 7T, or 9T allele) are present; the presence of a 5T allele will lead to splicing problems and to an increase of incomplete and nonfunctioning CFTR mRNA (Chu et al. 1993).

Chillon et al. (1995) studied the prevalence of CFTR mutations as well as of poly-T-polymorphisms in 102 men suffering from CBAVD. They described 28 mutations; 19 patients were compound heterozygotes. The prevalence of 5T alleles in intron 8 was significantly higher in the CBAVD population (21.1%) compared with the general population (5.2%). Forty-nine patients either showed no abnormality of the CFTR gene or had only one 5T allele. These men were proposed to have other, noncharacterized CFTR mutations or gene mutations outside the CFTR gene which led to a functional impairment of the CFTR gene product.

Another possibility of obstructive azoospermia similar to CBAVD is Young's syndrome. This seems to be a noninherited disease, perhaps linked to neonatal exposure to mercury, which is combined with bronchiectasia. A recent study showed that there is no increased risk of CFTR mutations in patients with Young's syndrome (Le Lannou et al. 1995).

Finally, about 20% of men suffering from CBAVD also suffer from other urinary tract abnormalities. In these patients no CFTR mutations are found, since here an entity distinct from CFTR-related CBAVD is present. In this subgroup of patients a damage of the wolffian ducts before the 7th week of embryonic development probably takes place, leading to malformations of both the urinary tract and the genital tract. CFTR mutations seem to have an influence on the embryonic development at a later time point, because only the genital tract is affected, which separates from the urinary tract after the 7th week of embryonic development. Therefore, this subgroup of patients need not be counseled about a risk of cystic fibrosis in their offspring (Lissens 1999).

Thus, especially in cases of obstructive azoospermia, genetic counseling and molecular genetic testing of CFTR mutations, as well as of T-polymorphisms in intron 8, are necessary to evaluate possible genetic risk factors in these patients. A careful clinical diagnosis must be undertaken to differentiate subtypes of obstructive azoospermia with a substantial genetic risk.

Y-Chromosome Microdeletions in Men with Male Factor Infertility

It is a well-known fact that not the whole Y-chromosome is necessary for determining a male phenotype. A typical example was males with the XX genotype with an apparent translocation of Y-chromosomal material to one of the two X-chromosomes (Sinclair et al. 1990). The question remained whether Y-chromosomal material has a function only in sex determination or also in spermatogenesis. In *Drosophila melanogaster* an X0 genotype leads to a sterile male, but in human beings the same karyotype will lead to a sterile female individual; this is known as Turner's syndrome (Vogt et al. 1996). A milestone along the road to answering this question was the work done by (Tiepolo and Zuffardi 1976), which included data on 1170 men. In six of these a deletion of the long arm of the Y-chromosome was present (Yq11), and all of these men presented with azoospermia. Therefore, the authors postulated the existence of an "azoospermia factor" (AZF) in this region of the Y-chromosome.

In 1995, Page and co-workers published a series of 89 patients presenting with nonobstructive azoospermia, who were studied together with 90 fertile controls; 84 Y-chromosomal sequence-tagged sites, i.e., small parts of the Y-chromosome, were studied using the polymerase chain reaction technique (PCR). In 12 of these 89 patients (micro-)deletions were identified which showed an overlapping in the distal part of the Y-chromosome in interval 6 at the location Yq11.23 (Reijo et al. 1995). A further analysis in this region, using another 30 sequence-tagged sites, lead to the identification of a gene called DAZ – deleted in azoospermia. The work by Reijo et al. (1995) was important, since here a large number of patients were investigated using a very high number of sequence-tagged sites. DNA samples from patients who had been investigated by others in the years before (Ma et al. 1992, Ma et al. 1993, Kobayashi et al. 1994) and showed deletions on another site of the Y-chromosome (YRRM gene) also showed deletions in the DAZ gene locus. Furthermore, there were no correlations between the size of the deletion and the testicular histology. However, most of the patients with Sertoli cell-only syndrome did not show a deletion of DAZ (88%). Recent publications have confirmed the results of Reijo et al. (1995) but also showed that deletions of Yq11 are not limited to men with azoospermia, since also men with severe oligozoospermia (Qureshi et al. 1996, Reijo et al. 1996a, Vogt et al. 1996, Foresta et al. 1997, 1998, In't Veld et al. 1997, Kremer et al. 1997, Pryor et al. 1997, Simoni et al. 1997, Vereb et al. 1997, Ludwig et al. 1998) as well as those with normozoospermia (Pryor et al. 1997) may present with deletions of DAZ.

In a recent review of the entire literature concerning DAZ deletions, a wide range of prevalence was shown, from 9% (96/1082) of men with azoospermia, to 6% (27/457) of men with severe oligozoospermia (< 5 million sperm/ml), to 2% (6/314) of men with oligozoospermia (5–20 million sperm/ml) and 0.5% (6/768) in fertile controls (Kuehl et al. 1998).

The DAZ protein has an RNA-binding region and may be involved in regulation of spermatogenesis. In *Drosophila* (Eberhart et al. 1996) and in the mouse (Reijo et al. 1996b) a similiar gene, called *boule* and *Dazh*, respectively, has been identified. Interestingly, boule is located autosomally and not gonosomally. This led to the suggestion that there might also be a human autosomal DAZ homologue. In fact, this has been identified and recently mapped to chromosome 3 (Saxena et al. 1996). Further investigations led to the assumption that a transposition of the DAZ gene took place during evolution from chromosome 3 to the Y-chromosome.

Vogt et al. (1996) reported on 370 men with idiopathic azoospermia or severe oligozoospermia. These men were investigated with 76 sequence-tagged sites, and deletions were found in 12. Three gene loci were identified: one of those was DAZ, called AZF c, one was YRRM, called AZF b, and the third was a new locus and called AZF a. Vogt et al. (1996) postulated that the three loci were correlated with testicular histology and that these AZF regions encoded genes which were involved in different steps of spermatogenesis. However, these findings were not in accordance with the results of (Reijo et al. 1995) and (Qureshi et al. 1996).

An interesting aspect was published by Kent-First et al. (1996), who screened 32 unselected men who had fathered sons following an ICSI treatment for Y-chromosome microdeletions. The DNA of the sons was also investigated. In three father-son combinations microdeletions were found. However, despite the presence of Y-chromosome deletions in two sons, these deletions were not present in their fathers. In only one father-son combination was the Y-chromosome microdeletion present in both. This must mean that the fathers have a mosaic regarding their Y deletions. Apparently, there was a postzygotic microdeletion on the Y-chromosome in one cell line, which was present in testicular tissue but not in the blood.

These observations limit the value of AZF screening for clinical use for several reasons:
1. In some studies, microdeletions were identified but did not map to the DAZ region (Qureshi et al. 1996, Vogt et al. 1996). This means that screening of the DAZ region alone is not sufficient.
2. Each analysis by PCR will be limited to a certain number of sequence-tagged sites. Therefore, deletions outside these sequence-tagged sites will not be detected. For clinical use, the number of sequence-tagged sites would have to be limited to far below the number used by Reijo et al. (1995) and by others. This would lead to a lower detection rate.
3. Until now, only one study has been done to identify point mutations of the DAZ gene. Vereb et al. (1997) were unable to find those alterations in a small number of patients with azoospermia. However, it cannot be excluded that the abnormalities might exist, and will also be inherited from father to son and lead to infertility in the son.
4. Since Kent-First et al. (1996) showed that mosaics are possible that cannot be detected by DNA analysis from genomic DNA prepared from blood cells, a high proportion of patients at risk may not be identified.
5. As described above, a DAZ homologue is located on chromosome 3, and other extragonosomal genes may also be involved in spermatogenesis and in the pathogenesis of azoospermia or severe oligozoospermia. This is very

likely, since more than 30% of men with fertility problems have the diagnosis of idiopathic male infertility – despite thorough clinical, genetic, and operative investigation. All these still unknown genetic causes cannot yet be investigated.

6. Finally, most patients will not draw any consequence from a Y-chromosome microdeletion. The only risk will be that a son born following ICSI will suffer from the same infertility problems as his father did. This is – from our clinical experience – in no case a cause to refrain from an ICSI treatment for these couples. Furthermore, if the information in this list is respected, *all* couples, even those with a negative result of AZF screening, must be counseled about the fact that there is still a risk of having sons with infertility problems because of unidentified deletions, Y-chromosomal point mutations, autosomal abnormalities, and mosaics.

Therefore, AZF screening does not seem to have the same value as CFTR screening and chromosome analysis for men with infertility. It is of scientific interest, but the clinical value is limited.

Androgen Receptor Gene Mutations and Male Infertility

During the embryonic and fetal development androgens must act by their receptors to enable normal development of the male phenotype. Androgen receptor mutations can lead to different abnormalities, depending on the degree of androgen function remaining in these patients. Besides patients with the full-blown clinical picture of the female phenotype there is a group of patients with infertile male syndrome. The prevalence of this abnormality is still unknown, since the data on androgen receptor mutations in the group of patients with male infertility are rare. These patients have normal male genitalia at birth but present with a more or less severe oligo-astheno-teratozoospermia or even azoospermia after puberty (Quigley et al. 1995).

In 1979, Aiman et al. published a report about three men with infertility and high mean plasma testosterone and LH levels. They suggested that these men might have androgen insensitivity, and that this insensitivity caused their fertility problems. However, due to the lack of molecular genetic testing at that time, they were not able to prove their thesis.

Puscheck et al. (1994) published their observation of exon 1 analysis of the androgen receptor gene in 16 oligozoospermic or azoospermic men. No abnormalities were found. Tincello et al. (1997) reported on six men suffering from male infertility and showing elevated LH and testosterone levels. These six were recruited from a cohort of 50 initially selected patients. In none of these six men was an androgen receptor mutation present. Therefore, the authors concluded that androgen receptor mutations seem not to be a common cause of male infertility. However, they were also aware that the sample size was small, and that further studies are necessary to prove their thesis.

Akin et al. (1991) published their finding of the first partial gene deletion of the androgen receptor gene in one of seven azoospermic males. Wang et al.

(1998) reported on one patient from a cohort of 234 subfertile men with a point mutation in the ligand-binding domain of the androgen receptor gene, leading to azoospermia in this patient. In vitro experiments showed an impaired *trans*-activation of androgen-regulated genes by this mutation.

Therefore, androgen receptor gene mutations as a cause of male infertility without further phenotypic abnormalities seem to be rare. However, it could be that by means of more detailed analysis, especially of point mutations in the different exons, more abnormalities can be found.

It is important to note that the identification of these men is of great clinical significance, since they represent one of the rare groups of men suffering from male infertility who really could be treated by the administration of high doses of testosterone (Yong et al. 1994). Most other patients would have deterioration of fertility when treated with androgens.

Is There an Increased Genetic Risk per se with the ICSI Technique?

The question of whether there may be a genetic risk connected with the ICSI technique itself was extensively reviewed by Engel and co-workers (Engel and Schmid 1995, Engel et al. 1996, 1998) as well as by others (Meschede et al. 1995). In 1995 and 1996, Engel et al. proposed some principle theses, which exclude the possibility that there might be an increased genetic risk related to the principle of ICSI itself: the selection of single sperms in an IVF laboratory.

First of all, there is no sperm selection against chromosome anomalies in the female tract under natural conditions. In fact, fertile men who carry balanced chromosome abnormalities have a 50% or more risk of producing offspring with an unbalanced translocation, which leads to an early abortion or to malformations at birth. There is, for example, a well-known risk of patients carrying robertsonian translocations of both chromosomes 21 to create a fetus with a nearly 100% chance of having a trisomy 21. Therefore, the chance of transmitting chromosome abnormalities in sperm should be the same under laboratory as under natural conditions.

In fact, there is to date no clear answer to the question of whether there is really an increased risk of chromosome abnormalities in the sperm of men with severe oligozoospermia – even without showing somatic chromosome abnormalities. The largest series of sperm nuclei of 45 infertile men did not show any increase in disomy or diploidy rates in this population compared with fertile controls (Guttenbach et al. 1997). There is no proof up to now that the morphology of sperm correlates with the genetic contents of their nuclei.

Furthermore, the mendelian laws clearly show that there is also no selection against monogenetic diseases in the female tract. Otherwise, there would not be 50% transmission of the affected genes.

Several studies have shown that the rate of chromosome abnormalities is highest in zygotes and embryos during the first cleavage stages (38%). They decrease subsequently by natural selection, i.e., nonimplantation and preclinical or clinical abortion later on, until it reaches 0.6% in newborn infants (Plachot et al. 1987; Plachot 1989). Therefore, the natural selection against chromosome abnormalities does not take place – even under natural conditions – in the gametes, but during the postimplantation phase. This stage is not influenced by the ICSI technique.

Finally, Engel et al. (1996) calculated that an increase from only 1.8% to 2.3% could be expected, even if all cases of male infertility had a genetic cause and all these men procreated with the help of ICSI. This increase would take about 600 years, i.e., 20 generations. Therefore, a dramatic increase in male infertility over the next few years cannot be expected if ICSI is widely used.

Meschede et al. (1995) added the problem of genomic imprinting to the possible genetic risks of ICSI. This might be a problem especially in cases where either epididymal or testicular sperm are used for microinjection (Devroey et al. 1994, 1995, 1996, Silber et al. 1994). The use of spermatids could imply even more risks of genetic disorders because of genomic imprinting. During development specific modification of genes controls the expression of differential genes of homologous chromosomes. Differential expression of the alleles of imprinted genes is related to the DNA methylation process (Fishel et al. 1996). Some studies reported that this fundamental genetic process of spermatogenetic cells is completed in the testes prior to the second meiotic division (in mouse cells) or within the cytoplasm of the mature oocyte after spermatid injection in human cells (Kimura and Yanagimachi 1995). However, some authors are have discussed the problem of genomic imprinting extensively (Tesarik et al. 1998a,b), since others have shown that the imprinting process in male gametes is not completed even with the fertilization process (Latham et al. 1995).

However, even if there is no theoretical risk using the ICSI technique itself, it is still proposed that children born after ICSI, and especially after the use of spermatids, must be carefully followed up to evaluate even small potential genetic risks.

Prenatal Diagnosis in Fetuses Conceived after ICSI

Several studies have been done so far to determine whether there is an increased number of chromosome abnormalities in fetuses conceived by an ICSI procedure. The data are summarized in Table 6.

The only reliable data were published by Bonduelle et al. (1998a), who included more than 1000 subjects with prenatal diagnostic testing in their study. The only anomaly observed was a slight increase in gonosomal aberrations compared with the rate in spontaneously conceived children. However, there were no data on the age of the mothers in these pregnancies, and no data on the origin of these abnormalities (paternal or maternal). Additionally, the data on chromosome abnormalities in spontaneously conceived and not preselected pregnancies are rare. Therefore, no real control group can be included in the analysis of these data.

Other studies listed in Table 6 do not reflect the real clinical situation in fetuses conceived with ICSI treatment. The data given by In't Veld et al. (1995)

Table 6. Collection of data on prenatal diagnosis following ICSI (from Ludwig and Diedrich 1999)

Reference	Source	Number	%
In't Veld et al. (1995)	De novo	5/15	33.3
	Inherited	0/15	–
ICSI Task Force 1994 (Bonduelle et al. 1995)	–	8/361	2.2
Testart et al. (1996)	De novo	0/108	–
	Inherited	5/7	71.4
Van Opstal et al. (1997)	De novo	9/71	12.7
Bonduelle et al. (1998)	De novo	2/70	2.9
Meschede et al. (1998)	Inherited	3/18	16.7
ICSI Task Force 1995 (Ludwig et al. 1996)	–	15/666	2.3
Palermo et al. (1998)	–	11/150	7.3
Bonduelle et al. (1998)	De novo	18/1082	1.7
	Inherited	10/1082	0.9
Ludwig et al. (1999a)	De novo	0/74	–
	Inherited	2/4	50

were based on a group of only 15 patients who were preselected. The same is true for the high prevalence reported by Van Opstal et al. (1997). Palermo et al. (1998) reported a prevalence of 7.3% of chromosome abnormalities in ICSI pregnancies. However, here also there seems to be a high and negative preselection of cases, since invasive genetic testing was reported in only 9% of all pregnancies.

These observations have led to the conclusion that couples who plan to undergo ICSI treatment should be counseled about the slight possibility of gonosomal aberrations in their children. However, most of these alterations will not lead to severe handicaps in the children born, and the advice to undergo invasive prenatal testing should therefore be considered carefully (Baschat et al. 1996, Meschede and Horst 1997, Meschede et al. 1998a, Ludwig et al. 1999a).

Conclusion

The data collected so far have led to the proposal to perform karyotyping in all men, and perhaps also in all female partners, who are candidates for ICSI treatment (Bundesärztekammer 1998). It should also become clinical practice to perform molecular genetic analysis for CFTR mutations in men with obstructive azoospermia. The value of screening for AZF microdeletions is a matter of debate, since despite a positive finding most couples will not refrain from ICSI treatment, the only consequence being that their child – if it is a boy – will suffer from the same problem as his father. Even if a negative finding is presented, a substantial genetic risk remains for male offspring, since most genes which control spermatogenesis or male fertility are currently unknown. Therefore, there cannot be 100% safety of this procedure regarding the fertility of especially male offspring. Androgen receptor mutations may become more important in the future, when more data are available on the expected prevalence of these abnormalities in collectives of men with male infertility.

A careful family history should be taken for all couples who plan to undergo ICSI treatment, in order to evaluate the presence of genetic risk factors. However, if genetic risk factors are not present, and molecular genetic analysis – especially of CFTR mutations – does not show any abnormality, there should be no increased risk of malformations for children born after ICSI. Whether there is really a substantially increased risk of gonosomal abnormalities in fetuses after ICSI must still be examined in a larger cohort of pregnancies.

References

Aiman J, Griffin JE, Gazak JM, Wilson JD, MacDonald PC (1979) Androgen insensitivity as a cause of infertility in otherwise normal men. N Engl J Med 300:223–227

Akin JW, Behzadian A, Tho SP, McDonough PG (1991) Evidence for a partial deletion in the androgen receptor gene in a phenotypic male with azoospermia. Am J Obstet Gynecol 165:1891–1894

Baschat AA, Schwinger E, Diedrich K (1996) Debate. Assisted reproductive techniques – are we avoiding the genetic issues? Hum Reprod 11:926–928

Bonduelle M, Legein J, Wilkins A et al (1995) Follow-up study of children born after intracytoplasmic sperm injection. Hum Reprod 10:52–54

Bonduelle M, Aytoz A, Wilikens A, Buysse A, Van Assche E, Devroey P, Van Steirteghem A, Liebaers I (1998a) Prospective follow-up study of 1987 children born after intracytoplasmic sperm injection (ICSI). In: Filicori M, Flamigni C (eds) Treatment of infertility:the new frontiers. Communications Media for Eduction, Inc, New Jersey, pp 445–461

Bonduelle M, Wilikens A, Buysse A, Van Assche E, Devroey P, Van Steirteghem AC, Liebaers I (1998b) A follow-up study of children born after intracytoplasmic sperm injection (ICSI) with epididymal and testicular spermatozoa and after replacement of cryopreserved embryos obtained after ICSI. Hum Reprod 13 [Suppl 1]:196–207

Bowen JR, Gibson FL, Leslie GI, Saunders DM (1998) Medical and developmental outcome at 1 year for children conceived by intracytoplasmic sperm injection. Lancet 351:1529–1534

Bundesärztekammer, W.B.d. (1998) Richtlinien zur Durchführung der assistierten Reproduktion. Dtsch Arztebl 95:A3166–A3177

Chillon M, Casals T, Mercier B, Bassas L, Lissens W, Silber S, Romey MC, Ruiz Romero J, Verlingue C, Claustres M et al (1995) Mutations in the cystic fibrosis gene in patients with congenital absence of the vas deferens. N Engl J Med 332:1475–1480

Chu CS, Trapnell BC, Curristin S, Cutting GR, Crystal RG (1993) Genetic basis of variable exon 9 skipping in cystic fibrosis transmembrane conductance regulator mRNA. Nat Genet 3:151–156

De Braekeleer M, Dao T-N (1991) Cytogenetic studies in male infertility: a review. Hum Reprod 6:245–250

Devroey P, Liu J, Nagy Z, Tournaye H, Silber SJ, Van Steirteghem AC (1994) Normal fertilization of human oocytes after testicular sperm extraction and intracytoplasmic sperm injection. Fertil Steril 62:639–641

Devroey P, Liu J, Nagy Z, Goossens A, Tournaye H, Camus M, Van Steirteghem A, Silber S (1995) Pregnancies after testicular sperm extraction and intracytoplasmic sperm injection in non-obstructive azoospermia. Hum Reprod 10:1457–1460

Devroey P, Nagy P, Tournaye H, Liu J, Silber S, Van Steirteghem A (1996) Outcome of intracytoplasmic sperm injection with testicular spermatozoa in obstructive and non-obstructive azoospermia. Hum Reprod 11:1015–1018

Eberhart CG, Maines JZ, Wasserman SA (1996) Meiotic cell cycle requirement for a fly homologue of human deleted in azoospermia. Nature 381:783–785

Engel W, Schmid M (1995) Gibt es genetische Risiken der mikroassistierten Reproduktion? Fertilitat 11:214–228

Engel W, Murphy D, Schmid M (1996) Are there genetic risks associated with microassisted reproduction? Hum Reprod 11:2359–2370

Engel W, Schmid M, Pauer H-U (1998) Genetik und mikroassistierte Reproduktion durch intrazytoplasmatische Spermieninjektion. Dtsch Arztebl 95:1548–1553

Ferguson-Smith MA, Lennox B, Mack WS, Stewart JSS (1957) Klinefelter's syndrome: frequency and testicular morphology in relation to nuclear sex. Lancet 2:167

Fishel S, Aslam I, Tesarik J (1996) Spermatid conception: a stage too early, or a time too soon? [editorial]. Hum Reprod 11:1371–1375

Foresta C, Ferlin A, Garolla A, Moro E, Pistorello M, Barbaux S, Rossato M (1998) High frequency of well-defined Y-chromosome deletions in idiopathic Sertoli cell-only syndrome. Hum Reprod 13:302–307

Foresta C, Ferlin A, Garolla A, Rossato M, Barbaux S, De Bortoli A (1997) Y-chromosome deletions in idiopathic severe testiculopathies. J Clin Endocrinol Metab 82:1075–1080

Giltay JC, Kastrop PM, Tuerlings JH, Kremer JA, Tiemessen CH, Gerssen-Schoorl KB, van d. V de Vries J, Hordijk R, Hamers GJ, Hansson K, van der Blij-Philipsen M, Govaerts LC, Pieters MH, Madan K, Scheres JM (1999) Subfertile men with constitutive chromosome abnormalities do not necessarily refrain from intracytoplasmic sperm injection treatment: a follow-up study on 75 Dutch patients [in process citation]. Hum Reprod 14:318–320

Gottlieb C, Plöen L, Kvist U, Strandvik B (1991) The fertility potential of male cystic fibrosis patients. Int J Androl 14:437–440

Govaerts I, Devreker F, Koenig I, Place I, Van den Bergh M, Englert Y (1998) Comparison of pregnancy outcome after intracytoplasmic sperm injection and in-vitro fertilization. Hum Reprod 13:1514–1518

Govaerts I, Koenig I, Van den Bergh M, Bertrand E, Revelard P, Englert Y (1996) Is intracytoplasmic sperm injection (ICSI) a safe procedure? What do we learn from early pregnancy data about ICSI? Hum Reprod 11:440–443

Guttenbach M, Martinez-Exposito MJ, Michelmann HW, Engel W, Schmid M (1997) Incidence of diploid and disomic sperm nuclei in 45 infertile men. Hum Reprod 12:468–473

In't Veld P, Brandenburg H, Verhoeff A, Dhont M, Los F (1995) Sex chromosomal abnormalities and intracytoplasmic sperm injection [letter] [see comments]. Lancet 346:773

In't Veld PA, Halley DJJ, van Hemel JO, Niermeijer MF, Dohle G, Weber RFA (1997) Genetic counselling before intracytoplasmic sperm injection. Lancet 350:490

Jacobs PA, Strong J (1959) A case of human intersexuality having a possible XXY sex-determining mechanism. Nature 183:302–303

Johanisson R, Schwinger E, Wolff HH et al (1993) The effect of 13:14 Robertsonian translocations on germ-cell differentiation in infertile males. Cytogenet Cell Genet 63:151–155

Kaplan E, Shwachman H, Perlmutter AD, Rule A, Khaw KT, Holsclaw DS (1968) Reproductive failure in males with cystic fibrosis. N Engl J Med 279:65–69

Kent-First MG, Kol S, Muallem A, Ofir R, Manor D, Blazer S, First N, Itskovitz-Eldor J (1996) The incidence and possible relevance of Y-linked microdeletions in babies born after intracytoplasmic sperm injection and their infertile fathers. Mol Hum Reprod 2:943–950

Kimura Y, Yanagimachi R (1995) Mouse oocytes injected with testicular spermatozoa or round spermatids can develop into normal offspring. Development 121:2397–2405

Kobayashi K, Mizuno K, Hida A, Komaki R, Tomita K, Matsushita I, Namiki M, Iwamoto T, Tamura S, Minowada S, Nakahori Y, Nakagome Y (1994) PCR analysis of the Y chromosome long arm in azoospermic patients: evidence for a second locus required for spermatogenesis. Hum Mol Genet 3:1965–1967

Kremer JA, Tuerlings JH, Meuleman EJ, Schoute F, Mariman E, Smeets DF, Hoefsloot LH, Braat DD, Merkus HM (1997) Microdeletions of the Y chromosome and intracytoplasmic sperm injection: from gene to clinic. Hum Reprod 12:687–691

Kuehl TJ, Sprague DCC, Brown ML, Yurchak MR, Wincek TJ (1998) PCR screening of human semen samples for the deleted in azoospermia locus (DAZ) of the Y chromosome (Abstract, 54th Annual meeting of the ASRM). Fertil Steril 70 [Suppl 1]:S8

Kurinczuk JJ, Bower C (1997) Birth defects in infants conceived by intracytoplasmic sperm injection: an alternative interpretation. Br Med J 315:1260–1266

Latham KE, McGrath J, Solter D (1995) Mechanistic and developmental aspects of genetic imprinting in mammals. Int Rev Cytol 160:53–98

Le Lannou D, Jezequel P, Blayau M, Dorval I, Lemoine P, Dabadie A, Roussey M, Le Marec B, Legall JY (1995) Obstructive azoospermia with agenesis of vas deferens or with bronchiectasia (Young's syndrome): a genetic approach. Hum Reprod 10:338–341

Lissens W (1999) Genetics of male reproductive dysfunction. In: Fauser BCJM (ed) Molecular biology in reproductive medicine, vol 1. Parthenon, New York, pp 479–504

Loft A, Ejdrup B, Pedersen K, Erb K, Mikkelsen L, Grindsted J, Hald F, Lundstrom P, Lenz S, Andersen AN, Society TDF (1998) Outcome after intracytoplasmic sperm injection (ICSI) – a Danish national cohort of 506 infants. Fertil Steril 70 [Suppl 1]:S350

Ludwig M. Al-Hasani S, Küpker W, Diedrich K (1996) Intrayztoplasmatische Spermatozoeninjektion (ICSI). Überblick über die aktuelle Situation. Frauenarzt 37:1624–1634

Ludwig M, Küpker W, Hahn K, Al-Hasani S, Diedrich K (1998) Klinische Bedeutung Y-chromosomaler Mikrodeletionen im Rahmen reproduktionsgenetischer Routinediagnostik bei schwerer männlicher Subfertilität. Geburtsh Frauenheilkd 58:73–78

Ludwig M, Geipel A, Mennicke K, Küpker W, Al-Hasani S, Ghasemi M, Gizycki U, Gembruch U, Diedrich K (1999a) Intrazytoplasmatische Spermatozoeninjektion – ICSI (I): Verlauf von 310 Schwangerschaften, Ergebnisse der Pränataldiagnostik und Diskussion eines non-invasiven Konzepts zur Pränataldiagnostik. Geburtsh Frauenheilkd 59:387–394

Ludwig M, Al-Hasani S, Ghasemi M, Gizycki U, Küpker W, Diedrich K (1999b) Intrazytoplasmatische Spermatozoeninjektion – ICSI (II): Geburt und Gesundheit von 267 Kindern. Geburth Frauenheilkd 59:395–401

Ma K, Sharkey A, Kirsch S, Vogt P, Keil R, Hargreave TB, McBeath S, Chandley AC (1992) Towards the molecular localisation of the AZF locus: mapping of microdeletions in azoospermic men within 14 subintervals of interval 6 of the human Y chromosome. Hum Mol Genet 1:29–33

Ma K, Inglis JD, Sharkey A, Bickmore WA, Hill RE, Prosser EJ, Speed RM, Thomson EJ, Jobling M, Taylor K, Wolfe J, Cooke HJ, Hargreave TB, Chandley AC (1993) A Y-chromosome gene family with RNA-binding protein homology: candidates for the azoospermia factor AZF controlling human spermatogenesis. Cell 75:1287–1295

Meschede D, De Geyter C, Nieschlag E, Horst J (1995) Genetic risk in micromanipulative assisted reproduction. Hum Reprod 10:2880–2886

Meschede D, Horst J (1997) Sex chromosomal anomalies in pregnancies conceived through intracytoplasmic sperm injection: a case for genetic counselling. Hum Reprod 12:1125–1127

Meschede D, Lemcke B, Exeler JR, De Geyter C, Behre HM, Nieschlag E, Horst J (1998a) Chromosome abnormalities in 447 couples undergoing intracytoplasmic sperm injection–prevalence, types, sex distribution and reproductive relevance. Hum Reprod 13:576–582

Meschede D, Lemcke B, Stüssel J, Louwen F, Horst J (1998b) Strong preference for noninvasive prenatal diagnosis in women pregnant through intracytoplasmic sperm injection (ICSI). Prenat Diag 18:700–705

Montag M, van d Ved S, Schmutzler A, Prietl G, Krebs D, Peschka B, Schwanitz G, Albers P, Haidl G (1997) Success of intracytoplasmic sperm injection in couples with male and/or female chromosome aberrations. Hum Reprod 12:2635–2640

Palermo G, Joris H, Devroey P, Van Steirteghem AC (1992) Pregnancies after intracytoplasmic injection of single spermatozoon into an oocyte. Lancet 340:17–18

Palermo G et al (1996) Evolution of pregnancies and initial follow-up of newborns delivered after intracytoplasmic sperm injection. JAMA 276:1893–1897

Palermo GD, Ergun B, Takeuchi T, Sills ES, Alonson L, Rosenwaks Z (1998) Maternal age as a factor in the embryonic and fetal abnormalities that occur following ICSI. In: Filicori

M, Flamigni C (eds) Treatment of infertility: the new frontiers. Communications Media for Education, Inc., New Jersey, pp 429–434

Patrizio P, Asch R, Handelin B, Silber S (1993a) Aetiology of congenital absence of vas deferens: genetic study of three generations. Hum Reprod 8:215–221

Patrizio P, Ord T, Silber SJ, Asch RH (1993b) Cystic fibrosis mutations impair the fertilization rate of epididymal sperm from men with congenital absence of the vas deferens. Hum Reprod 8:1259–1263

Plachot M (1989) Chromosome analysis of spontaneous abortions after IVF. A European survey. Hum Reprod 4:425–429

Plachot M, Junca A-M, Mandelbaum J, De Grouchy J, Salat-Baroux J, Cohen J (1987) Chromosome investigations in early life: II Human preimplantation embryos. Hum Reprod 2:29–35

Pryor JL, Kent-First M, Muallem A, Van Bergen AH, Nolten WE, Meissner L, Roberts KP (1997) Microdeletions in the Y chromosome of infertile men. N Engl J Med 336:534–539

Puscheck EE, Behzadian MA, McDonough PG (1994) The first analysis of exon 1 (the transactivation domain) of the androgen receptor in infertile men with oligospermia or azoospermia. Fertil Steril 62:1035–1038

Queißer-Luft A, Spranger J (1997) Fehlbildungen bei Neugeborenen: Mainzer Modell. Kinderarzt 3764:1–6

Quigley CA, DeBellis A, Marschle KB, El-Awady MK, Wilson EM, French FS (1995) Androgen receptor defects: historical, clinical, and molecular perspectives. Endocr Rev 16:271–321

Qureshi SJ, Ross AR, Ma K, Cooke H-J, Intyre MAM, Chandley AC, Hargreave TB (1996) Polymerase chain reaction screening for Y chromosome microdeletions: a first step towards the diagnosis of genetically determined spermatogenic failure in men. Mol Hum Reprod 2:775–779

Reijo R, Lee TY, Salo P, Alagappan R, Brown LG, Rosenberg M, Rozen S, Jaffe T, Straus D, Hovatta O, De LCA, Silber S, Page DC (1995) Diverse spermatogenic defects in humans caused by Y chromosome deletions encompassing a novel RNA-binding protein gene. Nat Genet 10:383–393

Reijo R, Alagappan RK, Patrizio P, Page DC (1996a) Severe oligozoospermia resulting from deletions of azoospermia factor gene on Y chromosome. Lancet 347:1290–1293

Reijo R, Seligman J, Dinulos MB, Jaffe T, Brown LG, Disteche CM, Page DC (1996b) Mouse autosomal homolog of DAZ, a candidate male sterility gene in humans, is expressed in male germ cells before and after puberty. Genomics 35:346–352

Saxena R, Brown G, Hawkin, T, Alagappan RK, Skaletsky H, Reeve MP, Reijo R, Rozen S, Dinulos MB, Disteche CM, Page DC (1996) The DAZ gene cluster on the human Y chromosome arose from an autosomal gene that was transposed, repeatedly amplified and pruned. Nature Genetics 14:292–299

Scholtes MC, Behrend C, Dietzel-Dahmen J, van Hoogstraten DG, Marx K, Wohlers S, Verhoeven H, Zeilmaker GH (1998) Chromosomal aberrations in couples undergoing intracytoplasmic sperm injection: influence on implantation and ongoing pregnancy rates. Fertil Steril 70:933–937

Silber SJ, Nagy ZP, Liu J, Godoy H, Devroey P, Van SAC (1994) Conventional in-vitro fertilisation versus intracytoplasmic sperm injection for patients requiring microsurgical sperm aspiration. Hum Reprod 9:1705–1709

Simoni M, Gromoll J, Dworniczak B, Rolf C, Abshagen K, Kamischke A, Carani C, Meschede D, BehreHM, Horst J, Nieschlag E (1997) Screening for deletions of the Y chromosome involving the DAZ (Deleted in Azoospermia) gene in azoospermia and severe oligozoospermia. Fertil Steril 67:542–547

Sinclair AH, Berta P, Palmer MS, Hawkins JR, Griffiths BL, Smith MJ, Foster JW, Frischauf A, Lovelladge R, Goodfellow PN (1990) A gene from the human sex-determining region encodes a protein with homology to a conserved DNA-binding motif. Nature 346:240–244

Steptoe PC, Edwards RG (1978) Birth after the reimplantation of a human embryo [letter]. Lancet 2:366

Tesarik J, Greco E, Mendoza C (1998a) ROSI, instructions for use: 1997 update. Round spermatid injection. Hum Reprod 13:519–523

Tesarik J, Sousa M, Greco E, Mendoza C (1998b) Spermatids as gametes: indications and limitations. Hum Reprod 13 [Suppl 3]:89–107

Testart J, Gautier E, Brami C, Rolet F, Sedbon E, Thebault A (1996) Intracytoplasmic sperm injection in infertile patients with structural chromosome abnormalities. Hum Reprod 11:2609–2612

Tiepolo L, Zuffardi O (1976) Localization of factors controlling spermatogenesis in the non-fluorescent portion of the human Y chromosome long arm. Hum Genet 34:119–124

Tincello DG, Saunders PTK, Hargreave TB (1997) Preliminary investigations on androgen receptor gene mutations in infertile men. Mol Hum Reprod 3:941–943

Van Assche E, Bonduelle M, Tournaye H, Joris H, Verheyen G, Devroey P, Van Steirteghem A, Liebaers I (1996) Cytogenetics in infertile men. Hum Reprod 11 [Suppl 4]:1–24

Van der Ven K, Messer L, Van der Ven H, Jeyendran RS, Ober C (1996) Cystic fibrosis mutation screening in healthy men with reduced sperm quality. Hum Reprod 11:513–517

Van Opstal D, Los FJ, Ramlakhan S, van Hemel JO, Van Den Ouweland AM, Brandenburg H, Pieters MH, Verhoeff A, Vermeer MC, Dhont M, In't VP (1997) Determination of the parent of origin in nine cases of prenatally detected chromosome aberrations found after intracytoplasmic sperm injection. Hum Reprod 12:682–686

Vereb M, Agulnik AI, Houston JT, Lipschultz LI, Lamb DJ, Bishop CE (1997) Absence of DAZ gene mutations in cases of non-obstructed azoospermia. Mol Hum Reprod 3:55–59

Vogt PH, Edelmann A, Kirsch S, Henegariu O, Hirschmann P, Kiesewetter F, Köhn FM, Schill WB, Farah S, Ramos C, Hartmann M, Hartschuh W, Meschede D, Behre HM, Castel A, Nieschlag E, Weidner W, Gröne HJ, Jung A, Engel W, Haidl G (1996) Human Y-chromosome azoospermia factors (AZF) mapped to different subregions in Yq11. Hum Mol Genet 5:933–943

Wang Q, Ghadessy FJ, Trounson A, de Kretser D, McLachlan R, Ng SC, Yong EL (1998) Azoospermia associated with a mutation in the ligand-binding domain of an androgen receptor displaying normal ligand binding, but defective trans-activation [in process citation]. J Clin Endocrinol Metab 83:4303–4309

Wennerholm UB, Bergh C, Hamberger L, Nilsson L, Reismer E, Wennergren M, Wikland M (1996) Obstetric and perinatal outcome of pregnancies following intracytoplasmic sperm injection. Hum Reprod 11:1113–1119

Yong EL, Ng SC, Ro AC, Yun G, Ratnam SS (1994) Pregnancy after hormonal correction of severe spermatogenic defect due to mutation in androgen receptor gene. Lancet 344:826–827

The Role of Endoscopy in Congenital Abnormalities: Diagnosis and Treatment

J. Donnez, M. Nisolle

Introduction

The endoscopic technique for the management of uterine septa was first proposed by Edström and Fernström in 1970 (Edström and Fernström 1970), but the method has only become widely used in recent years. In the past, whenever a patient presented with a müllerian fusion defect that was thought to be the cause of recurrent pregnancy loss, a Jones, Strassman, or Tompkins procedure would be performed by laparotomy. These procedures required lengthy anesthesia. Surgery could be complicated by infection or hemorrhage, necessitating antibiotic treatment and blood transfusions. Also, because the full thickness of the uterine fundus was surgically damaged, the patient would require cesarean section for future deliveries. Some women became infertile as a result of adhesions or tubal occlusion developing secondary to the procedure itself.

Many müllerian fusion defects are amenable to hysteroscopic treatment. Several different procedures have been adopted, with more or less similar results. The basic concept involves the transcervical observation of the uterine septum by means of hysteroscopy, followed by its resection (Chervenak and Neuwirth 1981, Valle and Sciarra 1986, Gallinat 1993; Nisolle and Donnez 1994; Donnez and Nisolle 1997). The use of an operative hysteroscope permits the passage of surgical instruments.

Uterine Septum: Partial and Complete

Prevalence and Diagnosis

Uterine septum is the most common müllerian fusion defect. Its incidence in the general population is estimated to be 1.8% (Ashton et al. 1988). Between 1986 and 1998 216 patients underwent hysteroscopic septoplasty in our department with the help of the Nd-YAG laser (Table 1). In 85% of cases (183/216) the uterine septum was partial (Fig. 1), and in 15% of cases (33/216) it was complete, with cervical duplication. A vaginal septum was noted in 22 cases (10%). The diagnosis of a complete uterine septum may be delayed, particularly if a vaginal septum is associated (Nisolle and Donnez 1995). Indeed, the vaginal septum can easily be misdiagnosed on gynecological examination, and at hys-

Table 1. Hysteroscopic septoplasty in 216 cases (1986–1998)

Partial uterine septum	Complete uterine septum
n=183 (85%)	n=33 (15%)
	11 (5%) no vaginal septum
	22 (10%) vaginal septum
10 cases (1986–1993)	23 cases (1994–1996)
Nd-YAG laser septoplasty in two steps	Nd-YAG laser septoplasty in one step

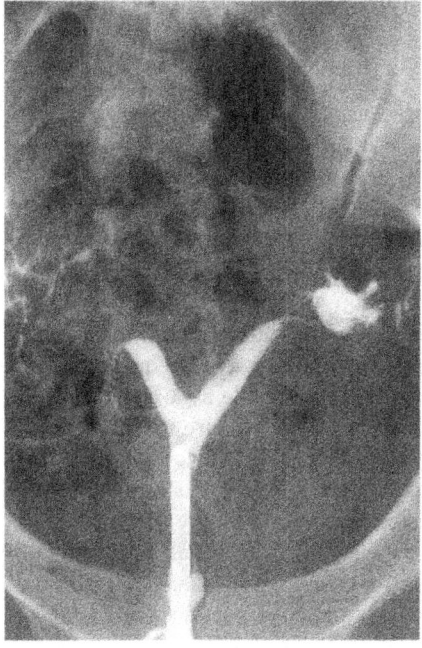

Fig. 1. Partial uterine septum: hysterography

terosalpingography, the uterus appears to be unicornous, except if there is a fistula between the two uterine cavities (Fig. 2). However, in the absence of a vaginal septum, the diagnosis is simple because two distinct external cervical orifices are clearly visible. The opacification through these two orifices allows the diagnosis of a septate uterus with cervical duplication.

The traditional liquid distention medium used to be dextran 70 or a solution of 5% dextrose; however, glycine is now preferred by most authors. This medium is not viscous, permits a clear visual field, and is not a conductor of electricity. If electricity is not used, saline or Ringer's lactate can be employed. These are well tolerated when absorbed into the system and represent an advantage of using the laser.

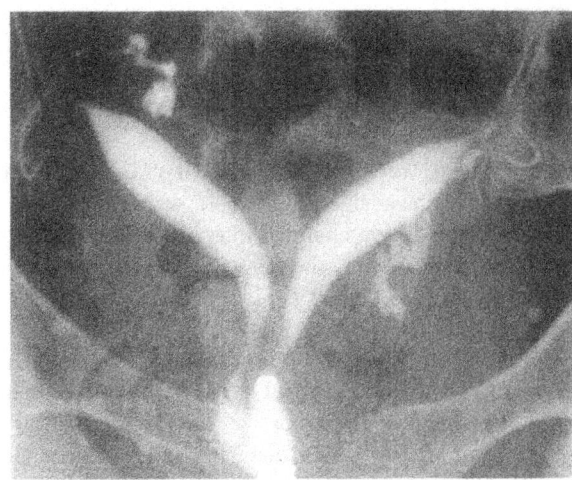

Fig. 2. Complete uterine septum (uterocervical septum) with a fistula between the two uterine cavities

Instruments

Various instruments can be used to resect the septum, i.e., miniature scissors or semirigid miniature scissors, which permit the required pressure but are small enough to pass through the hysteroscopic operating sheath and along the cervical canal with no difficulty or risk. The blades can be opened wide enough to allow resection of even thick septa. Some surgeons (De Cherney et al. 1986, Corson and Batzer 1986, Hamou 1993) prefer to use the resectoscope. High-frequency electric sources are advised for safety reasons.

The resectoscope has several advantages: it is inexpensive and readily available in most operating rooms, as well as being simple to operate and highly efficient at removing the septum. Finally, others (Daniell et al. 1987, Donnez and Nisolle 1989) have suggested the use of lasers for this type of hysteroscopic surgery.

Argon, krypton, KTP 532, and Nd-YAG lasers have all been successfully employed in the resection of uterine septa; however, certain limiting factors must be taken into consideration. First, hyskon should not be used because caramelization can prove troublesome and may damage the laser fiber, resulting in delay while fibers are replaced or repaired. Second, the surgeon must be thoroughly acquainted with the physics of the particular laser being used. Third, only bare fibers should be used: CO_2-conducting fibers may cause bubbling of the medium, which may lead to gas embolism, cardiovascular compromise, and even death.

The Nd-YAG laser uses a solid-state rig (garnet) in which the neodymium atoms play the active lasing role. The energy is supplied by a flashlight lamp which illuminates the rod. Both are housed in a container called the resonator.

The resonator is ellipsoid, and its inner surface is coated with a highly reflective material. The lamp and the rod are placed at the two focal points of the ellipsoid. The light emitted by the lamp is reflected by the internal coating of the resonator and it is collected, almost in its entirety, by the rod positioned at the opposite focal point.

In contrast to the CO_2 laser, Nd-YAG laser beams propagate well through commercially available glass fibers, very much like visible light. The propagation is effected by a chain of internal reflections occurring at the boundaries of the glass fiber. Hence, the delivery devices used with Nd-YAG lasers are a variety of fibers (see below) equipped with a connector that attaches to the output port of the laser system.

Manufacturers offer Nd-YAG laser units featuring maximum powers ranging from 40 to 100 watts. Nd-YAG laser systems are composed of:

1. A laser head or resonator
2. A power supply, which furnishes the flashlight lamp with the necessary electrical energy
3. A closed-circuit water-cooling system, further chilled by a radiator which removes excess heat from the resonator
4. A control system, based on a microcomputer
5. A He-Ne laser tube
6. An output-port optical assembly to which the external glass fiber is attached

The accessories offered with Nd-YAG systems are almost exclusively fibers. They fall into two categories:

1. Noncontact fibers, whose distal end is flat and highly polished. They operate at a short distance from the tissue, in order to create deep coagulation. A well-known example of their use is in the treatment of superficial bladder tumors, where the fibers are inserted through a cystoscope. Noncontact fibers have no incision capability. These fibers are usually reusable. However, after a limited number of surgical procedures, they must be repolished with the aid of a special polishing kit.
2. Contact fibers, featuring a sharpened, sculpted conical tip. The laser radiation is concentrated at the very narrow tip, and the fiber functions like a hot knife, capable of performing fine incisions when in contact with the tissue. Moreover, the tapered fiber prevents the rays from progressing forwards, while enabling their exit through the sides of the tip. The end result is that the forward penetration is reduced, much as in the case of the CO_2 laser. The side radiation, on the other hand, produces a hemostatic effect on the lateral surfaces of the wedge created by the incision. Contact fibers are used in a variety of configurations for freehand and endoscopic applications. They feature different shapes (conical, hemispherical) and different diameters (400, 600, 800, and 100 μm). They are offered as disposable, single-use, sterilized fibers.

New types of fibers have recently been introduced onto the market. These fibers possess a polished distal face which is inclined with respect to the fiber axis. This angle enables the fiber to emit the laser beam at right angles to its long axis. Employed transurethrally, these fibers are used to treat benign prostatic hypertrophy by coagulating the adenoma. Another type of fiber, emanating lateral diffusive radiation from an elongated segment located at its distal end, is used for the interstitial laserthermia of benign and malignant lesions.

Partial Uterine Septum

With the help of the "bare fiber", the surgeon begins the resection of the septum (Fig. 3), continuing until it has been resected almost flush with the surrounding endometrium. Regardless of the type of medium employed, the surgeon must be able to see the right and left cornual regions completely and keep the septum in view at all times. Concurrent laparoscopy at the time of hysteroscopic resection is recommended to confirm the diagnosis but is not mandatory if the diagnosis has previously been confirmed.

The septum is cut using the "touch technique" (Fig. 3). The hysteroscope with the laser fiber is advanced and melts away the septum, while visual contact is maintained with the right and left uterine ostia. The mean duration of hysteroscopic resection is <15 min. The risk of fluid overload is therefore minimal.

The most delicate part of the procedure is probably deciding exactly when the resection is sufficient, and when continuing would cause damage to the myometrium and immediate complications such as perforation, or more delayed complications such as uterine rupture during pregnancy. Almost all surgeons stop resection when the area between the tubal ostia is a line (Fig. 3). Simultaneous laparoscopic control is extremely useful for this purpose, especially for beginners. Querleu and associates (1990) use echography to distinguish the septum from the myometrium, and thus the decision to stop the resection is easily made.

Complete Uterine Septum

For many years, only partial septal defects were treated hysteroscopically, and wide (>2 cm) or complete septal defects were corrected via abdominal metroplasty. Donnez and Nisolle (Donnez and Nisolle 1989, Nisolle and Donnez 1995, 1996), however, described a method that allows even complete septal defects to be managed hysteroscopically. Rock and colleagues (Rock et al. 1987) proposed using the resectoscope for the lysis of a complete uterine septum by means of a new method which makes it possible to leave the cervical septum intact, thus avoiding any subsequent cervical incompetence. To treat a complete uterine septum, they described a one-stage method where the other cervical os is occluded with the balloon of a Foley catheter, in order to prevent loss of the distending medium. They believe that it is better not to remove the cervical canal, since this might lead to subsequent cervical incompetence. We do not agree with this hypothesis, and all complete uterine septa are removed using the following surgical procedure, previously done in two steps, but now in one.

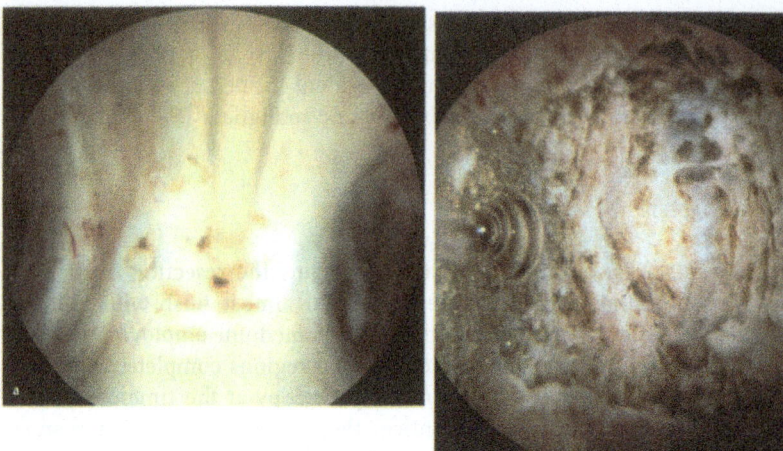

Fig. 3. a Resection of the uterine septum is carried out with the Nd-YAG laser. The septum is cut using the touch technique. The hysteroscope with the laser fiber is advanced. The septum is melted away by a simple advancement of the bare fiber. **b** Final view

In some cases, not only may a double cervical canal be observed, but a vaginal sagittal septum may also be present in the upper vagina or throughout its length (Fig. 4a). First, the vaginal septum (if present) is resected using a CO_2 laser or unipolar coagulation (Fig. 4b). The cervical septum is then incised with the scissors or with a CO_2 laser connected to a colposcope, until the lower portion of the uterine septum is seen. In the past, the second step was performed 2 months after the first operation. Now, however, Nd-YAG laser resection of the uterine septum is subsequently carried out (Fig. 5a,b). The hysteroscope is advanced while visual contact is maintained with the right and left uterine ostia. Because the septum is poorly vascularized, bleeding is usually minimal. When this procedure was carried out in two steps, hysterosalpingography demonstrated the presence of a normal, single cervical canal 2 months after the first step and a normal uterine cavity 2 months after the second step. Nowadays, all cases of complete uterine septa with or without a vaginal septum are managed in one step.

A double cervix and septate vagina with a normal uterus is an unusual müllerian anomaly, inconsistent with the current understanding of müllerian development (Candiani et al. 1996, Goldberg and Falcone 1996). In such cases, the vaginal septum and the cervical septum can be removed as previously described.

Pre- and Postoperative Management

Following excision of very wide septa, the surgeon's vision may be obscured by pieces of resected tissue and, at times, by uterine bleeding. The Nd-YAG laser produces no debris and carries a reduced risk of bleeding. Several authors have suggested preoperative treatment with danazol or LH-RH agonists (Parazzini et

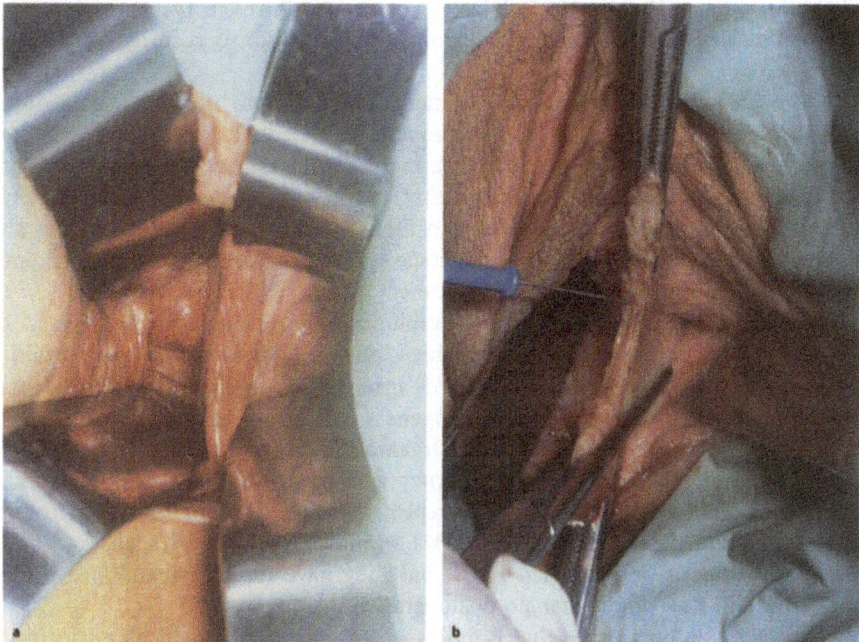

Fig. 4. a Vaginal sagittal septum; **b** Resection of the vaginal septum using unipolar coagulation

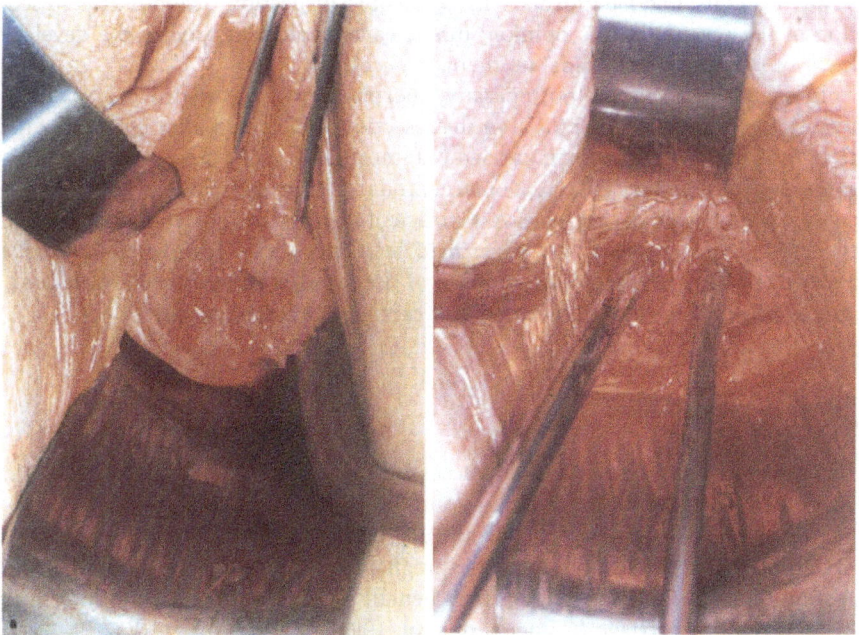

Fig. 5. a The external cervical os is completely normal; **b** dilatation of the cervical canal prior to the uterine septum resection

al. 1998); others (Hamou 1993) inject a solution of Pitressin (vasopressin) into the cervix. Neither Pitressin nor hormone administration is required with laser therapy.

Although preoperative hormone therapy causes atrophy of the endometrium and reduces vascularization and intraoperative bleeding, it also reduces the depth of the myometrium and therefore increases the risk of perforation and/or myometrial damage. It is suggested that surgery be performed immediately after the end of menstrual bleeding. In their literature review, Parazzini et al. (1998) pointed out that the only advantage to the preoperative use of hormone therapy was to decrease the operating time.

Postoperatively, a broad-spectrum antibiotic is administered for 3–4 days.

In order to avoid the risk of synechiae, an intrauterine device (IUD Multiload, Organon, GSS, The Netherlands) is inserted into the uterine cavity. Hormone replacement therapy with estrogens (100–200 µg ethinylestradiol) and progestogens (5–15 mg Lynestrenol, Orgametril, Organon, OSS, The Netherlands) is given for 3 months. De Cherney and co-workers (De Cherney et al. 1996), however, use neither hormone replacement therapy nor IUDs. Formerly, Perino and associates (Perino et al. 1987) administered both estrogens and medroxyprogesterone and inserted IUDs, but they have recently abandoned these measures and now administer no postoperative therapy.

Almost all authors agree that a follow-up examination should be performed 1–2 months after the operation, irrespective of the postoperative management. Inspection can be made either by means of hysterosalpingography or hysteroscopy. Hamou (1993) performs a hysteroscopic inspection 1 month after resection of the septum; in his opinion, this is early enough to prevent the development of synechiae or to separate them, if necessary.

In our department, the postoperative morphology of the uterine cavity is systematically evaluated 4 months after the resection. One month after removal of the IUD, hysterosalpingography is carried out; morphologically, the uterine cavity almost always resembles an arcuate uterus. Indeed, it is preferable not to resect the septum too extensively, but to leave a sufficient depth of myometrium at the top of the uterus. Hysteroscopy was performed in a first series (Donnez and Nisolle 1989) to confirm that reepithelialization of the resected endometrial area had occurred. Nowadays, this procedure is not carried out systematically.

Results and Complications

De Cherney et al. (1986) reported successful use of the urologic resectoscope in 72 women, with a term pregnancy rate of 89%. The full-term pregnancy rate reported in various studies ranges from 81% to 89%. Table 2 shows the results of hysteroplasty from the literature; the pregnancy rate is 86%. Hysteroscopic resection of an intrauterine septum may benefit patients suffering from infertility or recurrent miscarriage (Goldenberg et al. 1995).

Operative hysteroscopy is a safe and effective method of managing uterine septa associated with recurrent pregnancy loss, and makes future vaginal deliv-

Table 2. Results of hysteroscopic treatment for uterine septum

Reference	No. of patients treated	No. of pregnancies	No. of pregnancies > 1st trimester (%)	No. of miscarriages (%)
Corson and Batzer 1986	18	17	14 (82.3)	3 (17.6)
de Cherney et al. 1986	72	72	64 (89)	8 (11)
Fayez 1986	19	16	14 (87.5)	2 (12.5)
Valle and Sciarra 1986	12	13	11 (84.6)	2 (15.4)
March and Israel 1987	66	63	55 (87.3)	8 (12.7)
Blanc et al. 1994	45	31	25 (81)	6 (19.3)
Total	232	212	183 (86)	29 (13.7)

ery possible. In one of our series of 17 complete uterine septa, ten of the 17 women became pregnant and no signs of cervical incompetence were observed (Nisolle and Donnez 1996). The last patient is still being treated with a combination of estrogens and progestogens. Prophylactic cerclage was never performed after resection of a complete cervical and uterine septum. Following hysteroscopic metroplasty, cesarean section should be performed only for obstetric reasons.

In our series, peri- and postoperative complications were encountered in only three cases (1.4%). Classic perioperative complications such as fluid overload, hemorrhage, or perforation can result from the hysteroscopic procedure itself. In our series of 216 patients, no fluid overload or hemorrhage was encountered, and a perforation was noted in only one case. This was due to the fact that the patient had already undergone a uterine septum resection a few months earlier, which was considered to be insufficient. Postoperative hysterosalpingography revealed a persistent uterine septum which needed to be resected a second time. Upon diagnosis of the perforation, laparoscopy enabled us to exclude serious complications such as bowel damage or hemorrhage. Fedele et al. (1996) suggested that a remaining uterine septum of less than 1 cm after hysteroscopic metroplasty does not impair reproductive outcome and therefore does not require a second hysteroscopic surgical procedure.

Two postoperative complications encountered in another hospital were uterine ruptures during delivery. The two cases were twin pregnancies and the deliveries were very long, taking more than 24 h. The patients finally delivered by emergency cesarean section. The babies lived and the myometrium was sutured. In both cases, the rupture occurred at the fundus of the uterus. Obviously, under normal conditions, the delivery can be performed vaginally following a uterine septum resection, but in the case of multiple pregnancies, cesarean section should be considered.

Noncommunicating Rudimentary Horns

Pregnancy in a noncommunicating rudimentary horn (Fig. 6a) is uncommon and usually results in abortion or uterine rupture. At hysterography, a hemiuterus is diagnosed; indeed, the noncommunicating rudimentary horn is not opacified (Fig. 6b). Pregnancies in a noncommunicating rudimentary horn are due to transmigration of sperm into the fallopian tube of the affected horn. Most complications occur within the first 20 weeks: the most severe are uterine rupture and maternal death. Raman and colleagues (Raman et al. 1993) described a 17-week pregnancy occurring in a rudimentary horn, treated by laparotomy and excision. Recently, Dicker and colleagues described the laparoscopic management of rudimentary horn pregnancy at 8 weeks of amenorrhea (Dicker et al. 1998). In order to avoid maternal complications, we systematically perform an excision of the rudimentary horn. A laparoscopic hemihysterectomy

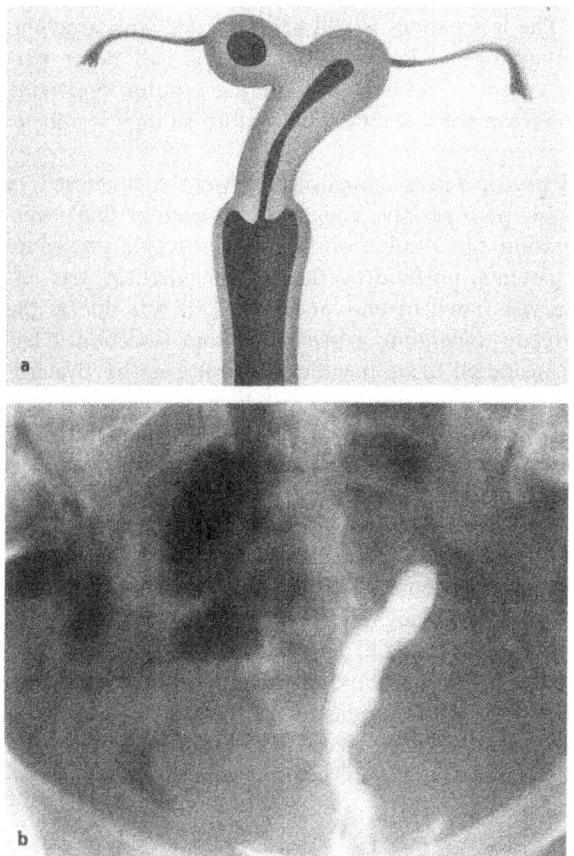

Fig. 6. a Noncommunicating rudimentary horn; right rudimentary horn. **b** Hysterography: normal left uterine horn

can easily be carried out using the same techniques as for laparoscopic hysterectomy.

In rare cases, such noncommunicating rudimentary horns can lead to dysmenorrhea and should then be laparoscopically removed. A Foley catheter is inserted during surgery to empty the bladder. Four laparoscopic puncture sites including the umbilicus are used: 10 mm umbilical, 5 mm right, 5 mm medial, and 5 mm left lower quadrant sites. These are placed just above the pubic hairline, and the lateral incisions are made next to the deep epigastric vessels. A cannula is placed in the single cervix for appropriate uterine mobilization. A bipolar forceps is used to compress and desiccate the fibrous tissue between the horns. The tissue is then cut with scissors and with a CO_2 laser. Bipolar coagulation is used to coagulate the pedicle. Scissor division is carried out close to the line of desiccation to ensure that a compressed pedicle remains. The mesosalpinx is then cut. If necessary, the peritoneum of the vesicouterine space is grasped and elevated with forceps, while the scissors dissect the vesicouterine space. Aqua dissection may be used to separate the leaves of the broad ligament, distending the vesicouterine space and defining the tendinous attachments of the bladder in this area, which are coagulated and cut. The tube of the affected horn is then removed.

The external tubal vessel is identified and exposed by applying traction to the adnexa with an opposite forceps. The dissection of the two horns is performed as follows: if there is true separation of the two horns, the fibrous tissue is coagulated with bipolar coagulation and then cut with scissors or with the CO_2 laser. If there is no external separation of the two horns, the dissection is more difficult; after coagulation, the myometrium must be cut in order to allow the removal of the rudimentary horn. For this purpose, bipolar coagulation and the CO_2 laser or the Nd-YAG laser fiber can be used to achieve coagulation and resection of the myometrium.

Earlier, the rudimentary horn was removed either through the trocar of the laparoscope, or through a posterior colpotomy in cases of larger rudimentary horns. For the past 2 years, the removal of large rudimentary horns has been carried out with the help of a morcellator (Steiner morcellator) (Storz, Tuttlingen, Germany), previously described for removal of the uterus in laparoscopic supracervical hysterectomy (Donnez and Nisolle 1993). This procedure has been successfully performed in our department on 20 women to date. Of the 14 who desired pregnancy, 11 became pregnant, and all had a normal vaginal delivery (>36 weeks) except for one woman on whom cesarean section was performed for fetal reasons.

References

Ashton D, Amin HK, Richart RM, Neuwirth RS (1988) The incidence of symptomatic uterine anomalies in women undergoing transcervical tubal sterilization. Obstet Gynecol 72:28–30

Blanc B, d'Ercole C, Gaiato ML, Boubli L (1994) Le traitement endoscopique des cloisons utérines. J Gynecol Obstet Biol Reprod 23:596–601

Candiani M, Busacca M, Natale A, Sambruni I (1996) Bicervical uterus and septate vagina: report of a previously undescribed müllerian anomaly. Hum Reprod 11:218–219

Chervenak FA, Neuwirth RS (1981) Hysteroscopic resection of the uterine septum. Am J Obstet Gynecol 141:351

Corson SL, Batzer FR (1986) CO_2 uterine distension for hysteroscopic septal incision. J Reprod Med 31:710

Daniell JF, Osher S, Miller W (1987) Hysteroscopic resection of uterine septa with visible light laser energy. Colpos Gynecol Laser Surg 3:217

De Cherney AH, Russel LJB, Graebe RA, et al (1986) Resectoscopic management of müllerian defects. Fertil Steril 45:726

Dicker D, Nitke S, Shoenfeld A, Fish B, Meizner I, Ben-Rafael Z (1998) Laparoscopic management of rudimentary horn pregnancy. Hum Reprod 13:2643–2644

Donnez J, Nisolle M (1989) Operative laser hysteroscopy in müllerian fusion defects and uterine adhesions. In: Donnez J (ed) Laser operative laparoscopy and hysteroscopy. Nauwelaerts Printing, Leuven, pp 249–261

Donnez J, Nisolle M (1993) Laparoscopic supracervical (subtotal) hysterectomy (LASH). J Gynecol Surg 9:91–94

Donnez J, Nisolle M (1997) Endoscopic laser treatment of uterine malformations. Hum Reprod 12:1381–1387

Edström K, Fernström I (1970) The diagnostic possibilities of a modified hysteroscopic technique. Acta Obstet Gynecol Scand 49:327

Fayez JA (1986) Comparison between abdominal and hysteroscopic metroplasty. Obstet Gynecol 70:399–406

Fedele L, Bianchi S, Marchini M, et al (1996) Residual uterine septum of less than 1 cm after hysteroscopic metroplasty does not impair reproductive outcome. Hum Reprod 11:727–729

Gallinat A (1993) Endometrial ablation using the Nd-YAG laser in CO_2 hysteroscopy. In: Leuken RP, Gallinat A (eds) Endoscopic surgery in gynecology. Demeter, Berlin, pp 109–116

Goldberg JM, Falcone T (1996) Double cervix and vagina with a normal uterus: an unusual müllerian anomaly. Hum Reprod 11:1350–1351

Goldenberg M, Sivan M, Sharabi Z, et al (1995) Reproductive outcome following hysteroscopic management of intrauterine septum and adhesions. Hum Reprod 10:2663–2665

Hamou J (1993) Electroresection of fibroids. In: Sutton C, Diamond M (eds) Endoscopic surgery for gynaecologists. Saunders, London, pp 327–330

March CM, Israel R (1987) Hysteroscopic management of recurrent abortion caused by septate uterus. Am J Obstet Gynecol 156:834–842

Nisolle M, Donnez J (1994) Müllerian fusion defects: septoplasty and hemihysterectomy of the rudimentary horns. In: Donnez J, Nisolle M (eds) An atlas of laser operative laparoscopy and hysteroscopy. Parthenon, Casterton Hall, pp 295–304

Nisolle M, Donnez J (1995) Letter to the editor. Fertil Steril 63:934–935

Nisolle M, Donnez J (1996) Endoscopic treatment of müllerian anomalies. Gynaecol Endoscopy 5:155–160

Parazzini F, Vercellini P, De Giorgi O, Pesole A, Ricci E, Crosignani PG (1998) Efficacy of preoperative medical treatment in facilitating hysteroscopic endometrial resection, myomectomy and metroplasty: literature review. Hum Reprod 13:2592–2597

Perino A, Mencaglia L, Hamou J, Cittadini E (1987) Hysteroscopy for metroplasty of uterine septa: report of 24 cases. Fertil Steril 48:321

Querleu D, Brasme TL, Parmentier D (1990) Ultrasound-guided transcervical metroplasty. Fertil Steril 54:995–998

Raman S, Tai C, Neom HS (1993) Non-communicating rudimentary horn pregnancy. J Gynecol Surg 9:59–62

Rock JA, Murphy AA, Cooper WH (1987) Resectoscopic technique for the lysis of a class V complete uterine septum. Fertil Steril 48:495

Valle RF, Sciarra JJ (1986) Hysteroscopic resection of the septate uterus. Obstet Gynecol 67:253

Endoscopic and Microsurgical Techniques in Reproductive Failure

M. Vandervorst, P. Devroey

Introduction

In the past decade there has been enormous progress in infertility treatment, especially in the field of assisted reproductive technology (ART). This evolution has resulted in a changing management of the infertile couple, putting surgery into the background.

Many articles with regard to microsurgery in the field of tubal infertility have been published. Operative laparoscopy, as an attempt to replace microsurgery, is rather new in this area. Almost no prospective data are known concerning fertility outcome after laparoscopic tubal reconstruction. Retrospective crude pregnancy rates after laparoscopy as well as after microsurgery fluctuate at around 30%. The frequency of tubal pathology resulting in distortion of ovum pick-up and transport is certainly increasing.

Infertility is often not due to one single factor. The indications for in vitro fertilization (IVF), initially developed to treat women with inoperable tubal pathology, have been extended. Particularly the introduction of intracyto-plasmic sperm injection as a means to treat severe male infertility has added a new dimension to infertility treatment.

This chapter analyzes the future strategies for tubal fertility treatment in the light of the retrospective results of microsurgey, laparoscopy, and ART.

Tubal Infertility

Disruption of the normal tubal anatomy and function accounts for 40% of female infertility (Speroff 1994). Pelvic inflammatory disease (PID), intra-abdominal infection (appendicitis), pelvic surgery, and less commonly endometriosis often result in distal tubal occlusion together with several degrees of dilatation and mucosal injury (Trimbos-Kemper 1982). Between 1960 and 1980 infertility as a result of infection increased by a factor 1.6, making PID the most common cause of tubal infertility (Westrom 1980). Midtubal occlusion, on the other hand, is seen most commonly after surgical sterilization or segmental tubal resection after an ectopic pregnancy (Urman 1992). An infectious process seldom results in a midtubal occlusion.

The role and etiology of proximal tubal occlusion (uterotubal junction) is unclear. It accounts for 10%–25% of tubal occlusions. Amorphous "plugs" stacked in the tubal lumen have been reported (Sulak 1987). Peritubal and periovarian adhesions without true occlusion can aggravate infertility (Gomel 1983; Fayez 1983). The mobility of the fallopian tube and ovary may be impaired by such adhesions, resulting in a poor ovum pick-up. Gomel (1983) states that adhesions are not an isolated problem but are probably associated with significant endothelial tubal damage. Bowman and Cooke (1994) confirm this. They found a strong correlation between the degree of tubal mucosal damage confirmed by salpingoscopy and the extent of pelvic adhesions in patients who have a history of PID. This correlation has not been demonstrated in patients with adhesive disease as a result of endometriosis.

The goal of surgery in cases of tubal infertility is to restore the salpingo-ovarian anatomy and tubal lumen in such a way that fertilization and passage of the zygote to the uterine cavity can take place with no problem. However, mucosal damage cannot be rectified by surgery.

Microsurgery Versus Laparoscopy

Microsurgery now extends far beyond the initial application of magnification techniques in conventional surgery. Its main purpose is to minimize tissue disruption and peritoneal trauma on the basis of a few rules. Magnification allows a careful hemostasis, constant peritoneal irrigation, and gentle tissue handling as a result of better recognition of various tissue structures.

The introduction of microsurgical principles into operative laparoscopy provides certain advantages (Gomel 1995). A closed peritoneal cavity prevents desiccation of the peritoneal surface. No foreign bodies are brought into contact with the peritoneal surface, and there is thus no foreign body reaction. Laparoscopy offers an excellent magnification with good visualization and illumination, while irrigation can expose bleeding vessels. Fine electrodes can be used to coagulate very small blood vessels.

Nomenclature

Various published reports on tubal surgery are difficult to compare because of the lack of universally accepted nomenclature and classification. At the Tenth World Congress of Fertility and Sterility held in Madrid (1980) a workable and acceptable classification was proposed to describe tubal reconstructive surgery techniques. This classification does not take into account the nature and extent of the pathology (Gomel 1980):

- Salpingolysis-ovariolysis: lysis of periadnexal adhesions
- Lysis of extra-adnexal adhesions
- Tubouterine implantation
- Tubotubal anastomosis

- Salpingostomy (salpingoneostomy): surgical creation of a new tubal ostium
- Fimbrioplasty: reconstruction of existing fimbria
- Other reconstructive tubal operations
- Combination of various types of operations

Ovariolysis and Salpingolysis

The role of adhesions in infertility is controversial. Tulandi et al. (1990) compared two groups of patients, with no significant differences in the extent of adhesions. One group of 69 patients underwent microsurgical adhesiolysis, while another group of 78 patients were not treated. Cumulative pregnancy rates after 1 and 2 years were, respectively, 32% and 45% in the treated group and 11% and 16% in the untreated group. This study reveals a conception rate after ovariosalpingolysis which is three times higher, suggesting that adhesions indeed play a role in infertility. Marana et al. (1995), on the other hand, found no correlation in a prospective study on 29 patients undergoing ovariosalpingolysis, either laparoscopical or microsurgical, between the extent of adhesions (AFS 1988) and the occurrence of a term pregnancy. The outcome was strongly associated with the tubal mucosal state.

Microsurgery

Microsurgical ovariosalpingolysis using scissors, electrocautery, and CO_2 laser have been reported.

Pregnancy rates vary between 36.7% (Frantzen 1982) and 75% (Fayez 1982). The latter was based on a very small cohort of eight patients undergoing the procedure. Analysis of the literature reveals a mean pregnancy rate after microsurgical adhesiolysis of 51.2% or intrauterine pregnancy rate of 47.6%.

Fayez (1982) and Donnez (1986) observe that two-thirds of pregnancies occur during the first year after the procedure. Tulandi et al. (1986) report a mean interval between intervention and conception of 9.9 months.

The effect of the various techniques has also been studied several times. Tulandi et al. (1986) could demonstrate no difference in pregnancy rates after microsurgical ovariosalpingolysis using the CO_2 laser or microdiathermy needle. Although the interval between the operation and conception is shortened by 3.2 months (13.1–9.9) with the use of the laser.

Watson et al. (1990) emphasize the role of expertise in this kind of surgery. They find a much lower pregnancy rate (21%) in two nonspecialized hospitals performing the procedure.

The outcome of microsurgical ovariosalpingolysis is listed in Table 1.

Table 1. Outcome after microsurgical ovariosalpingolysis

Reference	n	Pregnancy rate (%)	Intrauterine (%)	Ectopic (%)
Fayez (1982)	8	75	100	0
Frantzen (1982)	49	40.8	36.7	4.1
Donnez (1986)	42	66.7	64	2
Tulandi (1986)	63	57.1	52.4	4.8
Tulandi (1990)	69	49.3	42	7.2
Singhal (1991)	78	46.2	41	5.1
Total	309	51.2	47.6	4.9

Table 2. Outcome after laparoscopic ovariosalpingolysis

Reference	n	Pregnancy rate (%)	Intrauterine (%)	Ectopic (%)	Delivery (%)
Gomel (1983)	92	67.4	62	5.4	58.7
Fayez (1983)	50	60	56	4	46
Donnez (1989)	186	58	–	–	–
Total	328	61	59.8	4.9	54.2

Laparoscopy

Laparoscopic adhesiolysis can be carried out with scissors (Gomel 1983; Fayez 1983), electrocautery (Marana et al. 1995), or CO_2 laser (Donnez et al. 1989).

In 1983 Gomel published a retrospective series of 92 patients undergoing laparoscopic salpingo-ovariolysis by scissors. Fifty-seven (62%) achieved at least one intra-uterine pregnancy, while 54 patients (58.7%) had at least one term pregnancy. Ectopic pregnancy was observed in 5 patients (5.4%). Comparable results were reported by Fayez (1983), also using laparoscopic scissors. The authors state that the ectopic pregnancy rates are a reflection of endosalpingeal damage linked with the adhesions.

Using a CO_2 laser for adhesiolysis, Donnez (1989) obtained a pregnancy rate of 58%, suggesting that there is no difference between the use of various techniques. He failed to find a difference in conception interval. Results of laparoscopic salpingo-ovariolysis are listed in Table 2.

Fimbrioplasty

More frequently than in pelvic adhesions the underlying process of fimbrial agglutination turns out to be a PID. Endosalpingeal damage is a common finding associated with this fimbrial stenosis. If occlusion is present, it is usually partial (Lavy 1987; Benadiva 1995).

The aim of fimbrioplasty is to incise fibrotic fimbrial bands responsible for stenosis and to dilate fimbrial phimosis.

Microsurgery

Pregnancy rates after microsurgical fimbrioplasty are comparable to those observed after adhesiolysis, with a mean around 60% (Table 3).

Laparoscopy

Pregnancy rates after laparoscopic fimbrioplasty vary around 35%, with an ectopic pregnancy rate between 9.7% and 14% (Fayez 1983; Dubuisson 1990). Compared to salpingo-ovariolysis, these results are less favorable, probably reflecting the more serious salpingeal mucosal affection. The outcome of the procedure is described in Table 4.

Salpingostomy and Salpingoneostomy

Complete distal tubal occlusion with various degrees of hydrosalpinx formation are almost always a sequela of a serious PID. Owing to mucosal damage, tubal dysfunction is usually present. The goal of the operation is to create a new tubal ostium by incising the serosa and tubal wall. Eversion of the endosalpinx is maintained by electrocautery, laser, or microsurgical suturing.

Microsurgery

Gomel was one of the godfathers of microsurgical salpingo- and neosalpingo-stomy. In 1978 he published a series of 41 patients undergoing the procedure,

Table 3. Outcome after microsurgical fimbrioplasty

Reference	n	Pregnancy rate (%)	Intrauterine (%)	Ectopic (%)
Fayez (1982)	7	57.1	57.1	0
Donnez (1986)	132	61.4	59.8	1.5
Lavy (1987)	134	59.7	53.7	5.9
Total	273	60.4	56.8	3.7

Table 4. Outcome after laparoscopic fimbrioplasty

Reference	n	Pregnancy rate (%)	Intrauterine (%)	Ectopic (%)
Gomel (1983)	12	–	50	–
Fayez (1983)	14	35	21	14
Dubuisson (1990)	31	35.5	25.8	9.7
Total	57	35	30	11

Table 5. Outcome after microsurgical salpingostomy and neosalpingostomy

Reference	n	Pregnancy rate (%)	Intrauterine (%)	Ectopic (%)	Delivery (%)
Gomel (1978)	41	39	26.8	12.2	26.8
Fayez (1982)	20	40	35	5	35
Tulandi (1985)	67	26.9	22.4	4.5	–
Donnez (1986)	83	38.5	31.3	7.2	–
Schlaff (1990)	95	27.4	20	7.4	–
Singhal (1991)	97	40.2	34	6.2	28.8
Winston (1991)	323	42.7	32.8	9.9	22.9
Strandell (1995)	109	35.8	22.9	12.8	18.3
Total	835	37.8	28.9	8.9	23.7 [a]

[a] Calculated from a total of 590 patients

using microdiathermy and microsuturing. After 1 year 29% had had at least one intrauterine pregnancy, and the live birth rate was around 27%. Because all ectopic pregnancies and only 40% of intrauterine pregnancies occurred during the first year following the operation, Gomel concluded that a degree of restoration in the salpingeal mucosa and musculature with a reestablishment of patency and function is time dependent. Winston et al. (1991) also observed an increasing pregnancy rate after the first year.

A review of the literature reveals a pregnancy rate after microsurgical salpingo(neo)stomy between 27% and 43%. Almost one-quarter of pregnancies are ectopic, while in 58% a pregnancy comes to term. The outcome of microsurgical salpingo(neo)stomy is described in Table 5.

Tulandi (1985) compares the use of a CO_2 laser with electrodiathermy in a prospective trial. He did not demonstrate a difference in outcome except perhaps for a slight trend to a shorter interval between intervention and conception in favor of the laser. This difference was not statistically significant.

The benefit of repeat microsurgical salpingostomy was confirmed by Winston et al. (1991). They observed no difference in term pregnancy rates after primary and repeat salpingostomy in patients with limited tubal damage.

Laparoscopy

Laparoscopic salpingostomy can be carried out with scissors, needlepoint unipolar electrode, or CO_2 laser (Tulandi 1995).

Pregnancy rates after laparoscopic salpingo(neo)stomy after an interval of 6 months–2 years are around 29%. The intrauterine pregnancy rate is 24.2% and is comparable to the rate obtained after the microsurgical procedure. Almost 20% of the total number of pregnancies are ectopic. Table 6 describes the outcome after laparoscopic salpingo(neo)stomy.

Table 6. Outcome after laparoscopic salpingo(neo)stomy

Reference	n	Pregnancy rate (%)	Intrauterine (%)	Ectopic (%)
Fayez (1983)	19	11	0	11
Daniell (1984)	21	24	19	5
Donnez (1989)	25	20	–	–
Dubuisson (1990)	34	32.4	29.4	2.9
Canis (1994)	87	40.2	33.3	6.9
Dubuisson (1994)	81	37	32.1	4.9
Dlugi (1994)	113	20.4	15	5.3
Total	380	29.2	24.2	5

Discussion

The frequency of tubal infertility due to infectious causes is increasing, resulting in a growing interest in tubal reconstructive surgery. During the past decade a change in surgical treatment of tuboperitoneal disorders has been observed. Operative laparoscopy is tending to replace complete laparotomy with microsurgical techniques, as a decade earlier microsurgery did with macrosurgery (Fayez 1982). However, the evolution from microsurgery to laparoscopy took place without prospective randomized trials. The role of ART in tubal infertility has yet to be determined in a prospective controlled manner.

In comparing laparotomy with laparoscopy in general, the latter certainly has some benefits. Laparoscopy entails considerably lower peri- and postoperative morbidity. Avoiding laparotomy decreases both postoperative discomfort and analgetic requirements. Hospital stay, convalescence period, and interval to work resumption and normal physical activity are shortened. This results in socioeconomic arguments in favor of laparoscopy.

Therapeutic outcome, complication rate, and surgical experience naturally determine selection of the technique. However, if the outcomes of microsurgery with laparotomy and operative laparoscopy are similar, the least aggressive method must be chosen, which is laparoscopy.

The infertile couple even with a known tubal factor should undergo a thorough infertility investigation, including semen analysis, hormonal evaluation with basal day 3 measurements of follicle-stimulating hormone (Benadiva 1995), hysterosalpingography, and diagnostic laparoscopy. These investigations are decisive in referring the couple to a reconstructive tubal surgery program or ART program.

The role of adhesiolysis in promoting fertility has been demonstrated by Tulandi et al. (1990). They showed that ovariosalpingolysis promotes the ability to conceive by a factor of 3. No significant differences in outcome are found after microsurgical and laparoscopic ovariosalpingolysis. Cumulative pregnancy rates are between 50% and 60% after a follow-up of up to 2 years (Fig. 1). The laparoscopic approach results in an intrauterine pregnancy rate that is slightly higher, although does not reach statistical significance (Fig. 2). No differences are noted in ectopic pregnancy rates (Fig. 3). If adhesions are the only demon-

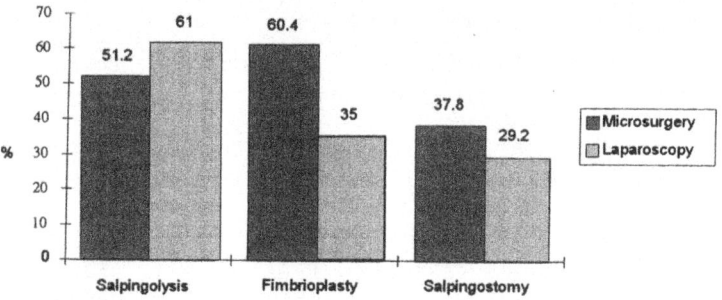

Fig. 1. Pregnancy rates by microsurgical and laparoscopic techniques. $p < 0.05$ in fimbrioplasty. (Student's t test)

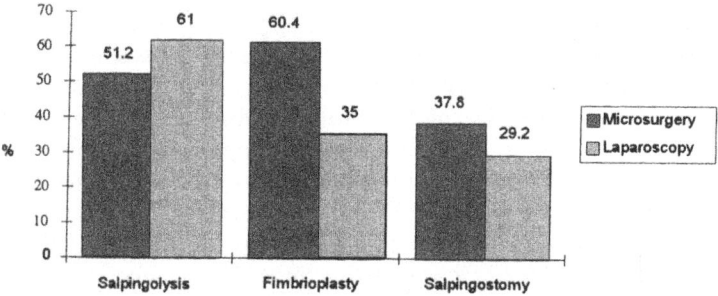

Fig. 2. Intrauterine pregnancy rates by microsurgical and laparoscopic techniques. $p > 0.05$ in the three groups. (Student's t test)

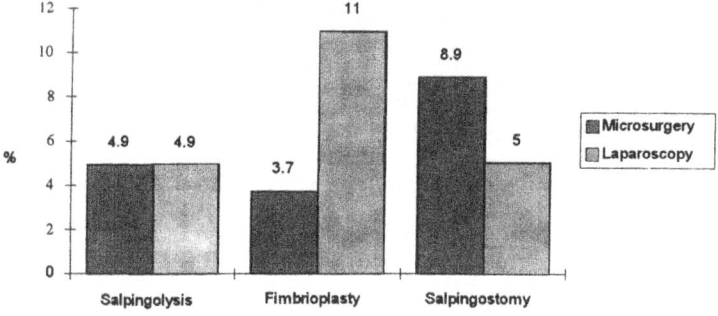

Fig. 3. Ectopic pregnancy rates by microsurgical and laparoscopic techniques. $p < 0.05$ in fimbrioplasty. (Student's t test)

strable factor in infertility, laparoscopic ovariosalpingolysis should be the treatment of choice. The results, however, are related to the extent of the adhesions. Hulka (1982) demonstrated a strong gradient in patients undergoing microsurgical adhesiolysis, with a 47% birth rate for minimal (avascular, filmy) adhesions, to 0% births with extensive (dense, vascular) adhesions. Endosalpingeal damage is a reflection of the adhesive state (Gomel 1983; Bowman and Coole 1994) explaining these results as well as an ectopic pregnancy rate of 4.9%. Surgery should be reserved for patients with mild and moderate adhesions.

Postoperative adhesion development after infertility surgery is another point of interest. Filmar et al. (1987), using a rat model, found no statistically significant difference in adhesion formation after uterine tissue injury, whether conducted by laparoscopy or laparotomy. The Operative Laparoscopy Study Group (1991) showed that adhesion reformation after laparoscopic adhesiolysis, occurred in 97% (66 of 68 patients) within 90 days. De novo adhesion formation, on the other hand, occurred in only 12% of patients (6/68), although the score reflecting the type of adhesions (from 0=no adhesions to 3=cohesive adhesions) decreased by 33%.

When partial distal tubal occlusion is present and associated with fimbrial agglutination or phimosis, the surgical approach involves fimbrioplasty. In our review we found a statistical increase in pregnancy rates in favor of microsurgery (Fig. 1). Results in terms of intrauterine pregnancy rate after microsurgical salpingolysis and fimbrioplasty are similar (Fig. 2). Ectopic pregnancies after fimbrioplasty occur almost three times more frequently in the laparoscopic group (Fig. 3). The reason for this difference is not clear. One would expect a large ectopic pregnancy rate in the two groups because endosalpingeal involvement together with fimbrial agglutination is frequently present. The difference in number of patients (273 vs. 57) may account for part of the diversity of results.

When a hydrosalpinx with partial or complete distal obstruction is present, salpingo- or neosalpingostomy should be carried out. Severe involvement of the tubal mucosa is almost always present, resulting in lower pregnancy rates. No difference has been found between the microsurgical and laparoscopic approaches in total, intrauterine, or ectopic pregnancy rates (Figs. 1–3).

Several classifications and prognostic factors for successful salpingostomy have been analyzed. Schlaff (1990) states that anatomical and functional integrity of the fallopian tubes is detrimental to the outcome after salpingostomy for distal tubal disease. Most classifications take these two factors into account. Mage et al. (1986) classify patients according to peri-adnexal adhesions and tubal state. This classification is based on the ovarian surface and type (filmy, vascular, dense) of adhesions. Tubal appearance is evaluated on the basis of the appearance of mucosal folds at hysterosalpingography, degree of distal tubal occlusion and aspect of the salpingeal wall (score I–IV, I being the best). Boer-Meisel et al. (1986) classify patients according to mucosal appearance. The American Fertility Society classification (1988), on the other hand, is based on tubal mucosa, tube walls, size of hydrosalpinx, type of adhesions, and area involved. De Bruyne et al. (1989) showed on the basis of a small cohort of 22 patients with hydrosalpinges the prognostic value of salpingoscopy following microsurgical salpingostomy. Intrauterine pregnancy rates in the group with and without intratubal adhesions were 0% and 59% respectively.

Dubuisson et al. (1994) found in a series of 81 patients undergoing laparoscopic salpingostomy a pregnancy rate inversely correlated with tubal score. According to Mage et al. (1986), this ranged from 60% in group I to 0% in group IV. They observed the same trend in pregnancy rates according to mucosal state using the Boer-Meisel criteria (1986). However, they failed to demonstrate a correlation between the intrauterine pregnancy rate and the appearance of pelvic adhesions. They recommended performing a salpingostomy on patients with mild and limited tubal damage, while patients with severely involved tubes should be counseled for IVF. Marana et al. (1995) come to the same conclusion in a prospective trial on 26 patients undergoing laparoscopic salpingoneostomy. They found a significant correlation between the salpingoscopic mucosal state (I and II) performed concomitantly to salpingoneostomy and the succes rate.

On the other hand, other authors point out that, similarly to ovariosalpingolysis, both the severity of preexisting tubal pathology and the extent of tubal adhesions plays a detrimental role in the succes rate. Strandell et al. (1995) state that adhesion formations influence all fertility operations negatively, although not significantly. They performed a retrospective study on 323 patients undergoing several fertility operations, of which 109 were microsurgical salpingo(neo)stomies. According to the Mage classification they found a delivery rate of 25.4% in groups I and II and one of 5.6% in groups III and IV. Dlugi et al. (1994) found in a prospective study of 113 patients a significant impact of pelvic and adnexal adhesions on pregnancy rates. They concluded also that tubal occlusion resulting from endometriosis is not as detrimental to the endosalpinx as an occlusion after an infectious process. Patients with endometriosis but without other infertility factors came to a crude pregnancy rate of 40.9% compared to 5.2% in patients without endometriosis and other infertility factors after laparoscopic salpingo(neo)stomy. The effect of uni- or bilateral occlusion was also examined. The presence of complete bilateral distal tubal occlusion has an adverse effect on the outcome. They suggested primary surgery in cases of unilateral complete or bilateral partial occlusion. In cases of bilateral total occlusion ART should be the treatment of choice.

The diameter of the hydrosalpinx is another important prognostic factor. Singhal (1991) found a significantly lower live-birth rate in patients with a hydrosalpinx larger 20 mm in diameter than in those with a diameter smaller than 20 mm. Donnez and Casanas-Roux (1986) came to a similar conclusion on the basis of a hydrosalpinx diameter of 25 mm. They concluded that this negative factor is a direct consequence of a decrease in the number of ciliated cells in the distal tubal lumen.

IVF with embryo transfer (ET) is a widely available alternative to tubal reconstructive surgery. The introduction of intracytoplasmic sperm injection in assisted reproduction has also certainly opened new fields, especially for couples with extreme male-factor infertility (Palermo 1992; Van Steirteghem 1994).

The question remains however, as to which couples should be offered fertility surgery or ART.

Pregnancy rates after IVF-ET on a tubal basis vary between 20% and 25% per transfer (FIVNAT 1993; Jones 1984). Alsalili et al. (1995) observed a cumulative pregnancy rate of 55% after six cycles of IVF-ET. Benadiva et al. (1995) studied retrospectively the cumulative pregnancy rates in couples with tubal-factor infertility. The overall delivery rate per transfer was 30.1% in 491 patients (673 retrievals) with exclusively tubal factor infertility. They showed that a secondary infertility diagnosis (anovulation, endometriosis, male factor, DES, immunological) does not affect the pregnancy rates (26%, 371 retrievals) significantly after IVF-ET. The cumulative pregnancy rates after four cycles were as high as >70% in both groups. An ectopic pregnancy rate of 2.4% was observed. Special care should be taken in the case of patients with large hydrosalpinges. IVF-ET results are adversely affected by retrograde flow of hydrosalpinx liquid to the uterine cavity. Implantation can be impaired because of the toxic effect on the endometrium (Meyer 1995; Strandell 1994; Andersen 1994). If tubal reconstructive surgery has a very bad prognosis, salpingectomy or salpingeal ligation should be carried out in these patients before starting ART.

When we consider the cumulative pregnancy rates after four cycles of ART or ovariosalpingolysis, fimbrioplasty or salpingo(neo)stomy (Fig. 1), then the former achieves better results on each front. Nevertheless it would be wrong to predict that reconstructive surgery will soon be history. First of all, if surgery is successful it offers the possibility of conceiving in multiple cycles and to achieve multiple consecutive pregnancies. The risk of multiple gestation is lower after surgical treatment.

Economic factors, on the other hand, can also influence decision-making. Lilford and Watson (1990) calculated the costs of ART and surgery in the United Kingdom and concluded that IVF-ET is less expensive than surgery once the small proportion of women with a good surgical prognosis are excluded. Naturally, the dilemma of how to select these patients remains.

The main goal is to determine the most efficacious technique with the fewest complications for each individual couple to achieve a pregnancy in the shortest time. Patients' age and basal level of follicle-stimulating hormone (Benadiva 1995) undoubtedly also play a crucial role in this decision.

The above results suggest that younger women with mild or moderate tuboperitoneal disturbance are primary candidates for tubal reconstructive surgery, while older patients with severe disease or frozen pelvis should be directed immediately to an assisted reproduction program. A comparable outcome is achieved with laparoscopic and microsurgical ovariosalpingolysis and salpingo(neo)stomy, making the endoscopic approach the most preferable. In cases in which fimbrioplasty should be carried out microsurgical laparotomy must be considered.

However, all of these conclusions are based on retrospective data. There is a great lack of randomized studies on a prospective base, comparing the pregnancy rates after microsurgical and laparoscopic surgery and ART in couples with a proven distal tubal obstruction and a normal semen analysis, according to WHO parameters (WHO 1992). The prognostic role of tuboscopy and salpingoscopy must yet be determined.

References

Alsalili M, Yuzpe A, Tummon I, Parker J, Martin J, Daniel S, Rebel M, Nisker J (1995) Cumulative pregnancy rates and pregnancy outcome after in-vitro fertilization: >5000 cycles at one centre. Hum Reprod 10:470–474

The American Fertility Society (1988) The American Fertility Society classifications of adnexal adhesions, distal tubal occlusion, tubal occlusion secondary to tubal ligation, tubal pregnancies, Müllerian anomalies and intrauterine adhesions. Fertil Steril 49:944–955

Andersen AN, Yue Z, Meng FJ, Petersen K (1994) Low implantation rate after in vitro fertilization in patients with hydrosalpinges diagnosed by ultrasonography. Hum Reprod 9:1935–1938

Benadiva CA, Kligman I, Davis O, Rosenwaks Z (1995) In vitro fertilization versus tubal surgery: is pelvic reconstructive surgery obsolete? Fertil Steril 64:1051–1061

Boer-Meisel ME, te Velde ER, Habbema JDF, Kardaun JWPF (1986) Predicting the pregnancy outcome in patients treated for hydrosalpinx: a prospective study. Fertil Steril 45:23–29

Bowman MC, Cooke ID (1994) Comparison of fallopian tube intraluminal pathology as assessed by salpingoscopy with pelvic adhesions. Fertil Steril 61:464–469

Canis M, Mage G, Pouly JL, Manhes H, Wattiez A, Bruhat MA (1991) Laparoscopic distal tuboplasty: report of 87 cases and a four year experience. Fertil Steril 56:616–621

Daniell JF, Herbert CM (1984) Laparoscopic salpingostomy utilizing the CO_2 laser. Fertil Steril 41:558–563

De Bruyne F, Puttemans P, Boeckx W, Brosens I (1989) The clinical value of salpingoscopy in tubal infertility. Fertil Steril 51:339–340

Dlugi AM, Reddy S, Saleh WA, Mersol-Barg MS, Jacobsen G (1994) Pregnancy rates after operative endoscopic treatment of total (neosalpingostomy) or near total (salpingostomy) distal tubal occlusion. Fertil Steril 62:913–920

Donnez J, Casanas-Roux F (1986) Prognostic factors of fimbrial microsurgery. Fertil Steril 46:200–204

Donnez J, Nisolle M, Casanas-Roux F (1989) CO_2 laser laparoscopy in infertile women with adnexal adhesions and women with tubal occlusion. J Gynecol Surg 5:47–53

Dubuisson JB, Bouquet de Jolinière J, Aubriot FX, Daraï E, Foulot H, Mandelbrot L (1990) Terminal tuboplasties by laparoscopy: 65 consecutive cases. Fertil Steril 54:401–403

Dubuisson JB, Chapron C, Morice P, Aubriot FX, Foulot H, Bouquet de Jolinière J (1994) Laparoscopic salpingostomy: fertility results according to the tubal mucosal appearance. Hum Reprod 9:334–339

Fayez JA (1983) An assessment of the role of operative laparoscopy in tuboplasty. Fertil Steril 39:476–479

Fayez JA, Suliman SO (1982) Infertility surgery of the oviduct: comparison between macrosurgery and microsurgery. Fertil Steril 37:73–78

Filmar S, Gomel V, Mc Comb PF (1987) Operative laparoscopy versus open abdominal surgery: a comparative study on postoperative adhesion formation in the rat model. Fertil Steril 48:486–489

Fivnat (1993) French national IVF registry: analysis of 1986 to 1990 data. Fertil Steril 59:587–595

Frantzen C, Schlosser HW (1982) Microsurgery and postinfectious tubal infertility. Fertil Steril 38:397–402

Gomel V (1978) Salpingostomy by microsurgery. Fertil Steril 29:380–387

Gomel V (1980) Classification of operations for tubal and peritoneal factors causing infertility. Clin Obstet Gynecol 23(4):1259–1260

Gomel V (1983) Salpingo-ovariolysis by laparoscopy in infertility. Fertil Steril 40:607–611

Gomel V (1995) From microsurgery to laparoscopic sugery: a progress. Fertil Steril 63:464–468

Hulka JF (1982) Adnexal adhesions: a prognostic staging and classification system based on a five-year survey of fertility surgery results at Chapel Hill, North Carolina. Am J Obstet Gynecol 144:141–148

Jones HW, Acosta AA, Garcia JE, Jones GS, Mayer J, Mc Dowell JS, Rosenwaks Z, Sandow BA, Veeck LL, Wilkes CA (1984) Three years of in vitro fertilization at Norfolk. Fertil Steril 42:826–834

Lavy G, Diamond MP, De Cherney AH (1987) Ectopic pregnancy: its relationship to tubal reconstructive surgery. Fertil Steril 47:543–556

Lilford RJ, Watson AJ (1990) Has in vitro fertilization made salpingostomy obsolete? Br J Obstet Gynaecol 97:557–560

Mage G, Pouly JL, Bouquet de Jolinière J, Chabrand S, Riouallon A, Bruhat MA (1986) A preoperative classification to predict the intrauterine and ectopic pregnancy rates after distal tubal microsurgery. Fertil Steril 46:807–810

Marana R, Rizzi M, Muzii L, Catalano GF, Carvana P, Mancuso S (1995) Correlation between the American Fertility Society classifications of adnexal adhesious and distal tubal occlusion, salpingoscopy and reproductive outcome in tubal surgery. Fertil Steril 64:924–929

Meyer WR, Beyler SA (1995) Deleterious effects of hydrosalpinges on in vitro fertilization and endometrial integrin expression. Ass Reprod Rev 5:201–203

The Operative Laparoscopy Study Group (1991) Postoperative adhesion development after operative laparoscopy: evaluation at early second look procedures. Fertil Steril 55:700–704

Palermo G, Joris H, Devroey P, Van Steirteghem AC (1992) Pregnancies after intracytoplasmic injection of single spermatozoa into an oocyte. Lancet 340:17–18

Patton GW (1982) Pregnancy outcome following microsurgical fimbrioplasty. Fertil Steril 37:150–155

Schlaff WD, Massiakos DK, Damewood MD, Rock JA (1990) Neosalpingostomy for distal tubal obstruction: prognostic factors and impact of surgical technique. Fertil Steril 54:984–990

Singhal V, Li TC, Cooke ID (1991) An analysis of factors influencing the outcome of 232 consecutive tubal microsurgery cases. Br J Obstet Gynaecol 98:628–636

Speroff L, Glass RM, Kase NG (1994) Female infertility. In: Clinical gynecologic endocrinology and infertility, 5th edn. Williams and Wilkins, Baltimore, pp 809–839

Strandell A, Bryman I, Janson PO, Thorburn J (1995) Background factors and scoring systems in relation to pregnancy outcome after fertility surgery. Acta Obstet Gynecol Scand 74:281–287

Strandell A, Waldenström U, Nilsson L, Hamberger L (1994) Hydrosalpinx reduces in-vitro fertilization/embryo transfer pregnancy rates. Hum Reprod 9:861–863

Sulak PJ, Letterie GS, Coddington CC, Hayslip CC, Woodward JE, Klein TA (1987) Histology of proximal tubal occlusion. Fertil Steril 48:437–440

Trimbos-Kemper T, Trimbos B, Van Hall E (1982) Etiological factors in tubal infertility. Fertil Steril 37:384–388

Tulandi T (1986) Salpingo-ovariolysis: a comparison between laser surgery and electrosurgery. Fertil Steril 45:489–491

Tulandi T, Bugnah M (1995) Operative laparoscopy: surgical modalities. Fertil Steril 63:237–245

Tulandi T, Collins JA, Burrows E, Jarrell JF, Mc Innes RA, Wrixon W, Simpson CW (1990) Treatment-dependent and treatment-independent pregnancy among women with periadnexal adhesions. Am J Obstet Gynecol 162:354–357

Tulandi T, Vilos GA (1985) A comparison between laser surgery and electrosurgery for bilateral hydrosalpinx: a 2 year follow-up. Fertil Steril 44:846–847

Urman B, Gomel V, Mc Comb P, Lee N (1992) Midtubal occlusion: etiology, management and outcome. Fertil Steril 57:747–750

Van Steirteghem AC, Nagy P, Liu J, Joris H, Smitz J, Camus M, Devroey P (1994) Intracytoplasmic sperm injection. Reprod Med Rev 3:199–207

Watson AJS, Gupta JK, O'Donovan P, Dalton ME, Lilford RJ (1990) The results of tubal surgery in the treatment of infertility in two non-specialist hospitals. Br J Obstet Gynaecol 97:561–568

Weström L (1980) Incidence, prevalance and trends of acute pelvic inflammatory disease and its consequences in industrialized countries. Am J Obstet Gynecol 138:880–892

Winston RML, Margara RA (1991) Microsurgical salpingostomy is not an obsolete procedure. Br J Obstet Gynaecol 98:637–642

World Health Organization (1992) Labarotory Manual for the Examination of Human Semen and Semen-Cervical Mucus Interaction. 3rd edn, Cambridge University Press, Cambridge

Micro- and Macroconsequences of Ooplasmic Injections of Early Haploid Male Gametes *

N. Sofikitis, N. Kanakas, I. Miyagawa

Spermatogenesis/Spermiogenesis

Spermatogenesis is the sequence of cytological events that result in the formation of mature spermatozoa from precursor cells. In most of the mammals, this process takes place within the seminiferous tubule throughout the reproductive life span of the male. The process of spermatogenesis involves a continuous replication of precursor stem cells to produce cells that can undergo successfully the subsequent changes. A reduction of the number of chromosomes to the haploid state occurs in spermatogenesis. The diploid state is restored on syngamy.

There are three fascinating events that together constitute spermatogenesis: (a) stem-cell renewal by the process of mitosis, (b) reduction of chromosomal number by meiosis, and (c) transformation of a conventional cell into the spermatozoon (spermiogenesis). During spermiogenesis no cell division is involved. This process is a metamorphosis in which a round cell is converted into a highly motile structure. The changes can be grouped (De Kretser and Kerr 1988) into:
1. Formation of the acrosome
2. Nuclear changes
3. Development of the flagellum
4. Reorganization of the cytoplasm and cell organelles

The acrosome structure arises from the Golgi complex. Proacrosomal granules are established in the Golgi complex. They coalesce to form a single, large granule that comes into contact with the nuclear membrane and spreads over approximately 25–60% of the nuclear surface. The caudal region of the acrosome is partly attenuated and is termed the equatorial segment. Although the reason for this specialization is unknown, this region of the acrosome persists after the acrosome reaction and it represents the region in which the spermatozoon binds to the plasma membrane of the oocyte during the normal fertilization process. Alterations in the final structure of the spermatid head occur during spermiogenesis. Coalescence of chromatin granules is accompanied by chemical changes in the DNA, which is stabilized and becomes resistant to digestion by the enzyme DNase. This stabilization occurs at a time when lysine-

* This paper was previously published in Hum Reprod Update (1998) 4: 197–212.

rich histones are being replaced by arginine-rich, testis-specific histones in the spermatid nuclei. During the chromatin condensation, there is a progressive reduction in nuclear volume with dramatic changes in cellular shape. At the stage of the elongated spermatid the histones of round spermatids are replaced by protamines. The transition proteins determined in elongated spermatids consist of two major types (Fawcett et al. 1971). They occupy the nucleus between the removal of histones and their replacement by protamines. After fertilization, the sperm DNA becomes devoid of protamines again and associated with histones of oocyte origin (Perreault and Zirkin 1982, Perreault et al. 1987).

The central core of the sperm tail, the axial filament, develops from the pair of centrioles lodged at the periphery of the spermatid cytoplasm and subsequently moves centrally, to be lodged at the caudal pole of the nucleus. Generation of spermatid flagella in vitro has been observed (Gerton and Millette 1984). The basic structure of the axial filament is common to flagella and cilia and consists of nine peripheral double microtubules. The last steps in spermiogenesis are characterized by additional changes in the relationship of the nucleus and cytoplasm and movement of organelles within spermatids (De Kretser and Kerr 1988, Sofikitis et al. 1997a).

Evolution of Round Spermatid Nuclei Injections (ROSNI) and Intact Round Spermatid Injections (ROSI)

Ogura and Yanagimachi (1993) have shown that round spermatid nuclei injected into hamster oocytes form pronuclei and participate in syngamy. DNA synthesis was found in these pronuclei. However, the developmental potential of the obtained zygotes was not evaluated in this study. In another study, Ogura et al. (1993) injected intact round spermatids into the perivitelline space of mature hamster or mouse oocytes and applied a fusion pulse, attempting to fuse the intact spermatids with the oocytes. They also studied the behavior of hamster and mouse round spermatid nuclei incorporated into mature oocytes by the above-mentioned electrofusion process. It was found that the spermatid nuclei commonly failed to develop into large pronuclei. In an additional study, Ogura et al. (1994) confirmed that it is difficult to fuse successfully intact round spermatids with mature oocytes via the above electrical pulse-fusion method. However, they showed that when mouse intact round spermatids are successfully fused with oocytes, some of the resulting zygotes develop into normal offspring. The overall success rate of the electrofusion of intact spermatids with oocytes was low, attributable to the difficulty to fuse large cells like oocytes with small cells like spermatids without lysis of the larger cells (Bates 1987, Ogura et al. 1993).

To avoid oocyte damage due to the fusion process, we chose a microsurgical approach to transfer round spermatid nuclei into rabbit ooplasm. By this method we achieved three pregnancies after ROSNI in rabbit oocytes (Sofikitis et al. 1994a). In that study the proportion of implanted embryos to the number of injected oocytes and the ratio of offspring to the number of injected oocytes were low. The low values of these parameters may be attributable to the low developmental potential of the injected oocytes due to inadequate mechanical stimulation applied to activate oocytes prior to ROSNI. For this reason we designed another study, the objective of which was to evaluate the effects of electrical stimulation of oocytes before ooplasmic ROSNI on oocyte activation and subsequent embryonic development (Sofikitis et al. 1996a). That study provided information on the optimal stimulation necessary for oocyte activation, fertilization, and normal embryonic development when ooplasmic ROSNI-embryo transfer procedures are scheduled. We showed that electrical stimulation of oocytes prior to ooplasmic ROSNI and ET has beneficial effects on oocyte activation, fertilization, and subsequent embryonic development and results in a 13% live birth rate per activated oocyte (Sofikitis et al. 1996a). We also assessed the possibility of achieving fertilization and embryonic development in vitro after ROSNI into the perivitelline space, speculating that ooplasmic injections may occasionally damage the oocytes and evaluating the possibility of increasing fertilization rates by avoiding injury to the oocytes. However, injections of two round spermatid nuclei into the perivitelline space of nonstimulated oocytes did not result in fertilization. The proportion of 2- to 4-cell stage embryos to the successfully injected oocytes after ROSNI was much lower in electrically stimulated oocytes treated with perivitelline space injections than in electrically stimulated oocytes treated with ooplasmic injections. Therefore, it was concluded that the entrance of the round spermatid nucleus into the ooplasm is more effective than nuclear injections into the perivitelline space for achieving fertilization.

The above successful attempts to produce offspring by microsurgical transfer of round spermatid nuclei into rabbit oocytes raised a question: Could round spermatid nuclei selected from subjects with various testicular disorders have similar fertilizing capacity? This was of great concern, because in our two previous studies the round spermatids had been harvested from healthy male rabbits. Furthermore, the probability that men/animals with primary testicular failure may not have anatomically and physiologically normal spermatids cannot be excluded. To answer the above question we induced an experimental varicocele model in the rabbit, isolated round spermatid nuclei from the testicles of varicocelized rabbits, injected the nuclei into healthy mature oocytes, and proved that these nuclei had fertilizing potential. The overall fertilization rate was 23%. However, embryo transfer procedures did not result in pregnancies (Sofikitis et al. 1996b). In contrast, Sasagawa and Yanagimachi (1997) achieved delivery of normal offspring after ooplasmic injections of round spermatid nuclei recovered from cryptorchid mice. Delivery of healthy offspring after ooplasmic injections of round spermatid nuclei in the mouse has also been reported by Kimura and Yanagimachi (1995a). However, healthy mice were used in that study.

Goto et al. (1996) examined the possibility of utilizing in vitro-derived spermatids for intracytoplasmic injection. There were no significant differences in the development of bovine oocytes injected with various types of male gametes (testicular spermatozoa, spermatids, or spermatids obtained after in vitro divisions of secondary spermatocytes). It was demonstrated that bovine oocytes injected with in vitro-derived spermatids were capable of developing to blastocyst stage. In another study, fertilization and embryo development in vitro were achieved after ooplasmic injections of nuclei extracted from frozen-thawed rabbit round spermatids (Ono et al. 1996).

Clinical Application of ROSNI/ROSI Techniques

Given the encouraging message from the above animal investigations, an attractive challenge was to apply ooplasmic injections of round spermatid nuclei selected from testicular biopsy material for the treatment of nonobstructed azoospermic men (Edwards et al. 1994, Sofikitis et al. 1994a). The first pregnancies via ROSNI techniques were achieved in 1994 and reported in the international literature in 1995 (Sofikitis et al. 1995a, Hannay 1995). However, these pregnancies resulted in abortions. A few months later, Tesarik et al. (1995) reported delivery of two healthy children after round spermatid injection into oocytes. The mean fertilization rate was 45% in that study. Fishel et al. (1995) reported a pregnancy and birth after elongated spermatid injections into oocytes. Vanderzwalmen et al. (1995) and Chen et al. (1996) reported successful fertilization of human oocytes by intracytoplasmic injections of late-stage spermatids or round spermatids, respectively.

The first ROSNI procedures in the USA were performed in California, Louisiana, and Florida (Sofikitis et al. 1995b). Fertilization and development up to 10-cell-stage embryos was achieved in nonobstructed American couples. The overall fertilization rate per injected oocyte was 31% in that study. The peak of the two-pronuclei (2PN) appearance curve in the group of oocytes injected with round spermatid nuclei was 9 h post injection. At that time all normally fertilized oocytes revealed 2PN, whereas 2 h later both pronuclei disappeared in 20% of the oocytes. Considering that the peak of 2PN appearance after intracytoplasmic sperm injection (ICSI) is 16 h post injection (Nagy et al. 1994), it appears that the speed of human embryo development is faster after ROSNI than after ICSI, and that oocytes injected with round spermatid nuclei should be checked for pronuclei earlier than oocytes injected with spermatozoa. This difference in the speed of embryo development is compatible with previous studies in the hamster (Ogura and Yanagimachi 1993) and the rabbit (Sofikitis et al. 1996a) and may be attributable to differences in the protein status of the nucleus (Perreault and Zirkin 1982, Ogura and Yanagimachi 1993).

Yamanaka et al. (1997) reported an oocyte cleavage rate of 61% following ROSNI procedures and confirmed that the appropriate time for assessment of fertilization after human ROSNI technique is 9 h post injection. Additional pregnancies achieved with ROSNI or ROSI techniques were recently reported by Tanaka et al. (1996), Mansour et al. (1996a,b), Antinori et al. (1997a,b), Vanderzwalmen et al. (1997), Amer et al. (1997), and Sofikitis et al. (1997b). Average fertilization rates were >25% in all of the above studies.

Nonobstructive Azoospermia and Indications for ROSNI/ROSI Procedures

Nonobstructive azoospermia may be due to secondary or primary testicular damage. Secondary endocrine and exocrine testicular dysfunction may be due to (a) defects in the hypothalamic-pituitary-testicular axis or (b) systemic organic disease (i.e., chronic renal failure, liver insufficiency, sickle cell anemia, diabetes mellitus). Primary testicular damage may be due to chromosomal abnormalities, orchitis, trauma, varicocele, cryptorchidism, gonadotoxins, or radiation, or it may be congenital (i.e., Sertoli cell-only syndrome, myotonic dystrophy). Furthermore, genetic abnormalities affecting the function of germ cells or Sertoli cells may be among the causes of animal or human nonobstructive azoospermia. Thus, mutations in the white spotting locus of the mouse (Chabot et al. 1988), the Sl locus encoding the c-kit ligand (Anderson et al. 1990), and genes encoding retinoic acid receptor a (Akmal et al. 1997) may impair spermatogenesis and result in azoospermia. Sex or autosomal chromosomal deletions are also involved in the etiology of nonobstructive azoospermia. Involvement of at least three Y-linked genes in spermatogenesis has been suggested (Chai et al. 1997). Several studies suggest that two gene families, RBM (RNA binding motif) and DAZ are present in Y-chromosomal regions that are deleted in some nonobstructed azoospermic men (Chai et al. 1997). Both gene families show specific testicular expression and encode proteins with RBMs. There is also increasing evidence for a putative human male infertility DAZ-like autosomal gene (Chai et al. 1997).

Recent studies have shown that a significant percentage of men with nonobstructive azoospermia have testicular foci of active spermatogenesis up to the stage of round spermatid, elongating spermatid, or spermatozoon (Sofikitis et al. 1995a, 1997b, 1998a, Silber et al. 1995a,b, Tesarik et al. 1995, Silber 1996; Mansour et al. 1996a, Antinori et al. 1997a, Vanderzwalmen et al. 1997, Yamanaka et al. 1997). Ooplasmic injections of spermatozoa offer a solution for men positive for spermatozoa in the therapeutic testicular biopsy material (Palermo et al. 1992, Silber et al. 1995b, Silber 1996). When spermatozoa are not present, ROSNI/ROSI techniques represent the only hope for treatment (Edwards et al. 1994, Sofikitis et al. 1994a).

Yamanaka et al. (1997) emphasized the need to collect an adequate amount of testicular tissue (>200 mg) for accurate demonstration of round spermatids by therapeutic testicular biopsy procedures in men who are negative for round spermatids in the routine diagnostic testicular biopsy specimen. It appears that some patients with a diagnosis of spermatogenic arrest at the primary spermatocyte stage or Sertoli cell-only syndrome may have rare foci of round spermatids somewhere in the testicles. Amer et al. (1997) used the term "complete spermiogenesis failure" for men in whom the most advanced germ cell present in the testicular biopsy material is the round spermatid and the term "incomplete spermiogenesis failure" for nonobstructed azoospermic men with a very limited number of elongated spermatids in testicular biopsy material. Several studies have shown clearly that in men with spermatogenic arrest at the primary spermatocyte stage or Sertoli cell-only syndrome a number of germ cells in a limited number of seminiferous tubules can break the barrier of the pre-meiotic spermatogenic block and differentiate up to the stage of the round or elongating spermatid (Mansour et al. 1996a, Tesarik et al. 1996, Amer et al. 1997, Antinori et al. 1997a, Vanderzwalmen et al. 1997, Yamanaka et al. 1997, Sofikitis et al. 1998a). Defects in the secretory function of the Leydig and Serto-li cells, or other factors, may not allow the round or elongating spermatids to complete the spermiogenesis. Silber et al. (1997) have demonstrated that nonob-structed azoospermic men have a mean of zero to six mature spermatids per seminiferous tubule seen on a diagnostic testicular biopsy, whereas four to six mature spermatids per tubule must be present for any spermatozoa to reach the ejaculate. In that study the authors claimed that there were no round sperma-tids in the therapeutic testicular biopsy material of men with maturation arrest if there was absence of elongated spermatids or spermatozoa. Thus, Silber et al. have objections to the ROSNI/ROSI techniques, supporting the thesis that when spermatozoa are absent in the therapeutic testicular biopsy specimen, round spermatids are also absent. However, the result of the latter study cannot be un-equivocally adopted because: (a) a limited number of participants were evalu-ated; (b) the authors attempted to identify round spermatids using a Nomarski or Hoffman lens, although they admit that they have difficulties in identifying round spermatids with this method; and (c) the most reliable method of round spermatid identification [i.e., transmission electron microscopy (TEM)] or an-other objective method [i.e., confocal scanning laser microscopy (CSLM) or flu-orescent in situ hybridization (FISH)] was not applied. To exclude the presence of round spermatids in testicular tissue, a large number of droplets of minced testicular tissue should be processed for the above microscopical techniques and the vast majority of the round germ cells should be examined. To the best of our knowledge, the above techniques were not employed by Silber et al. (1997). In contrast, as we mentioned above, several studies by independent groups clearly indicate that complete arrest in spermiogenesis is not rare in nonobstructed azoospermic men. In the latter men a large or small number of round spermatids represent the most advanced germ cells.

Several biochemical mechanisms may be responsible for the inability of the round spermatids to undergo the elongation process. O'Donnell et al. (1996) have shown that intratesticular testosterone concentration (ITC) suppression may be one of these mechanisms. Additional studies are necessary to clarify whether values of ITC below a given threshold cause failure of elongation of round spermatids. If this hypothesis is correct, testicular pathophysiologies af-fecting optimal ITC may result in complete spermatogenic failure. It should be emphasized that varicocele, the most frequent cause of male infertility and known to occasionally cause azoospermia, is accompanied by reduced ITC (Rajfer et al. 1987). A diagnostic testicular biopsy negative for round sperma-tids does not rule out the probability that few or many round spermatids will be found in the therapeutic testicular biopsy material. Furthermore, peripheral serum FSH levels and testicular size do not predict the presence/absence of round spermatids in the therapeutic testicular biopsy material. It should be stressed that the diagnostic testicular biopsy refers to the evaluation of a limited amount of tissue recovered from one testicular location. Diagnostic testicular biopsy material is exposed to various detergents during fixation/staining, and a number of cells are subsequently degenerated and their identity cannot be defined. In contrast, therapeutic testicular biopsy refers to the isolation of a larger amount of tissue from several areas of testicular tissue. Therapeutic testicular biopsy specimens are minced for hours into iso-osmotic solutions containing energy sources, and isolated, single cells can be observed. Therefore, the value of the diagnostic testicular biopsy in the management of nonobstructed azoospermic men should be questioned. The Tottori University International Research Group does not request diagnostic testicular biopsy in nonobstructed azoospermic men, except if there is a need to differentiate between obstructive and nonobstructive azoospermia.

Combined analysis of our studies in the management of nonobstructed azoospermic men (Sofikitis et al. 1995a, 1997b, 1998a, Yamanaka et al. 1997) showed that among the men who participate for the first time in an assisted reproduction program (regardless of positive or negative results for spermatozoa in the diagnostic testicular biopsy), a percentage of 39% have spermatozoa in their therapeutic testicular biopsy specimen. These men are candidates for ROSNI/ROSI techniques. It appears that nowadays only a small percentage of nonobstructed azoospermic men (ca. 18%) are excluded from assisted reproductive techniques. Among the men who are positive for spermatids and negative for spermatozoa in the therapeutic testicular biopsy, approximately 25% have a large number of round spermatids, whereas the biopsy specimen of the remaining men should be prepared for an extended period (occasionally longer than 5 h) to identify few spermatids.

Round spermatids are occasionally present in the seminal plasma of nonobstructed azoospermic men. These ejaculated round spermatids can be used for ooplasmic injections (Tesarik et al. 1996). Mendoza and Tesarik (1996) reported that 69% of non-obstructed azoospermic men have round spermatids in the ejaculate. However, the interesting results of that study may be criticized because the authors did not use standard, reliable methods for round spermatid identification (e.g., TEM, CSLM, or FISH techniques). A current study by the Tottori University International Research Group applying CSLM, FISH, and TEM on semen samples of >200 nonobstructed azoospermic men indicates that round spermatids are present in >20% of the latter men (Y. Yamamoto et al. unpublished observations). A landmark study by O'Donnell et al. (1996) provides strong evidence that testosterone withdrawal promotes stage-specific detachment of round spermatids from the seminiferous epithelium. It should be emphasized that even if round spermatids are present in the ejaculate of a nonobstructed azoospermic man, therapeutic testicular biopsy is indicated for the following reasons: (a) If spermatids are present in the ejaculate, spermatozoa may be found in the biopsy specimen. (b) The percentage of live spermatids in the biopsy specimen is significantly larger than that in the ejaculate of the same individual (Y. Yamamoto, unpublished observations). (c) Round spermatids from testicular biopsy have larger fertilizing capacity than round spermatids from the respective ejaculate (Fishel et al. 1997). (d) Primary testicular damage is often progressive. Therefore, collection of a large number of spermatids from a testicular biopsy specimen and subsequent cryopreservation offers the possibility of performing ROSNI/ROSI techniques in the future, even if testicular function deteriorates and the spermatogenic arrest at the round spermatid stage is replaced by spermatogenic arrest at the primary spermatocyte stage.

Criteria for Identification/Isolation of Human Round Spermatids

The gold standard for identification of round spermatids is TEM (Sofikitis et al. 1994a). Recently, Mendoza and Tesarik (1996) attempted to identify round spermatids by selective staining of the acrosin contained in the acrosomal granules. Another approach is to visualize proacrosin with the use of a monoclonal antibody (Mendoza et al. 1996). A drawback to all of the above techniques is that they result in cell death. Therefore, observed spermatids cannot be used in assisted reproduction programs. Indeed, one of the most perplexing problems in the laboratories applying human ROSNI/ROSI procedures is the difficulty of identifying alive, undisturbed, nonfixed, nonstained round spermatids. The following approaches are suggested for identification of undisturbed round spermatids in therapeutic testicular biopsy material or in cellular populations isolated from semen samples.

Observation of Samples by Confocal Scanning Laser Microscopy

Observation of testicular or semen samples via CSLM allows identification of round spermatids (Fig. 1). The CSLM is a relatively new instrument in the field of microscopy (Sofikitis et al. 1994b). Unlike the conventional light microscope, the CSLM produces sharp images, free of out-of-focus artifacts, that can be observed on a television monitor. It provides an automatic system for instantaneous measurement of distance. This technique has the capacity to provide three-dimensional images of cells up to ×10000 magnification without requiring staining of materials. Therefore, the observed cells can be processed for assisted reproduction techniques. Human and rabbit round spermatids are easily identified via laser microscopy by the presence of multiple granules or a single large (acrosomic) granule adjacent to the nucleus (Sofikitis et al. 1994a, 1996b, Yamanaka et al. 1997).

New models of CSLM computer-assisted systems (CAS) allow identification of round spermatids at stage 1 of spermiogenesis. These cells are negative for acrosomal granules. CAS analysis of images provided by CSLM differentiates between round spermatids at stage 1 and secondary spermatocytes. The size of round spermatids at stage 1 is <75% that of secondary spermatocytes (Sofikitis et al. 1997d). In addition, nuclei of stage 1 round spermatids show a finely granular texture, as opposed to the cloud-like texture exhibited by secondary spermatocytes. Another advantage of CSLM-CAS is that it allows identification and isolation of specific types of undisturbed primary spermatocytes. CSLM-

CAS recognizes specific characteristics of leptotene primary spermatocytes (i.e., sex vesicles). Diplotene primary spermatocytes can be identified easily because they are the largest germ cells.

Inverted Microscope–Computer-Assisted System (IM-CAS)

Application of quantitative criteria based on computer-assisted image analysis allows identification of round spermatids. "Round cells" with a minimum diameter between 6 and 10 μm that satisfy additional specific quantitative and qualitative criteria are considered to be spermatids (Yamanaka et al. 1997). The minimal cellular diameter of round spermatids is approximately equal to their average diameter (Yamanaka et al. 1997). In preliminary experiments human cadaveric germ cells with morphometric parameters satisfying Yamanaka's quantitative criteria were recovered and processed for TEM. It was found that 63% and 16% of the cells isolated were round spermatids of stages 2–5 and stages 6–8 of spermiogenesis, respectively (Yamanaka et al. 1997). These results were further confirmed by another study suggesting that cells <7.5 μm in diameter should be selected in assisted reproduction programs using round spermatids (Angelopoulos et al. 1997). However, the last approach excludes round spermatids with an average diameter of >7.5 μm.

Qualitative Criteria

IM-CAS and CSLM-CAS are not available in most IVF centers. Human round spermatids (Mansour et al. 1996a, Tesarik et al. 1996, Antinori et al. 1997a, Vanderzwalmen et al. 1997, Yamanaka et al. 1997) can be distinguished from other cell types according to their cellular shape, their size, and the form of the nucleus. A developing acrosomal granule can be recognized in the round spermatid as a bright/dark spot adjacent to the cell nucleus. A Nomarski lens is preferable to a Hoffman lens when qualitative criteria are applied for the identification of round spermatids.

ROSI Versus ROSNI

ROSI procedures ensure the transfer of all the cytoplasmic components of the male gamete into the maternal gamete and are less time consuming than round spermatid nucleus injection. Furthermore, manipulations of the nuclear matrix and envelope are avoided when ROSI techniques are applied. In contrast, ROSI procedures have two disadvantages: (a) injecting micropipettes of larger diameter are necessary, and consequently the probability of injuring oocytes during injections is greater, and (b) persistence of a large amount of cytoplasm around the round spermatid nucleus may impede its transformation into a male pronucleus. In the mouse (Ogura et al. 1993, Kimura and Yanagimachi 1995a,b) and the rabbit (Yamamoto et al. 1997), transferring the round spermatid nucleus into the oocyte is a far more efficient procedure for achieving fertilization and embryonic development than transferring the intact round spermatid cell. Embryonic development is faster after ROSNI than after ROSI techniques (Yamamoto et al. 1997). The Tottori University International Research Group applies ROSNI rather than ROSI because occasional inability of the ooplasm to digest the cytoplasm of the round spermatid and subsequent lack of exposure of the round spermatid nuclear membrane to ooplasmic factors have been considered causes of failure of fertilization after ROSI techniques (Ogura et al. 1993).

The number of pregnancies achieved via ROSI techniques (Tesarik et al. 1995, Mansour et al. 1996a, Antinori et al. 1997a,b, Vanderzwalmen et al. 1997) is larger than the number of ROSNI pregnancies (Hannay 1995, Sofikitis et al. 1995a, 1997b). This difference in favor of ROSI techniques is misleading, however, for two reasons: (a) ROSI techniques are relatively simple and applied by a large number of centers internationally. In contrast, ROSNI techniques are applied by Japanese centers only; (b) most of the Japanese centers applying ROSNI techniques cannot publish achieved ROSNI pregnancies because of recommendations by Japanese ethical committees.

Contributions of the Round Spermatid to the Zygote

The male gamete contributes several components important for the fertilization process and early embryo development to the zygote: the genetic material, the reproducing element of the centrosome (Schatten et al. 1986; Schatten 1994, Simerly et al. 1995), the microtubule organizer component of the centrosome (Schatten 1994), the oocyte-activating substance in the spermatozoon/spermatid (OASIS; Swan 1990, Parrington et al. 1996), nuclear proteins (Ogura and Yanagimachi 1993), and factors affecting early embryonic development and capacity for implantation.

Genetic Material

The deliveries of normal mouse and rabbit offspring (Sofikitis et al. 1994a, Ogura et al. 1994, Kimura and Yanagimachi 1995a) and healthy human newborns (Tesarik et al. 1995; Mansour et al. 1996a, Vanderzwalmen et al. 1997, Antinori et al. 1997, Sofikitits et al. 1997b) after ROSNI/ROSI indicate the maturity of the genetic material of the early haploid male gamete (i.e., the chromosomes of the round spermatid are capable of pairing with those of the oocyte and participate in syngamy, fertilization, and subsequent embryonic and fetal development).

OASIS

The male gamete-induced cascade of biochemical ooplasmic events that results in resumption of meiosis of the female gamete is referred to as oocyte activation. Oocyte activation is a prerequisite for male pronucleus development and fertilization. Therefore, an anatomical or functional defect of the OASIS may cause fertilization failure ICSI/ROSNI/ROSI procedures. It is generally agreed that the spermatozoon or spermatid triggers the embryonic development by increasing the Ca^{2+} ion concentration in the oocyte cytoplasm (Vitullo and Ozil 1992, Sousa et al. 1996, Yamanaka et al. 1997, Sofikitis et al. 1998a). These transient oscillatory or wave-form increases in Ca^{2+} ion concentration have been observed both after normal fertilization (Taylor et al. 1993) and ICSI/ROSI techniques (Tesarik et al. 1994, Sousa et al. 1996).

Injections of mouse round spermatids into oocytes do not result in oocyte activation, suggesting that the mouse OASIS has not been expressed at the round spermatid stage (Kimura and Yanagimachi 1995a,b). In contrast, ooplasmic injections of rabbit round spermatids lead to oocyte activation in a significant percentage (Sofikitis et al. 1994a). Electrical stimulation of the rabbit oocyte enhances the OASIS and benefits the activation process (Sofikitis et al. 1996a). Although electrical stimulation usually results in a monophasic ooplasmic Ca^{2+} response, it appears that there is a synergistic action of electrical stimulation and round spermatid OASIS which eventually produces Ca^{2+} oscillations. There is strong evidence that the human OASIS is activated at/before the round spermatid stage (Yamanaka et al. 1997, Sousa et al. 1996, Sofikitis 1998a). The achievement of human pregnancies via ROSNI/ROSI without application of an exogenous electrical or chemical stimulation supports the above thesis. The human oocyte activation after ROSNI/ROSI may not be attributed to parthenogenetic activation of the oocytes, since ooplasmic injections of medium only have not resulted in activation (Fishel et al. 1996, Yamanaka et al. 1997, Sofikitis et al. 1998a). Dozortsev et al. (1995) and Meng and Wolf (1997) have emphasized that human or monkey mechanical ooplasmic stimulation and/or oocyte exposure to a low or a relatively high extracellular calcium concentration of medium can alter intracellular Ca^{2+} but cannot, alone, cause activation. The human round spermatid OASIS should be nucleus associated, since nuclear injections are sufficient to cause activation (Yamanaka et al. 1997).

Human oocyte activation is faster after ROSNI techniques than after ROSI procedures Yamamoto et al. 1997). The faster speed of oocyte activation after ROSNI may be due to the presence of a smaller amount of male gamete cytoplasm facilitating the closer contact of the male gamete OASIS-nucleus complex with the cytoplasm of the oocyte.

Similar levels of OASIS activity have been demonstrated in human round spermatids and testicular spermatozoa using a quantitative assay (Sofikitis et al. 1997c). Whether the technique applied for ooplasmic injections of spermatids or spermatozoa influences the oocyte activation rates after ROSNI/ROSI techniques has been demonstrated after injections with minimal (Yamanaka et al. 1997, Sofikitis et al. 1998a) or vigorous ooplasmic stimulation (Tesarik et al.

1996). Tesarik et al. (1994) supported the idea of a positive role for vigorous oo-plasmic stimulation during ICSI techniques in the oocyte-activation process. In contrast, Mansour et al. (1996b) recommended a minimal ooplasmic stimula-tion. Recent studies have suggested that there may be an OASIS deficiency in selected subpopulations of nonobstructed azoospermic men (Sofikitis et al. 1997c). In the latter group, application of electrical (Sofikitis et al. 1995a) or chemical (Vanderzwalmen et al. 1997) stimulation prior, during, or immediately after ROSNI/ROSI techniques may (a) support the action of OASIS or (b) act synergetically with OASIS.

Mouse OASIS has not been expressed at the secondary spermatocyte stage (Kimura and Yanagimachi 1995b). We have recently shown that ooplasmic in-jections of human secondary spermatocytes with minimal ooplasmic stimula-tion do not activate oocytes and result in premature condensation of the chro-mosomes of the male gamete (Sofikitis et al. 1998b). However, when a second vigorous mechanical ooplasmic stimulation is applied 1–2 h after the secondary spermatocyte injection, human oocytes are activated in a significant percentage and both the oocyte and the secondary spermatocyte complete the second meiotic division (Sofikitis et al. 1998b).

Centrosomic Components: a Challenge to the Theory of Centrosomes

The zygote centrosome is a blend of paternal and maternal components. The re-storation of the zygote centrosome at fertilization requires the attraction of ma-ternal centrosomal components to the paternal reproducing element (Schatten et al. 1994, Simerly et al. 1995). The male gamete contributes to the zygote cen-trosome by transferring the reproducing element of the centrosome, the micro-tubule organizing center, and a g-tubulin-binding protein. However, the mater-nal γ-tubulin is necessary for the function of the zygote centrosome (Schatten et al. 1994).

The delivery of healthy babies after human ROSI/ROSNI tends to suggest that the centrosome components of the human round spermatid are normal, functional, and mature. Additional studies are necessary on the development of aster and the ooplasmic microtubule organization after ROSNI/ROSI proce-dures. Several studies have suggested that mammalian oocytes lose their centro-somes when they mature and that centrosome material is introduced into oo-cytes by the spermatozoa (see for review Palermo et al. 1994, Schatten 1994). However the normal embryonic and fetal development after ROSNI plus ET in the rabbit (nuclei were proven to be free of cytoplasmic and subsequently cen-trosome material; Sofikitis et al. 1994a, 1996a,b), the artificial parthenogenesis in several mammalian female gametes (Schatten et al. 1994), and the develop-ment of parthenogenetic rabbit fetuses up to day 10 of pregnancy (Ozil 1990) can be interpreted as a challenge to the theory of centrosomes and raise the probability that when paternal centrosome material is absent, novel maternal spindle-organizing centers can develop and previously denatured/nonfunctional/inactive female centrosome material can undergo renaturation/activation. However, the probability that paternal centrosome material is transferred during spermatid nuclear injections cannot be excluded (Navara et al. 1994), since the centrosome material is tightly anchored to the nuclear envelope in most of the cells (Schatten 1994).

Consideration of the centrosome as a cellular organ may be out of date (Mazia 1984). Observations by Mazia (1984) on the centrosome cycle refute any notion of the centrosome as an entity that is either present or not present and is always the same when it is present, and suggest that the centrosomes should be considered as flexible cyclical structures altering their shape and form. The flexible centrosome hypothesis has been further supported by Schatten et al. (1986). If unitary centrosomes can exist in a linear form, autoimmune methods might detect only nodes of higher concentration of the antigen. Furthermore, negative results on oocyte centrosome material obtained by TEM do not exclude the presence of centrosome material within mature oocytes, because of difficulties in locating centrioles and centrosomes at spindle poles by this method (Sathananthan et al. 1991) and the ability of centrosome material to change shape. In conclusion, negative results on oocyte centrosome material cannot be unequivocally accepted. As previously suggested by Sathananthan et al. (1991), a maternal contribution of centrosome material still needs to be considered and further investigation of centrosomes in both human oocytes and zygotes is clearly warranted.

Nuclear Proteins

Spermiogenesis is characterized by alterations in the protein composition of the nucleus. Testis-specific histones are replaced by spermatid-specific basic proteins. The latter are gradually replaced by protamines (Perreault et al. 1987). Following ROSNI/ROSI and disintegration of the round spermatid nuclear membrane within the ooplasm, the round spermatid DNA-nuclear protein complex is exposed to ooplasmic factors. Since the histones are proteins containing a reduced number of disulfide bonds, questions may be raised as to (a) how the round spermatid DNA that is not associated with disulfide bond proteins can survive within the ooplasm and how it is protected against an immediate action of ooplasmic factors, and (b) how a male gamete nucleus that has not undergone removal of spermatid-specific histones has the capacity to undergo the cascade of events that leads to normal male pronucleus development.

The answer to the first question is that activation of the oocyte can rescue the chromosomes of the round spermatid from premature condensation (Kimura and Yanagimachi 1995a,b). Therefore, in nonobstructed azoospermic men whose spermatids expose an impaired capacity for oocyte activation, application of an exogenous stimulus for ooplasmic activation is of paramount importance. In addition, it is possible that spermatid-specific histone removal is not a prerequisite for the formation of the male pronucleus.

Factors Affecting Early Development and Capacity for Implantation of ROSNI/ROSI Embryos

Janny and Ménézo (1994) have shown that the mission of the male gamete is not only to activate and fertilize the oocyte but also to contribute to the zygote potential to undergo the first mitotic divisions. It appears that there is a paternal effect on early embryonic development. This thesis has been further supported by Sofikitis et al. (1996b) and Ono and et al. (1997). The latter studies have shown a defect in the capacity for early development and implantation of embryos generated from the fertilization of oocytes by round spermatids or spermatozoa isolated from animals with varicoceles. Thus, embryos derived from the fertilization of human oocytes by spermatids recovered from men with primary testicular damage may have an impaired potential for further development and implantation. In addition, the round spermatid/elongating spermatid factors mediating the paternal influence on the embryonic development may be deficient, since the round or elongating spermatid represents an immature stage of the male gamete. The above speculation may explain why ROSNI/ ROSI techniques result in low pregnancy rates, although fertilization rates are relatively high (Antinori et al. 1997a, Yamanaka et al. 1997, Sofikitis et al. 1998a). Therefore, we may recommend transfer of all embryos generated from the fertilization of oocytes by spermatids (Sofikitis et al. 1998a).

Guidelines/Prerequisistes for ROSNI/ROSI Techniques

The Tottori University International Research Group achieved the first spermless pregnancies in 1994 (Hanay 1995, Sofikitis et al. 1995a). Later a number of other investigators achieved additional pregnancies. However, it is obvious that there is limited experienceon human ROSNI/ROSI techniques.

Quality Control for Identification of Round Spermatids

Several methods for identification of round spermatids have been discussed above. Furthermore, it should be pointed out that training is necessary for the staff of any assisted reproduction center applying ROSNI/ROSI. Even if a center has an excellent ICSI program, ROSNI/ROSI will result in a poor outcome if the staff have not spent many hours observing animal testicular tissue specimens and attempting to identify round spermatids via an inverted microscope. Technicians/embryologists/physicians performing ROSNI/ROSI should also confirm via TEM, FISH, or CSLM that the cells considered to be human round spermatids are indeed round spermatids.

Quality Control for Viability of Round Spermatids

An occasional finding in ROSNI/ROSI programs is the absence or a reduced number of live spermatids. Fractions of round spermatids retrieved from testicular tissue should be processed for assessment of viability Sofikitis et al. 1996a). Men with a percentage of live round spermatids <10% have a poor ROSNI outcome. Preliminary studies have shown that spermatids from these men cannot fertilize oocytes (N. Sofikitis et al., unpublished observations).

It should be mentioned that the trypan blue stain assesses plasma membrane and cytoplasmic viability but does not evaluate nuclear viability. Theoretically, a live nucleus of a round spermatid with partially degenerated cytoplasmic content may have the capacity to fertilize oocytes. Therefore, nuclear staining techniques are recommended for assessment of round spermatid viability.

Quality Control for the Capacity of Round Spermatids to Activate Oocytes

A previous study has shown that ICSI or ROSNI failure in a selected subpopulation of infertile men is attributable to subnormal OASIS profiles (Sofikitis et al. 1997c). Application of a recently reported quantitative assay is recommended to evaluate OASIS activity (Sofikitis et al. 1997c): Two round spermatids are injected into a hamster oocyte; if the percentage of activated hamster oocytes is <8%, fertilization is not anticipated after human ROSNI/ROSI. Alternatively, when OASIS deficiency is suspected, an exogenous stimulus (i.e., chemical or electrical) may be applied to support human oocyte activation and subsequently facilitate fertilization.

Stage of the Round Spermatid and Fertilization

When round spermatids are observed via an inverted microscope, the cells with the larger acrosomal (Golgi) bright/dark spots should be preferred for ooplasmic injections because they represent the most mature forms of the male gamete. A recent study has clearly indicated that round spermatids of stages 1 and 2 have smaller reproductive potential than round spermatids of stages 3–5 (Sofikitis et al. 1997d).

When both elongating and round spermatids are present in the testicular biopsy specimen, ooplasmic injections of elongating spermatids are considered preferable because they result in a higher fertilization rate (Fishel et al. 1997).

Media for Maintenance of Round Spermatids

Most of the popular media in assisted reproduction programs have been devised to maintain spermatozoa rather than spermatids. However, there are several anatomical and biochemical differences between the round spermatid and the spermatozoon. A medium has been developed by the first author (SOF medium) to prolong the viability of round and elongating spermatids (Sofikitis et al. 1998a). It has been already used for maintenance of human and rabbit round spermatids (Sofikitis et al. 1997d, Yamanaka et al. 1997). It contains lactate and glucose as energy substrates. Previous studies have demonstrated that lactate is the preferable energy substrate for round spermatids (Nakamura et al. 1978). Round spermatids have a larger amount of cytoplasm than spermatozoa. To protect round spermatids against environmental shock and to stabilize the spermatid membrane, cholesterol has been added to the SOF medium in a small concentration. We have also demonstrated that iron and vitamins influence spermatid viability. Therefore, vitamins and ferric nitrate are also components of the SOF medium (Sofikitis et al. 1998a).

Media for Culture of Oocytes Injected with Round Spermatids

Previous studies have shown that the addition of antioxidants to media used for culture of embryos generated from the fertilization of oocytes by spermatids has beneficial effects on embryonic development (Sofikitis et al. 1996a, 1997d).

The Importance of Preserving a Cytoplasmic Blanket Around the Round Spermatid Nucleus

During human ROSNI techniques round spermatids are treated with a variety of detergents to isolate nuclei surrounded by a thin cytoplasmic layer (cytoplasmic blanket; Yamanaka et al. 1997). Although ooplasmic injections of rabbit nude nuclei have resulted in delivery of healthy offspring, when human ROSNI techniques are scheduled, maintenance of a cytoplasmic blanket around the nucleus is preferred, to avoid exposure of the male gamete nuclear material to chemical and mechanical stimuli.

Time to Observe Pronuclei

Pronuclei should be observed 9 h after human ROSNI techniques (Sofikitis et al. 1995b, Yamanaka et al. 1997). When human ooplasmic injections of elongating spermatids are performed, the appropriate time for pronuclei observation is 13 h post injection (Sofikitis et al. 1998a).

How Many ROSNI/ROSI Embryos to Transfer

As we discussed in a previous paragraph, the implantation potential of human ROSNI/ROSI embryos is small; therefore, we recommend transfer of all the normally fertilized oocytes that subsequently cleave (Table 1; Yamanaka et al. 1997, Sofikitis et al. 1998a).

Table 1. Clinical pregnancies achieved via ooplasmic injection of spermatids or secondary spermatocytes

Reference	Ooplasmic injection of:	Clinical pregnancies	Abortions/ fetal losses	No. of offspring
Hannay et al. (1995)	Round spermatid nuclei	4	4	0
Tesarik et al. (1995)	Round spermatids	2	0	2
Fishel et al. (1995)	Elongated spermatid	1	0	1
Mansour et al. (1996a)	Round spermatids	1	0	1
Tanaka et al. (1996)	Round spermatids	1	1	0
Araki et al. (1997)	Elongated spermatids	3	0	4
Antinori et al. (1997a)	Round spermatids	2	0	2
Antinori et al. (1997a)	Elongating/elongated spermatids	3	1	2
Antinori et al. (1997b)	Round spermatids	1	0	1
Vanderzwalmen et al. (1997)	Elongating/elongated spermatids	3	0	3
Vanderzwalmen et al. (1997)	Round spermatids	1	0	1
Sofikitis et al. (1997b)	Round spermatid nuclei	3	0	3
Amer et al. (1997)	Elongating/elongated spermatids	2	0	No information
Sofikitis et al. (1998a)	Elongated spermatids	2	0	2
Sofikitis et al. (1998b)	Secondary spermatocyte nuclei	1	0	1

Cryopreservation of Round Spermatids

Antinori et al. (1997b) achieved the first human pregnancy via ooplasmic injections of frozen-thawed round spermatids. That study indicates the importance of cryopreserving round spermatids in all ROSNI/ROSI cycles.

Time to Perform the Second ROSNI/ROSI Trial

Testicular damage in nonobstructed azoospermic men with complete or incomplete arrest in spermiogenesis (Amer et al. 1997) may be progressive. Therefore, it is uncertain whether a man with a limited number of round spermatids in the therapeutic testicular biopsy material will still have round spermatids in his biopsy material 1 year later. Therefore, the second ROSNI/ROSI trial should be performed relatively soon after the first therapeutic testicular biopsy-ROSNI/ROSI cycle (4–9 months), regardless of the (female) partner's age. In contrast, a theoretical risk of damaging the testis exists if a second testicular biopsy is done early after the first. However, we believe that most clinical studies indicating testicular damage after a testicular biopsy are due to inappropriate technique, use of electrocautery, or damage of arteries by a needle during either administration of local anesthesia or tissue recovery, and cannot be unequivocally attributed to the testicular biopsy per se (N. Sofikitis, unpublished observations).

Adequate Counseling (see below)

Genetic Implications of ROSNI/ROSI Procedures

To evaluate the genetic risk of assisted reproductive technologies, one has to consider both the genetic risk inherent in the treatment population and the genetic risk inherent in the procedure performed (Baschat et al. 1996). Considering the limited number of full-term pregnancies achieved by ROSNI/ROSI procedures to date, we can only speculate on the safety/risks of these procedures.

Genetic risks inherent to ROSNI/ROSI procedures may involve (a) centrosome abnormalities resulting in aberrant spindle formation and subsequently in an increased risk of mosaicism, (b) injection of disomic/diploid genetic material which could give rise at fertilization to a trisomic/triploid embryo and fetus, (c) genomic imprinting abnormalities (see below), and (d) abnormalities due to the out-of-phase cycles of the round spermatid and the oocyte. The round spermatid is at the G1 stage, whereas the oocyte in the metaphase of the second meiotic division is in its M phase. However, the results of the studies by Kimura and Yanagimachi (1995a,b), Sofikitis et al. (1994a, 1996a, 1997b), Fishel et al. (1996), and Tesarik et al. (1996) indicate that the cell-cycle imbalance between the oocyte and the round spermatid does not affect fertilization, embryonic development, and fetal development. It must also be emphasized that the cell cycles of the spermatozoon and the oocyte are out-of-phase (Fishel et al. 1996). When spermatids are injected into oocytes the metaphase-promoting factor which maintains the oocyte in metaphase of the second meiotic division may also drive the spermatid nuclei to metaphase (Fishel et al. 1996). Genetic risks of ROSNI/ROSI inherent in a population of men with primary testicular damage are the same with the genetic risk of ICSI procedures (transferring sex chromosomal abnormalities, or reciprocal translocations associated with spermatogenic impairment). Inheritance of gene mutations/deletions of DNA sequences in specific regions of the Y-chromosome long arm represent additional risks.

Genomic Imprinting Abnormalities

Most genes are expressed equally from the two parental alleles, but a small subgroup of mammalian genes are differentially expressed, depending on whether they have been inherited from the mother or the father. The process which differentially marks the DNA in the parental gametes is termed genomic imprinting. Genes whose expression is inhibited after passage through the mother's germline are called maternally imprinted, whereas genes whose expression is inhibited when transmitted by fathers are called paternally imprinted.

Imprinted genes have been identified in mice and humans. Mouse insulin-like growth factor-II (IGF-II) gene is expressed only from the paternal allele. In contrast, the gene encoding a differentiation-related fetal RNA (H19) is expressed only from the maternal allele. IGF-II and H19 are also monoallelically expressed in the human. Additional imprinted genes have been characterized (Tycko 1997).

Several studies have shown that imprinted genes regulate the development of the embryo/fetus. It has also been suggested that DNA methylation maintains the imprinting of some genes. Abnormalities in genomic imprinting are associated with genetic diseases. Prader-Willi syndrome and Angelman syndrome are two examples of abnormal functional imprinting. Furthermore, abnormal functional imprinting is implicated in tumorigenesis. Although previous studies (Ogura et al. 1994, Sofikitis et al. 1994a, Kimura and Yanagimachi 1995a) suggest that genomic imprinting is complete at the rabbit and mouse round spermatid stage, additional studies are necessary in man. If genomic imprinting is incomplete in subpopulations of men with primary testicular damage, abnormalities may not become manifest at the early embryonic development, but they may be detectable in the fetus or during the postnatal life. A question of great clinical importance is whether genomic imprinting has been completed at the human round spermatid stage. To attempt to answer this question the imprinting of a gene should be divided into three stages: (a) erasure of the previous imprint, (b) re-imprinting, and (c) consolidation of the new imprint. There is strong evidence that erasure of the previous imprint occurs prior to meiosis and that re-establishment of the new imprint begins prior to the pachytene stage of meiosis (see for review Tycko 1997). In contrast, the fact that DNA methyltransferase enzyme is present in spermatids may be an argument against the thesis that genomic imprinting is complete at the round spermatid stage. However, it should be emphasized that waves of DNA methylation have been demonstrated during early embryonic development, the blastocyst stage, and the time of implantation (Fishel et al. 1996). These observations tend to suggest that even if genomic imprinting is not complete at the round spermatid stage, genomic reprinting may be completed after the transfer of the round spermatid within the ooplasm. The work of Kimura and Yanagimachi (1995a,b) supports the latter thesis. Fishel et al. (1996) claim that the genomic imprinting of mouse spermatogenic cells is complete in the testis prior to the male second meiotic division.

Is It Early to Perform ROSNI/ROSI Procedures? Ethical Issues

The first successful fertilization/pregnancy via ICSI was achieved accidentally (Palermo et al. 1992). Furthermore, prior to the first human ICSI pregnancy, there was a lack of studies in experimental animals evaluating the health/chromosomes/genes of offspring born after ICSI techniques. In contrast, prior to performance of human ROSNI/ROSI these techniques had been applied in rabbits (Sofikitis et al. 1994a) and mice (Ogura et al. 1994) and had resulted in delivery of healthy offspring, and human ROSNI/ROSI procedures were carefully scheduled before they were initially performed (Sofikitis et al. 1995a, Tesarik et al. 1995, Vanderzwalmen et al. 1995). Thus, it appears that ROSNI/ROSI procedures were designed more carefully than ICSI techniques had been prior to their initial clinical application.

ROSNI/ROSI techniques have been criticized by a number of scientists because of genetic risks, low pregnancy rates, and inherent technical difficulties (mainly regarding the identification of live round spermatids) that do not allow the majority of the assisted reproduction centers to perform these techniques. We feel that theoretical genetic risks should not be used to exclude men from appropriate infertility treatment. Rather, genetic risks should be extensively discussed with the ROSNI/ROSI or ICSI candidate. To date there has been no evidence of a major or minor abnormality in all ROSNI/ROSI human newborns and animal offspring. In addition, it is a fundamental human right for every couple to obtain therapy for relief of the disease of infertility. Thus, nonobstructed azoospermic men have the right to choose their treatment after adequate information. Furthermore, although specialized staff are necessary to perform ROSNI/ROSI, these techniques should be inexpensive. If fertilization is achieved, embryonic biopsy (preimplantation diagnosis) is recommended. Alternatively, couples should be advised to undergo prenatal monitoring after achievement of pregnancy. ROSNI/ROSI may not be criticized because of their low pregnancy rates since these techniques represent the only hope for nonobstructed azoospermic men to father their own children. During the 4 years that have passed since the first application of ROSNI/ROSI in human subjects, >20 pregnancies have been achieved worldwide via ooplasmic injections of spermatids, by seven different groups working independently (Fishel et al. 1995; Sofikitis et al. 1995a, 1997b, 1998a, Tesarik et al. 1995, Mansour et al. 1996, Tanaka et al. 1996, Amer et al. 1997, Antinori et al. 1997a, b, Araki et al. 1997, Vanderzwalmen et al. 1997). Additional research efforts are necessary to improve the outcome of ROSNI/ROSI. These efforts should be directed to the development/ discovery of (a) criteria for identification of round spermatids, (b) biochemical media prolonging the viability of spermatids, (c) exogenous stimuli to support oocyte activation in men with OASIS deficiency, (d) methodology to identify and purify human OASIS, and (e) methodology to study the metabolism and the implantation process of embryos generated by ooplasmic injections of spermatids. Finally, criticism of ROSNI/ROSI techniques based on their technical difficulties is not justified. Training and basic research in experimental animals are necessary for the staff of assisted reproduction centers applying ooplasmic injections of spermatids. The latter suggestion is supported by the fact that groups with excellent ICS results but without active basic research programs on testicular physiology have occasionally failed to demonstrate acceptable ROSNI/ ROSI outcomes.

Importance of ROSNI/ROSI Technique

The majority of clinicians worldwide may consider the ooplasmic injections of spermatids as important techniques because they have resulted in delivery of human newborns fathered by nonobstructed azoospermic men. Although a baby is the target in assisted reproduction programs we feel that ROSNI/ROSI techniques are important for an another reason; they can serve as a tool to investigate alterations in the viability, physiology, DNA integrity, and reproductive capacity of the early haploid male gamete as a response to a certain pathophysiology/toxic factor (Sofikitis et al. 1996b). Thus, various laboratories of different orientations and interests such as cellular biology, cellular metabolism, molecular biology, developmental physiology, and testicular physiology have a novel assay to investigate the influence of a physiological or nonphysiological stimulus on the early haploid male gamete (Sofikitis et al. 1996b).

Considerations for the Future: the Post-ROSNI Era

ICSI or ROSNI/ROSI procedures offer alternative solutions for men with nonobstructive azoospermia and testicular foci of spermatogenesis up to the spermatozoon or round spermatid stage, respectively. In addition, preliminary trials of human ooplasmic secondary spermatocyte injections (SECSI techniques) recently resulted in delivery of a healthy boy (Sofikitis et al. 1998b). In that study the human second meiotic division was completed within the ooplasm. However, clinical application of SECSI procedures may be limited, since most nonobstructed azoospermic men with secondary spermatocytes in the therapeutic testicular biopsy material have spermatozoa and/or spermatids. In contrast, men in whom the most advanced spermatogenic cells are primary spermatocytes cannot nowadays be candidates in assisted reproduction programs. For the latter group three recent achievements in basic research may offer new possibilities in assisted reproduction programs in the future.

Artificial Testis/In Vitro Culture of Germ Cells

An artificial testis may be considered as an in vitro culture system where primary spermatocytes or round spermatids will be cultured under biochemical conditions similar to testicular microenvironment, aiming to induce the human meiosis in vitro or to achieve generation of the spermatid flagella. The haploid products of an artificial testis may be used in assisted reproduction programs. To create a functional artificial testis more research efforts are necessary on the factors/second-messenger systems regulating meiosis in the testis. Few studies support the idea that utilization of an in vitro culture system in assisted reproduction may be possible in the future. Early studies by Gerton and Millette (1984) demonstrated generation of spermatid flagella in vitro. Furthermore, Gritsch et al. (1997) showed that human spermatogenic cells can survive long term under in vitro culture conditions. In a landmark study, Weiss et al. (1997) demonstrated generation of round spermatids from primary spermatocytes in vitro. Goto et al. (1996) achieved induction of the second meiotic division in vitro.

Transplantation of Human Spermatogenic Cells into a Host Testis

Results from transplantation of mouse spermatogenic cells into mouse seminiferous tubules and rat spermatogenic cells into mouse seminiferous tubules indicate that the donor germ cells are capable of differentiating to form spermatozoa morphologically characteristic of the donor species (Russell et al. 1996, Russell and Brinster 1996). Furthermore, recent findings in our laboratory (Tanaka et al. 1997) have shown that (a) spermatogenic cells isolated from hamsters with primary testicular damage are capable of transforming to hamster spermatozoa within the seminiferous tubules of host nonimmunosuppressed animals, indicating that the transluminal compartment of the seminiferous tubules is immunologically privileged; and (b) the above-mentioned cellular transformation of the donor cells is also inducible within the seminiferous tubules of immunosuppressed animals following macroscopic transfer techniques. If the above studies are applied successfully in man, primary spermatocytes of nonobstructed azoospermic men may be transformed into human spermatids or spermatozoa within a host testis, giving these men the opportunity to be candidates for ROSNI/ROSI or ICSI.

However, even if induction of human meiosis becomes possible within a host testis, application of human ROSNI or ICSI using human haploid male gametes generated in an animals testis is susceptible to genetic and immunological risks.

Gene Transfer for the Treatment of Nonobstructed Azoospermia

Gene therapy is an exciting and powerful technique capable of introducing novel genetic sequences to alter the cell phenotype. Recent data reported by Werthman et al. (1997) confirm successful gene transfer of a reporter gene to murine testicular tissue. This technique may have the potential to reverse the effects of genetic mutation which lead to nonobstructed azoospermia by reconstitution of the wild-type gene (Werthman et al. 1997).

Acknowledgements. The authors would like to express their gratitude to Toshiko Toda, MD, PhD, for participating in the development of ROSNI techniques; Manami Takenaka, BS, for significantly improving the technique of ooplasmic injection of round spermatids; and Ira Sharlip, MD, and Krinos Trokoudes, MD, for their contribution to the performance of the first ROSNI trials in the USA and Cyprus, respectively. Furthermore, we are thankful to our co-workers Panayiotis Zavos, PhD, Yasuyuki Mio, MD, PhD, Atsushi Tanaka, MD, Keiko Yamanaka, PhD, Katsuhiko Takahashi, MD, PhD, Martin Neil, PhD, George Mekras, MD, Jim Stein, PhD, Hiroshi Kawamura, PhD, Sspyros Antypas, MD, Emmanouel Agapitos, MD, Konstadinos Kalianidis, MD, Nikolaos Kanakas, MD, Fotini Dimitriadou, BS, Sanae Tsukamoto, BS, and Ritsa Bletsa, BS, for assisting us in improving ROSNI techniques.

References

Akmal KA, Dufour JM, Kim K (1997) Retinoic acid receptor a gene expression in the rat testis: potential role during the prophase of meiosis and in the transition from round to elongating spermatids. Biol Reprod 56:549, 556

Amer M, Soliman E, El-Sadek M et al (1997) Is complete spermiogenesis failure a good indication for spermatid conception? Lancet 350:116

Anderson DM, Lyman SD, Baird A et al (1990) Molecular cloning mast cell growth factor, a hematopoietin that is active in both membrane-bound and soluble forms. Cells 63:235-243

Angelopoulos T, Key L, McCullough A et al (1997) A single and objective approach to identifying human round spermatids. Hum Reprod 12:2208-2216

Antinori S, Versaci C, Dani G et al. (1997a) Fertilization with human testicular spermatids: four successful pregnancies. Hum Reprod 12:285-291

Antinori S; Versaci C, Dani G et al (1997b) Successful fertilization and pregnancy after injections of frozen-thawed round spermatids into human oocytes. Hum Reprod 12:554-556

Araki Y, Motoyame M, Yoshida A et al (1997) Intracytoplasmic injection of late spermatids: a successful procedure in achieving childbirth for couples in which the male partner suffers from azoospermia due to deficient spermatogenesis. Fertil Steril 22:559-561

Baschat A, Schwinger E, Diedrich K (1996) Assisted reproductive techniques – are we avoiding the genetic issues? Hum Reprod 11:330-333

Bates GW (1987) Electrofusion: principles and applications. In: Sowers AE (ed) Cell fusion. Plenum, New York, pp 367-395

Chabot B, Stephenson DA, Chapman VM et al (1988) The protooncogene c-kit encoding a transmembrane tyrosine kinase receptor maps to the mouse W locus. Nature 335:88-89

Chai N, Phyllips A, Fernandez A et al (1997) A putative human male infertility gene DAZLA: genomic structure and methylation status. Mol Hum Reprod 3:705-708

Chen S, Ho H, Chen H et al (1996) Fertilization and embryo cleavage after intracytoplasmic spermatid injection in an obstructive azoospermic patient with defective spermiogenesis. Fertil Steril 66:157-160

De Kretser DM, Kerr JM (1988) The cytology of the testis. In: Knobil E, Neil J (eds) The physiology of reproduction. Raven, New York, pp 837-866

Dozortsev D, Rybouchkin A, De Sutter P et al (1995) Human oocyte activation following intracytoplasmic sperm injection: the role of the sperm cell. Hum Reprod 10:403-407

Edwards RG, Tarin JJ, Dean NN et al (1994) Are spermatid injections into human oocytes now mandatory? Hum Reprod 9:2217-2219

Fawcett DM, Anderson WA, Phillips DM (1971) Morphogenetic factors influencing the shape of the sperm head. Dev Biol 26:220-251

Fishel S, Green S, Bishop M et al (1995) Pregnancy after intracytoplasmic injection of spermatid. Lancet 345:1641-1642

Fishel S, Aslam I, Tesarik J (1996) Spermatid conception: a stage too early, or a time too soon? Hum Reprod 11:1371-1375

Fishel S, Green S, Hunter A et al (1997) Human fertilization with round elongated spermatids. Hum Reprod 12:336-340

Gerton GL, Millette CF (1984) Generation of flagella by cultured mouse spermatids. J Cell Biol 98:619-628

Goto K, Kinoshita A, Nakanishi Y et al (1996) Blastocyst formation following intracytoplasmic injection of in-vitro derived spermatids into bovine oocytes. Hum Reprod 11:824-829

Gritsch H, Bruning C, Robels M (1997) Long term spermatogenic cell culture. J Urol 157 [Suppl]: abstract 654, p 169

Hannay T (1995) New Japanese IVF method finally made available in Japan. Nature Med 1:298-290

Janny L, Ménézo Y (1994) Evidence for strong paternal effect on human preimplantation embryo development and blastocyst formation. Mol Reprod Dev 38:36-42

Kimura Y, Yanagimachi R (1995a) Mouse oocytes injected with testicular spermatozoa or round spermatids can develop into normal offspring. Development 121:2397-2405

Kimura Y, Yanagimachi R (1995b) Development of normal mice from oocytes injected with secondary spermatocyte nuclei. Biol Reprod 53:855-862

Mansour RT, Aboulghar MA, Serour K et al (1996a) Pregnancy and delivery after intracyto-plasmic injection of spermatids into human oocytes. Middle East Fertil Soc 1. 223-225

Mansour RT, Aboulghar MA, Serour G et al (1996b) Successful intracytoplasmic sperm injection without performing cytoplasmic aspiration. Fertil Steril 66:256-259

Mazia D (1984) Centrosomes and mitotic poles. Cell Res 153:1, 23

Mendoza C, Tesarik J (1996) The occurrence and identification of round spermatids in the ejaculate of men with non-obstructed azoospermia. Fertil Steril 66:826-829

Mendoza C, Benkhalifa M, Cohen-Bacrie P et al (1996) Combined use of proacrosin immu-nochemistry and autosomal DNA in situ hybridization for evaluation of human ejacu-lated germ cells. Zygote 4:279-283

Meng L, Wolf DP (1997) Sperm induced oocyte activation in the rhesus monkey: nuclear and cytoplasmic changes following intracytoplasmic sperm injection. Hum Reprod 12:1062-1068

Nagy Z, Liu J, Joris H et al. (1994) Time course of oocyte activation, pronucleus formation, and cleavage in human oocytes fertilized by intracytoplasmic sperm injection. Hum Re-prod 9:1743-1748

Nakamura M, Romrell LJ, Hall P (1978) The effects of glucose and temperature on protein biosynthesis by immature (round) spermatids from rat testis. J Cell Biol 79:1-9

Navara C, First N, Schatten G (1994) Microtubule organization in the cow during fertiliza-tion, polyspermy, parthenogenesis, and nuclear transfer: the role of the sperm transfer. Dev Biol 162:29-40

O'Donnell L, McLachlan R, Wreford N et al (1996) Testosterone withdrawal promotes stage-specific detachment of round spermatids from the rat seminiferous epithelium. Biol Re-prod 55:895-901

Ogura A, Yanagimachi R (1993) Round spermatid nuclei injected into hamster oocytes form pronuclei and participate in syngamy. Biol Reprod 48:219-225

Ogura A, Yanagimachi R, Usui N (1993) Behavior of hamster and mouse round spermatid nuclei incorporated into mature oocytes by electrofusion. Zygote 1:1-8

Ogura A, Matsuda J Yanagimachi R (1994) Birth of normal young after electrofusion of mouse oocytes with round spermatids. Proc. Natl. Acad. Sci. U S A 91:7460-7462

Ono K, Sofikitits N, Miyagawa I (1996) Fertilization of rabbit oocytes with nuclei extracted from thawed round spermatids. Jpn J Urol 87 [Suppl 2]:393

Ono K, Miyagawa I, Sofikitis N et al (1997) Defects in genetic and epigenetic contributions of the male gamete to zygote affect early embryonic development and compromise em-bryonic capacity for implantation. Fertil Steril 68 [Suppl] abstract P-152, pp S165-166

Ozil JP (1990) The parthenogenetic development of rabbit oocytes after pulsatile electrical stimulation. Development 109:117-127

Palermo G, Joris H, Devroy P et al (1992) Pregnancies after intracytoplasmic injection of single spermatozoon into an oocyte. Lancet 340:17-18

Palermo G, Munné S, Cohen J (1994) The human zygote inherits its mitotic potential from the male gamete. Hum Reprod 9:1220-1227

Parrington J, Swann K, Shevchenko V et al (1996) Calcium oscillations in mammalian eggs triggered by a soluble protein. Nature 379:364-368

Perreault S, Zirkin BR (1982) Sperm nuclear decondensation in mammals: role of sperm-as-sociated proteinase in vivo. J Exp Zool 224:253-257

Perreault S, Naish S, Zirkin BR (1987) The timing of hamster sperm nuclear decondensa-tion and male pronucleus formation is related to sperm nuclear disulfide bond content. Biol Reprod 36:239-244

Rajfer J, Turner TT, Rivera F et al (1987) Inhibition of testicular testosterone synthesis fol-lowing experimental varicocele in rates. Biol Reprod 36:933-937

Russell LD, Brinster RL (1996) Ultrastructural observation of spermatogenesis following transplantation of rat testis cells into mouse seminiferous tubules. J Androl 17:615-626

Russell LD, Franca LR, Brinster RL (1996) Ultrastructural observations of spermatogenesis in mice resulting from transplantation of mouse spermatogonia. J Androl 17:603–614

Sasagawa I, Yanagimachi R (1997) Spermatids from mice after cryptorchid and reversal operations can initiate normal embryo development. J Androl 18:203–209

Sathananthan AH, Kola I, Osborne J et al (1991) Centrioles in the beginning of human development. Proc Natl Acad Sci U S A 88:4806–4810

Schatten G (1994) The centrosome and its mode of inheritance: the reduction of centrosome during gametogenesis and its restoration during fertilization. Dev Biol 165:299–335

Schatten G, Schatten H, Mazia D et al (1986) Behaviors of centrosomes during fertilization and cell division in mouse oocytes and sea urchin eggs. Proc Natl Acad Sci USA 85:105–109

Silber SJ (1996) Sertoli cell-only syndrome. Hum Reprod 11:229–233

Silber SJ, Nagy Z, Liu J et al (1995a) The use of testicular and epididymal spermatozoa for intracytoplasmic sperm injections: the genetic implications for male infertility. Hum Reprod 10:2031–2043

Silber SJ, Van Steirteghem AC, Devroey P (1995b) Sertoli cell only revisited. Hum Reprod 10:1031–1032

Silber SJ, Nagy Z, Devroey P et al (1997) Distribution of spermatogenesis in the testicles of azoospermic men: the presence or absence of spermatids in the testes of men with germinal failure. Hum Reprod 12:2422–2428

Simerly C, Wu G, Zoran S et al (1995) The paternal inheritance of the centrosome, the cell's microtubule-organizing center, in humans and the implications for infertility. Nature Med 11:47–52

Sofikitis NV, Miyagawa I, Agapitos E et al (1994a) Reproductive capacity of the nucleus of the male gamete after completion of meiosis. J Assist Reprod Genet 11:335–341

Sofikitis N, Miyagawa I, Zavos, PM et al (1994b) Confocal scanning laser microscopy of morphometric human sperm parameters: correlation with acrosin profiles and fertilizing capacity. Fertil Steril 62:376–386

Sofikitis N, Miyagawa I, Sharlip I et al (1995a) Human pregnancies achieved by intra-ooplasmic injections of round spermatid nuclei isolated from testicular tissue of azoospermic men. Presented at the American Urological Association 90th Annual Meeting in Las Vegas, April 23–28, 1995. J Urol 153 [Suppl]:258 A

Sofikitis N, Toda T, Miyagawa I et al (1995b) Application of ooplasmic round spermatid nuclear injections for the treatment of azoospermic men in USA. Fertil Steril 64 (Suppl]:S88–S89

Sofikitis NV, Toda T, Miyagawa I et al (1996a) Beneficial effects of electrical stimulation before round spermatid nuclei injections into rabbit oocytes on fertilization and subsequent embryonic development. Fertil Steril 65:176–185

Sofikitis NV, Miyagawa I, Incze P et al (1996b) Detrimental effect of left varicocele on the reproductive capacity of the early haploid male gamete. J Urol 156:267–270

Sofikitis NV, Yamamoto Y, Miyagawa I (1997a) The azoospermic father: fact or fiction? The reproductive potential of the early haploid male gamete. In: Waites GMH, Frick J, Baker JWH (eds) Current advances in andrology. Monduzzi Editore, Bologna, pp 189–195

Sofikitis NV, Mantzavinos T, Loutradis D et al (1997b) Treatment of male infertility caused by spermatogenic arrest at the primary spermatocyte stage with ooplasmic injections of round spermatids or secondary spermatocytes isolated from foci of early haploid male gametes. Presented at the 13th Annual Meeting of The European Society of Human Reproduction and Embryology in Edinburgh, June 22–25, 1997. Hum Reprod 12 [Suppl]:81–82

Sofikitis NV, Kanakas N, Mantzavinos T et al (1997c) Deficiency in the oocyte-activating substance in spermatozoa: a cause of ICSI failure. Presented at the 13th Annual Meeting of The European Society of Human Reproduction and Embryology in Edinburgh, June 22–25, 1997. Hum Reprod 12 [Suppl]:81

Sofikitis N, Yamamoto Y, Miyagawa I (1997d) The early haploid male gamete develops a capacity for fertilization after the coalescence of the proacrosomal granules. Hum Reprod 12:2713–2719

Sofikitis N, Yamamoto Y, Miyagawa I et al (1998a) Ooplasmic elongating spermatid injections for the treatment of non-obstructive azoospermia. Hum Reprod F13:F709–714

Sofikitis N, Mantzavinos T, Loutradis D et al (1998b) Delivery of a healthy male after ooplasmic injections of secondary spermatocytes. Presented at The 23rd Annual Meeting of The American Society of Andrology at Long Beach, Calif., USA, March 27–29, 1998. J Androl 19 [Suppl 1]:57 (abstract)

Sousa M, Barros A, Tesarik J (1996) Calcium responses of human oocytes after intracytoplasmic injection of leukocytes, spermatocytes, and round spermatids. Mol Hum Reprod 2:853–857

Swann K (1990) A cytosolic sperm factor stimulates repetitive calcium increases and mimics fertilization in hamster eggs. Development 110:1295–1302

Tanaka A, Nagayoshi M, Awata S et al (1996) Clinical evaluation of round spermatid injection into human oocytes. Fertil Steril 66 [Suppl]:abstract P 12, p S99

Tanaka A, Nagayoshi M, Sofikitis N (1997) Conclusions from transplantation of human or hamster spermatogonia/primary spermatocytes to rat or mouse testis. Fertil Steril 68 [Suppl]: abstract 0-122, p S61

Taylor CT, Lawrence YM, Kingsland CR et al. (1993) Oscillations in intracellular free calcium induced by spermatozoa in human oocytes at fertilization. Hum Reprod 8:2174–2179

Tesarik J, Sousa M, Testart J (1994) Human oocyte activation after intracytoplasmic sperm injection. Hum Reprod 9:511–518

Tesarik J, Mendoza C, Testart J (1995) Viable embryos from injection of round spermatids into oocyte. N Engl J Med 333:525

Tesarik J, Rolet F, Brami C et al (1996) Spermatid injections into oocytes. II: Clinical application in the treatment of infertility due to non-obstructive azoospermia. Hum Reprod 11:780–783

Tycko B (1997) Post-graduate course program of The American Society of Andrology, 22nd Annual Meeting, Baltimore, Maryland, February 22–25, pp 83–106

Vanderzwalmen P, Lejeune B, Nijs M et al (1995) Fertilization of an oocyte microinseminated with a spermatid in an in-vitro fertilization program. Hum Reprod 10. 502–503

Vanderzwalmen P, Zech H et al (1997) Intracytoplasmic injection of spermatids retrieved from testicular tissue: influence of testicular pathology, type of selected spermatids and oocyte activation. Hum Reprod 12:1203–1213

Vitullo AD, Ozil JP (1992) Repetitive calcium stimuli derive meiotic resumption and pronuclei development during mouse oocyte activation. Dev Biol 151:128–136

Weiss M, Vigier M, Hue D et al (1997) Pre- and postmeiotic expression of male germ cell-specific genes throughout 2-week-cocultures of rat germinal and Sertoli cells. Biol Reprod 57:68–76

Werthman P, Kaboo R, Peng S et al (1997) Adenoviral mediated gene transfer to murine testis in vivo. J Urol 157 [Suppl 1]: abstract 653, p 169

Yamamoto Y, Sofikitis N, Miyagawa I (1997) Round spermatid nuclear injections (ROSNI) versus intact round spermatid injections (ROSI) into the ooplasm. Int J Androl 20 [Suppl 1]:p a-133

Yamanaka K, Sofikitis N, Miyagawa I et al (1997) Ooplasmic round spermatid nuclear injections as an experimental treatment of non-obstructive azoospermia. J Assist Reprod Genet 14:55–62

Artificial Intrauterine Insemination: Noninvasive Management of Subfertile Couples

G. Prietl, H. van der Ven, D. Krebs

History of Artificial Insemination

Since time immemorial man has employed the "artificial transfer of seeds" through pollination to cultivate plants. Assyrians and Cretans already used pollination for systematic cross-breeding.

"Artificial insemination", i.e., the artificial introduction of semen into the female genital tract, was mentioned in writing for the first time in an Arab report dating back to 1322. As legend has it, the Arabs used artificial insemination to breed horses (Heiss 1972). Lazzaro Spallanzani (1729–1799), an Italian theologian, natural scientist, and eminent physiologist of his day, was able to provide experimental evidence of the ovum being fertilized by sperm. After initially experimenting with frogs and silkworms, he succeeded in artificially inseminating a warm-blooded mammal (dog) for the first time in 1780. However, it was not before the end of the 19th century, i.e., 100 years later, that the practical significance of Spallanzani's experiments for animal breeding was truly recognized. The era of modern animal breeding was ushered in by the Russian physiologist E. Iwanow with his comprehensive monograph "De la fécondation artificielle chez les mammifères", which he published in 1907.

The old Talmudists were the first to address the possibility of "fecundatio sine concubito" in theoretical terms. Documents dating back to the second and third centuries a.d. show that Jewish society studied the issue of conception without sexual intercourse. Ben Zoma (130 a.d.), for instance, discussed with students whether it would still be a case of virginity if a woman became pregnant without sexual intercourse (Kardinom 1942). "Fecundatio sine concubito" seemed to be a possibility in bathhouses where women took a bath in the same water that men had used first.

The first human artificial insemination is attributed to the English surgeon John Hunter (1728–1793; Fig. 1). As his nephew, E. Home, wrote in London in 1799, Hunter advised a husband who was infertile due to severe hypospadias to collect his ejaculate in a syringe and inject it into his wife's vagina. This report, however, did not attract particular attention at the time. In 1865, F. Dehaut published the first study in Paris that looked at the scientific basis of artificial insemination (Schlesinger 1870). In 1886, J. Girault reported ten cases that had been successfully treated with intracervical insemination (Holfelder 1953). Girault is also said to have been the first physician to transfer the semen directly into the

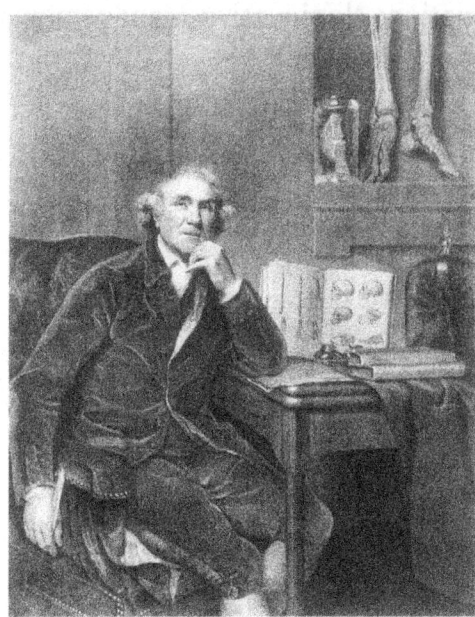

Fig. 1. John Hunter (1728–1793).
(Courtesy of F.R. Hau, Institute of the
History of Medicine, University of
Bonn)

uterine cavity (Kaiser 1966). J.M. Sims, an American gynecologist, intensively
studied the physiology and pathology of human reproduction as well as the
causes of sterility and the methods employed to diagnose it (Sims 1869). It was
Sims, too, who in 1866 performed the first successful homologous intrauterine
insemination in the United States of America. In 1884, artificial insemination
with donor sperm was introduced into sterility management by R.L. Dickinson
and W. Pankhurst from Philadelphia (Hard 1909; Glover 1948). In Europe at the
end of the last century, it was mainly in France that artificial insemination was
practiced, which led to heated public discussions about ethical issues. In 1871,
the medical faculty of Paris University had accepted a doctoral thesis by P.F. Gigon entitled "Essai sur la fécondation artificielle chez la femme dans certains
cas de stérilité"; in 1871, however, it declared artificial insemination to be "unnatural" and "immoral". A passionate debate was also engendered in the French
medical community about the social and ethical import of human artificial insemination, until in 1883 the French Society of Medicine finally declared homologous insemination acceptable as the ultimate possibility of ensuring reproduction. In Germany, the Cologne Higher Regional Court had to deal with artificial
insemination for the first time in 1905. Based on an expert opinion submitted
by H. Fritsch, director of the Bonn University Hospital of Obstetrics and Gynecology from 1893 to 1910, the case was initially dismissed. In the early twentieth century, the first medical, legal, and ethical studies on artificial insemination as a
method for treating involuntary childlessness were published in the German scientific literature (Bumm 1904; Fraenkel 1909; Döderlein 1912; Hirsch 1912; Rohleder 1912; Prochownik 1915; Sellheim 1924). In their articles, G. Döderlein and J.
Hirsch also warned about possible gonorrheal infection.

Since that time, artificial insemination (intravaginal, peri- and intracervical, or intrauterine) using husband or donor sperm has been performed for a wide range of indications. Indications for treatment included unexplained infertility, abnormal or hostile cervical mucus, abnormal semen parameters, and – more rarely – cases of anatomical malformation (e.g., severe hypospadias), neurological disorders (e.g., retrograde ejaculation), and psychological and psychogenic dysfunctions (e.g., loss of libido, vaginismus), as well as eugenic reasons due to the presence of genetic risks (e.g., rhesus incompatibility, hemophilia, Cooley's anemia, cystic fibrosis, Tay-Sachs disease, spinal muscular atrophy, Huntington's chorea, schizophrenia, and manic-depressive psychosis).

Direct intrauterine insemination, bypassing the cervical-mucus barrier with a catheter, has for many decades been performed with neat semen, i.e., not specifically prepared ejaculate. Due to frequent adverse side effects, above all uterine cramps caused by prostaglandins contained in seminal plasma and by microbial contamination of the inseminate, the method was practically abandoned (Hanson and Rock 1951; Russel 1960; Taylor and Kelly 1974; Barwin 1974; Kremer 1979; Stone et al. 1986). It was only after appropriate methods of semen washing and processing had been developed and were commonly applied that the rate of complications was reduced. Subsequently, painful uterine cramps rarely occurred, and the prevalence of pelvic infections following intrauterine insemination was lowered to 1.8 in 1000 treatment cycles (Sacks and Simon 1991). In addition, laboratory techniques for isolating capacitated high-quality spermatozoa resulted in significantly improved pregnancy rates. The most widely used techniques are the sperm-rise or swim-up method (Drevius 1971; Lopata et al. 1976; Harris et al. 1981; Makler et al. 1984b; Cohen et al. 1985; Russell and Rogers 1987) and density gradient centrifugation (Pertoft et al. 1977; Gorus and Pipeleers 1981; Lessley and Garner 1983; Berger et al. 1985). Some centers – like ours – have also gathered very positive experience with glass-wool filtration (Paulson and Polakoski 1977; Jeyendran et al. 1986). These semen processing and sperm isolation methods, in combination with improved ovulation induction protocols – developed primarily to meet IVF requirements – eventually led to the revival and widespread use of insemination treatment over the past 15 years.

General

Artificial intrauterine insemination using the husband's prepared spermatozoa (AIH) is a common procedure for the management of involuntary childlessness, even though in the literature there is no consensus on the effectiveness of such an approach. Especially in cases of male subfertility and persistent idiopathic fertility disorders, divergent views exist with regard to the therapeutic benefit of homologous insemination. Nevertheless, intrauterine insemination (IUI), both in spontaneous and, preferably, in ovulation induction cycles, is recommended as the first choice of assisted conception techniques, since – unlike gamete intrafallopian transfer (GIFT) or in vitro fertilization with embryo transfer (IVF/ET) – the procedure is noninvasive and also much more cost-effective.

Even though the cumulative pregnancy rates in normocyclic women under-going artificial intrauterine insemination with donor sperm (AID) due to their partners' infertility (e.g., azoospermia) are proof of the efficacy of artificial in-semination as such, the results of AIH vary considerably. A survey of the litera-ture published over the past 15 years shows a wide variation in the probability of conception per cycle after conventional IUI. This applies even to prospective randomized studies which break down the pregnancies achieved according to cause of subfertility (male factor, cervical factor, idiopathic factor) where rates are between 0% and 26% (Tables 2–3). In randomized, controlled studies, how-ever, that critically compare artificial insemination after ovarian stimulation with natural sexual intercourse in spontaneous cycles, pregnancy rates follow-ing conventional IUI still fluctuate between 3% and 15% (Table 4). Numerous factors may be considered as possible explanations for these variations. They include, most importantly, differences in the diagnostic groups and their defini-tion, the use of different protocols for ovarian stimulation, and different meth-ods of semen processing, as well as methodological variations between the studies themselves such, as the number of patients enrolled, treatment cycles performed, or the randomization procedure chosen. Moreover, many studies do not provide any information about previous pregnancies or treatment efforts, the duration of subfertility, tubal patency, or the number of mature follicles or of motile spermatozoa inseminated. Unfortunately, there are only few random-ized AIH studies that make a controlled comparison between therapy groups and untreated control groups (Table 4). However, it is such studies that are im-portant to assess the true benefit of treatment since with subfertile couples – in contrast to cases of sterility – there is still the possibility of pregnancy without therapy (Aafjes et al. 1978; Nachtigall et al. 1979; Glass and Ericsson 1979; Ha-ney et al. 1987; Bolton et al. 1989). Observations that 14% of the patients be-came pregnant spontaneously within a finite (3-year) time span after cessation of trials (e.g., Nachtigall et al. 1979; Bolton et al. 1989) should be borne in mind, as they justify the term "subfertility", which we prefer to use.

The choice of the most appropriate form of treatment is seldom as straight-forward as in cases where both fallopian tubes have been removed or are irre-parably damaged. Here, the only option available is IVF. For subfertility, how-ever, there are several possible courses of therapy. Working on the hypothesis that effective success (take-home baby) rates are the same in both cases, one could claim that IUI is doubtless superior and hence preferable to its invasive alternatives (IVF/ET, GIFT). In theory, it could not be precluded that for prop-erly selected patients, particularly those of younger age and limited duration of subfertility, under otherwise identical conditions (e.g., unexplained or mild male-factor disorders, stimulation with gonadotropins, comparable number/ quality of follicles, oocytes, or embryos, precise timing of ovulation, identical definition of success, consideration of former treatment efforts, cancellation rate of cycles initiated, as well as equivalent medical experience and diligence), the effective success rates of combined controlled ovarian hyperstimulation and intrauterine insemination (COH/IUI) are unlikely to differ significantly from those of the invasive methods (IVF, GIFT). In fact, some prospective randomized trials were reported where, in patients with unexplained subfertility, comparable pregnancy rates were obtained for all procedures (Crosignani et al. 1991; Abyholm et al. 1992; Wessels et al. 1992; Zayed et al. 1997; Goverde et al. 2000). From the scientific perspective, these peer-reviewed data from randomized studies cannot be ignored, and this also applies to the few randomized studies which documented the superiority of invasive methods for patients with the same condition (Iffland et al. 1991; Murdoch et al. 1991). In 1994, Petersen et al. compared a meta-analysis of 22 studies on COH/IUI with their own prospective, nonrandomized cohort study of IVF versus no treatment and the U.S. national data on IVF, zygote intrafallopian transfer (ZIFT), and GIFT: They found that for COH/IUI the pregnancy rates for one cycle were inferior to IVF, GIFT, or ZIFT, for two cycles comparable to IVF or ZIFT but inferior to GIFT, and for three cycles superior to IVF or ZIFT and comparable to GIFT. All in all, it can be said that as long as there is a lack of large-scale, prospective, randomized studies with well-defined populations as well as sufficient statistical power and confidence, it will be very difficult to identify objectively and in an evidence-based manner the superiority of one specific method (IVF or GIFT versus COH/IUI) or the equivalence of all methods. It is perhaps this want of convincing studies which can best explain the lack of consensus mentioned at the beginning on both effective success rates and valid cost-benefit considerations. Such a consensus still needs to be established regarding patients with idiopathic subfertility and a good prognosis. It is indispensable in this context to draw attention to remarkable results repeatedly obtained with fallopian tube sperm perfusion (Kahn et al. 1993; Fanchin et al. 1995; Mamas 1996; Trout and Kemmann 1999), which is actually a variant of noninvasive conventional IUI and will hence be discussed here in detail.

This chapter provides a topical overview of the use of noninvasive homologous IUI. We relied, to the best of our knowledge, on evidence-based data. Our emphasis is, of course, on traditional IUI, as it is still the most widely used technique, and also on fallopian tube sperm perfusion (FSP), which recently was found to be twice as effective (Trout and Kemmann 1999).

Fecundity of Fertile and Subfertile Couples

Expectations of therapeutic success should best be related to the probability of natural conception of fertile couples seeking pregnancy. The epidemiological data on human fecundity cited in this section were taken from Spira (1986) and are acknowledged reference figures (Hull 1992; Edwards and Brody 1995a). The fecundity of a couple is measured by their fecundability, i.e. the monthly probability of conception without any contraception. Figure 2 shows the distribution (beta or Pearson-I distribution; Schwartz 1980) of fecundability of young and fertile couples which, according to an estimation from several samples, ranges from 0% to more than 60%. The mean fecundability of the population studied is about 25–30%. At the first attempt at becoming pregnant, peak normal probability of conception is ~33% on average, but drops quickly in the following

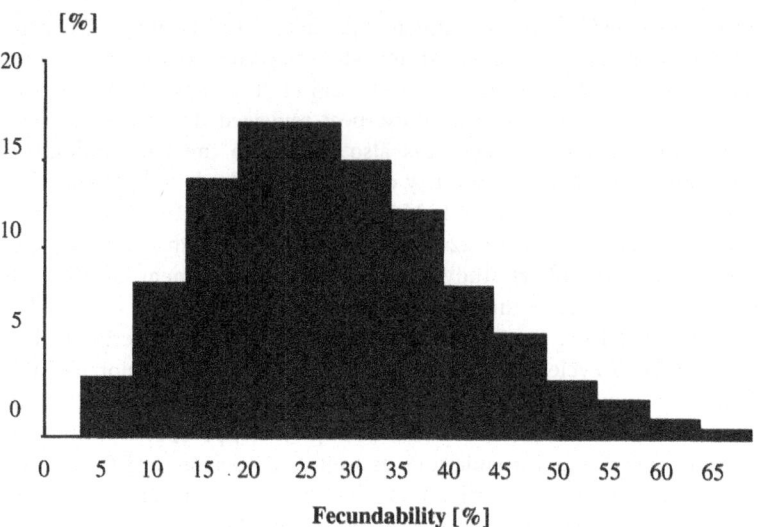

Fig. 2. Plausible distribution (Pearson-I distribution) of fecundability (monthly probability of conception) in young couples. Few couples have only a low mean fecundability (<10%), while an equally small percentage have a relatively great chance of conception per cycle (>35%). Average fecundability of the whole population is 20%–30%. (From Spira 1986)

months, settling to ~5% after 4 years. The mean fecundability of still infertile couples is 16% after 6 months, 12% after 12 months, 8% after 24 months, and ~5% after 48 months. In cumulative terms and based on a mean fecundability of 25–30%, the average statistical risk of non-conception is 25–20% after 6 months, 10–7% after 12 months, 3–2% after 24 months, and less than 1% after 48 months. The marked heterogeneity of human fecundability – as demonstrated in Fig. 2 – is reflected in the interindividual variability in the time required to conceive, and among couples desiring pregnancy there is a distinct selection process, with the most fertile couples conceiving first. It is estimated that in industrialized countries ~15% of newly married couples are subfertile and will take longer than they would like to conceive, while only 3–5% of couples are involuntarily sterile at the end of their reproductive life. The fecundability of subfertile couples, according to the distribution of time necessary to conceive, however, is four to five times lower than that of fertile couples, i.e., approximately 5%, and it may be assumed that in about 22% of these cases pregnancy will not have occurred after 3 years. This is also the mean length of time for unsuccessfully attempting pregnancy before undergoing specific diagnostic evaluation and treatment.

Patient Counseling, Defense of an "Algorithmic" Management

One of the most frequent questions asked by patients seeking advice during the first consultation is about the probability of becoming pregnant as the result of treatment and having a healthy child. Already at this point a trusting working relationship should be established between the two partners to the treatment agreement, the patient and the clinician, as this is indispensable on the road to success. One essential objective of close interpersonal cooperation is to protect the patient from an atmosphere of uncertainty, emotional stress, disappointed expectations, and lingering hope. A task as complex as this cannot be accomplished by clinicians alone, and "fertility counseling" has thus emerged as a new professional discipline. Fertility counseling, which can be briefly described as the process of assisting individuals or couples to make informed decisions about their bioreproductive state (Raeburn and Meniru 1997), should be provided at several different stages of treatment (Human Fertilisation and Embryology Authority (HFEA) 1990). For a couple facing the decision to undergo several – possibly stressful – treatment attempts it is of fundamental importance to receive precise information about their personal chance of success. Ideally, the most basic audit of treatment outcome would require birth rates per treatment cycles initiated to be calculated, so that the best statistical approximation to reality can be made. Since there are already major interindividual variations in fecundability and time-to-conception in any given population of young couples (Spira 1986), it is particularly important in infertility management to give preference to time-specific cumulative pregnancy rates over crude data collected on a per-patient basis (Hull 1992). While success rates of infertility treatment are highly empirical and may vary not only among centers but also by type of treatment, treatment success is primarily a function of the couples' intrinsic variables such as underlying disorders, age, and duration of infertility. For this reason, reliable cumulative probabilities must take these prognostic factors into account. In addition, the validity of life-table analysis depends on the reasons for some couples not continuing in treatment as long as others being unbiased. Also, experience has taught us that none of the assisted conception techniques precludes the possibility of failure. Couples should repeatedly be alerted to this fact. To prevent patients from developing too optimistic and hence counterproductive expectations, it seems advisable to mention – by way of example – the take-home baby rates of natural conception. As indicated above, these are 25% per cycle on average, and the cumulative rate after 6 months is about 75%. Because none of the methods of assisted conception can be expected to yield any higher rates even under favorable prognostic conditions, and the number of attempts at treatment should be limited if patients take a sensible attitude, the comparison with natural conception rates has turned out to be a particularly useful argument.

It is not uncommon to observe that after repeated therapy failures a latent psychopathological condition may even turn into what may be diagnosed as a "supervalent desire". The impending manifestation of such a condition – which needs to be recognized and prevented in time – is primarily a function of the duration of treatment as well as of the invasiveness of diagnosis and therapy. This is why the patients' emotional resources should be reviewed after failed attempts and fertility counseling should be offered. The choice of a treatment procedure should be the balanced result of several factors, such as diagnosis and treatment options, probability of success, and biological time span remaining for conception, as well as the patients' emotional and economic situation. Figuratively speaking, the weight of all means and methods has to be balanced against the couple's individual situation.

The Hippocratic principle of "nihil nocere" should guide medical intervention not only with regard to the highly sensitive issue of involuntary childlessness. This principle also makes it a sine qua non to protect the patients from any harm that might be caused by ovarian hyperstimulation and higher-order multiple pregnancy. However, provided all medical precautions are complied with (i.e., a maximum of three follicles for IUI or a maximum of three oocytes/ embryos for transfer), none of the currently used assisted reproductive techniques can guarantee a safe foreseeable success. Hence, when considering the problems involved – i.e., performing management under pressure to succeed while at the same time trying to apply a gentle procedure – it makes sense indeed to use primarily noninvasive methods of therapy in couples with a good prognosis in whom major causal factors of subfertility cannot be detected. In the light of this philosophy, patients should be referred to IVF (or GIFT) only after noninvasive procedures have failed, say after four cycles, thus providing an opportunity for techniques which might then be more successful. In fact, such a stepwise approach results in a distinct "skimming-off" of couples with the most favorable conditions for noninvasive treatment.

For more than 20 years our infertility management has followed such an "algorithmic" concept. During this time we have never abandoned the principle of indication-based and "nonaggressive" diagnosis and therapy, planning the treatment of our patients primarily with their individual situation in mind. Being a noninvasive and successful procedure, IUI is still an indispensable part of our treatment concept. It also enjoys a high level of acceptance on the part of our patients, as it is less stressful and is performed on an out-patient basis. In view of the positive experience gathered with IUI, we – like many others – do not agree with those who advocate IVF, GIFT, or even intracytoplasmic sperm injection (ICSI) as first-line treatments in couples with unexplained or mild male-factor disorders.

Conventional Intrauterine Insemination

Passage of Spermatozoa Through the Female Genital Tract, Rationale for IUI

The classic studies by Croxatto et al. (1973) and Ahlgren (1969) report that after coitus several thousand spermatozoa can be recovered in the entire fallopian tube and only a few hundred in its ampulla (Ahlgren 1975). Mortimer and Templeton (1982) established that a much higher number of spermatozoa was found in the peritoneal cavity after intracervical insemination (ICI) than after coitus. These authors also confirmed studies by Settlage et al. (1973) and Ahlgren et al. (1974), which pointed out that the number of motile sperm inseminated decreases over the length of the female genital tract by 5–6 orders of magnitude. Sperm transport has been described as occurring in two phases: a fast initial phase and a subsequent phase of sustained migration. During the initial "rapid transit phase" (Overstreet and Cooper 1978), a vanguard of sperm is capable of reaching the upper female reproductive tract within a surprisingly short period of time. As demonstrated by "immediate post-coital tests", sperm can travel from the vaginal pool to receptive mucus within 90 s of coitus (Sobrero and MacLeod 1962); Settlage et al. (1973) found sperm in the tubes as early as 5 min after intravaginal insemination. This rapid transit of sperm cannot be achieved by flagellar activity alone; rather, it is due to contractions of the uterus and the tubes (Overstreet 1996). However, this process is not closely linked to orgasm, because the rate of sperm transport is the same both after artificial insemination and after coitus (Overstreet and Cooper 1978). The biological role which rapid sperm transit plays in normal human reproduction is uncertain, and it is open to speculation whether these sperm are involved in the fertilization process directly or indirectly, e.g., through involvement in the suppression of the immune response of the female tract (Overstreet 1996). During the sustained migration phase, on the other hand, spermatozoa first accumulate in the cervical mucus and thereafter migrate by flagellar activity into the upper reproductive tract. Sperm are stored in receptive mucus and may retain their fertilizing capacity for a period of up to 80 h (Gould et al. 1984). It is also known that, under physiological conditions, the number of sperm in the mucus correlates with the concentration of sperm in the ejaculate (Gould et al. 1984). In a randomized study, Ripps et al. (1994) performed intrauterine and peri-/intracervical insemination (semen deposited at the external cervical os with a syringe) – both with a standardized number of 50×10^6 spermatozoa – and after 4 h examined the peritoneal fluid and cervical mucus. After IUI with a 0.5 ml suspension of washed sperm, they found between 2×10^3 and 30×10^3 spermatozoa; however, they did not detect any sperm intraperitoneally after ICI, using small volumes of ejaculate (volumes adjusted to the number of sperm inseminated). Interestingly enough, cervical mucus contained significantly more spermatozoa after IUI than after ICI. The lower colonization rate of cervical mucus by peri-/intracervically deposited spermatozoa was attributed to a high attrition rate associated with sperm transport from the vaginal pool to the entire mucus column. This attrition effect is likely to be particularly strong in the case of small peri-/intracervical deposits, and the sperm are likely to be more intensely exposed to the deleterious action of the acidic vaginal environment than in the case of normal ejaculate volumes. However, the authors concluded that one therapeutic mechanism for IUI is the delivery of larger numbers of sperm to the fertilization site by rapid transit, and that increased retrograde colonization of the mucus after IUI may be another mechanism of action, involving sustained release of sperm.

In functional terms, cervical mucus constitutes a physiological barrier, especially to sperm of impaired quality. The mucus retains not only morphologically abnormal spermatozoa (Hanson and Overstreet 1981) and those coated with antisperm antibodies (Bronson et al. 1984a,b, Naz and Menge 1994), but also low-motility sperm. In fact, almost 100% of the sperm found in the mucus of fertile women are viable, and over 90% have intact acrosomes (Zinaman et al. 1989).

This effective filtration by the receptive mucus explains why, in the case of poor-quality semen, too few functional spermatozoa may be available to fertil-

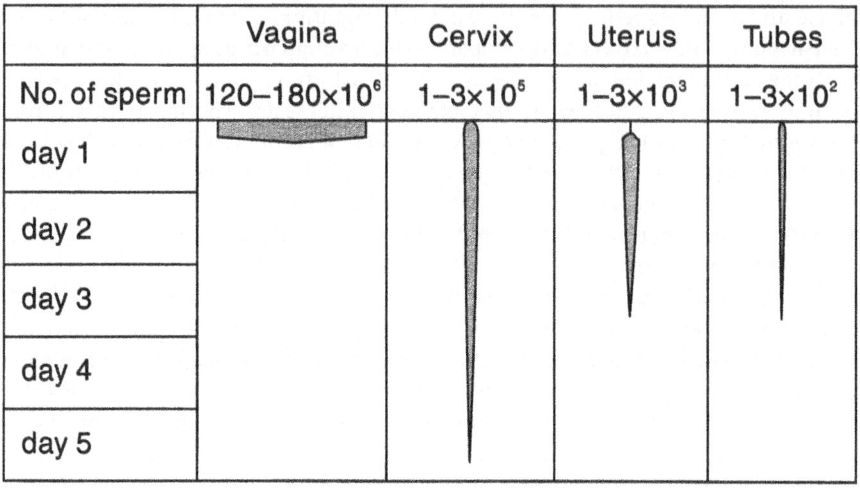

	Vagina	Cervix	Uterus	Tubes
No. of sperm	120–180×10⁶	1–3×10⁵	1–3×10³	1–3×10²
day 1				
day 2				
day 3				
day 4				
day 5				

Fig. 3. Passage of spermatozoa through the female genital tract after coitus. Drop in the number of spermatozoa between vagina and fallopian tubes. (From Diedrich et al. 1985)

ize the egg. On the other hand, even if semen quality is normal, hostile mucus or impaired mucus production (dysmucorrhea) may virtually reduce sperm concentrations to zero at the site of fertilization by blocking sperm entry.

The rationale for carrying out direct intracavitary insemination is that by circumventing the cervix the filtration effect of cervical mucus can be eliminated, thus increasing the concentration of vital and functional spermatozoa in the ampullary section of the fallopian tubes. Increased colonization of the fallopian tubes is often – and uncritically – cited as an argument for expecting higher pregnancy rates. However, in such general terms, this is not necessarily true if one considers, for instance, that semen preparation methods for IUI may produce sperm that are largely acrosome-reacted and less capable of zona binding and oocyte penetration; in addition, such sperm are also known to be subject to early senescence in the mucus.

Predictive Value of Sperm Parameters for Pregnancy Outcome

In individual cases it is almost impossible to predict the fertilizing potential of a semen sample (Devroey et al. 1998). The normal values of semen variables as given by the WHO (e.g., volume: ≥ 2.0 ml; sperm concentration: $\geq 20 \times 10^6$ spermatozoa/ml; total sperm count: $\geq 40 \times 10^6$ spermatozoa; motility: $\geq 50\%$ forward progression, or $\geq 25\%$ rapid progression; morphology: $\geq 30\%$; vitality: $\geq 75\%$) are empirical averages for which the fertility potential is known to be high in natural conception. However, as shown in Table 1, there is still a wide variability of semen characteristics which can lead to pregnancy. A comparison of fertile and infertile couples reveals considerable overlaps of the ranges of

Table 1. Semen characteristics of fertile and infertile patients. (From Barratt et al. 1995)

Characteristics	Fertile	Infertile
Volume	4 (1–8)	3 (0.5–5)
Sperm concentration ($\times 10^6$)	11 (11–241)	24 (10–337)
Progressive motility (%)	38 (9–86)	22 (0–86)

these variables (Barratt et al. 1995). This seems to indicate that sperm quality as determined by routine microscopy and fertility potential is not closely correlated with conception, and that it is only with a caveat that semen samples can be diagnosed as "normal" or "abnormal". Of course, if semen samples are extremely impaired, natural conception is unlikely. Nevertheless, conceptions have been recorded with sperm concentrations as low as 50 000/ml (Silber 1989), and attempts to achieve contraception by testosterone suppression of spermatogenesis are reported to have failed when sperm concentration remained as low as 3×10^6/ml (Wallace et al. 1992). Numerous prospective studies have shown that routine semen analysis is only a weak predictor of male fertility (e.g., Glazener et al. 1987; Polansky and Lamb 1988; Jouannet at al. 1988), and tests of sperm function suggest that there are men with low seminal sperm counts who have normal fertility, and vice versa (Hull 1992). This implies that it is sperm function which is of key importance for conception and not the commonly reported "male factor". In the final analysis, however, even complex in vitro tests of sperm function do not constitute safe predictors of fertility (Bolton et al. 1989). Jouannet et al. (1988) highlighted the problem when they said that the definition of normal and abnormal semen parameters was closely linked only to the biological end point of in vivo conception.

In day-to-day work, the WHO threshold values for normal semen samples are used to define the lower limits of male fertility. Because sperm is concentrated, introduced past the cervical mucus barrier, and may have immotile and abnormal forms removed by processing, the initial quality necessary for achieving pregnancy may be lower for IUI than the WHO normal values. Standards for initial sperm quality acceptable for IUI have not yet been established. Even though reference values are desirable from the practical point of view, they would be hard to define. Hence it is not surprising that the threshold values for performing IUI given in the literature differ widely. In a large cohort study, Campana et al. (1996) examined 332 infertile couples who underwent 1115 cycles of IUI with washed semen and in nonstimulated cycles identified a total motile sperm count of 20×10^6 spermatozoa as a threshold. On the other hand, in a study involving 1841 patients and 4056 cycles, Dickey et al. (1999) found for this combined seminal parameter a cut-off point before sperm preparation of only 5×10^6 motile sperm. For motility a critical level of 30% motile spermatozoa was identified. Above these threshold values the pregnancy rates per cycle given in these two studies were 8%. Almost no chance of success was reported when sperm values were lower. In their study of 61 patients that was specifically designed to establish threshold values for sperm used in IUI, McGovern et al. (1989) found that the only seminal sperm parameter significantly related to fecundity was progressive motility of ≥30%. Shulman et al. (1998) found none of the standard semen characteristics, such as volume, count, percentage motility, or percentage normal morphology, to correlate with cycle outcome after IUI and concluded that a spermatogram was not an accurate prognostic factor for therapeutic success. They also investigated standard parameters of the insemination specimen and found that the only variable to correlate significantly with the pregnancy rate was the degree of sperm motility following semen processing. Close to half (47.5%) of the couples studied conceived with most of the sperm presenting linear forward progression, whereas only 8% of the couples did so when sperm movement was slow. With regard to the morphology of spermatozoa to help predict the success or failure of IUI, different but probably not contradictory results are found in the literature (Toner et al. 1994; Matorras et al. 1995). Toner et al. (1994) examined the sperm parameters of the original semen specimens of 126 patients (40 of whom were donors) and found that percentage normal morphology assessed on the basis of strict Tygerberg criteria (Kruger et al. 1986; Menkveld et al. 1990) was the most significant predictor of pregnancy following COH/IUI. Linearity of movement significantly enhanced the predictive value of morphology alone. Overall, the pregnancy rates were significantly higher in cases with ≥14% normal morphology (15% per cycle) compared to cases with <14% normal morphology (7% per cycle). The threshold of 14% corresponded exactly with the results of studies published earlier by Kruger et al. (1986, 1987) on sperm morphology based on strict Tygerberg criteria and in vitro fertilization rates of human oocytes, according to which ejaculates with ≥14% normal forms are considered normal. Matorras et al. (1995), however, who also applied the Tygerberg criteria of normal sperm morphology, arrived at the conclusion that strict morphology analysis of the semen samples 1 month prior to IUI was not a useful prognostic factor in male subfertility. However, their conclusion probably does not contradict Toner et al. (1994), since in severe male-factor disorders the mean value of strict normal morphology should be lower than the predictive threshold value of 14% cited above. Indeed, the study of Matorras et al. (1995) presented no case with normal strict morphology ≥14% or a morphology index ≥30% (sum of normal and slightly amorphous forms), values which in the IVF studies mentioned above were shown to correlate with the highest fertilization and pregnancy rates and are therefore considered "normal" and excellent prognostic factors for semen specimens of men with normal sperm concentration and motility parameters. The fact that in their study Matorras et al. (1995) did not find any threshold levels for normal morphology or a morphology index indicates that in cases of male subfertility also other sperm variables relevant for the fertilization of oocytes, such as concentration and motility, have a predictive value. In IVF, motility parameters (% progressive motility and total motile sperm/ejaculate) were shown to have a profound influence on fertilization rates, thus adding to the predictive power of morphology (Grow et al. 1994). For IUI, it has been reported that an acceptable concentration of motile spermatozoa may offset the effects of abnormal sperm morphology (Irianni et al. 1993). No matter how critically one might view this statement, since intracorporeal fertilization results are not directly verifiable, it still seems worth mentioning in light of the above-average results of fallopian tube sperm perfusion (FSP), which is claimed to transport a larger number of motile sperm to the fertilization site than conventional IUI. In fact, in a prospective randomized study of IUI, using ejaculates from men with normal sperm concentrations and motility parameters and a morphology index <30% (mean 18.2±7.4) and normal strict morphology <10% (mean 3.6±2.8%), we did not find a single pregnancy, while with a morphology index ≥30% (mean 50.5±13.6) with strict normal morphology of 17.6±9.3% on average the ongoing pregnancy rate per patient and cycle was 21%. The difference between these two groups in terms of reproductive performance was statistically significant (Prietl and Haidl 1999, unpublished observation). Differential morphology was assessed on the basis of strict Düsseldorf criteria (Hofmann and Haider 1985). Our threshold limits of strict normal morphology and morphology index for IUI should be in keeping with the lower threshold limits for IVF defined by Kruger et al. (1988) in patients with normal morphology <14%. The authors broke this group down into two prognostic subgroups – a poor-prognosis pattern group (normal morphology <4%, morphology index <30%) and a good-prognosis pattern group (normal morphology 4–14%, morphology index ≥30%) – for which ongoing pregnancy rates of 7.6% and 18.7%, respectively, were identified. Interestingly, in IVF, application of Kruger's strict criteria has been shown to account for previously unexplained failed fertilization (Oehninger et al. 1988).

As yet, the literature offers only limited prospective data on the optimal number of motile spermatozoa in the insemination specimen and its correlation with pregnancies achieved. Considering the studies of Byrd et al. (1987, 1990), Horvath et al. (1989), Francavilla et al. (1990), Dodson and Haney (1991), and Campana et al. (1996), it is highly improbable that pregnancy can be achieved after homologous insemination of less than 1 million spermatozoa. Using a logarithmically transformed distribution of post-preparatory sperm numbers, Horvath et al. (1989) found a near-linear correlation of pregnancies per cycle in the range of 1×10^6 to 10×10^6 inseminated motile sperm after swim-up semen processing. However, in their studies using a double-wash technique Dodson and Haney (1991) did not establish any dependency of the pregnancy rate on the number of sperm inseminated. These authors account for the divergence of their results from those of Horvath et al. (1989) by arguing that the fertilization potential of spermatozoa could be influenced by the different methods used for semen preparation. Horvath et al. (1989) and Ho et al. (1992) suggest that among the routine parameters the total number of motile spermatozoa inseminated is the crucial criterion for conception. This was confirmed by Brasch et al. (1994) in a retrospective study involving 546 patients and more than 1200 IUI cycles. Huang et al. (1996) defined a cut-off level at a total motile sperm count of 5×10^6, with the success rate of IUI being significantly higher when this point is exceeded. This threshold agrees perfectly with the results of a discriminant analysis undertaken in our department of prospectively collected data on 494 couples and 840 cycles, where the women had patent tubes and had undergone ovulation induction and IUI. Logistic regression modeling involving the most relevant variables known to influence the outcome of assisted reproduction (e.g. 'couples' age, duration of subfertility, ovulation induction, number of follicles, estradiol concentration) revealed that the mean pregnancy rate achieved can be raised by an average of 7% ($p = 0.001$) by increasing the number of motile sperm in the inseminate by 1 million (Wilrodt-Klein 1999). There is no doubt, however, that linear forward progression is just as important (McGovern et al. 1989; Marshburn et al. 1992; Shulman et al. 1998), and that inseminates with an excellent degree of motility, higher than 80%, are highly successful (Arny and Quagliarello 1987; Horvath et al. 1989). As regards sperm morphology, there has so far been a lack of prospective data in the literature correlating the percentage of strict normal morphology of post-preparatory spermatozoa in the inseminates with treatment outcome. In the Bonn prospective randomized IUI study the thresholds of strict normal morphology according to the Düsseldorf criteria and of the morphology index were 6% and 25%, respectively, and were thus slightly lower than the thresholds prior to processing (Prietl 1998). As the total number of spermatozoa with normal morphology and linear progression in the inseminate constitutes the actual biologically relevant fraction, and post-preparatory results cannot be predicted for individual semen samples with sufficient accuracy, we use diagnostic spermatograms as a basis for our decisions on IUI; to this end, we apply the post-preparatory threshold values determined for our laboratory (total motile sperm count 5×10^6 spermatozoa, rapid forward progression 50%, normal morphology 6%, morphology index 25%). The experience thus gathered with conventional IUI led to a current overall birth rate of 20% per treatment cycle initiated in couples with unexplained subfertility (Prietl 1998).

Preparation of Semen Specimens

There is no doubt that the semen processing technique used and the care employed are crucial to the success of insemination. One objective of semen processing is to separate a high percentage of functional, progressively motile, and morphologically normal spermatozoa by removing defective and nonvital sperm as well as cells other than spermatozoa and debris. These cells include polygonal epithelial cells from the urethral tract, spermatogenic cells, and leukocytes. The other objective is to eliminate seminal plasma, which contains prostaglandins and cytokines, as well as possible antigenic or infectious matter. Regardless of the technique used, the preparation of the insemination specimen must be as gentle as possible in order not to affect the fertilizing potential of normal spermatozoa; during processing sperm function may be threatened by the secretion of cytotoxic cytokines and the generation of free oxygen radicals responsible for the initiation of a deleterious lipid peroxidation cascade in the sperm plasma membrane (Aitken and Clarkson 1987; Hill et al. 1987; Iwasaki and Gagnon 1992; Weese et al. 1993).

Semen is obtained by masturbation into a 60–100 ml wide-mouthed sterile container (glass or nontoxic polypropylene jar) after an optimal period of 3–5 days of sexual abstinence (Menkveld 1987; Menkveld and Kruger 1990). Ideally, the sample should be collected in the privacy of a room near the laboratory. The container should be warm, to minimize the risk of cold shock. If the sample is obtained at home it should be protected from extreme temperatures. Sperm motility and velocity are dependent upon cellular metabolism and are, therefore, temperature sensitive. Thus, sperm motility should be assessed at a standard temperature of 37 °C. Too long a period of abstinence may affect sperm count and motility and increase the proportion of contaminating cells and debris. In this regard it is important for each laboratory to comply with standards, since variability in this time period may increase the variability in the results and make comparisons between multiple specimens from individual patients virtually impossible (Centola 1993). After liquefaction, which normally occurs within 30 min at 37 °C, the semen sample should be thoroughly mixed, examined, processed, and inseminated immediately or within an hour of collection, at the latest. In cases of impaired liquefaction, increased consistency (often referred to as 'viscosity'), and inferior semen quality it may be useful to obtain split ejaculates (Perez-Pelaez and Cohen 1965). This means that the first three ejaculatory emissions are collected separately. In over 90% of all patients the concentration of spermatozoa is much higher in the first split fraction (up to 90% of all spermatozoa) than in the second fraction. This high concentration is usually combined with a markedly better motility (Farris and Murphy 1960; Elliasson and Lindholmer 1972). In addition, ejaculate consistency is lower in the first split fraction, as is prostaglandin concentration (Amelar and Hotchkiss 1965; Kremer 1979). However, in up to 10% of cases, the semen quality is superior in the second fraction. For this reason both the first and the second split fraction should be examined by means of simple microscopy to ascertain higher concentration and motility levels (Krebs 1989).

A variety of semen processing techniques are described in the literature that are recommended for IUI to produce a significantly higher percentage of functional spermatozoa. Each of these techniques has its specific advantages and drawbacks, and all methods may be suitable for normal semen samples. Accordingly, each laboratory has its own preferred routine method. Subnormal samples, however, may indeed represent a challenge. In such cases it is a crucial advantage to be able to draw on experience gathered with different techniques and to use them as circumstances require. The most widespread methods and their underlying principles are briefly described and discussed below.

Centrifugation and Washing

The traditional standard wash method uses centrifugation only to separate the cellular components of the semen specimen from the seminal plasma (Hanson and Rock 1951; Kaskarelis and Comninos 1959; Marrs et al. 1983; Wiltbank et al. 1985). To this end, the liquefied sample is first diluted with a suitable culture medium (e.g., supplemented Earle's medium, HEPES-buffered medium, commercial ready-to-use media), usually in a ratio of between 1:1 and 1:3. The suspension is then subjected to gentle centrifugation, preferably for 10 min at 200 × g or for 3(–5) min at 500 × g. The supernatant is decanted, and the resultant pellet is rediluted in a smaller volume (2 ml) of fresh medium. This wash procedure is repeated once (or twice). The final pellet is resuspended in the culture medium to achieve a total volume of about 0.5 ml for insemination. The spermatozoa are thus concentrated in a very small suspension volume. However, this method fails to separate motile and normally shaped sperm from immotile and morphologically poor spermatozoa and to eliminate other cells and debris (agglutinated sperm, immature spermatogenic forms, polygonal epithelial cells from the urethral tract, white blood cells, and particulate matter) commonly seen in the ejaculate. This technique may be considered in cases where sperm density is low, and the second centrifugation step may be omitted ("soft wash") for severely oligozoospermic samples, as this will result in higher sperm recovery. However, "incomplete" washing does not sufficiently reduce prostaglandin concentrations and possible microbial contaminants in the inseminates, thus causing painful cramps. This is why it is in exceptional cases only that we use centrifugation as the sole preparatory step for intrauterine inseminates, i.e., ejaculates which have surprisingly low sperm counts when leukocyte counts are low. In our day-to-day routine, however, we still perform gentle centrifugation of all normal and marginally subnormal semen samples prior to swim-up or glass-wool filtration, bearing in mind that vigorous centrifugal pelleting may impair the fertilizing ability of spermatozoa.

As a rule, both centrifugal force and centrifugation time should be kept as low as possible, since sperm and white blood cells in the ejaculate are rich in polyunsaturated fatty acids and are particularly sensitive to lipid peroxidation membrane damage induced by reactive oxygen species (ROS) (Aitken and Clarkson 1988). It is almost impossible to propose generally valid guidelines for optimal centrifuging, as effective separation of cellular components from seminal plasma requires the pellets to have a certain consistency while detrimental ROS activity should be avoided. However, the ROS patterns observed in many ejaculates vary widely and are often unpredictable. The centrifuging times and forces mentioned above of 10 min at 200 × g or 3(–5) min at 500 × g are recommendations resulting from one of our own prospective series involving 250 normal semen samples from different individuals in which, after satisfactory separation of the solid and liquid phases, the lowest average ROS activities were measured by chemiluminiscence (Noack and Prietl 1999, unpublished observation). While effects generated by ROS and other mechanisms potentially prejudicial to the functional capacity of a sperm sample may not be that strong and hence are unproblematic for most normal semen specimens, they may well be deleterious in male-factor cases (Aitken et al. 1989, 1992; Mortimer 1991; Quinn 1993; Alvarez et al. 1993). This applies in particular to ejaculates with a substantial proportion of membrane-defective and dead spermatozoa, as well as to leukocytospermic samples.

Swim-Up and Swim-Down Methods

The principle underlying the swim-up methods is that motile spermatozoa separate from liquefied semen, or alternatively from washed pellets, and swim up into supernatant culture media, leaving most of the immotile sperm, other cells, and debris behind (Drevius 1971; Lopata et al. 1976; Russell and Rogers 1987; Harris et al. 1981; Makler et al. 1984b; Cohen et al. 1985).

Swim-Up from Semen. With this method, several aliquots of liquefied semen are placed in round-bottom tubes underneath an overlay of culture medium. Preferably, small volumes of semen (0.5–1.0 ml) and 1.0 ml of culture medium should be used in 15-ml centrifuge tubes. This portioning process helps to maximize the combined total interface area between semen and culture medium. The tubes may also be prepared by gently layering culture medium over liquefied semen. After incubation for 30–60 min at 37 °C, all supernatants are carefully lifted; the separate preparations are combined, centrifuged once at $200 \times g$ for 10 min or at $500 \times g$ for 3(–5) min, and finally resuspended in culture medium to achieve a total of 0.5 ml for insemination.

Swim-Up from Washed Pellets. After the sperm have been gently washed and concentrated, as described above, 0.5–1.0 ml of culture medium is carefully layered over the final pellet and the sample is incubated for 30–60 min at 37 °C in a 5% CO_2-in-air atmosphere. It is recommended that the tube be held at an angle of 45 ° so that a larger interface is created. Slight turbidity of the supernatant is macroscopic evidence of the fact that the sperm are migrating into the diluent. The supernatant (swim-up specimen) is then collected, with care taken not to disturb the pellet at the bottom.

The swim-up techniques provide an excellent isolation of almost exclusively motile spermatozoa containing a high percentage of morphologically normal sperm (McDowell et al. 1985; Cruz et al. 1986; Hughes et al. 1987; Russell and Rogers 1987). The rate of sperm loss, however, tends to be high and may exceed 90%, depending on the sample consistency, sperm motility, and the volumes used for processing (Kerin et al. 1984; Arny and Quagliarello 1987). Using the swim-up method from semen, viscous samples should be blended with a small amount of culture medium prior to layering because otherwise too low a percentage of spermatozoa will enter the culture medium. Too dense pellets resulting from vigorous centrifugation will lead to low sperm yields in post-migration preparations, as many motile spermatozoa are retained in the compacted pellet and hence cannot reach the interface with the overlaying culture medium.

Swim-Down from Semen. It has been stressed in the literature that the problem with the swim-up procedure is that sperm have to migrate against gravitational force (Lopata et al. 1976; Russell and Rogers 1987; Makler et al. 1993). Thus, to enhance sperm recovery it has been recommended that the semen be layered directly over the medium and that the swim-down sperm be collected rather than the swim-up sperm (Urry et al. 1983; Aitken and Clarkson 1988; Gonzales and Pella 1993).

Glass-Wool Filtration

A glass-wool filter, trapping in its fabric a high percentage of immotile, membrane-defective, and agglutinated sperm, as well as leukocytes, immature germ cells, epithelia, and debris, is used to isolate high-quality spermatozoa (Paulson and Polakoski 1977; Jeyendran et al. 1986).

Ready-to-use glass-wool filtration kits are commercially available. However, we prefer a traditional self-made system using a tuberculin syringe, at the bottom of which we place 15 mg of glass wool (microfiber code 112; Manville Co., Denver, Colo.). The filter fabric should not be too close-meshed or rise more than 3–4 mm from the bottom of the syringe (0.06-ml mark). Just before use, the sterilized filter is rinsed twice with 2 ml medium to remove any loose glass-fiber particles. The rinsing medium is then examined microscopically for glass-wool fragments. Generally, it is recommended to filter well-liquefied semen or, in the case of viscous ejaculate, diluted semen. We subject normal semen samples to a pre-wash procedure before suspensions are placed upon the glass-wool column and allowed to pass through the filter solely by gravity. Finally, the filter is rinsed with 0.2–0.3 ml medium to ensure that as little sperm suspension as possible is left behind (Jeyendran et al. 1986; van der Ven et al. 1988). Compared with the original semen sample, the filtrate mostly contains a much higher percentage of motile spermatozoa combined with a morphologically superior selection. The sperm loss rate of average normal semen samples is generally lower (60–70%) than that usually associated with the swim-up technique, but other cellular and acellular matter is not completely eliminated. For IUI we prefer to use glass-wool filtration, especially in cases of moderate oligozoospermia and asthenozoospermia, since it may yield a satisfactory sperm recovery rate (Tünnerhoff et al. 1986; van der Ven et al. 1988; Rhemrev et al. 1989). This rate can be increased significantly by employing two filter columns operating in parallel (Prietl 1998). It was indicated in an earlier report that filtration by glass wool could induce damage to the sperm plasma membranes and acrosomes in spermatozoa (Sherman et al. 1981). However, Jeyendran et al. (1986) later demonstrated that sperm recovered from glass-wool columns retain the functional integrity of their membranes. Moreover, it has been shown that spermatozoa separated by means of glass-wool filtration are functionally superior to the original ejaculate and have a higher potential to penetrate zona-free hamster ova (Rana et al. 1989). In addition, Katayama et al. (1989) found that glass-wool filtration of sperm resulted in a higher percentage of in vitro fertilized human oocytes than did the swim-up procedure.

Density Gradient Separation Systems

Effective density gradient separation systems are widely used to prepare sperm for both extracorporeal (IVF and ICSI) and intracorporeal (GIFT and IUI) fertilization. Buoyant density gradient centrifugation provides for a substantial separation of progressively motile, high-quality spermatozoa by virtue of their enhanced velocity and relatively high density (Lessley and Garner 1983; Berger et al. 1985; Pousette et al. 1986; Gellert-Mortimer et al. 1988; Tanphaichitr et al. 1988; McClure et al. 1989; Serafini et al. 1990) and at the same time produces high-purity samples that are essentially free from microbial or other contaminants (Bolton et al. 1986; Punjabi et al. 1990). It has also been demonstrated that the density gradient systems keep lipid peroxidation of spermatozoa low by separating most of the ROS-producing cells from the normal and functional cells, and that spermatozoa prepared by this approach have an enhanced capacity for fertilization (Aitken and Clarkson 1988; Serafini et al. 1990; Jaroudi et al. 1993). The mechanisms underlying the selection of highly motile spermatozoa are not completely understood. It may be assumed that because of the density gradients, progressively motile sperm – yielding to the centrifugal force – tend to actively migrate to the bottom of the centrifuge tube (Rhemrev et al. 1989). Obviously, the recovery rate of the desirable subpopulation of functional spermatozoa is dependent largely on the quality of the original semen sample (Mortimer and Mortimer 1988). While the yield may be high in normal specimen, very low yields can frequently be seen in astheno- and oligozoospermic ejaculates. Unlike IVF or ICSI, this limits the range of semen samples eligible for density gradient processing for intrauterine insemination.

Ficoll, a synthetic sucrose polymer, was the first in a series of buoyant density gradient materials (Harrison 1976); the best known of these substances and the one most widely used in clinical applications has been Percoll (Pertoft 1977; Gorus and Pipeleers 1981). However, a few years ago, serious concern was expressed about the PVP component and endotoxin levels of Percoll, a colloidal polyvinylpyrrolidone (PVP)-coated silica particle preparation. This is why Percoll should definitely not be used anymore for human gametes. Other colloidal gradients, which were then developed for density separation and which are assumed to be less harmful, contain silica particles coated with silane instead of PVP (e.g., PureSperm, ISolate, Sil-Select). However, since it is well known that silica particles may cause tissue irritation, a caveat also applies to the use of silica-containing preparation media, especially for intracorporeal fertilization techniques (IUI, GIFT). Nycondenz (iohexol), an iodinated organic molecule dissolved in TRIS buffer, or Ixaprep, a combination of polysucrose and iodixanol, have been available for years as alternative silica-free gradient media. It was shown that a four-layer discontinuous iohexol gradient can indeed very effectively isolate functional long-lived motile sperm from oligo- and asthenozoospermic semen samples. Under the trade names of Omnipaque, Accupaque, and Visipaque, iohexol and iodixanol are used worldwide as radiopaque media for radiological diagnosis (e.g., angiography, arthrography, urography, hysterosalpingography) with a low incidence of adverse reactions.

There are two categories of density gradients: continuous and discontinuous. While with continuous gradients density increases gradually from the top to the bottom, discontinuous gradients are composed of several layers of different concentrations, typically in the 40–90% range. With both methods gradients are overlaid with semen and centrifuged. The discontinuous density gradient, usually consisting of two or three layers, is used most widely. A two-layer gradient column is prepared by placing, for example, 1 ml of a 90% solution on the bottom of a small conical tube and adding 1 ml of a 45% solution without disturbing the interface between the two concentrations. Alternatively, the 90% layer may be gently pipetted under the 40% layer. Finally, a maximum of 2.0 ml of well-liquefied ejaculate is layered over the gradient and the tube is centrifuged for 10–20 min at 200–300 × g. Following centrifugation, the bottom layer of the gradient, containing the highest percentage of motile sperm, is aspirated with a pipette and suspended in 2 ml of physiological medium. Following one to two wash runs, required to remove the gradient material, the final pellet is resuspended in culture medium to achieve a total volume of 0.5 ml for intrauterine insemination.

Other Semen-Processing Methods

As comparatively little use is made of the methods mentioned below, they are described only briefly. As regards other procedures such as the separation of sperm by means of semi-permeable membranes (Agarwal et al. 1991) and the migration of sperm through glass tubes (Wang et al. 1992), the interested reader is kindly requested to refer to the literature. In clinical use, albumin columns for gradient separation of motile sperm by means of human or bovine serum albumin (Ericsson et al. 1973; Glass and Ericsson 1978; Dmowski et al. 1979) should nowadays be of historical interest only.

The *Sperm Select* separation method is a modification of the swim-up technique where high-purity sodium hyaluronate (mean molecular weight 3 000 000 Da) is layered over the semen sample (Wikland et al. 1987). Hyaluronate is a linear polysaccharide whose composition is similar to that of cervical mucus, acting as a filter that motile spermatozoa can pass. The final concentration recommended for this purpose in a culture medium is 1 mg/ml. It would seem that spermatozoa selected with this technique are exposed to less oxidative damage and can be directly inseminated without any additional washing. This procedure has been reported to produce a significantly higher separation of motile spermatozoa and also higher pregnancy rates after in vitro fertilization than the conventional swim-up method using washed pellets (Huszar et al. 1990; Wikland et al. 1987). It is not known whether these favorable effects result mainly from the use of hyaluronate or from the fact that centrifugal pelleting is avoided.

With another method, semen is layered on top of *Sephadex gel columns* (Steeno et al. 1975; Graham et al. 1976; Drobnis et al. 1991; Zavos and Centola 1991) and is allowed to pass the gel solely by gravity. Sephadex gel is a filter consisting of a three-dimensional network which motile sperm can pass while immotile cells are retained. After the procedure, however, the filtrate still contains seminal plasma components and requires subsequent centrifugation in order to obtain pure preparations. A commercially available sperm separation kit based on the use of Sephadex beads (SpermPrep) may produce reasonable yields of motile and morphologically normal spermatozoa from the original semen samples (Zavos 1992).

There are many variants of each of the semen processing methods described, and the question arises as to which technique is best suited for IUI. Many publications have addressed this issue. Since their conclusions are quite divergent, it is not possible to give a single answer. This is why the sperm recovery rates cited above for the various methods should be regarded as reference values which may vary considerably, depending on semen quality. For this reason every laboratory should be able to perform several techniques (e.g., swim-up method, glass-wool filtration, density gradient separation) to select – based on their own experience – the most appropriate method for a specific semen sample. We would use the swim-up technique primarily for normozoospermia as a simple and quick way of producing a purified inseminate containing a high percentage of progressively motile spermatozoa. Given a normal ejaculate volume, the sperm loss rate to be expected would be acceptable. For the various manifestations of sperm disorders (oligozoospermia, asthenozoospermia, teratozoospermia), filtration and density gradient separation methods tend to be superior to the swim-up technique. However, since this is not true of every ejaculate and since every separation process may cause damage (e.g., to the acrosome or to the spermatozoal membranes), it is recommendable to prescreen with the method of choice and monitor long-term motility. Particular attention should be paid, however, to the presence of abundant leukocytes in ejaculates. The efficiency of antibiotic treatment of subfertile men showing symptoms of prostatitis, urethritis, or epididymitis is undisputed (Puris and Christiansen 1993). In subclinical chronic infections, a combined antiphlogistic and antibiotic treatment can effectively reduce leukocyte concentration and enhance sperm motility (Haidl 1990). Leukocytes – especially neutrophils – are a substantial source of ROS (Jones et al. 1979; Aitken et al. 1992; Kovalski et al. 1992). Studies indicate that as long as spermatozoa are surrounded by epididymal and seminal plasma, antioxidant factors (e.g., glutathione peroxidase, superoxide dismutase, catalase, ascorbate, and α-tocopherol) largely protect them from the harmful effects of oxidative stress (Alvarez et al. 1987; Alvarez and Storey 1989; Perry et al. 1992, 1993; Zini et al. 1993; Lewis et al. 1997). However, centrifuging high-leukocyte ejaculates prior to swim-up or glass-wool filtration will increase the risk of oxygen radicals causing oxidative damage and of initiating the lipid peroxidation cascade in the sperm plasma membranes. The oxidative attack of free radicals is directed against the double bonds of unsaturated fatty acids, resulting in a deleterious accumulation of lipid peroxides in those membranes. As a result of this self-propagating mechanism, sperm motility will be impaired and the acrosome will be damaged, and hence the ability of sperm-oocyte fusion will be lost. This is why semen samples with high leukocyte concentrations ($\geq 1 \times 10^7$/ml) should be processed using methods which either do not require centrifugation and pelleting (e.g., swim-up from semen, glass-wool filtration) or involve sperm washing only after cell separation (e.g., density gradient separation). We have already drawn attention repeatedly to the general need for gentle centrifugation of all samples, irrespective of their quality.

In summary, it should be emphasized that special care should be given to semen processing to optimize the recovery of progressively motile and – most importantly – functional spermatozoa from the ejaculates. Successful IUI, especially in the case of male subfertility, invariably requires high-quality semen processing in the laboratory.

Intrauterine Transfer of Spermatozoa

Standard Technique

It is characteristic of conventional IUI that motile spermatozoa obtained from the ejaculate are concentrated in low suspension volumes of 0.3–0.5 ml and deposited in the fundus of the uterus. The rationale for inseminating small volumes is to avoid reflux through the cervix into the vagina, or efflux through the tubes into the peritoneal cavity. Catheters of various sizes and diameters are commercially available for this purpose. It is important that the catheter material not have a toxic effect on the gametes; it should give the catheter a certain stiffness, but at the same time provide some flexibility at its distal end to ensure that the uterine flexion can be negotiated without any harm to the endometrium. The catheter tip should preferably be rounded, with side holes to prevent any injury to the site of embryo nidation. With the woman in the dorsal lithotomy position, the cervix is exposed with a moistened bivalve speculum and rinsed with physiological saline. Antiseptic solutions must be strictly avoided. The catheter is firmly connected to the cone of a 1-cc tuberculin syringe, the plunger is withdrawn slightly, and the sperm suspension is then aspirated from the test tube into the catheter without any air bubbles. If catheter passage through the cervical canal proves difficult the cervix may be grasped with a tenaculum to straighten the utero-cervical angle by gentle traction. Rough probing or dilatation of the cervical canal should be avoided, as any insensitive manipulation may cause bleeding, uterine contractions, and pain. If a cervical resistance cannot be overcome at first, it is advisable to bend the distal part of the catheter slightly or to use a catheter set with a curved guiding cannula. In most cases only a little patience will then be required to solve the problem. Once the internal os has been passed the catheter tip is advanced close to the fundus of the uterus and the inseminate is gently expelled. It is recommended to leave the catheter in place for a short while and then withdraw it slowly to avoid a suction effect and prevent reflux. After the procedure the patient should rest for 15 min. As simple as the procedure may seem, one cannot overstate the significance of an atraumatic sperm transfer, since a poorly performed technique is frequently responsible for low pregnancy rates – a problem which is also well known with IVF/ET.

Fallopian Tube Sperm Perfusion

Fallopian tube sperm perfusion (FSP) may be regarded as a special method of intrauterine insemination (Kahn et al. 1992, 1993). The essential difference between this procedure and conventional insemination is that the inseminate volume is typically 4 ml. As described by Kahn et al., the inseminate is prepared by adding culture medium to the sperm suspension after processing. This large volume is chosen to ensure that part of the suspension perfuses the tubes so that a greater number of spermatozoa are flushed passively into the oviducts. The catheter does not cause any tubal trauma in the process because the inseminate is transferred only into the uterine cavity. It is recommended to inseminate slowly, at a rate of 1 ml/min, to avoid adverse effects such as uterine and tubal contractions or vasovagal reactions. Having gathered experience with this method over several years we have not observed any patient discomfort caused by the larger inseminate volume, nor have we seen any pelvic infection. We did find, however, frequent reflux from the cervical canal since, unlike Kahn et al., we did not use Allis clamps to seal the external os. With FSP it seems to be particularly important that insemination is performed before ovulation occurs; since otherwise, the oocyte might be flushed out of the tube.

Timing and Number of Inseminations, Monitoring of Cycles

In natural intercourse, cervical mucus and cervical crypts act as a reservoir at midcycle, ensuring a gradual release and constant supply of long-lived sperm into the upper reproductive tract (Moghissi 1984). Where the mucus performs this physiological function, it is possible to postulate a biological "window of opportunity" with a higher probability of syngamy. It can be assumed that spermatozoa retain their fertilizing capacity in the female genital tract for a period of 40–80 h (Gould et al. 1994), while oocytes are likely to have a life-span of only 12–24 h after ovulation (Moghissi 1986; Weinberg and Wilcox 1995). The relatively short period of time during which oocytes retain their potential to be fertilized requires the presence – during that period – of a few hundred motile and functional sperm in the ampulla of the tubes. In fact, a vanguard of ejaculated spermatozoa is capable of leaving the cervical pool very rapidly and reaching the oocyte in a capacitated state. Basic studies conducted by Settlage et al. (1973) have demonstrated that rapid sperm transport to the oviducts can take place within only 5 min. Furthermore, it has been shown that even India ink particles placed in the cervix can reach the peritoneal cavity within 15 min (Boer 1972). It can be assumed that mechanical (and possibly also chemical) stimuli lead to reflex-mediated contraction of the uterus and the fallopian tubes, which perform the passive sperm transport. The (physiological) rationale for this rapid transit of an initial sperm cell population through the genital tract is still unclear, and the question as to whether it is really the primary biological function of these early sperm to fuse with the oocyte is still a matter of debate (Overstreet 1996). Unlike the initial phase of rapid sperm transport, there is an extended period during the subsequent phase in which the oocytes can become fertilized due to sustained sperm release from the cervical depot. However, the essential criterion for the optimum timing of natural intercourse is the receptivity of the cervical mucus, which undergoes cyclic changes in response to sex steroids and which has a major impact on the extent of mucus colonization. Favorable changes in the mucus occur only at the end of the follicular phase in the presence of maximum estrogen levels; optimum receptivity is reached with the onset of the luteinizing hormone (LH) surge in the serum or with the peak of LH secretion, which occurs 12 h later on average (Moghissi et al. 1982; Hoff et al. 1983). Subsequently, mucus receptivity decreases progressively in response to increasing progesterone secretion. However, sperm concentration and linear velocity are factors which are of similarly great importance for mucus colonization and which are indispensable for the penetration of sperm into the cervical mucus. The onset of the LH surge in the serum is regarded as an early reference point for the prediction of ovulation, which in the vast majority of women can be expected to occur only 37 h later (Testart and Frydman 1982; Edwards and Purdy 1982). The average time oocytes need for maturation is also 37 h (from the onset of the LH surge until metaphase II of the meiosis), both in vivo and in vitro (Seibel et al. 1982). Consequently, the optimum timing – for both natural intercourse and intracervical insemination (ICI) – is between 2 days before and the day of ovulation, with the conception rate being highest at the beginning of this period. On the day after ovulation, the probability of conception is virtually zero (Wilcox et al. 1995). Thus, in view of what has been said about the gamete's life span and about the receptivity of the cervical mucus, coitus does not necessarily have to be timed with ovulation as long as there is a constant supply of long-lived motile sperm in the oviducts (Moghissi 1986); furthermore, one would expect that the optimum timing of intercourse and ICI is earlier than that of IUI (Ford et al. 1997), for the reasons discussed below.

Unlike natural intercourse and intracervical insemination, it can be assumed in intrauterine insemination that the majority of the sperm deposited directly in the uterine cavity will reach the fallopian tubes within a very short period of time and that some of them will be discharged into the peritoneal cavity, where they will probably be phagocytized (Moghissi 1986). A delay in the release of spermatozoa from the mucus after intrauterine insemination is possibly of no major importance, because fewer functional sperm are stored in the cervix (Glezerman et al. 1984). This is why it is considered crucial to accurately predict the time of ovulation when insemination methods are used in which the cervical canal is bridged by a catheter (Allen et al. 1985; Moghissi 1986; Kemmann et al. 1987). Traditional methods used to this end include basal body temperature (BBT) records (Moghissi 1976), assessing the amount, spinnbarkeit, and ferning of the cervical mucus (Insler et al. 1972) and vaginal cytology. In order to be reliable, BBT measurements require two-phase temperature curves, reflecting the sensitivity of the hypothalamic temperature regulation center to the thermogenetic property of progesterone. The method can fail simply because the temperature center may be refractory to progesterone. It has been reported that over 10% of all actual ovulatory cycles are accompanied by a single-phase temperature profile (Moghissi 1976). However, limitations in predicting ovulation are usually due to the fact that the nadir of the BBT curve shows a wide range of scatter over time and that the diagnosis of ovulation can be made only retrospectively. Templeton et al. (1982) found the nadir of basal temperature within a period of 1 day before until 1 day after the day of the LH peak in only 55% of the ovulatory cycles. Mastroianni et al. (1957) found that if ovulation is determined on the basis of BBT charts, only 65% of inseminations are performed during the immediate periovulatory period. Multiple periovulatory inseminations, however, resulted in overall conception rates of up to 60% per patient (Barwin 1974; Glezerman et al. 1984). A method more reliable than BBT measurements in predicting impending ovulation is the determination of the cervical score according to Insler. Templeton et al. (1982) found that the score was optimum within a period of 1 day before to 1 day after the day of the LH peak in 92% of the ovulatory cycles. Although the temporal scatter of the optimum cervical score is much less pronounced than the scatter of the reference point of the BBT curve, it should be emphasized that the interpretation of the cervical score is very subjective. In addition, supraphysiological estrogen concentrations or local antiestrogenic effects caused by hormone stimulation (clomiphene citrate) can distort the cervical pattern, which makes it very difficult to predict ovulation. In modern reproductive medicine, the traditional methods used to predict the onset of ovulation have been largely discarded and replaced by monitoring hormones and follicles. Transvaginal ultrasonography is a standard practice today which is indispensable – in particular in ovarian induction cycles – in order to monitor the number of developing follicles and to avoid higher-order multiple pregnancies. However, there is a residual risk in hormone-stimulated cycles because it may be that not all the potentially ovulatory follicles are detected. For this reason, it is recommendable – especially if ultrasonography reveals polycystic ovaries – to measure estradiol (E_2) serum concentrations in addition, based on random samples. This also makes it easier to assess the risk of ovarian hyperstimulation syndrome (OHSS). Despite linear growth throughout the follicular phase, follicle size is not a reliable predictive parameter for the accurate timing of the onset of ovulation (Vermesh et al. 1987). This is due to the fact that the mean range of the ovulatory follicle size varies substantially (between 18 and 26 mm). Macnamee et al. (1988) reported that up to 20% of patients treated with clomiphene citrate (CC) and human menopausal gonadotropin (hMG) exhibited an endogenous LH surge before the leading follicles reached a diameter of between 18 and 20 mm. Unlike ultrasound monitoring, the endogenous onset of the LH surge is an early predictor of impending ovulation and a generally reliable reference point. As already mentioned, Testart et al. (1981) found in a large-scale study that follicular rupture occurred during natural cycles almost always after the 37th hour following the onset of the serum LH rise (range: 33–43 h). However, the timing of the LH onset is subject to wide intra- and interindividual variations. In this context, attention should be drawn to the findings of a study which showed that in 16% of the women, ovulation occurred prior to the LH peak (WHO 1980); this also suggests that the LH peak is a less reliable reference point than the onset of the LH surge. However, hormone measurements – in combination with ultrasonography – are the best predictors of ovulation. For economic reasons, combined monitoring is carried out only to provide orientation, also in patients receiving hormone stimulation. This means that only very few ultrasound and E_2 scans are sufficient in the majority of cycles in order to adjust the dose of medication (controlled ovarian stimulation). Experienced clinicians will use additional LH measurements only immediately before the onset of ovulation. For practical reasons – mainly for traveling convenience – patients themselves may use home-kit urinary LH assays to determine the onset of ovulation with sufficient accuracy (Martinez et al. 1991; Agarwal and Buyalos 1995; Deaton et al. 1997; Zreik et al. 1999). However, since these ovulation prediction kits have a lower detection limit for urinary LH concentrations of usually 20–40 IU/l (the color of the substrate changes as a function of the LH concentration), it must be borne in mind that false-negative results may be obtained in patients with a low ovulatory LH peak amplitude, short expression of the periovulatory LH concentration curve and in dilute urine (Zreik et al. 1999). Although LH enters the urine already 3–4 h after its initial discharge into the plasma (Edwards and Brody 1995c), a positive urine result is often found only 12 h after the onset of the LH surge in the serum (i.e., around the point of the serum LH peak), or even later if tests are performed only once or twice daily (Nulsen et al. 1987). This interval must be taken into account when timing the onset of the serum LH surge. This means that ovulation must be expected to occur on average as early as 25 h after a positive urine test. If one adds a fertilizing life span for the ovulated ovum of only 12 h to be on the safe side (Moghissi 1986), intrauterine insemination 37 h after the positive urine test may be very satisfactory. However, if one uses urinary LH detection kits for timing natural intercourse or intracervical insemination, both should be performed immediately or within a few hours after the positive LH result because, on average, the receptivity of the cervical mucus is optimum at the onset or the peak of the serum LH surge (Moghissi et al. 1982). Later on, increasing progesterone secretion leads to a hostile mucus, thus significantly reducing the probability of conception, which already decreases drastically on the day after the urine LH surge (Odem et al. 1991).

Considering that endogenous LH secretion is an event crucial to the maturation process of the follicles and the oocytes (resumption of meiosis), the question arises as to whether it is preferable to wait for the LH surge to occur spontaneously and for maturation to take place naturally, or whether it is also possible to induce ovulation with human chorionic gonadotropin (hCG). The exogenous hCG bolus mimics the endogenous LH surge and offers the advantage that the onset of the LH surge is known precisely. Based on their findings in a controlled crossover study conducted in 48 CC-stimulated patients, Martinez et al. (1991) recommend that one should wait for the onset of the endogenous LH surge and allow the natural maturation process to happen. They found a higher pregnancy rate (20%) in these cycles after IUI than in cycles in which ovulation had been induced with hCG (9%). An analysis of midcycle events showed that, based on sonographic criteria, hCG was administered significantly earlier when compared with the occurrence of a spontaneous LH surge. In addition, the mean diameter of the preovulatory follicles was significantly smaller and insemination was substantially earlier in the hCG-induced cycles. However, other investigators did not find any differences in the probability of conception between patients whose ovulation was triggered primarily by hCG and others who showed a spontaneous LH surge (Agarwal and Buyalos 1995; Deaton et al. 1997; Zreik et al. 1999). Nevertheless, hCG is widely used in most IUI programs to time ovulation and to promote the final maturation of follicles and oocytes. It is interesting to note that Fuh et al. (1997) observed improved pregnancy rates in IUI cycles in which the administration of hCG was delayed by 8–20 h after a spontaneous LH surge had been detected in the morning serum (20%), compared with cycles in which hCG was given before the onset of the LH rise (14%).

We generally perform intrauterine insemination in gonadotropin-stimulated cycles, usually beginning with 50–75 IU of FSH on day 4 of the cycle. Patients are stimulated on a daily basis, and the dose can be carefully increased after several days, if ultrasound and E_2 scans suggest that no more than three ovulatory follicles will develop in both ovaries. Monitoring is performed at an average interval of approximately 3 days, and routinely in the morning. When the dominant follicle has reached a diameter of 18–20 mm, we trigger ovulation in the evening, using 5000 IU of hCG. Insemination is performed 36–40 h after ovulation induction. In cases in which the endogenous serum LH concentration is significantly higher than on the previous day (doubling of LH concentrations), insemination is performed during the late morning of the following day. This time schedule is appropriate because most women have the onset of their natural LH surge at about 3 a.m., and they will ovulate on average 37 h later, at about 4 p.m. (Edwards et al. 1980). In cases where we detect elevated LH levels combined with a progesterone shift (1.5-fold increase in progesterone relative to basal levels), we perform insemination immediately, i.e., within a few hours of the blood test. No insemination is performed in patients who present more than three follicles >16 mm on the day of ovulation induction; these patients are administered gestagens in a transformation dose, and they are asked to abstain from sexual intercourse.

Andersen et al. (1995) closely studied the time elapsing between hCG administration and follicular rupture after stimulation with clomiphene citrate, by performing ultrasound checks at short intervals. They found that the mean time to ovulation was 37 h (range: 34–46 h). They also established that in 66% of the cycles studied, the largest follicle was the first to rupture. The pregnancy rate per cycle achieved after IUI was well over 16%. In ovulation induction cycles, follicles do not all rupture at the same time; instead, they rupture in waves and in the course of several hours (Abbasi et al. 1987). Theoretically, this provides a wide window for effective insemination. Since it can be assumed that a large number of spermatozoa leave the genital tract very soon after intracavitary insemination, multiple periovulatory inseminations performed at intervals should theoretically increase the probability of conception. However, there is no consensus in the literature on this matter. Silverberg et al. (1992) were the first to address this issue in a prospective, randomized study comparing single intrauterine insemination 34 h after hCG administration (periovulatory insemination) with double intrauterine insemination timed 18 and 42 h after hCG (one before and one after ovulation). The fecundity rate per human menopausal gonadotropin (hMG)-stimulated cycle achieved after double insemination was 50%, compared with 8.7% after single insemination, showing a difference of 600% between treatment groups. These results contradict those of another prospective, randomized study conducted by Ransom et al. (1994) who did not find any difference in pregnancy rates per cycle between single insemination performed 35 h after ovulatory hCG (11%) and double insemination timed 19 and 43 h after hCG (14%). The authors conclude from their data that a single well-timed insemination is sufficient in women undergoing controlled ovarian hyperstimulation (COH) and IUI therapy. It is difficult to explain the discrepancy between these two investigations, which have a fairly identical design. The third and so far latest prospective, randomized study on this subject was published only recently (Ragni et al. 1999). Based on the number of cycles included (449 cycles), the study claims a statistical power of 80% and a confidence level of 95% for its results. This three-arm, parallel study was conducted over a period of 2 years. Patients were stimulated with 100 mg clomiphene citrate per day for 5 days and 75–150 IU of pure FSH starting on day 6. When the dominant follicle had reached a size of 18–20 mm, ovulation was triggered by administering a dose of 5000 IU hCG. Couples with both male-factor infertility and couples with unexplained infertility were enrolled in the study (a total of 273 couples). Pregnancy rates following single insemination performed 34 h after hCG administration (group A) were statistically compared with rates achieved following double insemination after 12 and 34 h (group B) and double insemination 34 and 60 h after ovulation induction with hCG (group C). For both indications (male factor and unexplained infertility combined), the overall pregnancy rate per cycle was 8% for group A, 19% for group B, and 7% for group C. The authors suggest that the statistically superior results achieved in group B were attributable to the full utilization of the insemination window. In their discussion, they refer to a study by Templeton et al. (1996), pointing out that after clomiphene citrate "a certain number of oocytes can be fertilized as early as 12 h after hCG administration". The study does not explain why inseminations were performed in group C as late as 60 h after hCG administration, even though it is known that most patients ovulate much earlier. Thus, the lack of a statistical difference in the pregnancy rates between groups A and C seems to be in keeping with the correct timing of inseminations 34 h after hCG, and the higher pregnancy rate in group B must indeed be attributable to an optimized window, taking full advantage of sequential ovulations. However, this effect may have been caused by the fact that the authors refrained from insemination only if more than six follicles with a diameter of ≥16 mm (potentially preovulatory) were present at the time of hCG administration. Even though there was only one set of triplets among all multiple pregnancies (overall multiple pregnancy rate of 25%), we would emphatically warn against emulating the high dosage of ovarian stimulation given by Ragni et al. because of the unpredictable risk of higher-order multiple pregnancies. Instead, we recommend that insemination not be performed when a total of more than three preovulatory follicles are present in both ovaries at the time of hCG administration. If this principle is observed, we feel that the advantage of double insemination as described by Ragni et al. will be put into perspective because, on average, a much lower number of oocytes will be available for sequential ovulation. It should also be mentioned that the authors do not indicate whether and, if so, how many patients showed an endogenous LH surge prior to hCG administration. In the final analysis, it remains open whether individually timed single inseminations based on LH measurements would not have yielded equivalent rates.

In any case, we inseminate our patients with satisfactory success (mean viable clinical pregnancy rate per cycle is 20%) only once per treatment cycle, taking advantage of monitoring ovulations by hormone measurements and ultrasonography. Quite apart from the fact that double insemination is a stressful experience for the couple concerned and involves additional logistics and cost, we do not really believe in the adequacy of such a measure. Instead, we fear that a second catheterization of the uterine cavity increases the risk of injuring the endometrium and thus the site of embryo nidation. However, we feel that it does make sense to perform pelvic sonograms on the day after insemination to check whether ovulation has definitely occurred. In a prospective study, for instance, we found luteinized unruptured follicles (LUF) in the first treatment cycle in eight out of 94 patients (8.5%) with "idiopathic" subfertility, although ovulation had been induced with recombinant hFSH/hCG. In the succeeding treatment cycles, performed on average 3 months later, the recurrence rate was 50%. After analysis, elevated tonic LH concentrations were identified in six patients with LUF, corresponding to 31.6% of all patients with elevated basal LH levels. Twenty-one percent of patients with endogenously elevated LH concentrations definitely did not ovulate, even after the second insemination, in spite of ovulation induction attempts using 5000–10 000 IU hCG. Although the absolute figures obtained in this observation are relatively small, and larger numbers might have yielded lower percentages, one cannot fail to recognize the significance of sonographic ovulation control. It can help to avoid further futile insemination attempts and to refer patients in time to oocyte collection and in vitro fertilization (or optionally to gamete transfer).

Literature Survey and Results of Controlled Studies of Conventional AIH

The literature survey presented below is intended to provide information on the pregnancy rates achievable after artificial intrauterine insemination using the husband's spermatozoa (AIH). For the sake of clarity, this review is limited to prospective, randomized AIH studies conducted since 1984, which clearly indicated that the work focused on a single specific diagnostic group (male, idiopathic, or cervical subfertility) as well as on either spontaneous cycles or cycles stimulated with a single regimen only (clomiphene citrate or gonadotropins). Unlike the approach adopted in the first edition of this book, we have refrained here from listing any retrospective studies because of their well-known inherent weaknesses. In Tables 2–4, relevant prospective, randomized studies on male,

Table 2. Literature survey of prospective randomized trials of IUI for male-factor subfertility

Reference	Study design	Couples randomized	IUI		Controls
			Pregnancies/ cycles	Fecundity/ cycle	Fecundity/ cycle
Nonstimulated cycles					
Kerin et al. 1984	Crossover	35	8/39	0.21	0.00[a]
Thomas et al. 1986	Crossover	10	0/30	0.00	0.00[a]
Hughes et al. 1987	Parallel	20	0/32	0.00	0.11[a]
Ho et al. 1989	Crossover	47	0/114	0.00	0.01[a]
te Velde et al. 1989	Crossover	30	3/112	0.03	0.02[a]
Kirby et al. 1991	Crossover	188	24/397	0.06	0.03[a]
Arici et al. 1994	Crossover	30	1/26	0.04	0.04
Lähteenmäki et al. 1995	Crossover	46	9/108	0.08	0.01[a]
Cohlen et al. 1998	Crossover	74	13/155	0.08	0.14
Clomiphene-stimulated cycles					
Bolton et al. 1989	Crossover	29	5/158	0.03	0.00[a]
Arici et al. 1994	Crossover	30	1/26	0.04	0.04
Balasch et al. 1994	Parallel	60	3/58	0.05	0.13
Aribarg and Sukcharoen 1995	Crossover	50	8/253	0.03	0.004[a]
Gonadotropin-stimulated cycles					
Ho et al. 1992	Crossover	15	6/42	0.14	0.00[a]
Balasch et al. 1994	Parallel	60	7/56	0.13	0.05
Nan et al. 1994	Crossover	59	11/107	0.10	0.04
Melis et al. 1995	Parallel	81	11/103	0.11	0.11
Gregoriou et al. 1996	Parallel	62	15/130	0.12	0.04
Cohlen et al. 1998	Crossover	74	21/153	0.14	0.08

[a] Natural intercourse.

idiopathic, and cervical subfertility have been grouped on the basis of three criteria: Studies in which conventional intrauterine inseminations were performed in nonstimulated cycles were compared with studies in which inseminations were performed after hormonal stimulation, using either clomiphene citrate or gonadotropins. Studies comparing intrauterine insemination (IUI) with natural intercourse as a control variable in order to determine treatment efficacy are summarized again in Table 4. Table 5 shows the results of randomized trials of intrauterine insemination versus timed intercourse (TI), both following controlled ovarian hyperstimulation using gonadotropins in patients with unexplained subfertility.

Statistically representative infertility research – designed to generate information for the evidence-based practice of reproductive medicine – essentially requires investigations on a large number of patients. In order to give an impression of the number of randomized couples and treatment cycles in the prospective AIH studies published to date, figures are specified for each of the trials listed below. As the tables clearly indicate, the random samples are very small in nearly all studies. The largest study by far is the multicenter trial conducted by the European Society of Human Reproduction and Embryology (ESHRE) involving a total of 236 couples and 241 cycles (Crosignani et al. 1991). Currently, there are several – albeit very few – excellent meta-analyses of prospective, randomized AIH studies, providing the best evidence currently available to be used as a basis for giving advice and making clinical decisions. However, this must not hide the fact that there is an urgent need for more tightly controlled individual large-scale studies designed to assess specific infertility problems or a given treatment protocol. Because of increasingly rapid progress in the field of infertility management and the resulting need to define and update guidelines, the time available is limited. In conjunction with calls for basing treatment selection categorically on objective, statistically valid data (Mastroianni 1999), this is a challenge which in future can be tackled satisfactorily only by centers which have the capacity and the logistics needed for rapid multicenter evaluation. Hence, initiatives such as the National Cooperative Multicenter Reproductive Medicine Network established in the United States by the National Institutes of Child Health and Human Development – which are designed to tackle the objectives mentioned above – should be welcomed, not least because infertility and its causes pose a serious health problem in our society and because the public is aware of the fact that infertility management is cost-intensive.

Male-Factor Disorder

Roughly 50% of all subfertile couples are affected by the "male factor". In about 30% of the cases, a severe male-factor disorder is the sole cause of infertility, and in another 20%, causes of subfertility are diagnosed in both partners (Howards 1995). The relatively large contribution of the male factor to the overall problem of involuntary childlessness and the difficulties involved in overcoming this disorder call for intensive efforts on the part of physicians and understanding and patience on the part of couples undergoing therapy. Although high fertilization and pregnancy rates can be achieved even in hopeless cases by taking advantage of the possibilities offered by microinsemination into the oocyte (intracytoplasmic injection of spermatozoa), this highly invasive technique should not be used a priori in mild and moderate cases of male subfertility. Instead, it should be considered the last resort in the algorithm of infertility treatment.

Among all the causes leading to homologous intrauterine insemination, male-factor disorder is easily the most controversial one. Many colleagues categorically refuse to apply this treatment method for male subfertility, while others have used it successfully – at least in cases which they define as "mild" or "moderate". These contradictory views are also reflected in the diverging results of controlled AIH studies. If one tries to interpret the literature in terms of the conflicting results published, one soon comes across a multitude of confounding variables. To begin with, it is striking that even the definition of what constitutes male factor subfertility is anything but standardized. Moderate oligozoospermia alone, for instance, is not sufficient diagnostic evidence, because many fertile men have sperm counts of less than 20×10^6/ml. On the other hand, men with normal seminal sperm counts may be severely subfertile owing to impaired sperm function. Furthermore, the different methods employed for, and varying quality of, sperm preparation have a major impact on the results of IUI treatment. Finally, the precise timing of insemination in sync with ovulation is likely to be very advantageous, particularly in cases of male subfertility. Another aspect to be considered in a critical assessment of the reasons for different pregnancy rates is the number of oocytes available for fertilization. Differences between treatment results can often be explained by this variable alone. When assessing treatment effects, it must also be borne in mind that hormonal stimulation may correct hidden ovulatory dysfunctions, enhance the quality of oocytes, and improve the conditions for embryo implantation and development. Because of the lack of large-scale controlled trials, no satisfactory answer can be given to the question as to whether there are actually differences in the treatment outcome of intrauterine insemination after ovulation induction with clomiphene citrate and after stimulation with gonadotropins.

In the case of male subfertility, pregnancy rates in nonstimulated cycles vary between 0% and 8%, except for the study conducted by Kerin et al. (1984). In this group of studies, fecundity per cycle averaged over eight studies is 5% (50/974). For the four studies using CC stimulation, the mean pregnancy rate is 3% (17/495). In gonadotropin stimulation, however, the probability of pregnancy seems to be clearly higher, amounting to 12% (71/591) on average. Kerin et al. (1984) found significantly higher pregnancy rates after IUI (21%) than after timed intercourse (TI) in cases of oligozoospermia. This result, which is conspicuously different from the other results in this group, has never been confirmed by subsequent controlled trials and should therefore be viewed critically. Based on current WHO criteria, the Kerin trial used quite a liberal definition of male factor (sperm density $< 40 \times 10^6$/ml, motile sperm/ejaculate $< 60 \times 10^6$), and it can be assumed that the population studied consisted mainly of patients with unexplained subfertility. Neither the controlled trials conducted by Thomas et al. (1986) and Ho et al. (1989) nor the study by te Velde et al. (1989) demonstrated that IUI in nonstimulated cycles was superior to timed intercourse in cases of oligoasthenozoospermia (Table 4). The results obtained by Hughes et al. (1987) – while statistically not significantly different – showed even higher pregnancy rates after intercourse in spontaneous cycles than after insemination (11% versus 0%) and suggested that AIH was of no benefit in the treatment of oligoasthenozoospermia. On the other hand, in their study on male immunological infertility, Lähteenmäki et al. (1995) found a significant difference in pregnancy rates after IUI (8%) versus timed intercourse with administration of cortisone (1%). Bolton et al. (1989) and Aribarg and Sukcharoen (1995) studied the efficacy of IUI in CC-stimulated cycles by comparing this procedure with natural intercourse cycles, obtaining conception rates after IUI of only 3% while pregnancy rates were virtually zero in the control groups. Finally, Ho et al. (1992) reported a 14% pregnancy rate after IUI in gonadotropin-stimulated cycles, which was significantly different from that after natural intercourse (0%). Nan et al. (1994) and Gregoriou et al. (1996) investigated whether IUI in couples with male subfertility leads to a higher conception rate than timed intercourse, both in gonadotropin-stimulated cycles. Like the other authors, they found that gonadotropins combined with IUI considerably increased the probability of conception in cases of male subfertility. Later on, Cohlen et al. (1998) also came to the same conclusion; in couples with less severe semen defects (total motile sperm count $\geq 10 \times 10^6$) they achieved a significantly higher conception rate (17%) after stimulation with low-dose hMG and IUI than after IUI in natural cycles (8%), while such treatment did not improve the outcome if the total count was less than 10×10^6 motile sperm. On the other hand, insemination in cycles stimulated with clomiphene citrate did not provide a benefit compared with insemination in nonstimulated cycles (Arici et al. 1994). In a randomized AIH study, Balasch et al. (1994) made a direct comparison between clomiphene citrate and low-dose gonadotropins; in this study, the gonadotropins proved to be efficacious and safe, i.e., they were not associated with any substantial risk of higher-order multiple conceptions or hyperstimulation syndrome. Finally, the investigations performed in male subfertility by Arici et al. (1994) showed that – in spite of active ovulation management with clomiphene citrate, ultrasound monitoring, and hCG timing for ovulation – intrauterine insemination led to the same low success rate (4%) as urinary LH-timed insemination. However, mention should also be made – last but not least – of the study conducted by Melis et al. (1995), which did not demonstrate a significant difference in pregnancy rates between ovulation induction with gonadotropins alone and gonadotropins combined with intrauterine insemination, both in mild male factor and in unexplained cases.

Unexplained (Idiopathic) Subfertility

Unexplained infertility is a diagnosis which is usually given if – after 2 years of involuntary childlessness – standard tests of possible causes lead to normal results (Spira 1986). There is general agreement that these tests should show a gynecological and andrological status without pathological findings, including ovulatory cycles, patent tubes, and at least normal values in semen microscopy. If idiopathic infertility is defined more precisely, it is necessary in any case to exclude a sperm dysfunction. The need to test sperm function is as important in the definition of unexplained infertility as it is – conversely – in the diagnosis of sperm disorder (Hull 1992). The prevalence of unexplained infertility in couples seeking assisted conception is quite constant ($\sim 15\%$ on average; Collins et al. 1983; Spira 1986). Diverging rates quoted on prevalence in the literature tend to reflect multifactorial causes and the strictness of criteria used for the definition of idiopathic infertility. Given a stricter definition of unexplained infertility, the main factors determining the chance of conceiving naturally are the woman's age and the duration of infertility; life-table analyses show that most couples will conceive within 2 years without therapy (Hull et al. 1985). This suggests that most causes of this disorder are intermittent and that these patients probably represent a subgroup of the fertile population in whom the time to conception is prolonged. Therefore, this condition should be more properly designated as subfertility rather than infertility (Fisch et al. 1989). After more than 3 years of unexplained childlessness, the monthly chance of natural conception is very low (1–3%), i.e., about 25% per year (Hull et al. 1985; Crosignani et al. 1991; Murdoch et al. 1991), and calls for therapy. By definition, such a therapy is purely empirical after exclusion or correction of possible causes such as occult infection (Friberg 1980), transient hyperprolactinemia (Ben-David 1983), psychological stress (O'Moore et al. 1983), or antisperm antibodies (Bronson et al. 1984a). Placebo-controlled studies of hormone responses and conception rates have shown that, in idiopathic infertility, treatment with clomiphene citrate in natural intercourse cycles provides only a slight benefit (Fisch et al. 1989; Glazener et al. 1990). For instance, Fisch et al.(1989) registered a pregnancy rate of only 19% in the course of 4 months after CC stimulation, while no conception occurred in the placebo group. On the other hand, several investigators were able to show that ovulation induction with CC in combination with IUI increases the pregnancy rates in unexplained infertility (Kemmann et al. 1987; Deaton et al. 1990; Martinez et al. 1991; Arici et al. 1994). Sher et al. (1984) were the first to suggest empirical treatment of unexplained infertility with gonadotropins in combination with intrauterine insemination; in fact, a number of randomized studies conducted subsequently achieved very good and impressive success rates for this treatment modality (Crosignani et al. 1991; Karlström et al. 1993; Chung et al. 1995; Gregoriou et al. 1995b; Shalev et al. 1995; Arcaini et al. 1996). Active ovulation management, ovulation induction with clomiphene citrate, and superovulation with gonadotropins became popular based especially on the assumption that increasing the number of gametes could help to overcome nonidentified endocrinological disorders or subtle defects of fertilization and implantation.

Depending on whether IUI was performed in nonstimulated or stimulated cycles, cycle fecundity varies between 1% and 26% (with an average of 15%) in prospective, randomized studies on unexplained subfertility (Table 3). In male-factor subfertility, on the other hand, the pregnancy rate per cycle varies between 0% and 14%, with an average of only 7% (Table 2). While a summary analysis and a rough comparison of Tables 2 and 3 create the impression that there are no differences between male factor and unexplained subfertility in terms of the average success rates achieved in nonstimulated patients (5% and 3%, respectively), the question of whether pregnancy rates within the group of unexplained subfertility are actually better after stimulation with clomiphene citrate (10%) than without stimulation (3%) is debatable. In a randomized crossover comparison, at any rate, Arici et al. (1994) showed that intrauterine insemination in CC-stimulated cycles and after hCG timing of ovulation leads to significantly better pregnancy rates than insemination in nonstimulated urinary LH-timed cycles (26% versus 5%). According to the results obtained in a controlled study by Kirby et al. (1991), intrauterine insemination does not seem to offer any significant advantage over timed intercourse in natural cycles (4% versus 2%). The study conducted by Deaton et al. (1990), which showed improved conception rates in a randomized comparison with natural intercourse (10%

Table 3. Literature survey of prospective randomized trials of IUI for unexplained and cervi-cal-factor subfertility

Reference	Study design	Couples randomized	IUI		Controls
			Pregnancies/ cycles	Fecundity/ cycle	Fecundity/ cycle
Nonstimulated cycles					
Quagliarello and Arny 1986	Crossover	14	1/42	0.02	0.05
Kirby et al. 1991	Crossover	73	6/145	0.04	0.02[a]
Zikopoulos et al. 1993	Crossover	36	1/103	0.01	0.13
Arici et al. 1994	Crossover	26	1/20	0.05	0.26
te Velde et al. 1989[b]	Crossover	27	13/82	0.16	0.00[a,b]
Kirby et al. 1991	Crossover	24	7/58	0.12	0.08[a,b]
Clomiphene-stimulated cycles					
Deaton et al. 1990	Crossover	67	14/148	0.10	0.03[a]
Karlström et al. 1993	Parallel	148	1/17	0.06	0.20
Arici et al. 1994	Crossover	26	6/23	0.26	0.05
Balasch et al. 1994	Parallel	40	1/40	0.03	0.13
Check and Spirito 1995[b]	Parallel	80	17/80	0.21	0.04[b]
Gonadotropin-stimulated cycles					
Crosignani et al. 1991	Crossover	236	55/241	0.23	0.09
Karlström et al. 1993	Parallel	148	3/15	0.20	0.06
Zikopoulos et al 1993	Crossover	48	11/85	0.11	0.02[a]
Balasch et al. 1994	Parallel	40	5/38	0.13	0.03
Sengoku et al. 1994	Parallel	45	7/62	0.11	0.13
Chung et al. 1995	Parallel	100	24/110	0.22	0.08
Gregoriou et al. 1995	Crossover	23	19/74	0.26	0.09
Melis et al. 1995	Parallel	103	22/123	0.18	0.18
Shalev et al. 1995	Parallel	48	18/68	0.26	0.15
Arcaini 1996	Parallel	68	22/116	0.19	0.09

[a] Natural intercourse.
[b] Cervical factor subfertility.

versus 3%), may also underline the benefit of intrauterine insemination after CC stimulation. Using life-table analyses and the log-rank test, the difference in fecundity was statistically significant. However, the benefit no longer applied to the outcome of pregnancy. Finally, randomized studies have shown that excel-lent results can be achieved (20%) in cases of idiopathic subfertility if intrauter-ine insemination is combined with the administration of gonadotropins. The controlled study performed by Zikopoulos et al. (1993) confirmed the benefit of controlled ovarian hyperstimulation/IUI for couples with long-standing unex-plained infertility (Table 4) but failed to demonstrate any advantage of homolo-gous IUI over ovulation induction alone. Based on the criteria mentioned ear-lier, Table 5 provides a list of the randomized studies on unexplained infertility which compared intrauterine insemination after controlled ovarian hyperstimu-lation (COH/IUI) with timed intercourse after controlled ovarian hyperstimula-tion (COH/TI). Table 5 shows that – on a rough average – cycle fecundity is

Table 4. Efficacy of treatment for single indications only: IUI versus timed intercourse (TI) in natural cycles as untreated controls

Reference	Diagnosis	Study design	Couples randomized	IUI Pregnancies/cycles	Fecundity/cycle	TI Pregnancies/cycles	Fecundity/cycle	p-value[a]
Nonstimulated cycles								
Kerin et al. 1984	Male	Crossover	35	8/39	0.21	0/38	0.00	0.02
Thomas et al. 1986	Male	Crossover	10	0/30	0.00	0/30	0.00	
Ho et al. 1989	Male	Crossover	47	0/114	0.00	1/124	0.01	
te Velde et al. 1989	Male	Crossover	30	3/112	0.03	2/90	0.02	0.01
Kirby et al. 1991	Mucus	Crossover	27	13/82	0.16	0/61	0.00	
	Male	Crossover	188	24/397	0.06	10/331	0.03	
	Unexpl	Crossover	73	6/145	0.04	3/123	0.02	
	Mucus	Crossover	24	7/58	0.12	4/52	0.08	
Lähteenmäki et al. 1995	Male	Crossover	46	9/108	0.08	1/96	0.01	0.001
Clomiphene-stimulated cycles								
Bolton et al. 1989	Male	Crossover	29	5/158	0.03	0/?	0.00	
Deaton et al. 1990	Unexpl	Crossover	67	14/148	0.10	5/150	0.03	0.03
Aribarg and Sukcharoen 1995	Male	Crossover	50	8/253	0.03	1/242	0.004	0.05
Gonadotropin-stimulated cycles								
Ho et al. 1992	Male	Crossover	15	6/42	0.14	0/42	0.00	0.05
Zikopoulos et al. 1993	Unexpl.	Crossover	48	11/85	0.11	1/62	0.02	0.01

[a] Given only if statistically significant.

Table 5. Prospective randomized trials of COH/IUI versus COH/TI for unexplained subfertility

Reference	Study design	Couples randomized	IUI Pregnancies/ cycles	IUI Fecundity/ cycle	TI Pregnancies/ cycles	TI Fecundity/ cycle	p-value[a]
Crosignani et al. 1991	Crossover	236	55/241	0.23	9/106	0.09	0.05
Chung et al. 1995	Parallel	100	24/110	0.22	10/130	0.08	0.05
Gregoriou et al. 1995b	Crossover	46	19/74	0.26	6/67	0.09	0.05
Arcaini et al. 1996	Parallel	68	22/116	0.19	12/127	0.09	0.05
Karlström et al. 1993	Parallel	148	3/15	0.20	3/24	0.13	
Zikopoulos et al. 1993	Crossover	48	6/40	0.15	5/45	0.11	
Melis et al. 1995	Parallel	103	22/123	0.18	23/126	0.18	

[a] Given only if statistically significant.

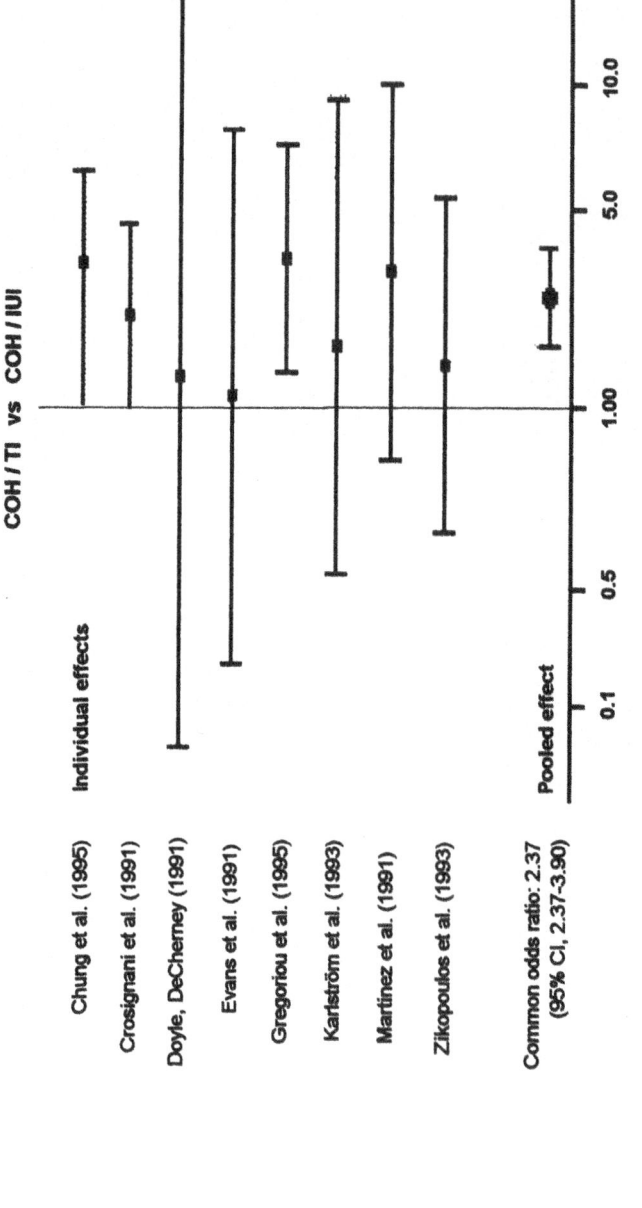

Fig. 4. Meta-analysis of prospective randomized trials comparing controlled ovarian hyperstimulation/intrauterine insemination (COH/IUI) with controlled ovarian hyperstimulation/timed natural intercourse (COH/TI). The pooled data show the results of the meta-analysis. (From Hughes 1997)

higher after COH/IUI (21%) than after COH/TI (11%). This impression is confirmed by a meta-analysis of prospective studies. Based on 5214 cycles reported in 22 trials, this meta-analysis examined the effectiveness of ovulation induction and intrauterine insemination in the treatment of persistent infertility (Hughes 1997). The findings – which for now are the best available evidence – indicate that average fecundity is more than two times higher in a cycle with either IUI or gonadotropins and approximately five times higher when both treatments are used in combination, compared with untreated cycles. The same paper also reported a meta-analysis of eight trials specifically examining FSH/IUI versus FSH/TI for unexplained infertility and showing a 2.4-fold significant increase in the probability of conception following FSH/IUI management when compared with superovulation alone (Fig. 4). A very similar meta-analysis, based on almost the same trials, was published only a short while later and arrived at the same result (Zeyneloglu et al. 1998).

Cervical-Factor Subfertility

In the literature, the prevalence of the cervical factor as a cause of infertility is cited as ranging between 2% and 10% (Spira 1986; Moghissi 1993). Mucus quantity and quality are most important in natural conception because – on their way to the ampullary site of the tubes – the sperm first of all penetrate into the mucus and will eventually have to pass the mucus. Optimal conditions are present at midcycle, just before the onset of ovulation. The production of cervical fluid is regulated largely by estrogens, and during the follicular phase estrogen receptors are prominent in the basal ectocervix layers (Edwards and Brody 1995b). The mucus controls sperm entry into the upper genital tract, protects the sperm against vaginal acidity, selects spermatozoa, initiates capacitation, and serves as a sperm reservoir. Furthermore, the mucus is a site of antibody-mediated reactions in genital infections or – rarely – in the immunological response against spermatozoa (so-called sperm allergy). Compromised mucus production is also found in hormone disorders and in antiestrogenic effects, as well as in cervical anomalies and in cervical stenosis due to infections and previous surgery. Guttmacher (1960) suggested that compromised production of cervical mucus or cervical stenosis were the only causes of sterility justifying IUI. Barwin (1974), White and Glass (1976), Glezerman et al. (1984), Sher et al. (1984), Wiltbank et al. (1985), and Allen et al. (1985) also pointed out that patients in whom the cervical factor was the sole cause of infertility would truly benefit from IUI, leading to pregnancy rates of up to 70%. However, it is not always easy to define a cervical factor reliably by means of the postcoital test (PCT), mainly because timing and repetition in different cycles are critical. Furthermore, the clinical value of the test is controversial because of the lack of standardization of the scoring system. Finally, a definite diagnosis of cervical factor is possible only when a male factor has been largely excluded. This aspect must be kept in mind, considering that differing success rates have been reported in the literature after intrauterine insemination. Unfortunately, there are only very few randomized studies on properly defined cervical-factor sub-fertility which have demonstrated – in an evidence-based manner – the as-sumed efficacy of direct intracavitary insemination (te Velde et al. 1989; Check and Spirito 1995).

Literature Survey and Results of Controlled Studies of Fallopian Tube Sperm Perfusion

Fallopian tube sperm perfusion was inaugurated in 1991 by Kahn et al. Accord-ing to this method, 4 ml of a sperm suspension is transferred into the uterine cavity, based on the assumption that a maximum number of sperm – most of them passive – are delivered into the fallopian tubes. The purpose of using ap-proximately eight times the volume of sperm applied in conventional intrauter-ine insemination is to perfuse the fallopian tubes so that a certain quantity of the inseminate will be flushed through the tubes and end up in the peritoneal cavity. Originally, an Allis clamp was used at the cervical os in order to prevent reflux of the insemination fluid from the cervix.

The first prospective randomized study in which this method was applied (Kahn et al. 1993) for couples with unexplained infertility, after ovarian stimu-lation with clomiphene citrate and human menopausal gonadotropins, led to a pregnancy rate of 27% per treatment cycle and 47% per patient. Following con-ventional IUI with an inseminate volume of ~0.5 ml, on the other hand, the pregnancy rate was only 10% per cycle and 18% per patient. In this trial, which was designed as a parallel study, the average number of follicles >15 mm on the day of ovulation induction with hCG was 2.7 in both randomization arms. Statistical differences between FSP and IUI treatment were observed in terms of the number of motile spermatozoa inseminated and the volume of the inseminate. The authors concluded that it was conceivable that the difference in the number of spermatozoa inseminated might have contributed to the ob-served difference in pregnancy rates, and in addition that the presence of sper-matozoa in the whole female genital tract had increased the probability of con-ception.

The promising results of this study, which was statistically excellent, subse-quently encouraged other investigators to conduct randomized controlled stud-ies comparing the efficacy of FSP treatment with that of standard IUI. All the studies conducted to date are listed in Table 6. They cannot be directly com-pared with each other because they use different study populations, stimulation protocols, sperm preparation methods, numbers of inseminations (single or double insemination), and perfusion techniques with different catheters. Gre-goriou et al. (1995) allocated 60 patients with unexplained infertility randomly to either FSP or IUI treatment. All of them underwent laparoscopy and demon-strated patent fallopian tubes. Only hMG was used for ovarian stimulation. Gre-goriou et al. (1995) used the same volumes of inseminate as Kahn et al. (1993); however, they used different catheters for FSP and IUI: the Makler device for IUI (Makler et al. 1984a) and a Frydman embryo transfer catheter for FSP. Like Kahn et al. (1993), they placed an Allis clamp on the cervix to prevent reflux.

There were no statistically significant differences between the two insemination methods in terms of the pregnancy rates achieved. They amounted to 16% per cycle and 40% per woman after FSP, and to 15% and 37%, respectively, after IUI. In conclusion, the authors suggested that the two methods were equally effective in the treatment of couples with unexplained infertility, but large-scale randomized studies were necessary to demonstrate that FSP offered a benefit. Karande et al. (1995) found no difference between FSP and IUI in a general unselected infertility population with different etiologies such as endometriosis, tubal, male, ovarian, and idiopathic factor. Semen for IUI and FSP underwent three routine sperm washes. IUI was performed with an inseminate volume of 0.5 ml, FSP was performed using a volume of 4 ml. Both methods were applied on 2 consecutive days after hCG administration. Ovulation induction was induced with different protocols, using either clomiphene citrate or gonadotropins. On the other hand, Fanchin et al. (1995) found – also in an unselected group of patients – a remarkably high pregnancy rate per cycle after FSP (40%) compared with IUI (20%) after stimulation with CC and hMG, hMG alone, or GnRH agonist and hMG or FSH. Treatment indications included partial tubal alterations (37%), idiopathic factor (32%), cervical factor (18%), and ovulatory dysfunction (13%). The sperm suspension was prepared by means of a discontinuous two-layer Percoll gradient. FSP was performed with 4 ml, IUI with 0.2 ml. Unlike Karande et al. (1995), Fanchin et al. (1995) performed only one timed insemination per cycle. It is important to note that they used an atraumatic catheter system, the Fallopian Sperm Transfer System (FAST System), specifically designed for sperm perfusion. According to the authors, this special device provides an efficient cervical seal (only two cases of reflux were observed). The authors suggest that there is a triple rationale for their results. First, the injection pressure with which the inseminate is transferred helps to remove and/ or circumvent any transitory or partial obstruction of the fallopian tubes which may be caused by intraluminal mucus or detritus. Second, they hypothesize that the concentration of sperm at the oocyte is higher after FSP than after IUI. Third, the overflow of the inseminate into the peritoneal cavity may lead to re-entry of the sperm into the tubes (Forrler et al. 1986). Mamas (1996) investigated the efficacy of a specifically developed cervical clamp, double nut, bivalve speculum used for FSP with 4 ml of the inseminate, in comparison with standard IUI using a volume of 0.5 ml. A total of 104 couples with unexplained infertility were enrolled in the trial and assigned randomly to either IUI or FSP. Various protocols were used for ovarian stimulation, all of them in combination with gonadotropins. The sperm was prepared by means of a discontinuous two-layer Percoll gradient. A commercially available intrauterine catheter (Wallace) was used, both for FSP and for IUI. In FSP, the cervix was securely clamped with the bivalve speculum, and no leakage was detected. In both treatment groups, the same number of motile spermatozoa was inseminated on average (40×10^6). A comparison between the two treatment groups shows that there is a significant difference in pregnancy rates per cycle (26% after FSP and 12% after IUI); these results are similar to the ones achieved by Kahn et al. (1993). In an unselected group of 100 patients, Nuojua-Huttunen et al. (1997) compared the efficacy of FSP utilizing a pediatric Foley catheter with that of standard IUI. They used CC and hMG for ovarian stimulation and a standard Percoll technique for sperm preparation. The Foley catheter was inserted into the uterine cavity, and the inflated balloon was pressed on the internal cervical os. The pregnancy rate per cycle after FSP was surprisingly low (8%), while a rate of 20% was achieved after IUI. However, the difference was not statistically significant. They explain their results primarily by suggesting that the endometrium may have been traumatized by the tip of the catheter or the inflated balloon. Furthermore, they contend that the catheter material may have also had a toxic effect. A third assumption of the authors is that the inseminate volume of 4 ml may have led to myosalpingeal contractions, and subsequently to the expulsion of the oocytes from the fallopian tubes. In another study conducted in unselected patients, El Sadek et al. (1998) – like Kahn et al. (1993) – used a Frydmann intrauterine catheter for both FSP and IUI, and also applied Allis clamps to seal the cervix. However, unlike the pioneers of FSP, they did not find any difference between the two methods in terms of pregnancy rates.

Finally, Fig. 5 presents the results of a meta-analysis of randomized trials recently published by Trout and Kemmann (1999); in the trials included in this analysis, FSP was compared with standard IUI. The analysis also covered a controlled study conducted by the authors themselves. Six trials were statistically evaluated; all of them have already been described in detail above. The meta-analysis showed

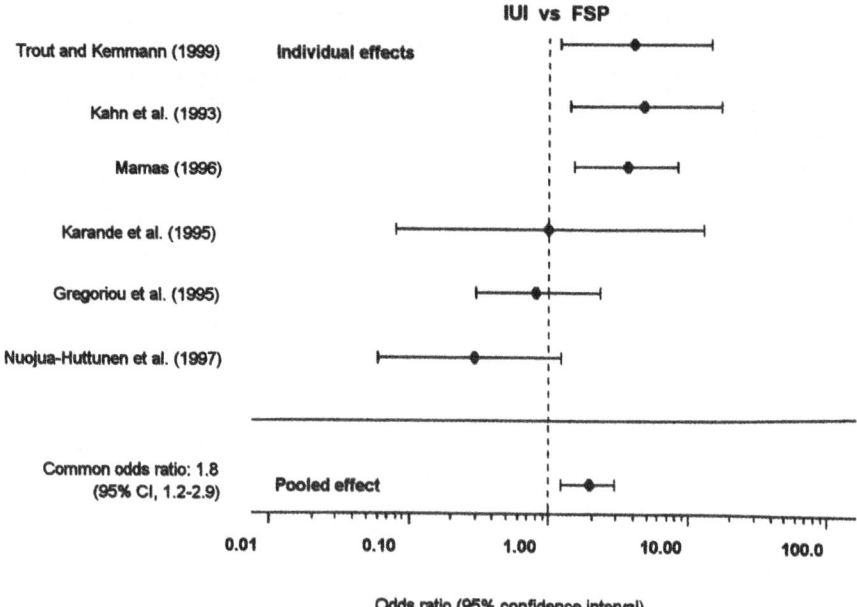

Fig. 5. Meta-analysis of prospective randomized trials comparing fallopian tube sperm perfusion (FSP) with standard intrauterine insemination (IUI). The pooled data show the results of the meta-analysis. (From Trout and Kemmann 1999)

Table 6. Prospective randomized trials of COH/IUI versus COH/FSP for different indications

Reference	Diagnosis	Study design	Couples randomized	COHIUI		COH/FSP		p-value[a]
				Pregnancies/ cycles	Fecundity/ cycle	Pregnancies/ cycles	Fecundity/ cycle	
Kahn et al. 1993	Unexpl.	Parallel	60	5/51	0.10	14/52	0.27	0.05
Gregoriou et al. 1995a	Unexpl.	Parallel	60	12/74	0.16	11/76	0.15	
Karande et al. 1995	Unselected	Parallel	Not stated	13/120	0.11	13/120	0.11	
Fanchin et al. 1995	Unselected	Parallel	74	10/50	0.20	20/50	0.40	0.04
Mamas 1996	Unexpl.	Parallel	104	11/92	0.12	29/110	0.26	0.001
Nuojua-Huttunen et al. 1997	Unselected	Parallel	100	10/50	0.20	4/50	0.08	
El Sadek et al. 1998	Unselected	Parallel	96	8/50	0.16	9/50	0.18	
Trout and Kemmann 1999	Unselected	Parallel	268	14/137	0.10	18/131	0.14	
Prietl 1998	Unexpl.	Parallel	101	4/49	0.08	14/52	0.27	0.05
	Unexpl.	Parallel	95	16/110	0.15	30/93	0.32	0.005

[a] Given only if statistically significant.

that only patients with unexplained infertility benefited from FSP. For patients in this diagnostic group who were stimulated with gonadotropins, the pooled data show a twofold probability of conception after FSP compared with after IUI. Based on the currently best available evidence, this result suggests that couples with unexplained infertility should be treated with FSP rather than with IUI.

Concluding Remarks

Modern therapy of involuntary childlessness offers a number of highly effective treatments, which can generally be subdivided into noninvasive and invasive methods. Both intrauterine insemination and fallopian tube sperm perfusion after ovarian stimulation with gonadotropins are without any doubt successful and efficacious, and pregnancy rates of roughly 20% in couples with unexplained or cervical-factor infertility seem to be quite realistic, based on the published literature. However, the methodological requirements are complex and need to be followed precisely. This applies not only to the diagnostic exploration of infertility but also to the careful preparation of the inseminates and the exact timing of insemination in sync with ovulation. Great attention should be paid to the selection of the couples who qualify for insemination treatment. Cases with a pronounced male factor are undeniably unsuitable candidates for insemination. In the case of couples with long-standing infertility and older women, the patients' individual circumstances should be the primary factor in deciding whether treatment should be attempted using mainly noninvasive methods, and if so, how many. However, since the probability of conception is generally highest during the first three or four treatment attempts, the number of inseminations should be limited especially in these patients, and extracorporeal fertilization should be recommended at an early point in time. At present, insemination treatment is experiencing a revival; as already mentioned, such a treatment is certainly justified as a reasonable first-line therapy for an elective part of the infertility population.

"What is reasonable is real, and what is real is reasonable."

Georg Wilhelm Friedrich Hegel (1770–1831)

References

Aafjes JH, v d Vijver JCM, Schenck PE (1978) The duration of infertility: an important datum for the fertility prognosis of men with semen abnormalities. Fertil Steril 30:423–429

Abbasi R, Kenigsberg D, Danforth D, Falk RJ, Hodgen GD (1987) Cumulative ovulation rate in human menopausal/human chorionic gonadotropin-treated monkeys: "step-up" versus "step-down" dose regimens. Fertil Steril 47:1019–1024

Abyholm T, Tanbo T, Dale PO, Magnus O (1992) In vivo fertilization procedures in infertile women with patent fallopian tubes: a comparison of gamete intra-fallopian transfer, combined intrauterine and intraperitoneal insemination, and controlled ovarian hyperstimulation alone. J Assist Reprod Genet 9:19–23

Agarwal A, Manglona A, Loughlin KR (1991) Filtration of spermatozoa through L membrane: a new method. Fertil Steril 56:1162–1167

Agarwal SK, Buyalos RP (1995) Corpus luteum function and pregnancy rates with clomiphene citrate therapy: comparison of human chorionic gonadotrophin-induced versus spontaneous ovulation. Hum Reprod 10:3218–3231

Ahlgren M (1969) Migration of spermatozoa to the fallopian tubes and the abdominal cavity in women, including some immunological aspects. Dissertation, University of Lund, Sweden

Ahlgren M (1975) Sperm transport and survival in the human fallopian tube. Gynecol Invest 6:206–214

Ahlgren M, Boström K, Malmquist R (1974) Sperm transport and survival in women, with special reference to the fallopian tube. In: Hafez ESE, Thibault CG (eds) Sperm transport, survival and fertilizing ability in vertebrates. INSERM, Paris 26:183–200

Aitken RJ, Clarkson JS (1987) Cellular basis of defective sperm function and its association with the genesis of reactive oxygen species by human spermatozoa. J Reprod Fertil 81:459–469

Aitken RJ, Clarkson JS (1988) Significance of reactive oxygen species and antioxidants in defining the efficacy of sperm preparation techniques. J Androl 9:367–376

Aitken RJ, Clarkson JS, Hargreave TB, Irvine DS, Wu FCW (1989) Analysis of the relationship between defective sperm function and the generation of reactive oxygen species in cases of oligozoospermia. J Androl 10:241–250

Aitken RJ, Buckingham D, West K, Wu FC, Zikopoulos K, Richardson DW (1992) Differential contribution of leucocytes and spermatozoa to the generation of reactive oxygen species in the ejaculates of oligozoospermia patients and fertile donors. J Reprod Fertil 94:451–462

Allen NC, Herbert CM III, Maxson WS, Rogers BJ, Diamond MP, Wentz AC (1985) Intrauterine insemination: a critical review. Fertil Steril 44:569–580

Alvarez JG, Storey BT (1989) Role of glutathione peroxidase in protecting mammalian spermatozoa from loss of motility caused by spontaneous lipid peroxidation. Gamete Res 13:77–90

Alvarez JG, Touchstone JC, Blasco L, Storey BT (1987) Spontaneous lipid peroxidation and production of hydrogen peroxide and superoxide in human spermatozoa. Superoxide dismutase as major enzyme protectant against oxygen toxicity. J Androl 8:338–348

Alvarez JG, Lasso JL, Blasco L, Nuñez RC, Heyner S, Caballero PP, Storey BT (1993) Centrifugation of human spermatozoa includes sublethal damage: separation of human spermatozoa by a dextran swim-up procedure without centrifugation extends their motile lifetime. Hum Reprod 8:1087–1092

Amelar RD, Hotchkiss RS (1965) The split ejaculate: its use in the management of male infertility. Fertil Steril 16:46–48

Andersen AG, Als-Nielsen B, Hornnes PJ, Franch Andersen L (1995) Time interval from human chorionic gonadotrophin (HCG) injection to follicular rupture. Hum Reprod 10:3202–3205

Arcaini L, Bianchi S, Baglioni A, Marchini M, Tozzi L, Fedele L (1996) Superovulation and intrauterine insemination vs. superovulation alone in the treatment of unexplained infertility. A randomized study. J Reprod Med 41:614–618

Aribarg A, Sukcharoen N (1995) Intrauterine insemination of washed spermatozoa for treatment of oligozoospermia. Int J Androl 18 [Suppl 1]:62–66

Arici A, Byrd W, Bradshaw K, Kutteh WH, Marshburn P, Carr BR (1994) Evaluation of clomiphene citrate and human chorionic gonadotropin treatment: a prospective, randomized, crossover study during intrauterine insemination cycles. Fertil Steril 61:314–318

Arny M, Quagliarello J (1987) Semen quality before and after processing by a swim-up method: relationship to outcome of intrauterine insemination. Fertil Steril 48:643–648

Balasch J, Ballesca JL, Pimentel C, Creus M, Fabregues F, Vanrell JA (1994) Late low-dose pure follicle-stimulating hormone for ovarian stimulation in intra-uterine insemination cycles. Hum Reprod 9:1863–1866

Barratt CLR, Naeeni M, Clements S, Cooke ID (1995) Clinical value of sperm morphology for in-vivo fertility: comparison between World Health Organization criteria of 1987 and 1992. Hum Reprod 10:687–693

Barwin BN (1974) Intrauterine insemination with husband's semen. J Reprod Fertil 36:101–106

Ben-David M, Schenker J (1983) Transient hyperprolactinemia: a correctable cause of idiopathic female infertility. J Clin Endocrinol Metab 57:442

Berger T, Marrs RP, Moyer DL (1985) Comparison of techniques for selection of motile spermatozoa. Fertil Steril 43:268–273

Boer CH (1972) Transport of particulate matter through the human female genital tract. J Reprod Fertil 28:295–297

Bolton VN, Warren RE, Braude PR (1986) Removal of bacterial contaminants from semen for in vitro fertilization or artificial insemination by the use of buoyant density centrifugation. Fertil Steril 46:1128–1132

Bolton VN, Braude PR, Ockenden K, Marsh SK, Robertson G, Ross LD (1989) An evaluation of semen analysis and in vitro tests of sperm function in the prediction of the outcome of intrauterine AIH. Hum Reprod 4:674–679

Brasch JG, Rawlins R, Tarchala S, Radwanska E (1994) The relationship between total motile sperm count and the success of intrauterine insemination. Fertil Steril 62:150–154

Bronson R, Cooper G, Rosenfeld D (1984a) Sperm antibodies: their role in infertility. Fertil Steril 42:171

Bronson RA, Cooper GW, Rosenfeld DL (1984b) Autoimmunity to spermatozoa: effect on sperm penetration of sperm cervical mucus as reflected by postcoital testing. Fertil Steril 41:609–614

Bumm E (1904) Über die Behandlung und Heilungsaussichten bei der Sterilität der Frau. Dtsch Med Wochenschr 30:1756

Byrd W, Ackermann GE, Carr BR, Edman CD, Guzick DS, McConnel JD (1987) Treatment of refractory infertility by transcervical intrauterine insemination of washed spermatozoa. Fertil Steril 48:921–927

Byrd W, Bradshaw K, Carr B, Edman C, Odom J, Ackerman G (1990) A prospective randomized study of pregnancy rates following intrauterine and intracervical insemination using frozen donor sperm. Fertil Steril 53:521–527

Campana A, Sakkas D, Stalberg A, Bianchi PG, Comte I, Pache T, Walker D (1996) Intrauterine insemination: evaluation of the results according to the woman's age, sperm quality, sperm count per insemination and life-table analysis. Hum Reprod 11:732–736

Centola GM (1993) Conventional semen analysis. In: Schlaff WD, Rock JD (eds) Decision-making in reproductive endocrinology. Blackwell Scientific, Boston, pp 433–437

Check JH, Spirito P (1995) Higher pregnancy rates following treatment of cervical factor with intrauterine insemination without superovulation versus intercourse: the impact of a well-timed postcoital test for infertility. Arch Androl 35:71–77

Chung CC, Fleming R, Jamieson ME, Yates RW, Coutts JR (1995) Randomized comparison of ovulation induction with and without intrauterine insemination in the treatment of unexplained infertility. Hum Reprod 10:3139–3141

Cohen J, Edwards RG, Fehily CB, Hewitt J, Purdy JM, Rowland RF, Steptoe PC, Webster JB (1985) In vitro fertilization: a treatment for male infertility. Fertil Steril 43:422–432

Cohlen BJ, te Velde ER, van Kooij RJ, Looman CW, Habbema JD (1998) Controlled ovarian hyperstimulation and intrauterine insemination for treating male subfertility: a controlled study. Hum Reprod 13:1553–1558

Collins JA, Wrixon W, Janes LH, Wilson EH (1983) Treatment-independent pregnancy among infertile couples. N Engl J Med 309:1201

Crosignani PG, Walters DE, Soliani A (1991) The ESHRE multicentre trial on the treatment of unexplained infertility; a preliminary report. Hum Reprod 6:953–958

Croxatto HB, Faundes A, Medel M, Avendano S, Croxatto HD, Vera C, Anselmo J, Pastene L (1973) Studies on sperm migration in the human female genital tract. In: Hafez ESE, Thibault CG (eds) Sperm transport, survival and fertility ability in vertebrates. INSERM Paris 26:162–182

Cruz RI, Kemmann E, Brandeis VT, Becker KA, Beck M, Beardsley L, Shelden R (1986) A prospective study of intrauterine insemination of processed sperm from men with oligoasthenospermia in superovulated women. Fertil Steril 46:673–677

Deaton JL, Gibson M, Blackmer KM, Nakajima ST, Badger GJ, Brumsted JR (1990) A randomized controlled trial of clomiphene citrate and intrauterine insemination in couples with unexplained infertility or surgically corrected endometriosis. Fertil Steril 54:1083–1088

Deaton JL, Clark RR, Pittaway DE, Herbst P, Bauguess P (1997) Clomiphene citrate ovulation induction in comparison with a timed intrauterine insemination: the value of urinary luteinizing hormone versus human chorionic gonadotropin timing. Fertil Steril 68:43–47

Dehaut F De la fécondation artificielle dans l'espèce humaine comme moyen de remédier à certaines causes de stérilité chez l'homme et chez la femme. Paris, 1865–1872 [cited in Schlesinger W (1870) Über künstliche Befruchtung beim Weib, eine französische Studie des Dr. Girault. Wien Med Wochenschr 20:499]

Devroey P, Vandervorst M, Nagy P, Van Steirteghem A (1998) Do we treat the male or his gamete? Hum Reprod 13 [Suppl 1]:175–185

Dickey RP, Pyrzak R, Lu PY, Taylor SN, Rye PH (1999) Comparison of sperm quality necessary for successful intrauterine insemination with World Health Organization threshold values for normal sperm. Fertil Steril 71:684–689

Diedrich K, van der Ven H, Krebs D (1985) Physiologie der Reproduktion. In: Wulf K-H, Schmidt-Matthiesen H (eds) Klinik der Frauenheilkunde und Geburtshilfe: Reproduktion-Störungen der Frühgravidität. Urban & Schwarzenberg, München, pp 33–83

Dmowski WP, Gaynor L, Lawrence M, Rao R, Scommegna A (1979) Artificial insemination homologous with oligospermic semen separated on albumin columns. Fertil Steril 31:58–62

Döderlein G (1912) Über künstliche Befruchtung beim Menschen. Münch Med Wochenschr 59:1081, Berl Klin Wochenschr 49:721, Arztl Zentralztg 24:67–411

Dodson WC, Haney AF (1991) Controlled ovarian hyperstimulation and intrauterine insemination for treatment of infertility. Fertil Steril 55:457–467

Drevius L-O (1971) The 'sperm-rise' test. J Reprod Fertil 24:427–429

Drobnis EZ, Zhong CQ, Overstreet JW (1991) Separation of cryopreserved human semen using Sephadex columns, washing or Percoll gradients. J Androl 12:201–208

Edwards RG, Brody SA (1995a) Human fecundity and assisted conception. In: Edwards RG, Brody SA (eds) Principles and practice of assisted human reproduction. Saunders, Philadelphia, pp 1–15

Edwards RG, Brody SA (1995b) Human menstrual and ovarian cycles. In: Edwards RG, Brody SA (eds) Principles and practice of assisted human reproduction. Saunders, Philadelphia, p 189

Edwards RG, Brody SA (1995c) Natural cycle and ovarian stimulation in assisted conception. In: Edwards RG, Brody SA (eds) Principles and practice of assisted human reproduction. Saunders, Philadelphia, p 235

Edwards RG, Purdy JM (eds) (1982) Human conception in vitro. Proceedings of the first Bourn Hall Meeting; Sept 3–5, 1981, Bourn Hall, Cambridge. Academic, London

Edwards RG, Steptoe PC, Purdy JM (1980) Establishing full-term human pregnancies using cleaving embryos grown in vitro. Br J Obstet Gynaecol 87:737–756

El Sadek MM, Amer MK, Abdel-Malak G (1998) Questioning the efficacy of fallopian tube sperm perfusion. Hum Reprod 13:3053–3056

Elliasson R, Lindholmer C (1972) Distribution and properties of spermatozoa in different fractions of split ejaculates. Fertil Steril 23:252–256

Ericsson RJ, Langevin CN, Nishino M (1973) Isolation of fractions rich in human Y sperm. Nature 246:421–424

Evans J, Wells C, Gregory L, Walker S (1991) A comparison of intrauterine insemination, intraperitoneal insemination, and natural intercourse in superovulated women. Fertil Steril 56:1183–1187

Fanchin R, Olivennes F, Rhigini C, Hazout A, Schwab B, Frydman R (1995) A new system for fallopian tube sperm perfusion leads to pregnancy rates twice as high as standard intrauterine insemination. Fertil Steril 64:505–510

Farris EJ, Murphy DP (1960) The characteristics of the two parts of the partitioned ejaculate and the advantages of its use for intrauterine insemination. Fertil Steril 11:465–469

Fisch P, Casper RF, Brown SE, Wrixon W, Collins JA, Reid R, Simpson C (1989) Unexplained infertility: evaluation of treatment with clomiphene citrate and human chorionic gonadotropin. Fertil Steril 51:828–833

Ford WC, Mathur RS, Hull MG (1997) Intrauterine insemination: is it an effective treatment for male factor infertility? Baillieres Clin Obstet Gynecol 11:691–710

Forrler A, Badoc E, Moreau L, Dellenbach P, Cranz CL, Clavert A, Rumpler Y (1986) Direct intraperitoneal insemination: first results confirmed. Lancet 2:1468

Fraenkel PL (1909) Über die künstliche Befruchtung beim Menschen und ihre gerichtsärztliche Bedeutung. Arztl Sachv Ztg 15:169

Francavilla F, Romano R, Santucci R, Poccia G (1990) Effect of sperm morphology and motile sperm count on outcome of intrauterine insemination in oligozoospermia and/or asthenozoospermia. Fertil Steril 53:892–897

Friberg J (1980) Mycoplasmas and ureoplasmas in infertility and abortion. Fertil Steril 33:351

Fuh KW, Wang X, Tai A, Wong I, Norman RJ (1997) Intrauterine insemination: effect of the temporal relationship between the luteinizing hormone surge, human chorionic gonadotrophin administration and insemination on pregnancy rates. Hum Reprod 12:2162–2166

Gellert-Mortimer ST, Clark GN, Baker HWG, Hyne RV, Johnston WIH (1988) Evaluation of Nycodenz and Percoll density gradients for the selection of motile human spermatozoa. Fertil Steril 49:335–341

Gigon PF (1871) Essai sur la fécondation artificielle chez la femme dans certains cas de stérilité. Inaugural dissertation, University of Paris

Girault J (1886) Etude sur la génération artificielle dans l'espèce humaine. L'abeille médicale 25:403–417

Glass RH, Ericsson RJ (1978) Intrauterine insemination of isolated motile sperm. Fertil Steril 29:535–538

Glass RH, Ericsson RJ (1979) Spontaneous cure of male infertility. Fertil Steril 31:305–309

Glazener CMA, Kelly NJ, Weir MJA (1987) The diagnosis of male infertility – prospective and time-specific study of conception rate to seminal analysis and post coital sperm-mucus penetration in otherwise unexplained infertility. Hum Reprod 2:665–671

Glazener CM, Coulson C, Lambert PA (1990) Clomiphene treatment for women with unexplained infertility: placebo-controlled study of hormonal responses and conception rates. Gynecol Endocrinol 4:75–83

Glezerman M, Bernstein D, Insler V (1984) The cervical factor of infertility and intrauterine insemination. Int J Fertil 29:16–19

Glover WK (1948) Artificial insemination among human beings, medical, legal and moral aspects. Inaugural dissertation, University of Washington, Washington

Gonzales FG, Pella RE (1993) Swim-down: a rapid and easy method to select motile spermatozoa. Arch Androl 30:29–34

Gorus FK, Pipeleers DG (1981) A rapid method for the fractionation of human spermatozoa according to their progressive motility. Fertil Steril 35:662–665

Gould JE, Overstreet JW, Hanson FW (1994) Assessment of human sperm function after recovery from the female reproductive tract. Biol Reprod 31:888–894

Goverde AJ, McDonnell J, Vermeiden JPW, Schats R, Rutten FFH, Schoemaker J (2000) Intrauterine insemination of in-vitro fertilisation in idiopathic subfertility and male subfertility: a randomised trial and cost-effectiveness analysis. Lancet 355:13–18

Graham EF, Vasquez IA, Schmehl MKL, Evensen BK (1976) An assay of semen quality by use of Sephadex filtration. International Congress of Animal Reproduction and Artificial Insemination 8:896–899

Gregoriou O, Pyrgiotis E, Konidaris S, Papadias C, Zourlas PA (1995a) Fallopian tube sperm perfusion has no advantage over intra-uterine insemination when used in combination with ovarian stimulation for the treatment of unexplained infertility. Gynecol Obstet Invest 39:226–228

Gregoriou O, Vitoratos N, Papadias C, Konidaris S, Gargaropoulos A, Louridas C (1995b) Controlled ovarian hyperstimulation with or without intrauterine insemination for the treatment of unexplained infertility. Int J Gynecol Obstet 48:55–59

Gregoriou O, Vitoratos N, Papadias C, Konidaris S, Gargaropoulos A, Rizos D (1996) Pregnancy rates in gonadotrophin-stimulated cycles with timed intercourse or intrauterine insemination for the treatment of male subfertility. Eur J Obstet Gynecol Reprod Biol 64:213–216

Grow D, Oehninger S, Seltman HJ, Kruger TF, Swanson RJ, Muasher SJ (1994) Sperm morphology as diagnosed by strict criteria: probing the impact of teratozoospermia on fertilization and pregnancy outcome in a large IVF population. Fertil Steril 62:559–567

Guttmacher AF (1960) The role of artificial insemination in the treatment of sterility. Obstet Gynecol Surv 15:767–771

Haidl G (1990) Macrophages in semen are indicative of chronic epididymal infection. Arch Androl 25:5

Haney AF, Hughes CL, Whitesides DB, Dodson WC (1987) Treatment independent, treatment associated, and pregnancies after additional therapy in a program of in vitro fertilization. Fertil Steril 47:634–638

Hanson FW, Overstreet JW (1981) The interaction of human spermatozoa with cervical mucus in vivo. Am J Obstet Gynecol 140:173–178

Hanson FM, Rock J (1951) Artificial insemination with husband's sperm. Fertil Steril 2:162–166

Hard AD (1909) Artificial impregnation. Med World 27:253

Harris SJ, Milligan MP, Masson GM, Dennis KJ (1981) Improved separation of motile sperm in asthenospermia and its application to artificial insemination homologous (AIH). Fertil Steril 36:219–221

Harrison RAP (1976) A highly efficient method for washing mammalian spermatozoa. J Reprod Fertil 48:347–353

Heiss H (1972) Geschichte der künstlichen Insemination. In: Heiss H (ed) Die künstliche Insemination der Frau. Urban & Schwarzenberg, Munich, pp 6–9

Hill JA, Haimovici F, Politch JA, Anderson DJ (1987) Effects of soluble products of activated lymphocytes and macrophages (lymphokines and monokines) on human sperm motion parameters. Fertil Steril 47:460–465

Hirsch J (1912) Schwangerschaft nach künstlicher Befruchtung. Berl Klin Wochenschr 49:1361, Verhandl Berl Med Ges 43:293, MMW 28:1580

Ho P-C, Poon IML, Chan SYW, Wang C (1989) Intrauterine insemination is not useful in oligoasthenospermia. Fertil Steril 51:682–684

Ho P-C, So W-K, Chan Y-F, Yeung WS-B (1992) Intrauterine insemination after ovarian stimulation as a treatment for subfertility because of subnormal semen: a prospective randomized controlled trial. Fertil Steril 58:995–999

Hoff JD, Quigley ME, Yen SSC (1983) Hormone dynamics at midcycle: a re-evaluation. J Clin Endocrinol Metabol 57:792–796

Hofmann N, Haider SG (1985) Neue Ergebnisse morphologischer Diagnostik der Spermatogenesestörungen. Gynakologe 18:70–80

Holfelder W (1953) Die künstliche Befruchtung beim Menschen nach deutschem und kanonischem Recht. Inaugural dissertation, law, University of Heidelberg

Home E (1799) An account of the dissection of an hermaphrodite. Dog Philos Trans Roy Soc London 1:158

Horvath PM, Bohrer MK, Shelden RM, Kemmann E (1989) The relationship of sperm parameters to cycle fecundity in superovulated women undergoing intrauterine insemination. Fertil Steril 52:288–294

Howards SS (1995) Treatment of male subfertility. N Engl J Med 332:312–317

Huang HY, Lee CL, Lai YM, Chang MY, Wang HS, Chang SY, Soong YK (1996) The impact of the total motile sperm count on the success of intrauterine insemination with husband's spermatozoa. J Assist Reprod Genet 13:56–63

Hughes EG (1997) The effectiveness of ovulation induction and intrauterine insemination in the treatment of persistent infertility: a meta-analysis. Hum Reprod 12:1865–1872

Hughes EG, Collins JP, Garner PR (1987) Homologous artificial insemination for oligoasthenospermia: a randomized controlled study comparing intracervical and intrauterine techniques. Fertil Steril 48:278–281

Hull MGR (1992) Infertility treatment: relative effectiveness of conventional and assisted conception methods. Hum Reprod 7:785–796

Hull MGR, Glazener CMA, Kelly NJ, Conway DI, Foster PA, Hinton RA, Coulson C, Lambert PA, Watt EM, Desai KM (1985) Population study of causes, treatment, and outcome of infertility. Br Med J 291:1693–1697

Human Fertilisation and Embryology Authority (1990) Code of practice. London, pp 28–29

Huszar G, Willets M, Corrales M (1990) Hyaluronic acid (Sperm Select) improves retention of sperm motility and velocity in normozoospermic and oligozoospermic specimens. Fertil Steril 54:1127–1134

Iffland CA, Reid W, Amso N, Bernard AG, Buckland G, Shaw RW (1991) A within-patient comparison between superovulation and intra-uterine artificial insemination using husband's washed spermatozoa and gamete intrafallopian transfer in unexplained infertility. Eur J Obstet Gynecol Reprod Biol 39:181–186

Insler V, Melmed H, Eichenbrenner I, Serr DM, Lunenfeld B (1972) The cervical score: a simple semiquantitative method for monitoring the menstrual cycle. Int J Gynecol Obstet 10:223–228

Irianni FM, Ramey J, Vaintraub MT, Oehninger S, Acosta AA (1993) Therapeutic insemination improves with gonadotropin ovarian stimulation. Arch Androl 31:55–62

Iwanow E (1907) De la fécondation artificielle chez les mammifères. Arch Sci Biol 12:377

Iwasaki A, Gagnon C (1992) Formation of reactive oxygen species in spermatozoa of infertile patients. Fertil Steril 57:409–416

Jaroudi KA, Carver-Ward JA, Hamilton CJCM, Siek UV, Sheth KV (1993) Percoll semen preparation enhances human oocyte fertilization in male-factor infertility as shown by a randomized crossover study. Hum Reprod 8:1438–1442

Jeyendran RS, Perez-Pelaez M, Crabo BG (1986) Concentration of viable spermatozoa for artificial insemination. Fertil Steril 45:132–137

Jones R, Mann T, Sherins RJ (1979) Peroxidative breakdown of phospholipids in human spermatozoa, spermicidal properties of fatty acid peroxides and protective action of seminal plasma. Fertil Steril 31:531–537

Jouannet P, Ducot B, Feneux D, Spira A (1988) Male factors and the likelihood of pregnancy in infertile couples. 1. Study of sperm characteristics. Int J Androl 11:379–394

Kahn JA, Sunde A, von Düring V, Sørdal T, Molne K (1991) Intrauterine insemination. Ann NY Acad Sci 626:452–460

Kahn JA, von Düring V, Sunde A, Sørdal T, Molne K (1992) Fallopian tube sperm perfusion: first clinical experience. Hum Reprod 7 [Suppl 1]:19–24

Kahn JA, Sunde A, Koskemies A, von Düring V, Sørdal T, Christensen F, Molne K (1993) Fallopian tube sperm perfusion (FSP) versus intra-uterine insemination (IUI) in the treatment of unexplained infertility: a prospective randomized study. Hum Reprod 8:890–894

Kaiser G (1966) Künstliche Insemination und Transplantation. Juristische und rechtspolitische Probleme. In: Göppinger H (ed) Arzt und Recht. München

Karande VC, Rao R, Pratt DE, Balin M, Levrant S, Morris R, Dudkeiwicz A, Gleicher N (1995) A randomized prospective comparison between intrauterine insemination and fallopian tube sperm perfusion for the treatment of infertility. Fertil Steril 64:638–640

Kardinom S (1942) Artificial insemination in the Talmud. Heb Med J 2:162

Karlström PO, Bergh T, Lundkvist O (1993) A prospective randomized trial of artificial insemination versus intercourse in cycles stimulated with human menopausal gonadotropin or clomiphene citrate. Fertil Steril 59:554–559

Kaskarelis E, Comninos A (1959) A critical evaluation of homologous artificial insemination. Int J Fertil 4:38–41

Katayama KP, Stehlik E, Jeyendran RS (1989) In vitro fertilization outcome: glass wool-filtered sperm versus swim-up sperm. Fertil Steril 52:670–672

Kemmann E, Bohrer M, Shelden R, Fiasconaro G, Beardsley L (1987) Active ovulation management increases the monthly probability of pregnancy occurrence in ovulatory women who receive intrauterine insemination. Fertil Steril 48:916–920

Kerin JFP, Peek J, Warners GM, Kirby C, Jeffrey R, Matthews CD, Cox LW (1984) Improved conception rate after intrauterine insemination of washed spermatozoa from men with poor-quality semen. Lancet 1:533–534

Kirby CA, Flaherty SP, Godfrey BM, Warnes GM, Matthews CD (1991) A prospective trial of intrauterine insemination of motile spermatozoa versus timed intercourse. Fertil Steril 56:102–107

Kovalski NN, de Lamirande E, Gagnon C (1992) Reactive oxygen species generated by human neutrophils inhibit sperm motility: protective effect of seminal plasma and scavengers. Fertil Steril 58:809–816

Krebs D (1989) In vitro-Fertilisation, intratubarer Gametentransfer (GIFT) und intrauterine Insemination. In: Bettendorf G, Breckwoldt M (eds) Reproduktionsmedizin. Fischer, Stuttgart, pp 513–532

Kremer J (1979) A new technique for intrauterine insemination. Int J Fertil 24:53–56

Kruger TF, Menkveld R, Stander FSH, Lombard CJ, Van der Merwe JP, van Zyl JA, Smith K (1986) Sperm morphologic features as a prognostic factor in vitro fertilization. Fertil Steril 46:1118–1123

Kruger TF, Acosta AA, Simmons KF, Swanson RJ, Matta JF, Veeck LL, Morshedi M, Brugo S (1987) A new method of evaluating sperm morphology with predictive value for IVF. Urology 30:248–251

Kruger TF, Acosta AA, Simmons KF, Swanson RJ, Matta JF, Oehninger S (1988) Predictive value of abnormal sperm morphology in in vitro fertilization. Fertil Steril 49:112–117

Lähteenmaki A, Veilahti J, Hovatta O (1995) Intra-uterine insemination versus cyclic, low-dose prednisolone in couples with male antisperm antibodies. Hum Reprod 10:142–147

Lessley BA, Garner DL (1983) Isolation of motile spermatozoa by density gradient centrifugation in Percoll. Gamete Res 7:49–54

Lewis SEM, Sterling ESL, Young IS, Thompson W (1997) Comparison of individual antioxidants of sperm and seminal plasma in fertile and infertile men. Fertil Steril 67:142–147

Lopata A, Patullo MJ, Chang A, James B (1976) A method for collecting motile spermatozoa from human semen. Fertil Steril 27:677–684

Macnamee MC, Edwards RG, Howles CM (1988) The influence of stimulation regimes and luteal phase support on the outcome of IVF. Hum Reprod 3 [Suppl 2]:43–52

Makler A, De Cherney A, Naftolin F (1984a) A device for injecting and retaining a small volume of concentrated spermatozoa in the uterine cavity and cervical canal. Fertil Steril 42:306–308

Makler A, Murillo O, Huszar G, Tarlatzis B, DeCherney A, Naftolin F (1984b) Improved techniques for collecting motile spermatozoa from human semen. A self-migratory method. Int J Androl 7:61–65

Makler A, Stoller J, Blumenfeld Z, Feigin PD, Brandes JM (1993) Investigation in real time of the effect of gravidation on human spermatozoa and their tendency to swim-up and swim-down. Int J Androl 16:251–257

Mamas L (1996) Higher pregnancy rates with a simple method for fallopian tube sperm perfusion, using the cervical clamp double nut bivalve speculum in the treatment of unexplained infertility: a prospective randomized study. Hum Reprod 11:2618–2622

Marrs RP, Vargyas JM, Saito H, Gibbons WE, Berger T, Mishell DR jr (1983) Clinical applications of techniques used in human in vitro fertilization research. Am J Obstet Gynecol 146:477–481

Marshburn PB, McIntire D, Carr BR, Byrd W (1992) Spermatozoal characteristics from fresh and frozen donor semen and their correlation with fertility outcome after intrauterine insemination. Fertil Steril 58:179–186

Martinez AR, Bernadus RE, Voorhorst FJ, Vermeiden JP, Schoemaker J (1991) A controlled study of human chorionic gonadotrophin-induced ovulation versus urinary luteinizing hormone surge for timing of intrauterine insemination. Hum Reprod 6:1247–1251

Mastroianni L jr (1999) Statistically valid infertility research. Fertil Steril 72:398–400

Mastroianni L, Laberge JL, Rock J (1957) Appraisal of the efficacy of artificial insemination with husband's sperm and evaluation of insemination techniques. Fertil Steril 8:260–266

Matorras R, Corcostegui B, Perez C, Mandiola M, Mendoza R, Rodriguez-Escudero FJ (1995) Sperm morphology analysis (strict criteria) in male infertility is not a prognostic factor in intrauterine insemination with husband's sperm. Fertil Steril 63:608–111

McClure R, Nunes L, Tom R (1989) Semen manipulation: improved sperm recovery and function with a two-layer Percoll gradient. Fertil Steril 51:874

McDowell JS, Veeck LL, Jones HW jr (1985) Analysis of human spermatozoa before and after processing for in vitro fertilization. J In Vitro Fertil Embryo Transf 2:23–26

McGovern P, Quagliarello J, Arny M (1989) Relationship of within-patient semen variability to outcome of intrauterine insemination. Fertil Steril 51:1019–1023

Melis GB, Paolett AM, Ajossa S, Guerriero S, Depau GF, Mais V (1995) Ovulation induction with gonadotropins as sole treatment in infertile couples with open tubes: a randomized prospective comparison between intrauterine insemination and timed vaginal intercourse. Fertil Steril 64:1088–1093

Menkveld R (1987) An investigation of environmental influences on spermatogenesis as evidenced in seminal cytology and experimental production of these deviations. Dissertation, Faculty of Medicine, University of Stellenbosch, South Africa

Menkveld R, Kruger TF (1990) Basic semen analysis. In: Acosta AA, Swanson RJ, Ackerman SB, Kruger TF, van Zyl JA, Menkveld R (eds) Human spermatozoa in assisted reproduction. Williams & Wilkins, Baltimore, pp 68–84

Menkveld R, Stander FSH, Kotze TJvW, Kruger TF, van Zyl LA (1990) The evaluation of morphological characteristics of human spermatozoa according to stricter criteria. Hum Reprod 5:586–592

Moghissi KS (1976) Accuracy of basal body temperature for ovulation detection. Fertil Steril 27:1415–1421

Moghissi KS (1984) The function of the cervix in human reproduction. Curr Probl Obstet Gynecol 7:1

Moghissi KS (1986) Some reflections on intrauterine insemination. Fertil Steril 46:13–15

Moghissi KS (1993) Diagnosis classification of disturbed sperm-cervical mucus interaction. In: Insler V, Lunenfeld B (eds) Infertility: male and female, 2nd edn. Churchill Livingstone, Edinburgh, 335–351

Moghissi KS, Segal S, Meinhold D, Agronow SJ (1982) In vitro cervical mucus penetration studies in human and bovine cervical mucus. Fertil Steril 37:823–827

Mortimer D (1991) Sperm preparation techniques and iatrogenic failure of in-vitro fertilization. Hum Reprod 6:173–176

Mortimer ST, Mortimer D (1988) Percoll selection of human spermatozoa is dependent upon motility not concentration. J Reprod Fertil Abstr Ser 1:65

Mortimer D, Templeton AA (1982) Sperm transport in human female reproductive tract in relation to semen analysis characteristics and time of ovulation. J Reprod Fertil 64:401–408

Murdoch AP, Harris, M, Mahroo M, Williams M, Dunlop W (1991) Gamete intrafallopian transfer (GIFT) compared with intrauterine insemination in the treatment of unexplained infertility. Br J Obstet Gynaecol 98:1107–1111

Nachtigall RD, Faure N, Glass RH (1979) Artificial insemination of husband's sperm. Fertil Steril 32:141–147

Nan PM, Cohlen BJ, te Velde ER, van Kooij RJ, Eimers JM, van Zonneveld P, Habbema JDF (1994) Intra-uterine insemination or timed intercourse after ovarian stimulation for male subfertility? A controlled study. Hum Reprod 9:2022–2026

Naz RK, Menge AC (1994) Antisperm antibodies – origin, regulation, and sperm reactivity in human infertility. Fertil Steril 61:1001–1013

Nulsen J, Wheeler C, Ausmanas M, Blasco L (1987) Cervical mucus changes in relationship to urinary LH surge. Fertil Steril 48:738–736

Nuojua-Huttunen S, Tuomivaara L, Juntunen K, Tomas C, Martikainen H (1997) Comparison of fallopian tube sperm perfusion with intrauterine insemination in the treatment of infertility. Fertil Steril 67:939–942

Odem RR, Durso NM, Long CA, Pineda JA, Strickler RC, Gast MJ (1991) Therapeutic donor insemination: a prospective randomized study of scheduling methods. Fertil Steril 55:976–982

Oehninger S, Acosta AA, Morshedi M, Veeck LL, Swanson RJ, Simmons K, Rosenwaks Z (1988) Corrective measures and pregnancy outcome in in vitro fertilization patients with severe sperm morphology abnormalities. Fertil Steril 50:283–287

O'Moore AM, O'Moore RR, Harrison RF, Murphy G, Carruthers ME (1983) Psychosomatic aspects in idiopathic infertility; effects of treatment with autogenic training. J Psychosom Res 27:145

Overstreet JW (1996) Physiological changes in sperm during transport through the female reproductive tract. In: Acosta AA, Kruger TF (eds) Human spermatozoa in assisted human reproduction, 2nd edn. Parthenon, New York, pp 19–31

Overstreet JW, Cooper GW (1978) Sperm transport in the reproductive tract of the female rabbit. I. The rapid transit phase of transport. Biol Reprod 19:101–14

Paulson JD, Polakoski KL (1977) A glass wool column procedure for removing extraneous material from the human ejaculate. Fertil Steril 28:178–181

Perez-Pelaez M, Cohen MR (1965) The split ejaculate in homologous insemination. Int J Fertil 10:25–28

Perry AC, Jones R, Niang LS, Jackson RM, Hall L (1992) Genetic evidence for an androgen-regulated epididymal secretory glutathione peroxidase whose transcript does not contain a selenocysteine codon. Biochem J 285:863–870

Perry AC, Jones R, Hall L (1993) Isolation and characterization of a rat cDNA clone encoding a secreted superoxide dismutase reveals the epididymis to be a major site of its expression. Biochem J 293:21–25

Pertoft H, Rubin K, Kjellen L, Laurent TC, Klingeborn B (1977) The viability of cells grown or centrifuged in a new density gradient medium, Percoll (TM). Exp Cell Res 110:449–457

Petersen CM, Hatasaka HH, Jones KP, Poulson AM, Carrell DT, Urry RL (1994) Ovulation induction with gonadotropins and intrauterine insemination compare with in vitro fertilization and no therapy: a prospective, nonrandomized, cohort study and meta-analysis. Fertil Steril 62:535–544

Polansky FF, Lamb EJ (1988) Do the results of semen analysis predict future fertility? A survival analysis study. Fertil Steril 49:1059–1065

Pousette A, Akerlof E, Rosenborg L, Fredricsson B (1986) Increase in progressive motility and improved morphology of human spermatozoa following their migration through Percoll gradients. Int J Androl 9:1–13

Prietl G (1998) Die homologe intrauterine Insemination: klinische und klinisch-experimentelle Untersuchungen zur Optimierung der Methode und ihre gesundheitsökonomische Evaluierung. Habilitationsschrift, University of Bonn

Prochownik L (1915) Ein Beitrag zu den Versuchen mit künstlicher Befruchtung beim Menschen. Zentralbl Gynakol 10:145

Punjabi V, Gerris J, Van Bijilen J, Delbeke L, Giles M, Buytaert P (1990) Comparison between different pre-treatment techniques for sperm recovery prior to intrauterine insemination, GIFT or IVF. Hum Reprod 5:75–78

Puris K, Christiansen E (1993) Infection in the male reproductive tract, impact, diagnosis and treatment on relation to male infertility. Int J Androl 16:1

Quagliarello J, Arny M (1986) Intracervical versus intrauterine insemination: correlation of outcome with antecedent postcoital testing. Fertil Steril 46:870–875

Quinn P (1993) Sperm processing in assisted reproductive technology: male factor. Semin Reprod Endocrinol 11:49–55

Raeburn AR, Meniru MO (1997) Fertility counselling. In: Meniru GI, Brinsden PR, Craft IL (eds) A handbook of intrauterine insemination. Cambridge University Press, Cambridge, pp 46–55

Ragni G, Maggioni P, Guermandi E, Testa A, Baroni E, Colombo M, Crosignani PG (1999) Efficacy of double intrauterine insemination in controlled ovarian hyperstimulation cycles. Fertil Steril 72:619–622

Rana N, Jeyendran RS, Holmgren WJ, Rotman C, Zaneveld LJD (1989) Glass wool-filtered spermatozoa and their oocyte penetrating capacity. J In Vitro Fertil Embryo Transf 6:280–284

Ransom MX, Blotner MB, Bohrer M, Corsan G, Kemmann E (1994) Does increasing frequency of intrauterine insemination improve pregnancy rates significantly during superovulation cycles? Fertil Steril 61:303–307

Rhemrev J, Jeyendran RS, Vermeiden JPW, Zaneveld LJD (1989) Human sperm selection by glass wool filtration and two-layer, discontinuous Percoll gradient centrifugation. Fertil Steril 51:685–690

Ripps BA, Minhas BS, Carson SA, Buster JE (1994) Intrauterine insemination in fertile women delivers larger numbers of sperm to the peritoneal fluid than intracervical insemination. Fertil Steril 61:398–400

Rohleder H (1912) Normale, pathologische und künstliche Befruchtung beim Menschen. Monographien über die Zeugung beim Menschen. Leipzig

Russel JK (1960) Artificial insemination (husband) in the management of childlessness. Lancet 2:1223

Russell LD, Rogers BJ (1987) Improvement in the quality and fertilization potential of a human sperm population using the rise technique. J Androl 8:25–33

Sacks PC, Simon JA (1991) Infectious complications of intrauterine insemination: a case report and literature review. Int J Fertil 36:331–339

Schwartz D (1980) La notion de fécondabilité dans l'approche étiologique, diagnostique et thérapeutique de linfécondité. J Gynecol Obstet Biol Reprod (Paris) 9:607–612

Seibel MM, Smith DM, Levesque L et al (1982) The temporal relationship between the luteinizing hormone surge and human oocyte maturation. Am J Obstet Gynecol 142:568–572

Sellheim H (1924) Befruchtung, Unfruchtbarkeit und Unfruchtbarkeitsbehandlung. Z Arztl Fortbildg 19:573, 20:605, 21:636, 22:699

Sengoku K, Tamate K, Takaoka Y, Morishita N, Ishikawa M (1994) A randomized, prospective study of gonadotrophin-releasing hormone agonist for treatment of unexplained infertility. Hum Reprod 9:1043–1047

Serafini P, Blank W, Tran C, Mansourian M, Tan T, Batzofin J (1990) Enhanced penetration of zona-free hamster ova by sperm prepared by Nycodenz and Percoll gradient centrifugation. Fertil Steril 53:551–555

Settlage DSF, Motoshima M, Tredway DR (1973) Sperm transport from the external cervical os to the fallopian tubes in women: a time and quantitation study. Fertil Steril 24:655–661

Shalev E, Geslevich Y, Matilsky M, Ben Ami M (1995) Induction of pre-ovulatory gonadotrophin surge with gonadotrophin-releasing hormone agonist compared to preovulatory injection of human chorionic gonadotrophins for ovulation induction in intrauterine insemination treatment cycles. Hum Reprod 10:2244–2247

Sher G, Knutzen VK, Stratton CJ, Montakhab MM, Allenson SG (1984) In vitro sperm capacitation and transcervical intrauterine insemination for the treatment of refractory infertility: phase I. Fertil Steril 41:260–264

Sherman JK, Paulson JD, Lui KC (1981) Effect of glass wool filtration on ultrastructure of human spermatozoa. Fertil Steril 36:643–647

Shulman A, Hauser R, Lipitz S, Frenkel Y, Dor J, Bider D, Mashiach S, Yogev L, Yavetz H (1998) Sperm motility is a major determinant of pregnancy outcome following intrauterine insemination. J Assist Reprod Genet 15:381–385

Silber SJ (1989) The relationship of abnormal semen parameters to male fertility. Hum Reprod 4:947–953

Silverberg KM, Johnson JV, Olive DL, Burns WN, Schenken RS (1992) A prospective, randomized trial comparing two different intrauterine insemination regimes in controlled ovarian hyperstimulation cycles. Fertil Steril 57:357–361

Sims JM (1869) On the microscope as an aid in the diagnosis and treatment of sterility. NY J Med 8:393

Sims JM (1886) Clinical notes on uterine surgery with special reference to the management of the sterile condition. Harolwiche, London

Sobrero AJ, MacLeod J (1962) The immediate post-coital test. Fertil Steril 13:184–189

Spira A (1986) Epidemiology of human reproduction. Hum Reprod 1:111–115

Steeno O, Adimoel JA, Steeno J (1975) Separation of X- and Y-bearing human spermatozoa with the Sephadex gel-filtration method. Andrologia 7:95–97

Stone SC, de la Maza LM, Peterson EM (1986) Recovery of microorganism from the pelvic cavity after intracervical or intrauterine insemination. Fertil Steril 46:61–66

Tanphaichitr N, Millette CF, Agulnick A, Fitzgerald LM (1988) Egg penetration ability and structural properties of human sperm prepared by Percoll-gradient centrifugation. Gamete Res 20:67–81

Taylor PL, Kelly RW (1974) 19-OH E prostaglandins as the major prostaglandin of human semen. Nature 250:665

te Velde ER, van Kooy RJ, Waterreus JJH (1989) Intrauterine insemination of washed husband's spermatozoa: a controlled study. Fertil Steril 51:182–185

Templeton A, Penney GC, Lees MM (1982) Relation between the luteinizing hormone peak, the nadir of basal temperature, and the cervical mucus score. Br J Obstet Gynaecol 89:985–987

Templeton AA, Van Look P, Angell BD, Aitken RJ, Lumsden MA, Baird DT (1996) Oocyte recovery and fertilization rates in women at various times after the administration of hCG. J Reprod Fertil 76:771–778

Testart J, Frydman R (1982) Minimum time lapse between luteinizing hormone surge or human chorionic gonadotrophin administration and follicular rupture. Fertil Steril 37:50–53

Testart J, Frydman R, Feinstein MC (1981) Interpretation of plasma luteinizing hormone assay for the collection of mature oocytes from women: definition of a luteinizing hormone surge-initiation rise. Fertil Steril 36:50–54

Thomas EJ, McTighe L, King H, Lenton EA, Harper R, Cooke ID (1986) Failure of high intrauterine insemination of husband's semen. Lancet 2:693–694

Toner JP, Mossad H, Grow DR, Morshedi M, Swanson RJ, Oehninger S (1994) Value of sperm morphology assessed by strict criteria for prediction of outcome of artificial intrauterine insemination. Andrologia 27:143–148

Trout SW, Kemmann E (1999) Fallopian sperm perfusion versus intrauterine insemination: a randomized controlled trial and meta-analysis of the literature. Fertil Steril 71:881–885

Tünnerhoff A, van der Ven H, Al-Hasani S, Jeyendran RS, Diedrich K, Hamerich U, Krebs D (1986) Effectiveness of various sperm preparation techniques for human in vitro fertilization. Hum Reprod 1 [Suppl]:46

Urry RL, Middleton RG, McNamara L, Vikari CA (1983) The effect of single density bovine serum albumin columns on sperm concentration, motility and morphology. Fertil Steril 40:666–669

van der Ven HH, Jeyendran RS, Al-Hasani S, Tünnerhoff A, Hoebbel K, Diedrich K, Krebs D, Perez-Pelaez M (1988) Glass wool column filtration of human semen: relation to swim-up procedure and outcome of IVF. Hum Reprod 3:85–88

Vermesh M, Kletzky OA, Davajan V, Israel R (1987) Monitoring techniques to predict and detect ovulation. Fertil Steril 47:259–264

Wallace EM, Aitken RJ, Wu FCW (1992) Residual sperm function in oligozoospermia induced by testosterone enanthate administered as a potential steroid male contraceptive. Int J Androl 15:416–424

Wang FN, Lin CT, Hong CY, Hsiung CH, Su TP, Tsai HD (1992) Modification of the Wang tube to improve in vitro semen manipulation. Arch Androl 29:267–269

Weese DL, Peaster ML, Himsl KK, Leach GE, Lad PM, Zimmern PE (1993) Stimulated reactive oxygen species generation in the spermatozoa of infertile men. J Urol 149:64–67

Weinberg CR, Wilcox AJ (1995) A model for estimating the potency and survival of human gametes in vivo. Biometrics 51:405–412

Wessels PH, Cronje HS, Oosthuizen AP, Trumpelmann MD, Grobler S, Hamlett DK (1992) Cost-effectiveness of gamete intrafallopian transfer in comparison with induction of ovulation with gonadotropins in the treatment of female infertility: a clinical trial. Fertil Steril 57:163–167

White RM, Glass RH (1976) Intrauterine insemination with husband's semen. Obstet Gynecol 47:119–121

Wikland M, Wik O, Stehen Y, Qvist K, Soderlund B, Janson PO (1987) A self-migration method for preparing of sperm for in-vitro fertilization. Hum Reprod 3:191–195

Wilcox AJ, Weinberg CR, Baird DD (1995) Timing of sexual intercourse in relation to ovulation – effects on the probability of conception, survival of the pregnancy and sex of the baby. N Engl J Med 333:1517–1521

Wilrodt-Klein A (1999) Die intrauterine Insemination – eine Analyse prospektiv erfaßter Daten. Dissertation, University of Bonn

Wiltbank MC, Kosasa S, Rogers B (1985) Treatment of infertile patients by intrauterine insemination of washed spermatozoa. Andrologia 17:22–25

World Health Organization (1980) Temporal relationships between ovulation and defined changes in the concentrations of plasma estradiol-17β, luteinizing hormone, follicle-stimulating hormone, and progesterone. Am J Obstet Gynecol 138:383–430

World Health Organization (1992) Collection and examination of human semen. In: WHO laboratory manual for the examination of human semen and sperm-cervical mucus interaction, 3rd edn. Cambridge University Press, Cambridge

Zavos PM (1992) Preparation of human frozen-thawed seminal specimens using the Sperm-Prep filtration method: improvements over the conventional swim-up method. Fertil Steril 6:1326–1332

Zavos PM, Centola GM (1991) Selection of sperm from oligozoospermic men for ARTA: comparisons between swim-up and Spermprep filtration. ARTA 1:338–345

Zayed F, Lenton EA, Cooke ID (1997) Comparison between stimulated in-vitro fertilization and stimulated intrauterine insemination for the treatment of unexplained and mild factor infertility. Hum Reprod 12:2408–2413

Zeyneloglu HB, Arici A, Olive DL, Duleba AJ (1998) Comparison of intrauterine insemination with timed intercourse in superovulated cycles with gonadotropins: a meta-analysis. Fertil Steril 69:486–491

Zikopoulos K, West CP, Thong PW, Kacser EM, Morrison J, Wu FCW (1993) Homologous intra-uterine insemination has no advantage over timed natural intercourse when used in combination with ovulation induction for the treatment of unexplained infertility. Hum Reprod 8:563–567

Zinaman M, Drobnis EZ, Morales P, Brazil C, Kiel M, Cross NL, Hanson FW, Overstreet JW (1989) The physiology of sperm recovered from the human cervix: acrosomal status and response to inducers of acrosomal reaction. Biol Reprod 41:790–797

Zini A, de Lamirande E, Gagnon C (1993) Reactive oxygen species in semen of infertile patients: levels of superoxide dismutase- and catalase-like activities in seminal plasma and spermatozoa. Int J Androl 16:183–188

Zreik TG, Garcia Velasco JA, Habboosh MS, Olive DL, Arici A (1999) Prospective, randomized, crossover study to evaluate the benefit of human chorionic gonadotropin-timed versus luteinizing hormone-timed intrauterine inseminations in clomiphene citrate-stimulated treatment cycles. Fertil Steril 71:1070–1074

Subject Index

A

acridine orange staining 231, 245
acrosin 230
  activity 230, 240
acrosome 575
acrosome reaction 1, 4, 6, 230, 234, 242
activin 46, 90
add-back therapy 159
adhesiolysis 563
adhesions 562, 563
adrenal 66
adrenocorticotropin 39
algorithmic management 608
alpha-glucosidase 230, 233
alpha receptor blockers 256
androgen microenvironment 13
androgenes 16, 60, 263
androgen-estrogen ratio 17
androgen receptor gene mutations 539
andrology 223
  medical history 224
  physical examination 225
  ultrasonography 226
  semen analysis 227
androstendione 16
aneuploidy 455, 524
  maternal 478
Angelman syndrome 593
angiotensin-renin system 203
aniline blue 230, 231
  staining 231, 245
antibiotics 259
anticoagulant therapy 211
antiestrogens 167
antiphlogistic drugs 259
antisperm antibodies 259
apoptosis 13
Arachis hypogaea agglutinin 234
artificial testis 596

ascites 197
  aspiration 211
assisted hatching 474
assisted reproductive technology (ART) 449, 456, 489, 561
asthenozoospermia 229
atresia 12
autosomal dominant disorder 491
axial filament 576
azoospermia 229, 378
  factor (AZF) 240, 537
  nonobstructive 249, 579

B

bacteriospermia 246
basal body temperature, nadir 627
biopsy
  blastomere 478
  embryo 519
  laser-based 478
  polar body 478, 519
  techniques 476
  testicular 580, 581, 592
blastocyste culture
  benefits 312
  pitfalls 312
blastomere 517, 520
B2 medium 379
bromocriptine 265
brompheniramine 265
bunazosin 255

C

calcium 513
capacitation 230
captopril 256
cauterization 13

cell response   19
central nervous system (CNS)   25
centrosome   587
ceruloplasmin   232
cervical mucus   609, 623, 624, 626
cetrorelix   147, 178
children
  outcome born after IVF and ICSI   461
chlamydia trachomatis   247
chlortetracycline   234
chromatin condensation   231, 505
chromosomal abnormalities   449, 518
  in men   529
  in femal partners   532
ciliary dyskinesia   457
citric acid   233
clomiphene citrate   96, 167, 254
clotting abnormalities   204
cohort   12
collagenase   19
component Ĉ3   232
concanavalin A   234
confocal scanning laser microscopy
  (CSLM)   580, 582, 589
congenital
  absence of the vas deference
  (CBAVD)   233, 249, 378, 457, 520, 523,
  534
  abnormalities   452
  malformations   119
  postnatal development   468
  rate   466
  Mainz model   467
  major   384, 450, 466
  minor   384, 450, 466
corpus luteum   13, 215, 219
cortical cytoplasm   308
corticotropin-releasing hormone
  (CRH, CRF)   26, 35
cryoconservation   339
  freezing method   358
  microtubules   348
  oocytes   339
  ovarian tissue   350
  pregnancy rate   360
  protectants   343, 357
  slow freezing   346
  sperm   355
    functions   359
  testicular tissue   359
  ultrarapid freezing   346
  zona pellucida   349
cryopreservation   248, 339, 463
  of single Spermatozoa   480

cryptozoospermia   454
cumulativ embryo score (CES)   316
cumulus cells   19
cumulus oophorus   303
cumulus-oocyte complexe   379
cycle cancellation   184
cyclic AMP   508
cyclin   511
cystic fibrosis   249, 522, 523, 524
cystic fibrosis transmembrane-conductance regulator   450, 534
cytogenetic information   451
cytokines   203
cytoplasmatic blanket   590
cytostatic factor (CSF)   512

D

DAZ-deleted in azoospermia   537, 579
decapeptide   134
dimethylsulfoxide   343
diuretic agents   209
DNA   292, 521, 576, 593
  difference   290
dominance   13ff
dominant follicle   13ff
donor eggs   489
  guidelines   491, 493
  protocol for preparation of recipi-
    ent   496
  outcome   497
down-regulation   136, 174
Duchennes' muscular dystrophy   523,
  524

E

Earles' medium   379
ectopic pregnancy   561
edema   197
ejaculatory disorders   247
  retrograde ejaculation   247
  anejaculation   247
  anorgasmia   247
elastase   230, 232
electroejaculation   248
embryo
  classification   382
  grading   311
  number of transferred embryos   316
  transfer   438
endogenous opioids   30

endometrial biopsy 216, 495
endometriosis 561
endometrium 216, 220
endoscopy 549
  instruments 551
  noncommunicating rudimentary
  horns 558
  postoperative therapy 556
  pregnancy rate 556
  preoperative hormone therapy 556
  septum 549, 553
epididymis 233
Escherichia coli 247
estradiol 13, 215, 378
estrogen 13, 44, 54, 60, 93, 104, 107,
  207
estrogen/androgen ratio 16
estrogen microenvironment 13
estrone 16
extracellular matrix 19

F

fallopian tube sperm perfusion
  (FSP) 605, 613, 623, 640, 644
fecundatio sine concubito 601
fecundity 605
fertilin 5
fertility counseling 607
fertilization 506
  assessment 309
  capacity 577
  cascade 308
  rates 238, 361, 362
fetal reduction 120
ficoll 619
fimbrioplasty 564
flare-up effekt 136
flow-cytometric sorting 296
fluorescent in situ hybridization
  (FISH) 517, 524, 580, 589
folic acid 259
follicle
  development 52
  midsize 205
  intermediate-size 207
  preantral 12ff, 200
  primordial 11, 52, 350
follicle-stimulating hormone (FSH) 12,
  26, 39, 56, 57, 81, 90, 215, 491, 580
  highly purified 114, 168, 261
  recombinant 111, 171, 261, 514
  urinary 111, 171

follicular aspiration 389
  maturation 11
  phase 14ff
  selection 165
follitropin 171
forskolin 509
freezing method 358
French protocol 154, 178
fructose 230, 233
FSH gate 165
gamete intrafallopian transfer
  (GIFT) 81
ganirelix 178
gene therapy 597
genetic disease 522, 579
  X-linked 523
genomic imprinting
  maternally 593
  paternally 593
germ cells 51
germinal vesicle (GV) 504
  breakdown (GVB) 504
globozoospermia 230
glutathione 259
glycerol 357

G

GnRH agonists 136, 173, 176, 202, 206
  combined gonadotropin therapy 175
  combined hMG treatment 176, 378
GnRH antagonists 144, 177
  combined gonadotropin therapy 97,
  98, 177
gonadotropin 13, 25, 40, 54, 57, 79, 167,
  221
  chemistry 82
  clearance 82
  combined GH stimulation 181
  therapy 88, 90
    combined 96–98, 101
    complications 119
    effective daily dose 90, 105
    long-term safety 121
    monitoring 103
    pregnancy rate 93, 108
    outcome of pregnancies 117
    schemes 94
  pharmacokinetics 82
  secretion 41
gonadotropin-releasing hormone
  (GnRH) 26, 133, 215, 262, 512
  dopaminergic modulation 33

endogenous opioids   30
  pulsatile secretion   23, 27, 28
  regulation of secretion   30
  steroids   30
  surge-inhibiting factor   218
  synthesis   26
gonadotropin surge   13
gonosomal disorders   466
granulosa cell   11, 215, 507
  compartiment   49
  luteinization   16
growth factors
  epidermal (EGF)   512
  transforming (TGF)   512
growth hormone (GH)   26, 101, 181, 257
growth hormone-releasing hormone
  (GRH)   26, 35, 101
guidelines for egg donation   491, 493

H

Hams' F10   414, 513
haploid state   575
hatching   475
hemizona   480
hemizona assay (HZA)   234, 244, 480
hemoconcentration   203
hemophilia A   524
heterologous (hamster) ovum penetration test (HOP)   236
high-order gestations   451
histones   231, 576, 587
Hoechst 33342 stain   292
host testis   596
human albumin   208
human chorionic gonadotropin
  (hCG)   18, 207, 215, 260, 377, 504,
  507, 514
human menopausal gonadotropin
  (hMG)   79, 167, 197, 261
  treatment monitoring   206
hydrocortisone   208
hydrothorax   197
hydroxyethyl starch (HES)   208
hyperandrogenism   66
hyperinsulinemia   205
hyperprolactinemia   49, 265
hyperstimulation   81, 89, 93, 101
  controlled   80, 167, 199, 604, 637
hypogonadism   260, 261, 263
hypo-osmotic swelling test (HOS)   229,
  244
hypospadia   601, 603

hypothalamic dysfunction   36
hypothalamic-pituitary
  failure   88
  dysfunction   88
hypothalamic-pituitary-ovarian axis   11
hypothalamic-pituitary-testicular
  axis   579
hypothalamus   25, 26, 64
hypothyreoidism   64, 66
hypovolemia   197, 203

I

idiopathic fertility disorders   603
imipramine   265
implantation   219, 475
  failed   475
incipient ovarian failure   490
indomethacin   211, 259
infertility
  cervical factor   644
  etiology   456
  male factor   646
  management   607
  unexplained   640, 644
inhibin   46, 90, 167, 219
insemination of oocytes   435
insemination
  artificial   601, 603
    history   601
    husbands' prepared sperm
      (AIH)   603
    indication   603
    with donor sperm (AID)   602, 604
  intracervical   601, 608, 624, 626
  intrauterin   236, 608
    homologous   602
  periovulatory   627
insulin-like growth factor-I, -II (IGF-I, II)
  62, 102, 182
insulin resistance   205
intercourse, natural   624, 626, 630, 632,
  634
interferon alpha   259
interleukin-1, -6 (IL-1, IL-6)   203
intracytoplasmic sperm injection
  (ICSI)   81, 239, 377, 449, 461, 517, 594
  fertilisation   381
  malformation rate   384
  pregnancy rate   383
  prenatal diagnosis   383
intrafollicular pressure   18
intraovarian regulators   11

inverted microscope-computer-assisted system (IM-CAS) 583
in vitro fertilisation 80, 96, 107, 165, 175, 217, 237, 377, 389, 449, 475, 517
air conditioning 404
building materials 405
clothing 407
cocultures 417
2-deoxyadenosine 432
disinfection/sterilization 400
embryo transfer 438
follicular aspiration 389
glassware 411
glass-wool filtration 432
Hams' F10 414
incubators 408
insemination of oocytes 435
maintenance and cleaning 410
media 412
microinjection procedure 433
oocyte and embryo culture 436
pentoxyfylline 432
percoll gradient technique 427
preparation of testicular sperm 432
quality assurance 414
sperm collection and preparation 424
swim-up technique 430
water 412
workplace 407
in vitro maturation 306

K

Kallmans' syndrome 37
kallikrein 260
Kartageners' syndrome 457
karyotypes 451
trisomie 21 383, 451
trisomie 18 451
chromosome 18 translocation 451
Klinefelders' syndrome 451, 529
ketotifen 255

L

laparoscopy 561
laparotomy 209
laser 549
assisted hatching 476
biopsy techniques 476
contact 473
energy 482
immobilization of spermatozoa 482
indium-gallium-arsenic-phosphorus 474
noncontact 473
permeabilization of the sperm membrane 482
thermal effect 482
l-carnitine 258
leading follicle 12
leukocytes 246
LH/FSH ratio 64
lipid peroxydation 232
Lübeck protocol 147, 178
luteal phase 12, 222
defect 216
support 108, 143, 154
luteectomy 13
luteinizing hormone (LH) 17, 26, 39, 56, 59, 215, 504
peak 134
receptor 13
surge 16, 173, 215, 217, 221, 505, 507, 624
premature 97, 173, 175

M

Mainz model 467
male genital tract inflammation 232
male factor 611, 631
male factor cases 618
male-factor infertility 377, 517
drugs 224
male subfertility 603, 612, 622
mild 604, 608
unexplained 604, 608
male urogenital infection 246
mast cell blockers 255
master gland 11
maturation-promoting factor (MPF) 511
meiosis 503, 575
metaphase II 304
prophase I 304
meiotic prophase 11
melanocyte-stimulating hormone 39
melatonin 38
menstrual cycle 23
mesterolone 264
meta-analysis 605, 639, 642
methylprednisolone 259

microinjection
  procedure 239, 380, 433
  technique 450
microsurgery 561
microsurgical epididymal sperm astpiration (MESA) 223, 249, 461
microtool preparation 380
microtubule 348, 506
midodrin 229, 264
mitochondrial diseases 518
mitotic index 12
modulators 46
müllerian fusion defect 549
multiple follicular
  development 167
  growth 81
multiple pregnancies 81, 117, 119, 450, 608
mycoplasma 247

N

neovasculogenesis 200
neurophysin 48
noninvasive management 601
nuclear envelope 505, 511
nucleolus 327
nycondenz 619

O

OASIS 585, 586, 589
offspring 289
oligo-astheno-teratozoospermia 379
oligozoospermia 454
oocyte 11, 19, 55, 321, 339, 503
  activation 585, 586, 588
  grading 306
  In vitro maturation 306
  maturation 504, 626
oocyte and Embryo Culture 436
oocyte-cumulus complex 18, 505
oogenesis 503
oogonia 51
ooplasm 304
ooplasmic injektions 579
ooplasmic membrane 377
ovaries 49, 66
  development 51
ovarian
  cyclicity 13
  function 11

  pathophysiology 63
  reserve 180
  stimulation 165, 167, 217
    combined 181
ovarian hyperstimulation syndrome
  (OHSS) 113, 119, 153, 176, 197
  classification 198
  risk factors 204
  treatment schedule 205
ovariolysis 563
ovulation 12, 18, 56
  induction 183
    with hCG 184
ovulatory quota 12ff
ovum 11
oxidative stress 231
oxytocin 48

P

paracentesis, abdominal 210
partial zona dissection (PZD) 377
parenting, quality of 462
patient counseling 606
pelvic clock ("Zeitgeber") 11
pelvic inflammatory disease (PID) 561
penile vibratory stimulation (PVS) 248
pentoxyfylline 253, 432
percoll gradient technique 380, 427, 621
permeabilization of the sperm
  membrane 482
peroxidase-positive cells 232
phenotype 455
phosphodiesterase (PDE) 509
  inhibitor 509
pineal gland 38
  endocrine function 38
Pisum sativum agglutinin 234
pituitary 26, 39, 64
  pathophysiology 49
plasma expanders 209
plasmin 19
plasminogen 19
pleural effusions 210
polar body 478
polycystic ovarian syndrome (PCO) 63, 81, 88, 95, 101, 514
  LH/FSH ratio 64
polymerase chain reaction (PCR) 517, 521
polymorphonuclear granulocytes
  (PMN) 232

polyspermic block   308
poly-T-polymorphism   536
pool ejaculate   229
poor responder   179, 181
Prader-Willi syndrome   593
pregnancy
   rates   238, 360, 362
   outcome   316
preimplantation genetic diagnosis   517
   indications   518
   pregnancy rate   524
   selection of embryos   517
   take home baby rate   524
preimplantation genetic technique   491
preimplantation genetic testing   457
premature ovarian failure   63, 490
prenatal diagnosis   465
primary testicular failure   577
proacrosin   582
probability of conception
   monthly   605
   peak normal   605
progesterone   16, 45, 62, 93, 107, 215,
   220, 511
   exogenous   222
   luteal phase support   108, 379
prolactin   17, 26, 47
prolactinoma   49
pronuclear
   embryo transfer   309
   morphology   325
pronucleus   309, 576
   alignment   309
propanediol   343
prostaglandin   18, 48, 202
prostate   233
prostatic acid phosphatase   233
prostatitis   246
protamines   231, 576, 588
protease inhibitors   19
protein kinase   508
proteoglycan   18
protocol
   fast   175
   long   141, 175
   short   139, 175
      monitoring   140
   ultra-short   139, 175
      monitoring   140
   fixed stimulation   179
PSA   233
pulse generator   133
purines   510

R

reactive oxygen species (ROS)   230, 231,
   245, 616, 619, 621
recruitment   12
recurrent pregnancy loss   549
renal perfusion   203
reproductive cyclicity   11
RNA binding motif (RBM)   579
round spermatid (nuclei) injection
   (ROSNI/ROSI)   252, 576
   fertilization rate   578, 588
   genetic risk   592, 594
   indications   579

S

salpingolysis   563
salpingoneostomy   565
salpingostomy   565
secondary follicles   12
secondary spermatocyte injections   595
selection   12
   of embryos   517
semen analysis   227, 229, 379
   abstinence   228
   split ejaculate   228
   volume   229
semen
   origin   449
   parameters   449, 454
   processing technique   614
seminal vesicles   233
seminiferous tubules   580
sex   289
   preselection   289
   ratio   293
sex-chromosomal aberrations   383
sex-linked recessive disorder   491
Sheehan syndrome   49
SOF medium   590
sperm
   collection and preparation   424
   computer aided analysis
      (CASA)   238
   concentration   236
   cryoconservation   355
   flow-cytometric sorting   296
   human   294
   isolation   605
      density gradient centrifugation   603,
      618

glass-wool filtration   603, 616, 618
Sephadex gel columns   620
sperm-rise   603
sperm select   620
swim-up   603, 616, 620, 621
maturation   2, 6
morphology   229, 237, 360, 379
  "strict criteria"   229
motility   2, 237, 359, 379
oocyte fusion   5
parameters, predictive value   612
penetration test (SPA)   244
viability   229
spermatozoa
  ejaculated   378
  epididymal   378, 449
  immobilization   482
  maturity   456
  testicular   1, 378, 449
spermiogenesis   1, 231, 575
  complete failure   579
  incomplete failure   579
spindel formation   506
split ejakulate   615
spontaneous cycles   173
Steiners' myotonic dystrophy   523
steroids   13, 30, 57
stigma   18
stimulation
  combined   172
  poor responder   179
  protocols   172
    fixed   179
subfertility
  cervical factor   604, 629, 639
  idiopathic factor   604, 605, 629, 635
  male factor   604, 629, 634
  unexplained   605, 614, 630, 633
subzonal insemination (SUZI)   377
synchronisation   495
systemic organic disease   579

T

tail stump syndrome   240
tamoxifen   253
testicular damage   579
testicular sperm extraction (TESE)   223, 251, 461
  biopsy   251
testicular tissue   251
testolactone   255

testosterone   16
  intratesticular concentration (ITC)   580
testosterone undecanoate   263
theca cell   215
  compartment   50
thyroid   66
thyroid-stimulating hormone (TSH)   82
thyrotropin   39
thyrotropin-releasing hormone (TRH)   26, 36
translocation   518
  balanced   491, 524, 529
  unbalanced   524
transmission electron microscopy (TEM)   580, 582, 587, 589
triple staining   234
trisomie   383, 451, 455
tubal embryo transfer (TET)   81
tubal fertility treatment   561
tubal infertility   561
  adhesions   562
  ectopic pregnancy   561
  endometriosis   561
  microsurgery   562
  mucosal dammage   562
  pelvic inflammatory disease (PID)   561
tumorigenesis   593
two-cell theory   57

U

up-regulation   136
Ureaplasma urealyticum   247
urine   248
uterine lavage   519
uterine septum, partial/complete   549, 553

V

vaginal septum   549
varicocele   223, 580
vascular bed   202
vascular endothelial growth factor (VEGF)   200, 203
vasopressin   48
virilism   66
vitamin E   255
viteline membran   1

W

weight gain   204
WHO Laboratory manual   224
womans' age   489

X

X-chromosome   522, 524
X-chromosome-bearing sperm   289
X-linkes genetic diseases   523
X-linked recessive disorders   290

Y

Y-chromosome   522, 524
Y-chromosome microdeletions   240

Y-chromosome-bearing sperm   289
Youngs' syndrome   536

Z

zinc   233, 257
zona
  binding   2
  drilling   473
  glycoprotein   3
  hardening   475
    measuring   483
    fertilization-induced   483
  pellucida   230, 306, 308, 349, 377, 519
    empty   480
  receptor   3
ZP 3   308
zygote scoring   326

The manufacturer's authorised representative in the EU is Springer
Nature Customer Service Centre GmbH, Europaplatz 3, 69115 Heidelberg,
Germany. If you have any concerns regarding our products, please
contact ProductSafety@springernature.com

Printed and bound by CPI Group (UK) Ltd, Croydon, CR0 4YY
28/04/2026
02098453-0014